Pathophysiology

A Self-Instructional Program

Mary V. Burns, DVM
Adjunct Instructor
University of Nevada, Reno
Health Science Department
Reno, Nevada

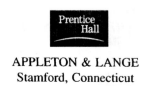
Prentice
Hall

APPLETON & LANGE
Stamford, Connecticut

Copyright © 1998 by Appleton & Lange
A Pearson Education Company
Upper Saddle River, NJ 07458

www.appletonlange.com

98 99 00 01 02 / 10 9 8 7 6 5 4 3

Prentice-Hall International (UK) Limited,London
Prentice-Hall of Australia Pty. Limited, Sydney
Prentice-Hall Canada Inc., Toronto
Prentice-Hall Hispanoamericana, S.A., Mexico
Prentice-Hall of India Private Limited, New Delhi
Prentice-Hall of Japan, Inc., Tokyo
Pearson Education Asia Pte. Ltd., Singapore
Editora Prentice-Hall do Brasil, Ltda., Rio de Janeiro

Library of Congress Cataloging–in–Publication Data

Burns, Mary 1956–
    Pathophysiology : a self-instructional program / by Mary Burns.
      p.   cm.
    ISBN 0-8385-8084-X (pbk. : alk. paper)
    1. Physiology, Pathological—Programmed instruction.   I. Title.
    [DNLM: 1. Disease—programmed instruction. 2. Pathology-
-programmed instruction. 3. Physiology—programmed instruction.
    QZ 18.2 B967p 1998]
    RB113.B87   1998
    616.07'07'7—dc21   97–41936
                                         CIP

Editor-in-Chief: Cheryl L. Mehalik
Acquisitions Editor: Lin Marshall
Production Editor: Lisa M. Guidone
Art Coordinator: Eve Siegel
Artist: Laura Duprey
Designer: Janice Barsevich Bielawa

ISBN 0-8385-8084-X

Knowledge is of two kinds—
We know a subject ourselves,
Or we know where we can find information upon it.

Samuel Johnson

Contents

Preface

The inspiration for this book came from two of my professional experiences. The first was teaching a principles of disease course as an associate professor of clinical laboratory science at the University of Nevada, Reno (UNR). The second was facilitating an independent study course in medical terminology through the Correspondence Study Division at UNR. It occurred to me that an introductory course in pathophysiology (the study of disease processes) is one that could also be presented in an independent study format. However, this unique approach to the study of basic disease principles demands carefully constructed features so students can grasp these often challenging principles on their own.

The most important of these features is *readability*. In independent study, the student spends his or her time with the textbook instead of with the instructor. This book must therefore *be* the instructor. For that reason, I have attempted to present the material in a relatively colloquial fashion. By this, I mean I have strived to produce a book written in a relatively informal, conversational manner that also guides the student through the concepts in a professional manner. I believe this text achieves a balance between "plain English" and proper medical language.

Other features that are designed to help the student learn the material include:

- Definitions of highlighted medical terms as the words are used to explain concepts.
- Division of information into sections within each chapter, with further division into individual numbered frames.
- Questions within each frame about the information just presented, along with answer columns on every page for immediate feedback.
- Many original line drawings and tables carefully created to reinforce understanding of the concepts. Included are illustrations in the form of flowcharts or conceptual maps that walk the student through the causes, development, and effects of various disease processes.
- Review questions and answers at the end of each chapter section to serve as the "take-home message."

Pathophysiology: A Self-Instructional Program is also an excellent adjunct to the traditional classroom course. An instructor can use text assignments to build a foundation of knowledge so time spent in the classroom can be used efficiently to accomplish more. The instructor can deepen the student's understanding of basic material by focusing on complex principles, in which further explanation can be beneficial. Thought-provoking classroom activities, such as case studies and problem-solving exercises, will help train students in the process of critical thinking and elevate their comprehension to higher levels.

The intended audience for this text is wide ranging. All pre-professional students in the medical fields (such as medicine, physician assistant, veterinary medicine, physical therapy, occupational therapy, pharmacy, and dentistry) can build on their education by gaining a basic understanding of disease principles at this level, before becoming inundated by more complex principles in professional school. Nursing students and students of allied health sciences, such as medical technology and radiologic technology, also require this knowledge as part of their education. With all of these students in mind, I worked to create a fundamental text that is user-friendly and understandable, yet comprehensive for diverse use. It is my sincere wish that students will be able to easily grasp these principles of disease, either on their own or in conjunction with a classroom course.

Mary V. Burns, DVM

Acknowledgments

First and foremost, I would like to express my deepest appreciation to the dedicated editors at Appleton & Lange. To Cheryl Mehalik, thank you for taking a chance on me, a first-time author with a crazy idea for a self-study book. And to Linda Marshall, you have my gratitude for your long-suffering patience (I thought I would *never* be finished) and for teaching this novice the ropes.

I would like to thank the reviewers for generously taking the time from their busy schedules to read completed chapters and provide helpful comments and suggestions. Appreciation for their insights goes to: Mary Jane Lofton, MA, RN, Belmont Technical College; Kent Thomas, PhD, Wichita State University; Sheri Innerarity, PhD, RN, CSN, University of Texas; Mark Weber, PhD, EdD, Grove City College; Mary Neiheissel, EdD, RN, University of Southwestern Louisiana; Allen Waldo, PhD, Texas Woman's University; Melanie Truesdell, RN, BSN, University of Texas at Austin; Kay Sackett, EdD, RN, Winona State University; Linda Ramge, MT, CMA, King's College; James Brennan, MEd, RRT, St. Louis Community College; and Patricia Finder-Stone, MS, RN, Northeast Wisconsin Technical College. My thanks also include my students who bravely volunteered to read and work through several chapters and offer useful feedback.

To Kent Thomas, PhD, I send my utmost appreciation for his work on the pedagogy, which greatly contributed to the completion of this book. Bless you!

And to Laura Duprey, many thanks for her beautiful work of turning my hand-drawn stick figures into lively illustrations.

How to Use This Book

DO NOT PROCEED THROUGH THIS BOOK UNTIL YOU READ
AND UNDERSTAND THESE INSTRUCTIONS FOR ITS USE!

Welcome to the challenging and rewarding world of independent study! This method of learning requires commitment and self-discipline on your part. Like so many aspects of life, what you gain from this course will depend on what you invest in it. The benefits of independent study include the satisfaction of knowing you have completed this task yourself and know the material well. The programmed format of this book is a well-established method of learning basic material on your own. This book is primarily designed as an independent study course, but also makes an excellent supplement for a classroom course. Since this is a study of disease mechanisms (abnormal function), you will benefit more if you have completed a course in anatomy and physiology (normal function).

0–2

Key words are presented to you in **boldface** type. This is to emphasize their importance and aid you in their retention. The **programmed** approach to learning is a method of self-study where you will supply missing information about previously read material. Supplying this information correctly will demonstrate that you understand and are learning the material. The material is presented in small to medium-sized blocks of text called **frames.** Each frame is numbered, first with the chapter number and then with the frame number. For example, 4–15 is Frame number 15 in Chapter 4. (This is the second frame you are reading.) The first part of a frame presents the information. At the end of a frame are a series of blanks in several sentences (occasionally these blanks will be found earlier in the frame). Fill in each blank with the correct word or words. The missing information will be found somewhere within that frame. BEFORE BEGINNING each page, cover up the **answer column** on the margin of the page with the answer mask provided. Check your answers by moving the paper down ONLY as far as the answer you are looking for. _____(1) learning is a manner of self-study where you supply missing _____(2) after reading the material. The material is presented in numbered blocks called _____(3). At the end of the frame, or within it, are a series of _____(4) which you must fill in. You will know what information is missing because you have just _____(5) the frame. The answers are in a _____(6) in the _____(7) of each page. You must _____(8) the answer column before beginning each page. When ready, uncover only the answer you are _____(9) for.

1. Programmed
2. information
3. frames
4. blanks
5. read
6. column
7. margin
8. cover
9. looking

------- O-3 -------

1. look
2. written
3. study
4. next

You will learn much more if you do not look first at the answer column before beginning a page. You will also learn more if you use this book in the intended manner. That is, make a sincere effort to write in the answers *before* checking them, instead of looking at the answer column. An added advantage of writing the answers instead of thinking them is that it will help you greatly in studying for the material. Frames that are relatively long will often have their programmed sections in the very next frames. In that case, you must look to the previous frame for the information. If you are not able to supply the answers correctly, you should study that frame again. Always read and work through the frames in the order they are presented, because you will be learning in a sequence that builds upon previous information. To learn as much as possible, do not _____(1) at the answer column before beginning a page. Answers should be _____(2) in the blanks before checking the answer column. Completing the blanks in writing will help you _____(3) the material. Long frames may have their programmed sections in the _____(4) frame.

------- O-4 -------

Non-programmed text is material that is presented for your information (FYI). It will help to complete a certain picture for you and further your understanding. Some terms are still presented in boldface text to facilitate your learning. In the interest of length of this book, and the burden placed upon you in this course, FYI material has been arbitrarily designated less critical so that you are not required to answer questions about it. Non-programmed information does not appear in the review questions. In keeping with the format of non-programmed text, this frame is not programmed.

------- O-5 -------

Another kind of information that is non-programmed is review of anatomy and physiology. It is expected you will have completed a study of normal structure and function before studying abnormal structure and function. The review of normal is found at the beginning of most chapters. A few chapters do not contain a review and are programmed from the beginning. That is because the material in those chapters is not traditionally presented in depth in an anatomy and physiology course.

------- O-6 -------

1. objectives
2. review questions
3. chapter summary
4. major
5. answer
6. alright
7. review

You will find the study aids valuable in this course. The study aids are the **objectives,** the **review questions,** and the **chapter summary.** The review questions appear at the end of each programmed section within a chapter. It is important that you answer the review questions. They emphasize the major points of the material you have learned. Do your best to answer the questions without looking up the answers. If you sincerely do not know the answer, it is acceptable to look back through the chapter. Your areas of weakness may be revealed by the review questions. Use them to repeat your study of a particular topic. At the end of each chapter is the summary. It serves as an excellent brief review of the major topics presented in that chapter.

The study aids in this course are the _____(1), _____(2), and the _____(3). Review questions emphasize _____(4) points, and you should always _____(5) them. It is _____(6) alright/not alright (choose one) to look up the answer to a review question. You should read the chapter summary because it is a good _____(7) of the topics in that chapter.

Knowledge is built in steps. It is expected that you retain basic concepts to be able to add to your knowledge in stepwise fashion. Frequently, you must answer a question that pertains to an earlier chapter because those earlier concepts are now incorporated into the new information. For example, when discussing autoimmune disease (Chap. 4), you will learn that a common result of this disease is widespread inflammation. You are expected to remember the general concepts of inflammation you learned in Chapter 2. Study the chapters in the order they are presented, since Part II is founded on Part I. No system or body part functions alone. When disease affects one part, its effects ripple through other parts. That is why your understanding must include an ability to tie several mechanisms or processes together.

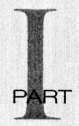

General Disease Processes

An Overview of Disease Processes and Fundamental Terminology

▶ OBJECTIVES

SECTION II
Define all highlighted terms.

I. AN OVERVIEW OF DISEASE PROCESSES

◀ SECTION
1-1

From your studies of anatomy and physiology, you have surely gained an appreciation of the complex and intricate workings of the human body. In this book you will be introduced to the remarkable mechanisms through which the body fights disease and attempts to restore harmony. A state of wellness or health requires a steady state of constant balance in our internal environment. The process of maintaining this normal balance, in spite of constant "knocks" off balance, is called **homeostasis** (this concept is explored in Chap. 3). A significant disruption in homeostasis often leads to disease. This book addresses concepts of **pathophysiology,** which can be literally defined as the study ("logy") of the function ("physio") of disease ("patho"). In other words, it is the study of how disease processes work to cause dysfunction in the body. As anatomy and physiology courses study normal function, pathophysiology studies abnormal function. Knowledge of abnormal physiology leads to an understanding of the signs and symptoms of disease, and of appropriate treatments. A solid understanding of fundamental disease mechanisms is necessary for every individual who desires a career in any aspect of the many health-care professions.

1-2

There are many **predisposing factors** that may allow disease to develop. Predisposing factors increase an individual's vulnerability or susceptibility to a particular disease. These factors help set the stage to make a particular disease more likely than in those people who do not experience these factors. **Age** is one factor. Newborn babies have an immature immune system, which causes them to be more susceptible to infection. Their liver enzymes necessary for detoxification of some substances are often lacking. They have fewer nutritional reserves, and less body fat to insulate against cold. The elderly are another age-susceptible population. They experience a decrease in immune function, which decreases their resistance to infectious disease. There is also a decline in homeostatic mechanisms, which impairs their ability to withstand temperature extremes. The general degeneration of the elderly may result in diseases of a degenerative nature. Their lifestyle (near-poverty economics, isolation, and alcoholism) can lead to malnutrition and debilitation. A person who is debilitated is "run down" and more prone to disease.

1–3

Sex sometimes plays a role as a predisposing factor. Some diseases are more prone in one gender than the other. Men are more likely to develop gout, while osteoporosis and rheumatoid arthritis occurs more frequently in women. An individual's **genetic makeup** can predispose to several disease processes, as you will see in later chapters. The advantage of this association is that when risk factors are known, lifestyle choices can help decrease the risk. For example, people who are at a genetic risk for diabetes can incorporate weight control, a healthy diet, and exercise into their lifestyle. **Stress** has been implicated as a factor in developing several disorders. Stress increases the body's production of steroid, which decreases immune system function. Stress can also worsen existing conditions. **Lifestyle** greatly influences the development of some diseases. Personal habits in regard to diet, exercise, weight control, smoking, and excessive alcohol consumption can have a positive effect or a negative effect on one's health. Finally, the **environment** can predispose to disease depending on exposure to pollution, chemicals, or other occupational hazards. Some of these hazards can lead to traumatic injury, chronic back pain, or carpal tunnel syndrome.

1–4

There are many ways to classify disease mechanisms. The first half of this book introduces you to some of these classifications. These classifications are:

1. **Inflammatory.** Inflammatory diseases are usually secondary to a primary disease, such as infection or autoimmune disease.
2. **Ischemic.** Interference in blood supply, and therefore oxygen, robs cells of their fuel and causes injury or death of cells and tissues.
3. **Immunologic.** Overreaction by the immune system (hypersensitivity), underreaction by the immune system (immune deficiency such as AIDS), and autoimmune disease are the three categories of immunologic disease. Autoimmune disease is the destruction of one's own tissues by antibodies produced by one's own immune system.
4. **Infectious.** Disease is caused by invasion and colonization with pathogenic microorganisms. The most common pathogens are bacteria, viruses, and fungi.
5. **Neoplastic.** This is uncontrolled growth of an abnormal cell line. A neoplasia ("new growth") may be benign or malignant. Malignant neoplasia is commonly called cancer, and its fatality is related to its spread or metastasis.
6. **Metabolic.** This is an upset in the biochemical reactions that govern the body processes, or metabolism. Metabolic diseases may be subclassified as nutritional because the upset is often in carbohydrate, fat, or protein metabolism.
7. **Nutritional.** Malnutrition can create disease because of insufficient resources for the body. Deficient protein means a decrease in osmotic pressure, a decrease in healing or formation of new body tissue, or a decrease in antibody production. Vitamin or mineral deficiencies can lead to interference in tissue integrity or in biochemical reactions of metabolism.
8. **Genetic.** Inherited or hereditary diseases are due to transmission of defective genes or chromosomes from one or both parents.
9. **Congenital defect.** Sometimes called developmental disease, this is a defect in embryonic or fetal development that may create a physiologic (functional) disorder, or a physical (structural) abnormality. A congenital defect may be genetic; may be induced by chemicals, drugs, or viruses; or may be a spontaneous event.

1–5

Additional classifications of disease that do not have entire chapters devoted to them in this text include:

1. **Trauma.** Trauma is physical force that mechanically disrupts the structure of the body, and therefore often disrupts function. The result of trauma is often commonly called an injury.

2. **Physical agents.** Temperature extremes, electrical shock, radiation, and poisons are examples of physical agents that cause disorder.
3. **Idiopathic.** Idiopathic diseases cannot be classified as to cause, because their cause is unknown.
4. **Iatrogenic.** An iatrogenic disorder is the result of a treatment. For example, high levels of steroids given for a variety of reasons can create iatrogenic Cushing's syndrome.

II. FUNDAMENTAL TERMINOLOGY ◄ SECTION

1-6

Before studying specific disease processes, it is important that you know many of the terms that relate to the general concepts of disease. Be certain you learn these terms before proceeding with the remaining chapters, because this knowledge will be assumed when disease mechanisms are explained. Occasionally, these definitions will be reinforced in later chapters.

1-7

Disease is defined as a change in normal body function that leads to abnormal function or structure. Another term sometimes substituted for disease is **disorder.** Disease may result from a direct insult, such as trauma or infection, or it may be an indirect result of a disturbance in metabolism. **Pathology** is the study of disease processes (their causes, typical characteristics, and effects). This word comes from the Greek language, where "pathos" means disease and "logos" means the science or study of. Pathology also describes a medical specialty that analyses body tissues and fluids to reach a diagnosis. Anatomic pathologists perform autopsies and examine tissue samples microscopically from cadavers or from living patients (biopsies). Clinical pathologists specialize in laboratory medicine, which is divided into several areas of study. **Pathogenesis** is the development or creation of disease. Pathogenesis refers to the established stages through which a disease progresses. The sequence of major events in pathogenesis is (1) cause, (2) abnormal function, and (3) manifestation. Manifestation refers to how the disease becomes visible or shows itself. Signs and symptoms are part of manifestation. The pathogenesis helps answer the question "How has this disease come about?" Abnormal function or structure is the result of the changes caused by _____(1). The study of disease processes is called _____(2). Pathogenesis describes the _____(3) or _____(4) of a specific disease. It includes the _____(5) through which a disease progresses, and this is seen as the events of _____(6), _____(7), and _____(8).

1. disease
2. pathology
3. development
4. creation
5. stages
6. cause
7. abnormal function
8. manifestation

1-8

The **etiology** of a disease is its cause, although the term literally means the study of causes. In some cases, the cause of a disease has never been discovered. When we don't know what causes a disease, we call it **idiopathic.** The manifestation of a disease is referred to as its **clinical presentation.** This phrase stems from the actions of a sick individual presenting himself or herself to a physician (clinician) for help. The clinical presentation of a disease is its signs and visible features or appearance. It describes what is seen in the patient by the examining health care professional. In this text, the phrase "clinical presentation" is often shortened to "clinically" to describe what is seen. The cause of a disease is medically referred to as the _____(1). Idiopathic is the term used when the cause is _____(2). The signs and appearance of a patient as seen by the examining health care professional is called the _____(3) of a disease.

1. etiology
2. unknown
3. clinical presentation

1-9

1. perception
2. symptom
3. measurable
4. sign
5. history
6. physical examination
7. noticeable
8. subclinical

The clinical presentation includes both the signs and symptoms of the disease. A **symptom** is a subjective complaint from a patient. Subjective means it is open to interpretation or not measurable. A symptom is the patient's perception of discomfort. Examples of symptoms are pain, nausea, weakness, fatigue, and dizziness. Symptoms are part of the patient's **history,** which is a written record of what has transpired before the patient presented himself or herself. A **sign** is an objective finding by the examining health care professional. Objective means it is not open to interpretation and it is measurable. These measurable findings include body temperature, pulse and respiratory rate, organ enlargement, abnormal heart sounds, edema (fluid swelling), and a change in body weight. Signs are part of the **physical examination,** a written record of the examiner's physical findings. Some sources include diagnostic test results as part of the signs. Some disease processes may be **subclinical** or **asymptomatic.** The prefix "a" means without. This means that even though a disease is present, it does not produce symptoms that are noticeable by the patient. Asymptomatic means without symptoms. A complaint based on the patient's _____(1) of discomfort is called a _____(2). A symptom is not _____(3). A measurable objective finding is called a _____(4). Symptoms are generally part of the _____(5), while signs are revealed from the _____(6). Asymptomatic means the disease does not cause _____(7) symptoms. Another term for this is _____(8).

1-10

1. signs
2. symptoms
3. together
4. not
5. generalized
6. nonspecific

When a disease process always has a specific set of signs and symptoms that occur together, this is called a **syndrome.** This combination may define a specific disease, such as Down's syndrome, or it may be a disorder caused by several different diseases, such as nephrotic syndrome. In Down's syndrome, mental retardation and abnormal facial features always occur together. In nephrotic syndrome, protein loss into the urine and edema always occur together, but nephrotic syndrome is a finding common to several specific kidney diseases. Some signs and symptoms are so common to many diseases that they are called **generalized** or **nonspecific.** This means that by themselves they do not indicate any particular disease. General signs and symptoms include anorexia (loss of appetite), malaise (a general feeling of unwellness), lethargy (mental drowsiness), and fatigue (tiredness or lack of energy). A syndrome is when a group of _____(1) and _____(2) always occur _____(3). A syndrome may or may _____(4) be associated with a specific disease. Common signs and symptoms that do not implicate a specific disease are called _____(5) or _____(6).

1-11

1. primary
2. secondary
3. complication
4. sequela

The **complications** of a disease are additional abnormalities that develop as the result of the disease. The first or initial disease is described as a **primary** dysfunction. Other dysfunctions that occur on top of the primary condition, and especially because of the primary condition, are **secondary** dysfunctions. Patients confined to bed for a long while because of a primary disease can develop pneumonia as a secondary disease or complication. Obstruction in the urinary tract can lead to secondary bacterial infection. A **sequela** (like the word "sequel") is what can come after a disease. Pelvic inflammatory disease (inflammation of the female reproductive tract) can leave the individual sterile afterwards. A disease that occurs first is a _____(1) disease, and one developing in addition to the primary condition is a _____(2) disease. A secondary disease is also described as a _____(3). The aftermath of a disease may be called a _____(4).

1-12

1. acute
2. gradual or slow
3. long
4. confined
5. systemic
6. generalized

The course of a disease may be acute or chronic. **Acute** means a sudden onset of signs and symptoms, which can be severe. Acute disorders are of a relatively short duration. Acute diseases either resolve completely (are eliminated) or may result in death. A **chronic** disease has a gradual onset, which can sometimes be described as insidious (in a slow, creeping manner). Chronic also describes the duration of the disorder, which is long (longer than 6 months). The symptoms of a chronic disorder are usually milder than an acute one, but elimination is more difficult. The effects of a disease may be confined to one area (be **localized**), or may spread to many parts of the body (be **systemic** or **generalized**). A disease of sudden onset with a relatively short course is described as _____(1). A chronic disease has a _____(2) onset and runs a _____(3) course. A localized disorder is _____(4) to one area of the body, while a _____(5) or _____(6) disorder affects many parts of the body.

-- 1-13 ------

The **diagnosis** of a disease is the *process* of identifying the manifestations so that the disease can be named. The *name* of the disease that the patient has is also called the diagnosis (this is the noun form of the word). The advantage of having a specific diagnosis is that the physician then knows what course the disease will follow and what treatment should be used. A diagnosis is arrived at using the history, physical examination, and a multitude of test procedures (including both laboratory and x-ray techniques). Two terms that are part of the physical examination are **palpation** (to feel and determine with the hands) and **auscultation** (to listen to sounds with a stethoscope). Having a specific diagnosis also allows the physician to state a **prognosis,** or most likely outcome of the disease. The process that leads to a name for a disease is called the _____(1). Diagnosis also means the _____(2) of the disease. A diagnosis is determined through the _____(3), _____(4), and _____(5) procedures. Feeling a body part to make a finding is called _____(6), while auscultation relies on _____(7) to sounds. A prognosis is the most probable _____(8) of a disease.

1. diagnosis
2. name
3. history
4. physical examination
5. test
6. palpation
7. listening
8. outcome

-- 1-14 ------

The treatment of a disease should be as specific as possible so that a cure is likely. In some cases there is no specific treatment or cure. Often **supportive therapy** is the only course of action. This is support of the body's needs to make it as strong as possible so that it may overcome the disease. Supportive therapy includes rest and supplying optimal nutrition, fluids to support hydration, and antibiotics to prevent a secondary infection while the immune system is stressed. **Palliative therapy** is also not curative, but it provides relief from signs and symptoms. Examples include anti-inflammatory medication, steroids, pain relievers, and surgical removal of a large tumor. If a disease does not require treatment to be cured, that is, it resolves on its own, it is referred to as **self-limiting.** The common cold is an example of a self-limiting disease. Supportive therapy and palliative therapy are applied in cases where there is no specific _____(1) or _____(2) for a disease. Strengthening the body so that it may heal itself is the goal of _____(3) therapy. Relief from the discomfort of a disease can be achieved with _____(4) therapy. A disease that doesn't need treatment to achieve healing is described as _____(5).

1. treatment
2. cure
3. supportive
4. palliative
5. self-limiting

-- 1-15 ------

The remaining terms that you need to learn relate to the body itself. The prefix **"intra-"** means within, such as intracellular (inside a cell) or intravascular (inside a vessel). The prefix **"extra-"** means outside of, such as extracellular (outside of a cell) or extravascular (outside of a vessel). **Endogenous** means coming from within the body, while **exogenous** means coming from the outside. Diabetes is a disease of endogenous origin, while infection is disease originating from the outside of the body. The **matrix** of the body is the structural ground substance that houses the **parenchymal** cells. The parenchymal cells are those cells that perform a function. Within an organ, the parenchyma is the functional tissue that is supported by the surrounding matrix (usually collagen-based connective tissue). Intracellular refers to something _____(1) a cell and extravascular refers to something _____(2) a vessel. Disease that results from an environmental insult to the body is _____(3) in origin. An endogenous disease is produced _____(4) the body itself. Functional cells make up the _____(5) tissue of an organ, and they are supported by the nonfunctional _____(6).

1. inside
2. outside
3 exogenous
4. within
5. parenchymal
6. matrix

1-16

1. structural
2. functional
3. space-occupying lesion
4. enlarged
5. Hypertrophy
6. cells
7. decrease
8. shrink
9. compensation

A **lesion** is either a disruption in the continuity of the tissues caused by disease or trauma, or the loss of function of a part. It is from the Latin language and means "to hurt." A lesion is either a structural or functional injury. A lesion that has mass and takes up space is a **space-occupying lesion.** Examples of a space-occupying lesion are a tumor, abscess, or cyst. An organ that is enlarged is described by the suffix **"-megaly."** An example is hepatomegaly (enlargement of the liver). Several diseases cause organ enlargement in response to the injury. Another term that describes enlargement is **hypertrophy.** This is when individual cells increase in size, and this is frequently seen in muscle cells. A skeletal muscle group may enlarge or hypertrophy in response to work or exercise. Cardiac muscle fibers can also enlarge, and this cardiac hypertrophy creates an overall enlargement of the heart, called cardiomegaly. Tissues and organs of the body can also react in an opposite manner and decrease in size. This shrinking or withering away is called **atrophy.** Atrophy is caused by disuse of a body part or organ. The last term is **compensation.** This is when the body attempts to make up or compensate for the effects of a disorder. Compensation is effort to restore balance that is upset by disease. In cardiovascular disease, the heart undergoes several changes to try to maintain normal cardiac output. Loss of one kidney causes the remaining kidney to enlarge and increase its workload to make up for the loss. A lesion is a _____(1) or _____(2) injury. A lesion that has mass is called a _____(3). The suffix "-megaly" describes an organ that has _____(4). _____(5) is another term for enlargement, and it applies to individual _____(6). Atrophy is when tissues or organs _____(7) in size or _____(8). When the body undergoes changes to counter the effects of a disease and tries to restore balance, this is called _____(9).

II. REVIEW QUESTIONS

1. The manner in which a disease develops through established stages is referred to as the:
   a. etiology
   b. pathogenesis
   c. pathology
   d. syndrome

2. A symptom is:
   a. the same as the clinical presentation
   b. a secondary result of a primary disease
   c. an objective finding during the physical examination
   d. a subjective complaint based on perception of discomfort

3. The science that studies disease processes is:
   a. pathology
   b. etiology
   c. pathogenesis
   d. diagnosis

4. A disease that has spread to affect many parts of the body is described as:
   a. asymptomatic
   b. a complication
   c. generalized or systemic
   d. chronic

1. b–pathogenesis

2. d–a subjective complaint based on perception of discomfort

3. a–pathology

4. c–generalized or systemic

5. Etiology means:
   a. of unknown cause
   b. the probable outcome of a disease
   c. the cause of a disease
   d. a physical or structural injury

6. A physical examination reveals the:
   a. signs of a disease
   b. symptoms of a disease
   c. history of a disease
   d. all of the above

7. A group of signs that always occur together may be described as:
   a. subclinical
   b. generalized or nonspecific
   c. the clinical presentation
   d. a syndrome

8. _____ describes a disease that develops rather quickly and does
   not last a long time.
   a. Acute
   b. Complication
   c. Sequela
   d. Chronic

9. Please match the terms in the left column with their meanings in the right column:
   a. endogenous   1. ____ increased cell size
   b. extra-   2. ____ outside of
   c. hypertrophy   3. ____ inside of
   d. intra-   4. ____ decreased cell size
   e. atrophy   5. ____ originating within the body
   f. exogenous   6. ____ organ enlargement
   g. -megaly   7. ____ originating outside of the body

10. The parenchyma of an organ is its:
    a. complication as the result of a primary disease
    b. functioning cells
    c. compensation for disease
    d. supporting matrix

5. c–the cause of a disease

6. a–signs of a disease

7. d–a syndrome

8. a–Acute

9. 1. c–hypertrophy
   2. b–extra-
   3. d–intra-
   4. e–atrophy
   5. a–endogenous
   6. g—megaly
   7. f–exogenous

10. b–functioning cells

CHAPTER 2

Principles of Cellular Injury and Response

► OBJECTIVES

SECTION I

Define all highlighted terms.
Define inflammation, explain its purpose, and cite its goal.
Relate each sign of inflammation with each phase of response to injury.
Explain how cell death is diagnosed.
Explain the difference between cell death and necrosis.
Characterize the differences between the types of necrosis, cite the most common causes, and explain the effect of necrosis on surrounding tissue.
Explain the relationship between hypoxia, ischemia, anoxia, and infarct.
List the three phases of response to injury and state the result of each.

SECTION II

Define all highlighted terms.
Describe all of the changes in blood vessels and blood flow that make up the vascular response.
Explain how fluid and cells escape from vessels.
Explain the term "exudate," state its purpose, and list its usual contents.
Describe the activities of white blood cells during the vascular response and exudation.
State the purpose of fibrin in an exudate.
Explain how a clot is formed and state its purpose.

SECTION III

Define all highlighted terms.
List the cells of acute inflammation and characterize each, including their secretions.
Explain the purpose of each cellular activity.
Explain the purpose of demolition.
Describe the role of the myofibroblast.
Define a chemical mediator, explain its mechanism of action, and list the major effects of chemical mediators.
List all of the events of acute inflammation in the order in which they occur.

SECTION IV

Define all highlighted terms.

Describe the process of regeneration and its final outcome.

Describe the process of fibrous connective tissue repair and its final outcome.

State the common term for fibrosis and explain its significance in a vital organ.

Explain how wound contraction is accomplished, and state its purpose.

Compare debridement with demolition.

Compare the different features and results of primary versus secondary intention wound healing.

Describe the complications of healing and their associated results.

List the factors that influence successful healing.

SECTION V

Define all highlighted terms.

Describe the microscopic appearance of chronic inflammation, including specialized cell types, their function, and the amount of fibrosis.

List the causes of chronic inflammation.

Describe granuloma, epithelioid cell, and giant cell formation.

Identify the components of chronic suppurative inflammation.

List systemic changes that can result from inflammation.

SECTION ▶ I. AN OVERVIEW OF DAMAGE AND REPAIR IN THE HUMAN BODY

2–1

1. cell
2. biochemistry

In discussing the mechanisms of injury and the response of healing, it is important to relate the events occurring at the level of the whole organism to the events occurring at the cellular level. What we see as disease in an individual usually has its basis at the level of the cell, or even lower, in the area of biochemistry. To understand what is happening when a person is ill, one must first comprehend the events at the basic level of the _____(1) or sometimes in the area of _____(2).

2–2

1. specialized
2. tissue
3. organ
4. system

The human body is structured in a building block fashion, of which the **cell** is the foundation. The cell can be seen as a self-sustaining factory that carries on all the processes of life. Some of these processes are respiration, the use of energy, the production of energy in other forms, and reproduction. There are many different types of cells, each type being referred to as **specialized.** A large group of cells of the same and other types joined together is called a **tissue.** The purpose of this union is to begin to perform a function in common. An **organ** is the combination of different tissues to perform a larger function. Finally, a **system** is composed of organs whose individual functions work together to produce a final process of life, such as digestion. Cells of all the same type are called _____(1). The first level where different cells begin to function together is called a _____(2), and this leads to the formation of an _____(3), which performs a larger function. What we consider to be a bodily process is accomplished by different organs working together in a _____(4).

2–3

By examining injury and response first at the cellular level, we can lay the framework for a better understanding of a disease process affecting an entire system. **Most signs of disease can be traced back to damage to individual cells and the attempts at repair. Make certain that you grasp the principles of this chapter before advancing to the systemic diseases.** We will be referring back to these fundamental principles often during the study of specific diseases.

▶ PRINCIPLES OF CELLULAR INJURY

Inflammation is a term familiar to most people, yet it is a very complex process. By definition, inflammation is the body's response to injury that results in characteristic visible signs produced by vascular and chemical changes. (**Vascular** pertains to blood vessels.) The purpose of inflammation is to contain or destroy the offending agent. Inflammation is not the same as infection. Infection, which we will study later, is the invasion of living tissue by microorganisms. An infection causes inflammation. However, inflammation may exist without the presence of microbes, as you will see when we look at some causes. The purpose of inflammation is to _____(1) or _____(2) the agent of injury. This reaction to damage produces visible _____(3) because of changes in blood _____(4) and _____(5).

2–4

1. contain
2. destroy
3. signs
4. vessels
5. chemicals

The suffix "-itis," when joined with a root word, usually means inflammation or an inflammatory process. An example is gastritis. **Gastric** is the root word and refers to the stomach. Therefore **gastritis** means inflammation of the stomach. Appendicitis, tonsillitis, and bronchitis are other familiar examples, indicating inflamed appendix, tonsil, or bronchi. These terms do not always mean a specific diagnosis but more often refer to a general process. The cause is not indicated. "Gastritis" is only a partial diagnosis, because it could be due to toxins, diet, stress, or chemicals such as alcohol or drugs. A term indicating inflammation of an organ is not a complete diagnosis because the _____(1) is not indicated. "Bronchitis" simply means _____(2) of the _____(3).

2–5

1. cause
2. inflammation
3. bronchi

There are two major categories of inflammation, **acute** and **chronic.** You will remember from Chapter 1 that acute means a condition of _____(1) onset, and, if resolved, lasts a relatively _____(2) time. Chronic refers to a _____(3) duration, and may arise from an acute condition where the cause of damage was not removed. We will study acute inflammation first and end with the events of chronic inflammation.

2–6

1. sudden
2. short
3. long/longer

The characteristic signs that accompany inflammation were first described centuries ago using Latin terms. There are four classic signs, with some sources referring to a fifth. (You will not be asked to remember the Latin terms.) These are:

1. Redness (from the Latin *rubor*).
2. Swelling (tumor).
3. Pain (dolor).
4. Increased warmth or heat (calor).
5. Loss of function (*functio laesa*).

2–7

1. redness
2. swelling
3. pain
4. heat
5. loss of function

Each sign can be explained in terms of vascular and chemical response to the injury. These visible signs were first described from skin inflammation. An example is shown to you in Figure 2–1. Some tissues may respond differently without all the described changes, but the process is the same. If you were asked to relate the signs most associated with inflammation, you would list _____(1), _____(2), _____(3), _____(4), and _____(5).

2–8

This reaction to injury we call inflammation is intended as a defense mechanism that serves to protect the body. It is supposed to be beneficial, but this is not always the case. Some of the products may accumulate in areas that interfere with vital functions. Fluid in the lungs may interfere with the exchange of oxygen. The inflammation itself, as it contacts adjacent normal tissue, may cause a reaction to the chemicals involved. Severe pain can produce spasms that decrease blood flow to an adjacent area. If this damages the area it will respond with more inflammation. Visualize a domino effect to depict how inflammation can become a cycle of injury in itself. Even though inflammation is intended to

1. defense
2 beneficial
3. damage

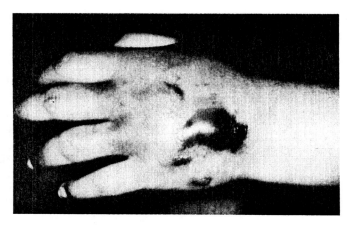

Figure 2–1. Cardinal signs of acute inflammation. Note swelling and redness of the skin around an infected burn. Marked tenderness, increased local temperature, and loss of function were also present. *(From Chandrasoma and Taylor,* Concise Pathology, *2nd ed., Appleton & Lange.)*

be a _____(1) mechanism with _____(2) effects, it can become a cycle of _____(3). Often in the course of treatment of an inflammatory disease, medications such as anti-inflammatories are used to help bring the process itself under control.

There are some tissues in the body that cannot respond to injury with inflammation. A basic requirement for response is vascularity, that is, an adequate number of blood vessels present for the vascular portion of the response. The cornea of the eye is clear to allow for vision; therefore there are no blood vessels, and this tissue cannot respond to injury with _____(1).

Over the next several frames you will be introduced to some terms needed to discuss the inflammatory process and also to terms used in explaining more generalized disease processes. **Do not proceed with this study until you are familiar with these terms.** Injury to cells may occur first at the biochemical level, depending on the causative agent. The result is an upset of normal chemical processes. This may lead to structural changes in the cell, such as nuclear breakdown, or the injury may begin with structural changes. If these changes are mild or reversible the term **degeneration** is applied. Degeneration is a breakdown that leaves some loss of function. **Adaptation** can also be used here, because the cell undergoes responses to counter and repair the injury. The structure of a cell can be seen microscopically and therefore can be described. This is referred to as **morphology,** and can be thought of as the appearance of a cell as shown in Figure 2–2. If injury to a cell can be reversed, the associated changes are called _____(1) or _____(2). By looking at the cell, the structure or _____(3) can be described to help determine the extent of injury.

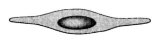

A   B

Figure 2–2. Cell morphology. **A.** Rounded and grainy. **B.** Spindle-like and smooth.

2–11

If the cell cannot recover from the injury, the damage is irreversible and **cell death** is the result. Specific structural changes in the cell, usually in the nucleus, are used to diagnose cell death. An entire chapter can be written on these pathologic changes, but for our purposes you need only recognize the terms and know they diagnose cell death. These visible signs are **pathognomonic,** which means when they are present, there is no doubt as to the diagnosis. A pathognomonic sign is very specific for one diagnosis. The first change in the nucleus following death is **pyknosis,** which means the nucleus has undergone condensation or becomes very dense. This is followed by **karyorrhexis,** which is the fragmentation or breaking up of the nucleus. The final change is **karyolysis** or fading away due to lysis (dissolving). _____(1) is diagnosed by looking at changes in structure or _____(2) (appearance) of a cell. These extremely specific or _____(3) signs include a dense nucleus or _____(4), a fragmented nucleus or _____(5) and a dissolving nucleus or _____(6).

1. Cell death
2. morphology
3. pathognomonic
4. pyknosis
5. karyorrhexis
6. karyolysis

2–12

Autolysis is the self-digestion of a cell following death. It is accomplished by the degeneration of the organelles' lysosomes, which contain lytic enzymes whose function is to digest substances. As more cells die, the area becomes large enough to be differentiated from living tissue. The area is described as necrotic. **Necrosis** is a section of dead tissue, diagnosed according to the structural changes of cell death. As cell death becomes widespread enough to be visible in a section of tissue, the section is described as _____(1). A diagnosis of _____(2) is arrived at when the structural changes of cell death are evident.

1. necrotic
2. necrosis

2–13

There are various types of necrosis. We will examine just a few that are most relevant to your understanding. **Coagulation necrosis** occurs when the proteins in a cell denature, that is, lose their configuration when chemical bonds holding the shape of the protein break down. The classic example of protein denaturation is cooking an egg. As the protein in an egg white is subjected to heat, the bonds holding the molecule together break apart. The molecule then falls apart and this is visible as the egg white changes from clear to white. In the case of necrosis these changes are due to lysosomal enzymes. The most common cause of this type of necrosis is deprivation of oxygen. In the next frame you will learn several terms associated with oxygen deprivation. Necrosis associated with denatured cellular proteins is classified as _____(1) and is usually due to lack of _____(2).

1 coagulative
2. oxygen

2–14

The most common cause of either localized or generalized tissue injury is deprivation or lack of oxygen. Coagulation _____(1) is the type of widespread cell death seen here. **Hypoxia** refers to less than the normal amount of oxygen reaching the cells. Since oxygen reaches cells through the circulation or blood supply, hypoxia is the result of decreased blood supply to an area. We call this diminished blood supply **ischemia.** Therefore, hypoxia is a result of ischemia or decreased _____(2). **Anoxia** is complete deprivation of oxygen due to no blood supply at all to a tissue. The necrosis that results from this complete absence of oxygen is called an **infarct.** The term "infarct" is also associated with sudden lack of blood supply, because this causes anoxia. Understand the difference between the terms referring to the amount of oxygen present (hypoxia, anoxia) and those meaning the amount of blood supply to transport oxygen to cells (ischemia, infarct). Hypoxia and anoxia are *secondary* to, or the *result* of ischemia or an infarct. This is shown in Figure 2–3. Impaired circulation to an area leads to less oxygen than normal, which is called _____(3). This impairment in circulation is termed _____(4). In complete lack of oxygen, or _____(5), the resulting necrotic area is called an _____(6), which may also describe absence of circulation. Mechanisms that cause ischemia and infarcts will be discussed in Chapter 9.

1. necrosis
2. blood supply
3. hypoxia
4. ischemia
5. anoxia
6. infarct

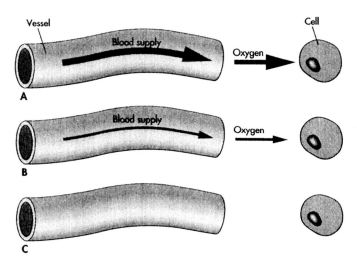

Figure 2–3. A comparison of normal blood and oxygen supply with decreased and absent supply. **A.** Normal blood and oxygen supply to the cells, as shown by large arrows. **B.** Decreased supply (**ischemia** and **hypoxia**), as shown by small arrows. **C.** Absent supply (**infarction** and **anoxia**), as shown by no arrows.

2–15

1. liquefaction
2. amorphous
3. cheesy

Liquefaction necrosis occurs when pyogenic (pus-producing) bacteria are the cause of tissue injury and death. In addition to the autolytic changes of coagulation necrosis, the bacteria attract a type of white blood cell that releases enzymes to destroy them. The combination of dead cells, bacteria, and associated debris forms the thick yellow fluid commonly known as pus. When bacteria and pus are involved in producing tissue death, this is known as _____(1) necrosis. Liquefaction necrosis may also follow an infarct, as seen in Figure 2–4. **Caseous necrosis** is very often associated with damage produced by the bacteria that cause tuberculosis. It looks different from coagulative necrosis because the tissue structure is typically lost. The tissue is described as **amorphous** (without shape or structure), and is characteristically firm and has a cheesy consistency. In caseous necrosis, the tissue loses its structure and is described as _____(2) or without shape. It has a firm and _____(3) consistency.

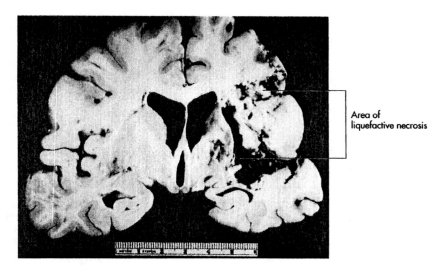

Area of liquefactive necrosis

Figure 2–4. Cerebral infarct, showing liquefactive necrosis of the cerebral hemisphere. The involved area has been converted to a fluid-filled cyst that collapsed when the brain was cut and the fluid drained out. *(From Chandrasoma and Taylor,* Concise Pathology, *2nd ed., Appleton & Lange.)*

2-16

Regardless of the type, necrosis itself incites an inflammatory response. This is because as dead tissue it is unnatural or foreign to the body. This is helpful when performing post-mortem studies. If an area of dead tissue is surrounded by a zone of acute inflammation, the area can be classified as a premortem change, that is, occurring before death of the individual. Autolysis due to death of the individual would not be accompanied by inflammation. Finding necrosis accompanied by a zone of inflammation would add something to the list of possible causes that resulted in death. For example, such a finding in heart muscle would put "heart attack" on the list of suspected causes.

2-17

The causes of injury to living tissue are of two broad categories, internal and external. Internal agents of damage include:

1. Genetic defects where an enzyme vital to normal metabolism is missing or defective.
2. Lack of necessary nutrients, hormones, or other essential chemicals vital to normal metabolism.
3. Deficiency of blood supply and therefore oxygen.
4. Autoimmune disease where antibodies attack the host's own tissues (the antibodies are called "autoantibodies").
5. The presence of free radicals or oxidants, which are unstable, imbalanced molecules that interact with normal molecules and damage cell membranes.

2-18

External agents of injury to cells are those you would more readily recognize, such as:

1. Pathogenic microorganisms (bacteria, viruses, fungi).
2. Chemicals such as poisons or caustic (burning) substances.
3. Physical injury, which includes trauma, radiation, ultraviolet rays, and temperature extremes.
4. Some would list nutritional deficiency as external, since the deficiency is coming from the outside.

2-19

In this frame please classify these agents of injury as internal or external:

1. Ischemia _____
2. Bacteria _____
3. Trauma _____
4. Hypoxia _____
5. Autoantibodies _____
6. Vitamin deficiency _____ or _____

1. internal
2. external
3. external
4. internal
5. internal
6. internal, external

2-20

General principles of cellular injury must include a survey of the cascade of events that occur following harm to the tissues. The word "cascade" is used to signify the relationship of one event leading to another, which is an important concept. All of the parts or events work together. The various events will be referred to as "responses," which are the reactions living tissue has to injury. The first response is termed **vascular** because it pertains to changes in blood _____(1). These changes will be presented in more detail later in this chapter. The two most important results of the vascular response are **vasodilation** and an increase in **permeability** of the vessels. **Dilation** is the increase in diameter of a tubular or rounded structure. When pupils of the eyes dilate, they become larger. When vessels _____(2) they become larger. The increase in size allows the vessels to provide to the area more ammunition to fight the injury. Thus the first response, or the _____(3) response, is the first line of supply of substances needed to reverse the effects of injury and allow healing. After providing an increase in various cells and chemicals to an area, there must be a mechanism for these materials to leave the vessels and reach out into the tissues where the damage is occurring. This is accomplished through an increase in vessel permeability.

1. vessels
2. dilate
3. vascular

2–21

1. permeability

Permeability is the degree of selectivity a membrane shows in allowing substances to pass through or in preventing passage. This concept can be thought of in terms of "leakiness." For example, if you were to pour a cup of water into a paper bag and some into a plastic bag, the paper bag would be permeable to the water (it would allow water to pass through or leak) and the plastic would be impermeable. If changes in blood vessels allowed more substances to pass through than normal, the vessels would be showing an increase in _____(1). Refer to Figure 2-5, which illustrates vasodilation and increased permeability.

2–22

1. white blood
2. phagocytosis

The second reaction is a cellular response. What are the materials or substances the vessels have provided? The answer is the cells of the inflammatory response. The source for these cells is the circulation itself, where they are classified as **white blood cells (WBCs).** A WBC is also called a **leukocyte,** whose name means white cell. The function of each type is specific and will be described later. The main objective is to isolate the offending agent, destroy it or remove it, and clean up the aftermath of battle to allow healing. The cell type that predominates early in an acute inflammation is the **polymorphonuclear WBC (PMN)** or **neutrophil.** These are the cells that engulf or **phagocytize** foreign particles, bacteria, dead material, or other debris. **Phagocytosis** is a process in which a cell takes particles and substances into itself for destruction. A PMN or neutrophil is a type of _____(1) cell or WBC that "swallows" and digests foreign agents in a process called _____(2). (The word element "phag" means eating or swallowing and "cyto" means cell.)

2–23

1. macrophage
2. eater
3. phagocytosis
4. debris

As the inflammatory process continues another type of WBC becomes more numerous in the area. That is the **monocyte** as it is called in circulation, or the **macrophage** as it is called in tissue. The function is similar to the PMN. The difference is in the slower reaction time and larger quantity of intake of the macrophage. The name "macrophage" means large ("macro") eater ("phage"). The macrophages finish what the neutrophils begin, joining in on the attack a little later. This type of WBC also is important in cleaning up the debris that is a result of the destruction of a foreign agent. A slower-moving WBC is the _____(1), whose name means big _____(2). This process of cellular "eating" is called _____(3). Macrophages are also important in cleaning up _____(4).

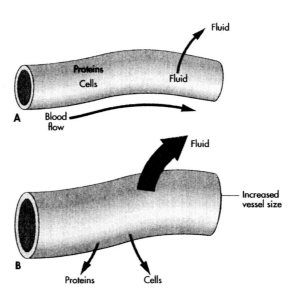

Figure 2–5. Vasodilation and increased permeability. **A.** Normal vessel size and permeability, as depicted by the small arrow. **B.** Vasodilation and increased permeability, as depicted by the additional and large arrows.

Following removal of the harmful agent by WBCs and cleanup in preparation for repair, the next major cellular participant is the **fibroblast.** The fibroblast is not of the circulation but is a tissue cell. It is responsible for producing some of the new tissue in the repair process. The term **myofibroblast** has also been used to describe these cells because of the contractile movement they display during the weaving process of repair. "Myo" is a term relating to muscles and contractile movement is similar to muscle contraction. A cell of tissue origin that spins new tissue in the process of _____(1) is called a _____(2) or _____(3), since its movements have been compared to muscular contractions.

2-24

1. repair
2. fibroblast
3. myofibroblast

A third important part of the acute inflammatory response involves substances often referred to as **chemical mediators.** They are indeed chemicals, not cells. **Humoral** is sometimes used to indicate action by chemicals instead of cells, so this part of the events is sometimes called the **humoral response.** These chemicals are secreted by various cells and the damaged tissue. One example of which you are probably familiar is histamine. The living organism uses chemicals in some instances as messengers to "tell" the target tissue what to do or how to react. As a mediator is a "go between," the chemical mediators of inflammation go from their origin to their target with very specific instructions. The target "reads" the message when the chemical binds or joins to a **receptor** that resides on the membrane of the target cell. A receptor is a molecular structure that binds only to certain chemicals, like a lock being specific for a key. The result is a particular reaction by the target tissue to the chemical. Figure 2–6 diagrams these events. In describing the effect of _____(1) mediators on _____(2) tissue, a lock-and-key analogy helps to explain the binding between a _____(3) and its _____(4). This joining causes a particular _____(5) by the target to the chemical.

2-25

1 chemical
2. target
3. receptor or chemical
4. receptor or chemical
5. response or reaction

▶ RESPONSE TO INFLAMMATION AND HEALING

The signs we associate with inflammation are the direct result of the vascular, cellular, and chemical changes that are occurring. The production of these signs will be explained as each response is studied in more detail in the next section. We mentioned earlier that **containment,** or the holding of a damaging agent in check, is a desired result of the _____(1) process. This can also be described as the destruction of the agent. Successful containment is affected by several conditions. Most can be divided into two classifications. The first is the nature of the injury. In the example of trauma, an _____(2) cause of injury, the severity is of critical importance. A paper cut is easily resolved, whereas a stab wound may resist the body's defensive mechanisms. In the case of infection, also an _____(3) cause of injury, numbers of microorganisms are an important determining factor in whether the body can successfully contain the invasion.

2-26

1. inflammatory
2. external
3. external

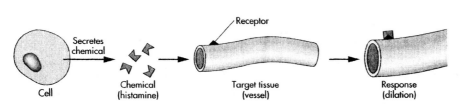

Figure 2–6. Target tissue response to chemical mediators. When the chemical mediator binds to the receptor on its target, the message is received and the target reacts.

2–27

1. vascular
2. mediator or messenger

The second classification of conditions that affect the success of containment is the ability of the host organism to produce an effective inflammatory response. There must be an adequate number of mature cells in the response and their function must be normal. Blood vessels that make up the _____(1) response and the appropriate chemical _____(2) must be working according to plan. In short the host should not be debilitated (run down), immunosuppressed, or otherwise compromised for effective containment to take place. (Immunosuppression is when the immune system is not fighting foreign invaders as it should. The reasons for this poor response are discussed in Chapter 4.)

2–28

1. demolition
2. macrophages
3. big
4. eater

If an injury can be successfully contained and stabilized, the final act of the inflammatory process can begin. Healing of the area is then able to proceed. An activity does, however, exist in between containment and healing that is necessary before healing takes place. That activity is **demolition.** This term indicates a cleaning up process prior to healing. During the course of inflammation some products are produced that become waste. Dead cells and necrotic tissue resulting from the injury itself are present, and dead inflammatory cells fill the area. If the injury is due to a living agent, there are now dead agents in the wound. All of this debris must be removed before new tissue can be generated during healing. It is very difficult to build a new structure if the demolished remains of the old structure still exist on the foundation. The phase of inflammation that removes or resolves the remaining waste just prior to healing is called _____(1). As previously mentioned, the inflammatory cells most responsible for demolition (clean up) are called monocytes in circulation or _____(2) when they are phagocytizing material in the tissues. The name macrophage literally means _____(3) _____(4).

2–29

1. parenchymal
2. regeneration
3. parenchymal

The terms most frequently associated with the healing process are **regeneration** and **repair.** **Regeneration** is the replacement of lost cells and tissue whose function is so similar to the original lost cells, that the replacements may be considered identical. For all intents and purposes, regeneration reproduces the same tissue that was lost. The intents and purposes we are most interested in are metabolic functions, especially in the tissue that makes up the vital organs of the body. As you will recall from Chapter 1 the cells in an organ that are responsible for the functions we associate with an organ are called _____(1) cells. Therefore the process of _____(2), which reproduces original function, is most important when _____(3) cells are injured.

2–30

1. regeneration
2. function
3. regeneration
4. function

Besides restoring function, an additional aspect to regeneration is related to the ability of the injured cells to reproduce. If a cell can't reproduce how can a functioning "clone" be generated? Obviously it can't. Two examples of tissues in adults that don't regenerate are neurons and cardiac muscle. When these tissues are damaged, healing occurs in the form of repair, not regeneration. The difference is that the repair tissue does not function as the original. Other cells of the body have great capacity to regenerate or restore function. Some types, such as epithelial cells, undergo a large turnover normally. The skin is an organ of the body that is constantly subject to minor trauma, so the capacity for regeneration must be great. Epithelial tissue heals through the process of _____(1) because original function must be restored. Regeneration allows for healing in such a manner that reproduced cells carry out the original activity or _____(2). Other types of cells do not normally have a large turnover, but if injured have the ability to regenerate. Cells of the liver and kidney are of this type. This is related to the importance of the work of these organs in maintaining the health and life of the individual. Cells of vital organs heal through _____(3) because it is important that original _____(4) be restored.

2–31

1. repair
2. function

Repair tissue is generally referred to as **fibrous connective tissue repair.** This mechanism differs from regeneration in that original function is not restored. Connective tissue serves as a structural framework for support of vital tissues. It is the matrix or foundation that holds everything together. Following an injury that results in tissue loss, as most do, the body is left with a defect or hole that must be filled. Connective tissue repair patches the hole or bridges the gap to rejoin the remaining tissue. There is no function associated with connective tissue repair. The process of patchwork healing called _____(1) does not restore original _____(2). Repair occurs where regeneration is not possible or is very limited.

2-32

Repair tissue is frequently called _____(1) _____(2) _____(3) _____(4). The term **fibrous** means made up of fibers, which are threadlike structures. Fibrous tissue is stringy, dense, tough collagen that makes a strong repair. (Collagen is a supportive protein.) Fibrous repair as seen in the skin is what is commonly known as **scar** tissue. **Fibrosis** is the abbreviated term for fibrous connective tissue repair, and is commonly called **scarring.** In some parts of the body healing by scar formation is perfectly acceptable and does not compromise the function of the body as a whole. The common term for fibrous repair is _____(5). Two tissues mentioned in frame 2–30 that have no ability to regenerate are _____(6) and _____(7). When injury occurs to these tissues, healing is by repair, not regeneration. The significance here is that the healed area has lost original _____(8) or activity. This area of fibrous _____(9) would be called a _____(10). To illustrate this significance, consider the patient who has had a "heart attack" or myocardial infarction. Infarction means complete loss of _____(11) to an area resulting in dead tissue or _____(12). The cardiac muscles heal through what we commonly call scarring or _____(13). The probable outcome of this patient's condition, or the _____(14) (Chap. 1) depends directly on the amount of functioning heart tissue remaining compared to the amount of nonfunctioning scar tissue or _____(15).

1. fibrous
2. connective
3. tissue
4. repair
5. scar
6. neurons or cardiac muscle
7. neurons or cardiac muscle
8. function
9. repair
10. scar
11. blood supply
12. necrosis
13. fibrosis
14. prognosis
15. fibrosis

2-33

Many injuries heal through a combination of regeneration and fibrosis or _____(1). An important early feature of the healing process is the activity of **contraction.** Contraction is the shrinking inward of the tissue surrounding a defect. The result is a decrease in the size of the defect or a smaller wound for the body to heal. The cells responsible for contraction are those that produce some of the new tissue and show muscle-like contractions. These cells are called _____(2). Figures 2–7 and 2–8 diagram these healing activities. The final phase of healing is called **remodeling.** These are changes the new tissue undergoes as it is put to the same use as the old tissue. An example would be a scar on the skin developing wrinkles over time.

1. scarring
2. myofibroblasts

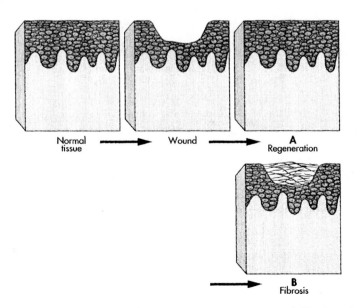

Figure 2–7. A comparison between regeneration and repair. **A.** Regeneration. **B.** Fibrosis repair.

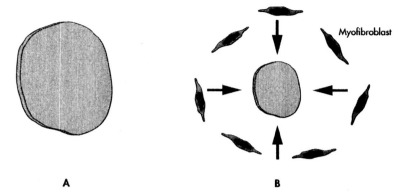

Figure 2–8. Wound contraction. **A.** Tissue gap before contraction. **B.** Tissue gap after contraction.

I. REVIEW QUESTIONS

1. List, from the smallest to the largest, the building blocks of the human body:
   a. _____ b. _____ c. _____
   d. _____

2. List five characteristic signs of inflammation: a. _____
   b. _____ c. _____ d. _____
   e. _____

3. True or false: Inflammation is a reaction to injury that is a defense mechanism and is never harmful by itself. _____

4. A sign that is specific for one diagnosis is called:
   a. pathognomonic
   b. histologic
   c. microscopic
   d. any of the above

5. Please match the terms in the left column with their meanings or descriptions in the right column:
   a. necrosis
   b. coagulation
      necrosis
   c. hypoxia
   d. anoxia
   e. ischemia
   f. infarct
   g. liquefaction necrosis
   h. caseous necrosis

   1. _____ necrosis due to total lack of blood supply
   2. _____ dead tissue
   3. _____ no oxygen present
   4. _____ cheesy consistency
   5. _____ low amounts of oxygen present
   6. _____ associated with pyogenic bacteria
   7. _____ caused by anoxia
   8. _____ less than normal blood supply necrosis

6. The two major phagocytic cells of the cellular response are the a. _____
   and the b. _____.
   1. eosinophil
   2. neutrophil or PMN
   3. macrophage
   4. lymphocyte
   5. myofibroblast

7. Phagocytosis means:
   a. attraction of WBCs to the site of injury
   b. WBCs swallow or engulf foreign material
   c. WBCs digest foreign material
   d. answers a. and b. are correct
   e. answers b. and c. are correct

8. The cell responsible for producing collagen during healing is the:
   a. monocyte
   b. myofibroblast
   c. macrophage
   d. PMN

9. A chemical mediator:
   a. initiates and controls the process of healing
   b. binds to receptors on target cells
   c. can produce chemotaxis
   d. initiates and controls the inflammatory process
   e. all are correct except d.
   f. all are correct except a.
   g. all are correct except c.

10. Briefly describe what it means for an injury to be contained or stabilized:
    _____
    _____

11. Please complete these sentences: Removal of all debris after inflammation is called a.
    _____. This activity must occur before the process of b._____ can begin.
    1. phagocytosis
    2. chemotaxis
    3. healing
    4. opsonization
    5. demolition

12. What is the fundamental difference between the outcome of regeneration and fibrous connective tissue repair?
    _____
    _____

13. Two terms that mean fibrous connective tissue repair are: (choose two)
    a. scar tissue
    b. necrosis
    c. autolysis
    d. fibrosis
    e. containment

II. VASCULAR RESPONSE TO INJURY ◄ SECTION

2-34

At this time we will begin to look at the individual parts of the inflammatory process, now that you have a basic understanding of how the parts fit together. One of the first changes to occur after cellular damage is the reaction by the blood vessels or the _____(1). In describing these responses it is helpful to first define the associated terms. **Vasodilation** is the increase in size, or in the diameter, or a blood vessel. The vessel becomes larger. Because of this it can hold more blood. When an area of tissue is perfused or supplied with a greater vol-

---

7. e—answers b. and c. are correct

8. a—myofibroblast

9. f—all are correct except a.

10. The agent of damage has been isolated and removed or destroyed. There is no ongoing injury. The cause of injury has stopped or been stopped.

11. a—5. demolition;
    b—3. healing

12. After regeneration most of the original function has been restored and the organ may carry out normal activity. After fibrosis, scar tissue replaces functioning cells with an inert patch material. Overall activity of the organ may be adversely affected, depending on the extent of scarring.

13. a—scar tissue;
    d—fibrosis

1. vascular response

2. vasodilation
3. hyperemia
4. stasis or hemostasis
5. stasis or hemostasis

ume of blood than normal, this condition is **hyperemia.** "Hyper" means increased and "emia" refers to blood. Therefore an increase in vessel size, called _____(2), leads to increased blood supply to an area or _____(3). Another event in this process is **stasis,** which essentially means stopping. Since what is stopping or slowing down is the speed of blood flow through the area it can also be referred to as **hemostasis.** ("Hemo" is another word part that means blood.) Some of this slowing down is due to the blood becoming thicker, as we will see in the next frames. _____(4) or _____(5) is how we describe the reduction in velocity or speed of blood flow through an area.

► CHANGES IN THE FLOW PATTERNS OF BLOOD

2-35

1. hyperemia
2. vasodilation
3. stasis

Under normal circumstances there is a major channel of blood flow through a location called a thoroughfare channel. It is similar to the main street in a small town experiencing most of the traffic with several small side streets not used as frequently. In inflammation the thoroughfare partially closes and blood is diverted or detoured to the lesser-used capillaries in the location. Capillaries are the smallest part of the vascular system, compared to arterioles and venules, arteries and veins. Circulation through capillaries is named **microcirculation.** While blood is diverted to the microcirculation, the arterioles or supply end of the system also dilate to increase the amount of blood available. Increased blood in a location is termed _____(1). This is made possible by increased vessel size or _____(2). Hyperemia provides for more fluid, nutrients, and agents of defense to the injured site. Vasodilation and the slowing of blood flow or _____(3) are important aspects of hyperemia. Vasodilation produces some degree of stasis according to a basic law of physics. You know that a river flows fastest through a narrow passage and slows down if the passage becomes wider. In the same manner, blood flow velocity is dependent upon vessel size.

2-36

1. stasis
2. permeability
3. mediator

Once the microcirculation is engorged with excess blood, fluid begins to leak from the vessels. As fluid is removed from whole blood, the blood becomes more viscous or thick. This also contributes to slowing or _____(1) of the blood flow. This leaking occurs due to the capillaries becoming more permeable to fluid passing through the walls. Capillaries are lined with endothelial cells whose edges contact each other. This point of contact is named a **junction** because it has the ability to open and provide a small space between the endothelial cells. Figure 2–9 shows how the cells contract, or pull inward, and create holes through which fluid, molecules such as protein, and WBCs may pass out into the tissue to reach the site of injury. The material that has escaped the microcirculation is an exudate and will be discussed shortly. **Histamine** is a substance that carries the message to the microcirculation that helps to produce vasodilation and increased leakiness or _____(2). By our previous definition histamine is therefore a chemical _____(3).

2-37

1. margination of WBCs
2. pavementation of endothelium
3. adhesion receptors

The next sequence of events is actually a cellular response, but it is important to present it as still a part of the vascular response because it involves both aspects. WBCs normally occupy the center of the blood flow stream. During the vascular response the WBCs leave the center and begin to line up along the capillary walls in preparation for escape. The walls are made up of endothelial cells whose junctions will soon open to help the WBCs squeeze through. This lining up of WBCs along endothelial cells is called **margination of WBCs** or **pavementation of endothelium.** The walls of the capillaries have become sticky and the WBCs stick like barnacles on the bottom of a ship. This sticking of WBCs to endothelium is called _____(1) or _____(2). On the membranes of the WBCs are specific molecules that bind with or join to other molecules called **adhesion receptors** on the endothelium. In a sense the WBC "docks" onto the endothelial cell. The molecules on the endothelium that interact with WBCs to produce adhesion between the two are referred to as _____(3).

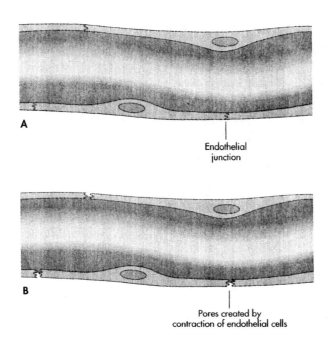

A

Endothelial
junction

B

Pores created by
contraction of endothelial cells

Figure 2–9. Endothelial contraction. **A.** Normal endothelial junctions. **B.** Pores created by contraction of endothelial cells.

▶ EXUDATE FORMATION

2–38

The net result of the vascular response is the formation of an exudate outside of the vessel at the damaged site. An **exudate** is a fluid accumulation outside of a vessel that has a high protein content, and in the case of inflammation, contains various types of inflammatory cells. Chemical mediators may also be a part of the exudate. Other conditions cause fluid accumulation in the tissues that is not considered an exudate. If there is increased hydrostatic pressure, which is related to high blood pressure, then more fluid than normal is squeezed out of the vessels. Or if there is decreased osmotic pressure, which is related to protein (albumin) content, then more fluid than normal is lost out of the vessels. Fluid buildup in these cases is a **transudate,** because the presence of proteins, cells, and other substances is minimal. This is because there is *not* an increase in permeability when inflammation is not the cause of the loss. Transudates differ from exudates in that the protein content is low. Transudates are thin and watery compared to the thicker, protein-rich exudate. A fluid accumulation outside a vessel that contains proteins and perhaps cells is an _____(1) while a _____(2) does not have these components. Exudate formation is the result of the _____(3) response. It is made possible by the increased leakiness of the vessels to proteins. This is properly referred to as increased vascular _____(4).

1. exudate
2. transudate
3. vascular
4. permeability

2–39

An exudate can be classified in three ways. **Serous exudate** has the least amount of protein and is seen in cases of minimal damage. (Usually the degree of response and change in permeability is directly proportional to the amount of injury.) A skin blister as a result of a burn contains a serous (serum-like) exudate. A **fibrinous exudate** contains fibrinogen, which is converted to fibrin, an important player in containment and healing. A **purulent exudate** is commonly known as pus, and is associated with infected inflammations. Pus is made up of thousands of neutrophils and other blood cells most of which are dead due to lysosomal activity. Also contained in pus are bacteria. The infectious process is **suppuration.** Bacteria that cause pus to be formed are **pyogenic.** If pus is confined or localized in one area, this is an **abscess** (Fig. 2–10). If the infection is not in a pocket but spread through the tissues, this condition is called **cellulitis.** All of these situations will be thoroughly examined in Chapter

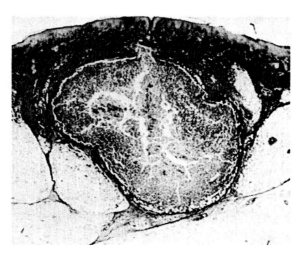

Figure 2–10. Histology of an abscess of the skin with localized collection of purulent exudate. *(From Kent and Hart,* Introduction to Human Disease, *3rd ed., Appleton & Lange.)*

1. fibrinous
2. purulent
3. suppurative

5 on bacterial infections. An infected inflammation producing a purulent exudate is called a **suppurative inflammation**, instead of an infected inflammation. An exudate that has a lot of fibrin is a _____(1) exudate, while an exudate primarily made of pus is a _____(2) exudate. A purulent exudate is formed during infected or _____(3) inflammations.

2–40

1. antibodies (antiglobulins)
2. drugs

The composition of an exudate can be compared to plasma although it is not exactly the same. **Plasma** is the fluid component of whole blood. (The term "whole blood" comes from the fact that blood can be separated into its parts during testing procedures.) Plasma has everything except blood cells. This includes many kinds of proteins, such as albumin, antiglobulins, and fibrinogen. Circulating fats, glucose, electrolytes, enzymes, and other substances compose plasma. You have learned that an exudate contains proteins that may include fibrinogen. Another important protein of exudates is antiglobulin, which is made up of antibodies of the immune system (Chap. 4). Antibodies are vital in the neutralization and destruction of many foreign agents. Therapeutic drugs such as antibiotics are commonly found in exudates. This is a mechanism for the drug to reach the site of action. Now you know two more components that can make up an exudate. These are _____(1), which neutralize foreign agents, and _____(2), such as antibiotics.

2–41

1. fibrin
2. fibrinogen
3. fibrin
4. engulf or "eat"
5. capture or contain
6. connect
7. phagocytosis

Fibrinogen is a soluble (dissolved) blood protein in an exudate that undergoes chemical changes in the tissue to become the solid **fibrin**. Fibrin is a threadlike protein that forms a **fibrin clot.** This is a network or mesh of fibers that forms a structural foundation for several activities. A clot is made of protein fibers called _____(1). The soluble or dissolved precursor of fibrin is _____(2). There are several functions of a clot (Fig. 2–11). One is to act as a net and capture or contain the damaging agents. This serves to prevent further spread of the agent, as with bacteria that invade or spread into surrounding tissue. A _____(3) clot also connects the area of severed tissue as an early stage of healing. The activity of phagocytosis, in which cells _____(4) materials, is physically supported by the threadlike mesh. This may be thought of in terms of the cells working on a scaffold to accomplish their purpose. Three functions of a fibrin clot are to _____(5) damaging agents, close or _____(6) a gap in injured tissue, and to support the cellular activity of _____(7).

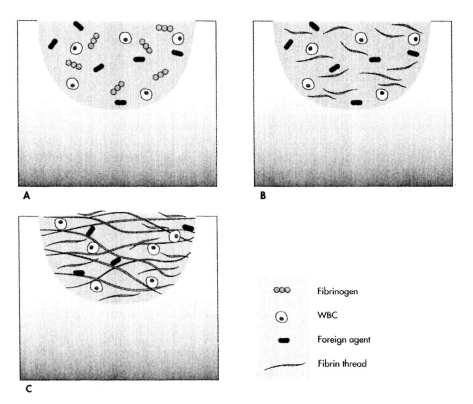

Figure 2–11. Formation of a fibrin clot. **A.** Wound containing exudate with dissolved fibrinogen, white blood cells, and foreign agents. **B.** Formation of fibrin threads. **C.** Scaffold structure of the clot, which traps foreign agents, supports white blood cells, and connects the gap.

2–42

The purposes of exudate in general are to:

1. Cause a diluting effect in the area, which is helpful in cases where irritating chemicals or toxins are present.
2. Provide a mechanism by which agents of defense reach the site.
3. Help the process of phagocytosis, as we will see in the next section.

▶ RELATIONSHIP OF THE VASCULAR RESPONSE TO SIGNS

2–43

Most of the hallmark signs of inflammation can be attributed to the vascular response. Hyperemia, which means increased _____(1) in the area, accounts for the redness and heat. Blood is responsible for the pink pigment of living tissue and carries much of the body's heat. Hyperemia is assisted by the process of _____(2) or increase in vessel size. Increased capillary permeability allows _____(3) and other materials to escape and build up outside of the vessels. Swelling is due to this fluid buildup in tissues. The presence of this exudate also contributes to pain as the tension in the tissues increases. Nerve endings are irritated by the pressure and probably by some of the chemicals involved in the process. The amount of exudate that can be formed is eventually limited by the degree that the tissue can be stretched. The presence of pain in a mobile part of the body causes the individual to limit its activity, thereby causing some loss of function. Vasodilation and hyperemia cause inflamed tissue to become _____(4) and _____(5). Exudate produces _____(6) and _____(7), which leads to a loss of _____(8).

1. blood
2. vasodilation
3. fluid
4. red or hot
5. red or hot
6. swelling
7. pain
8. function

II. REVIEW QUESTIONS

1. a–vasodilation; b–hyperemia; c–hemostasis; d–permeable; e–exudate; f–vascular

2. True

3. d–margination or pavementation

4. 1. d–purulent exudate
   2. c–fibrinous exudate
   3. a–exudate
   4. b–serous exudate

5. c–the network of fibrin fibers acts as an opsonin for phagocytosis

6. a–exudate formation; c–hyperemia; e–pressure in tissues

1. Please complete these sentences: An increase in the size of a blood vessel is called a. _____. This results in more than the normal amount of blood in an area, which is called b. _____. Increased vessel size and fluid loss contribute to the slowing down of blood through the vessel, and this is called c. _____. Fluid, cells, and proteins leak out of the vessels because the vessels have become leaky or more d. _____. This extravascular fluid accumulation in the tissues is referred to as an e. _____. All of this describes the first part of inflammation, which is called the f. _____ response.

2. True or false: Capillaries are lined with endothelial cells that contract during inflammation to create tiny holes called junctions. It is through these junctions that cells, proteins, and fluid leave the vessels. _____

3. Interaction between WBCs and capillary endothelial cells through adhesion receptors produces:
   a. vasodilation
   b. hemostasis
   c. phagocytosis
   d. margination or pavementation

4. Please match:
   a. exudate   1. _____ suppurative inflammation
   b. serous exudate   2. _____ fibrinogen and fibrin
   c. fibrinous exudate 3. _____ proteins, cells, fluid, drugs, antibodies
   d. purulent exudate   4. _____ minimal protein

5. Which of the following statements if INCORRECT?
   a. the dissolved protein in an exudate that changes to solid form is fibrinogen
   b. the solid form of this protein is fibrin
   c. the network of fibrin fibers act as a opsonin for phagocytosis
   d. the network of fibrin fibers acts as a net to capture foreign agents
   e. the network of fibrin fibers provides physical support for phagocytosis

6. The characteristic signs of inflammation are produced by which of the following activities? (choose all that are correct)
   a. exudate formation
   b. the presence of bacteria
   c. hyperemia
   d. necrosis
   e. pressure in the tissues
   f. karyorrhexis

III. CELLULAR AND CHEMICAL RESPONSE TO INJURY ◀ SECTION

▶ ACTIVITIES OF INFLAMMATORY CELLS

There are many terms to be learned in studying the role of WBCs in inflammation. "WBC" stands for _____(1). These terms involve the activities of the WBCs. We will look at the particular cells shortly. **Phagocytosis** is a process you have already learned, and you know it means for a _____(2) to engulf or swallow particles. You also know that **margination of WBCs** or **pavementation of** _____(3) is when WBCs _____(4) along capillary endothelium. The sticking process is greatly assisted by _____(5) receptors. A new activity is **diapedesis.** Once margination is complete, the WBCs are ready to travel to the site of injury. Diapedesis is the process whereby the cells push themselves through the opened endothelial junctions by moving like amoeba. This is illustrated in Figure 2–12. Once this is accomplished, the WBCs head for where they are needed. Travel to the site is called **emigration** or **migration.** Both diapedesis and migration are under the influence of **chemotaxis.** "Chemo" means chemical and "taxis" is moving, especially toward a particular destination. Chemotaxis is a phenomenon that guides and attracts WBCs to the injury. The cells do not "know" where to go. Chemicals, molecules, cellular secretions, and other substances act as a homing signal that WBCs find irresistible. Specific chemotactic agents include some of the chemical mediators, antibodies that have neutralized their foreign targets, products from bacteria, and dead tissue in some cases. The act of WBCs arriving at the site of inflammation is the result of being drawn by the presence of specific substances, and this is known as _____(6). This influential pull begins when the cells are still inside the vessels. To get outside the vessel the WBCs squeeze through junctions, and this is referred to as _____(7). Once outside the vessel, the cells travel or _____(8) to the damaged tissue.

1. white blood cell
2. cell
3. endothelium
4. line up
5. adhesion
6. chemotaxis
7. diapedesis
8. emigrate or migrate

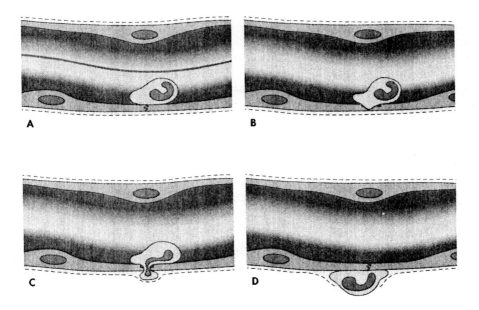

A   B

C   D

Figure 2–12. Diapedesis. **A.** Margination by WBCs (pavementation of endothelium). **B., C.** Diapedesis. **D.** WBC ready for emigration (migration).

2-45

1. phagocytosis
2. lysosomes
3. lysis
4. coated
5. opsonin
6. easier

Two important terms that are part of phagocytosis are **opsonization** and **lysis.** Before being ingested by WBCs, bacteria and other particulate material may be coated with a plasma protein called an **opsonin.** An opsonin makes phagocytosis easier, like the coating on a pill to be swallowed. Sometimes an antibody itself becomes an opsonin after complexing with its foreign agent. An opsonin is also a signal to the phagocytic cell in recognizing what needs to be engulfed. The engulfing process or _____(1) is accomplished by the WBC wrapping pseudopods (temporary arm-like projections) around the foreign material. Once inside, the material is digested through the act of **lysis.** Organelles in the cytoplasm called **lysosomes** release enzymes and break down the ingested material. It should be noted that lysis specifically refers to the rupture of a cell membrane along with spillage of the intracellular contents. The action of the lysosomal enzymes is the final stage in the destruction of particulate agents. The enzymes inside the cell that digest engulfed materials come from organelles ("little organs") called _____(2) in a process specifically referred to as _____(3). Before being phagocytized the foreign matter may be _____(4) with a protein called an _____(5). Coating by an opsonin makes phagocytosis _____(6).

2-46

1. four
2. two
3. seven
4. one
5. six
6. three
7. five
8. eight

Please take a few minutes to look at the illustration in Figure 2–13. The activities we have studied are shown in the order in which they occur. After studying this visual presentation, **number** the following activities in the **order** in which they occur:

exudation _____(1)   opsonization _____(5)
margination _____(2)   diapedesis _____(6)
phagocytosis _____(3)   migration _____(7)
vasodilation _____(4)   lysis _____(8)

▶ TYPES OF INFLAMMATORY CELLS

2-47

1. PMN
2. lysis
3. inflammation
4. chemotaxis
5. first or early
6. fastest
7. hours

The cells that make up whole blood are of two categories: erythrocytes, which literally means "red cells," and leukocytes, which means "white cells." The cells of inflammation are of the leukocyte category. There are five different kinds of leukocytes, three of which are part of inflammation. The neutrophil or _____(1) has been mentioned as a WBC that plays a crucial role in the defensive inflammatory reaction. All leukocytes are very mobile, which contributes to the success of diapedesis and migration. The neutrophil is part of the first line of defense and specializes in phagocytosis and digestion or _____(2) of foreign materials. The material is usually particulate, which means solid but microscopic. Bacteria are an excellent example, and make up a large portion of the diet of the "eating" cells. Two common types of bacteria that neutrophils are well programmed to destroy are the staphylococcus and streptococcus organisms that are a part of our environment. Polymorphonuclear cells respond first and fastest in the body's defense mechanism against injury that we call _____(3). This cell type dominates the scene early after injury. It responds well to chemical signals that attract it to the injury. This attraction is called _____(4). The cytoplasm of the PMN is loaded with lysosomes. The large numbers of lysosomes make neutrophils very effective in destroying their targets. Because of the release of all the lytic enzymes, the neutrophil sacrifices itself and is dissolved away along with its ingested material. You will recall the many dead neutrophils we said were present in pus. From the time the neutrophils leave the vessels on active duty to the time of their death is just a few hours. When we speak of the timing involved in the response to injury, the neutrophil arrives _____(5) on the scene, so its response time is _____(6) in comparison to other cells. The lifespan of an active neutrophil in the tissues is a few _____(7).

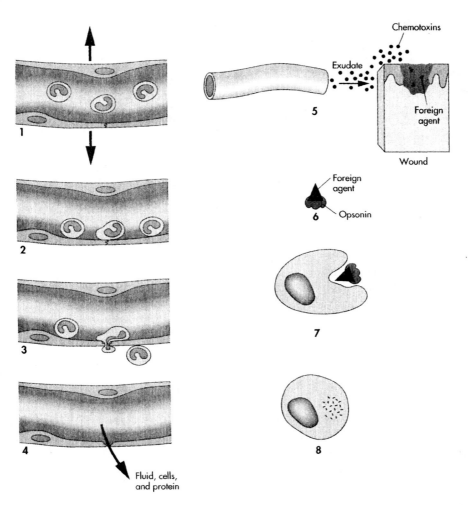

Figure 2–13. The order of activities in the vascular and cellular response **1.** Vasodilation. **2.** Margination. **3.** Diapedesis. **4.** Exudation. **5.** Migration. **6.** Opsonization. **7.** Phagocytosis. **8.** Lysis.

2–48

An interesting aspect of the destructive activity of the PMN is the production of H_2O_2, or **hydrogen peroxide.** You are probably familiar with the **bacteriocidal** or bacteria killing effect of H_2O_2 when it is used to clean wounds. When they are active, PMNs change the way they normally oxidize or metabolize glucose. A compound called a peroxide or a free radical is produced. This is also known as an oxidant. These unstable molecules have an unpaired electron that upsets the balance of other molecules through their interaction with them. The result is severe damage to the cell membrane that contacted the peroxides. The cell is destroyed if the membrane damage is complete or through the entire thickness of the membrane. H_2O_2 destroys bacteria in this manner. H_2O_2 or _____(1) has an effect on bacteria that is described as bacteriocidal or bacteria _____(2). Unstable molecules known as _____(3) cause severe damage to cell _____(4), thereby destroying the cell.

1. hydrogen peroxide
2. killing
3. peroxides, free radicals, or oxidants
4. membranes

2–49

The next cell to be examined is a second kind of leukocyte called a **monocyte** or a **macrophage.** When this cell is intravascular, or inside the blood vessels, it is called a monocyte. Once the monocyte leaves the vessels and is extravascular, it is known as a macrophage. You will recall the name "macrophage" means _____(1). When this cell is intravascular and inactivated, it is called a _____(2). When a monocyte is activated and moves out to the tissues it is a _____(3). As the

1. big eater
2. monocyte
3. macrophage

4. demolition
5. more
6. cells
7. slowly
8. after
9. longer
10. macrophage

name implies, macrophages are very phagocytic and engulf dead cells as well as bacteria. They are the mainstay in clearing away post-destructional debris. They clean up the dead PMNs and dead tissue. They are vultures or scavengers on the scene. This particular phagocyte is much longer lasting than the neutrophil and may stay in the area indefinitely. Macrophages move slowly toward the injury and arrive after the PMNs. They are lumbering giants that take the lion's share of debris removal. This is the important cleanup process of _____(4) that must occur prior to healing. The slower response of the macrophage causes a change in the population of cells at the site over time. You will recall that neutrophils arrive first and die quickly. They are then replaced by macrophages. When comparing the amount of work between neutrophils and macrophages, we can say macrophages phagocytize _____(5) than neutrophils. They not only ingest particles but entire dead _____(6) as well. Macrophages move _____(7) compared to PMNs and arrive _____(8) the PMNs. The life span of the macrophage is much _____(9) than that of the neutrophil. Another distinguishing feature of the macrophage is response to injury that is not due to infections, where bacteria are not present. An example would be blunt trauma that damaged or destroyed inner tissue. The macrophage would be activated as part of demolition. In injury not due to infection the phagocyte responsible for cleanup is the _____(10).

2-50

1. enzymes
2. dissolve
3. enzymes
4. hydrogen peroxide
5. interleukin

In addition to phagocytosis, macrophages produce a number of secretions that play an important role in inflammation. Some of these are part of the chemical mediators or humoral response. Only a few will be discussed here. One type of secretion is a class of enzymes that digest or breakdown extracellular substances such as collagen and elastin. These compounds make up the matrix or ground substance that provides the structural framework for living cells. Collagen and elastin can be compared to the mortar between bricks in a wall. By releasing an enzyme such as collagenase or elastase, the mortar is somewhat dissolved and the macrophages can move more easily toward the work site. This is like clearing a path through a jungle. Movement by macrophages through solid tissue is helped by the secretion of _____(1), which _____(2) extracellular collagen and elastin. Macrophages also produce enzymes from their lysosomes to digest engulfed material and cells. Hydrogen peroxide is formed as in the case of the neutrophil. **Interleukin** is another secreted chemical that stimulates a third cell, the lymphocyte. Three additional secretions from macrophages are lysosomal _____(3), the bacteriocidal _____(4), and the lymphocyte-stimulating _____(5). The macrophage, then, is a major defensive cell that serves to isolate and ingest a damaging agent and provide the basis for healing via demolition.

2-51

1. oxygen
2. macrophages
3. attract
4. lymphokine
5. viral

The third leukocyte involved in inflammation is the **lymphocyte.** Lymphocytes are the main cells of the immune response and there is much to learn about them in Chapter 4. The role they play in inflammation is less prominent but all contributions, even minor ones, lead to the success of the total process. Lymphs produce antibodies against specific foreign agents called antigens. Any time an injury is due to an antigen that the lymph has produced an antibody against, that cell will be closely involved in the destruction. For the most part, lymphs play a lesser role in inflammation due to trauma, hypoxia [which means decreased _____(1) to cells], toxins, or other non-antigen causes. Lymphs release substances that are chemotactic for neutrophils and monocytes [which are also called _____(2)]. Chemotactic means that certain chemicals _____(3) inflammatory cells to the site. Chemotaxins from lymphs are **lymphokines.** If an injury is specifically due to a viral infection, then lymphs do act as the early predominant cell in containing and destroying the invaders. Their part in the healing process will be discussed shortly. A chemical secreted by lymphs that attracts other cells is called a _____(4). The type of infection where lymphs are the early predominant cell is a _____(5) infection.

2-52

1. vasodilation
2. permeability
3. histamine
4. allergy or parasite
5. allergy or parasite
6. myofibroblast
7. tissue

We will conclude our study of the inflammatory cells with three last cells: the **mast cell,** the **eosinophil,** and the **fibroblast.** The mast cell is found *along* capillaries in all tissues, not in the circulation. It is activated earliest in response to injury. From the mast cell comes a very important chemical mediator called **histamine.** Histamine sends the messages that help produce vasodilation and an increased vascular permeability. As you now know, these are two pivotal events that allow for the recruitment and mobilization of the defensive forces, which are the cells. A chemical mediator released from mast cells that causes _____(1) and an increased _____(2) is _____(3). The eosinophil is a WBC of the circulation and contains granules of substances that are active in allergic responses. Therefore eosinophils are prominent in inflammations caused by allergies. A specific type of antibody is bound to the surface of the mast cell. When this antibody contacts the corresponding antigen in an allergic response, a chemotaxin is released that signals the presence of eosinophils to the site. Any type of inflammation due to a parasite also attracts eosinophils. Two causes of the presence of eosinophils at the site of inflammation are _____(4) and _____(5). The last cell is the fibroblast, which you know is also named a _____(6) because of its contractile movement. The myofibroblast is important in healing. This cell produces new _____(7) in a spinning-like process.

► CHEMICAL MEDIATORS

2-53

Let us now turn our attention to the last aspect of the response to injury by the body. Chemical mediators are secretions from cells that act as messengers to different parts of the body to produce the coordinated process of inflammation. It is important to note that the process is very well orchestrated and controlled most of the time. The initiation (start of) and control is due primarily to the actions of these chemical conductors. In particular, histamine from mast cells is the most important, primary initiator of the vascular response.

2-54

There are ten major substances that can play a part as chemical mediators during inflammation. Their names are:
1. Histamine
2. Bradykinin
3. Complement
4. Lysosomal enzymes
5. Prostaglandin
6. Leukotrienes
7. Platelet-activating factor
8. Cytokines
9. Serotonin
10. Fibrin

What is important for your understanding is to know the most significant effects that are produced because of their messages. These include:

1. Vasodilation
2. Increased vascular permeability
3. Chemotaxis
4. Acting on other cells to cause their activation or the release of other chemical mediators

Because of the effects of chemical mediators, these substances both **initiate** (begin) and **control** the process of acute inflammation.

2-55

1. initiate
2. control
3. vasodilation
4. vascular permeability
5. chemotaxis
6. vascular
7. cellular

It should be noted here that histamine and bradykinin are both part of the earliest phase of response and their effects are short lived. The red line, flare, and wheal reactions by histamine are named for the visible events occurring in the skin after an injection of histamine. These three effects together are called the Triple Response, which will be discussed under the topic of allergy. Two major functions of chemical mediators are to _____(1) and _____(2) acute inflammation. Chemical mediators that cause vessels to enlarge are producing _____(3). Those that increase the leakiness of vessels are increasing _____(4). Chemical signals that attract inflammatory cells to a site are causing _____(5). All chemicals causing vasodilation and increased vascular permeability, which produce the exudate, are mediators of the _____(6) response during inflammation. Chemicals producing chemotaxis are part of the _____(7) response to injury.

2-56

One practical application of our knowledge of chemical mediators is in the treatment of an undesired inflammatory response. There are several conditions where it is helpful to control, minimize, or even prevent inflammation. Pain, loss of function, and the prevention of healing during an exaggerated response can be good reasons to intervene. By knowing the mechanism of production and the effects of the chemicals involved, anti-inflammatory drugs can and have been synthesized to control the process. A drug called an anti-histamine is a familiar example. Aspirin acts as an anti-prostaglandin. The prefix "anti" in this instance means that the drugs decrease the production of the chemicals or that they inhibit their activity. Steroid medications at lower doses are also anti-inflammatories by a variety of mechanisms. In this instance, the controllers are controlled themselves. We can modify the body's level of response to injury through the use of drugs.

2-57

1. short
2. longer

To this point our study has focused on the **acute** condition. Acute means of _____(1) duration. If the offending agent can be completely contained and destroyed, healing may take place as an end to injury. If for various reasons the damaging agent is not contained and persists within the body, then complete healing cannot take place. The efforts of inflammation will then continue over time. This is considered **chronic** inflammation. By definition a chronic condition lasts _____(2) than an acute condition. Before we begin our study of chronic inflammation, it is necessary to learn about the repair process, since some of the repair efforts become part of the chronic condition.

III. REVIEW QUESTIONS

1. 1. d–lysis
   2. e–opsonization
   3. a–phagocytosis
   4. b–diapedesis
   5. c–emigration
   6. f–margination of WBCs

2. True

3. d–neutrophil

1. Please match the terms in the left column with their definitions in the right column:

   a. phagocytosis
   b. diapedesis
   c. emigration
   d. lysis
   e. opsonization
   f. margination of WBCs

   1. ____ digestion by lysosomal enzymes
   2. ____ coating foreign material with a protein that eases phagocytosis
   3. ____ to engulf foreign material
   4. ____ WBC movement through endothelial junctions
   5. ____ travel by WBCs to injury site
   6. ____ adhesion receptors

2. True or false: To this point, the order of activities of the inflammatory response begins first with vasodilation and ends with lysis. _____

3. The WBC that acts quickly in response to phagocytizing foreign material and dies quickly is the:
   a. eosinophil
   b. macrophage
   c. lymphocyte
   d. neutrophil

4. Another term for neutrophil is _____ WBC.

5. True or false: Attraction of cells to the injured site by chemicals is called opsonization.
   _____

6. A product of neutrophils and macrophages that is bacteriocidal by causing oxidizing damage to cell membranes is:
   a. interleukin
   b. lymphokines
   c. hydrogen peroxide
   d. histamine

7. The slow-responding scavenger cell that phagocytizes most of the dead cells and debris, and is present a long time, is the:
   a. eosinophil
   b. macrophage
   c. neutrophil
   d. lymphocyte

8. Inflammation due to a viral agent presents this cell as the early predominant defense:
   a. neutrophil
   b. eosinophil
   c. macrophage
   d. lymphocyte

9. Histamine is a chemical mediator secreted by the:
   a. fibroblast
   b. lymphocyte
   c. mast cell
   d. macrophage

10. Eosinophils are WBCs that are actively involved in inflammation due to
    a. _____ and b. _____.

11. True or false: Chemicals causing chemotaxis are part of the vascular response, while those causing increased permeability are part of the cellular response.
    _____

12. What is the role of chemical mediators in inflammation?
    _____
    _____

13. Knowledge of chemical mediators is important so that drugs can be synthesized to:
    a. begin the process of inflammation in a debilitated individual
    b. initiate healing activities
    c. control the production of chemical mediators
    d. intensify the activities of chemical mediators

4. polymorphonuclear
5. false
6. c–hydrogen peroxide
7. b–macrophage
8. d–lymphocyte
9. c–mast cell
10. a–parasites or allergy
    b–parasites or allergy
11. false
12. They initiate or begin the process of inflammation and act as controllers for the various activities. This control occurs as a result of sending messages to cells and tissues by interacting with receptors.
13. c–control the production of chemical mediators

SECTION ▶

1. material
2. outcome
3. cells
4. function
5. scar
6. function

IV. PRINCIPLES OF HEALING

There are two mechanisms of healing that differ from each other in the replacement material and in the final outcome. The replacement material may be new cells or it may be connective tissue. The outcome may be return of loss of function of the injured area. Replacement with new cells preserves function while replacement with connective tissue leaves an area relatively inert. **Regeneration** is the healing method that produces cells almost identical to the original cells that were destroyed. This is different from **fibrous connective tissue repair,** where scar tissue is the end result. Regeneration restores original function while fibrous repair does not. In the following frames we will look at these two mechanisms in detail. Remember, they differ from each other in their replacement _____(1) and final _____(2). Regeneration produces new _____(3) and restores _____(4), while fibrous connective tissue repair leaves _____(5) tissue and loss of _____(6).

▶ REGENERATION

1. regeneration
2. function
3. organ

The purpose of regeneration is return of original function. The extreme importance of this is seen when considering healing in a vital organ such as the liver or kidney. There are specific injuries that can occur to these organs such as hepatitis or kidney failure due to a toxin. But widespread injury can occur as a result of systemic causes such as hypoxia. Shock is a good example of generalized hypoxia (Chapter 9). The liver and kidney have a relatively high metabolic rate because of the amount of work they do. Because of this their need for oxygen is great and they are especially sensitive to being deprived of the normal amount of oxygen. It is fortunate that cells of some vital organs have the ability to be reproduced, especially when considering their sensitivity to injury. The primary purpose of _____(1) is to restore original _____(2). This is especially important after injury to a vital _____(3).

1. death
2. amount
3. division
4. mitosis
5. regeneration
6. function

The basic requirement for regeneration is that the remaining live cells have the ability to undergo cell division or mitosis and produce new replacement cells. One vital organ that does not have the ability to reproduce its cells is the heart. Following necrosis or tissue _____(1), healing occurs by fibrous repair or scarring. Permanent loss of function is directly proportional to the amount of injury. That is why the prognosis depends on the amount of injury after a heart attack. For the victim of a heart attack, the prognosis depends on the _____(2) of injury, because cardiac cells do not have the ability to undergo cell _____(3) or _____(4). Replacement in this manner is the basic requirement for the healing process of _____(5), which restores original _____(6).

1. oxygen

The body's tissues vary in their ability to undergo cell division and reproduction. It was previously thought that regenerative ability was strictly related to how specialized the tissue was. The more specialized, the less power for cellular division and replacement. Neurons are a good example of a sophisticated tissue that cannot replace itself. The central nervous system and the heart are unable to regenerate after an irreversible injury. (Necrosis occurs after irreversible injury.) However, both the liver and kidney could certainly be considered specialized in the work they perform. Because we know their regenerative powers are very good, then other factors must come into play. Likelihood of injury is a recent theory to explain the differences in healing mechanisms. We have mentioned the sensitivity of the liver and kidney to hypoxia, which is a deprivation of _____(1). Consider also the fact that these two organs act as a processing center and giant filter, respectively, for the entire blood supply. All circulating injurious agents such as chemicals and bacteria make their way to these organs, so the likelihood of injury is relatively high. Two factors that govern regenerative ability are how _____(2) the tissue is and how likely it is to be _____(3).

2-62

Epithelial cells of the skin and the lining of the intestinal, respiratory, and urogenital tracts have a great ability to regenerate themselves. This makes complete sense when considering how likely it is that this tissue will be subject to injury (especially physical injury). The skin is directly subject to contact with the outside world, and the other systems are subject to some form of access by damaging agents through their openings to the outside. It is interesting to note that the composition of the liver and kidney is based in epithelial tissue, and this certainly contributes to their regenerative powers. The central nervous system (brain and spinal cord) is encased in bone (the skull and spinal column) and is not exposed to the general circulation in a clearing house fashion. Likelihood of injury to this tissue ranks at the bottom of the list. One might think that the heart is fairly susceptible to injury, as indicated by the prevalence of heart disease, and should be able to regenerate. However, most cardiac disease today is related to lifestyle choices and the stress of our fast-paced society rather than more natural injury.

2-63

Originally, the ability to regenerate was thought to only be related to how _____(1) the tissue was. Highly specialized tissue, such as a neuron, does not undergo cell _____(2) to replace itself. A more recent theory is that regeneration is related to likelihood of _____(3). One example of tissue that is very likely to be injured by contact with the outside is _____(4) tissue. The examples presented in the last few frames are at the opposite ends of the spectrum of regeneration ability, being either very good or poor. The remaining tissues fall somewhere in between.

1. specialized
2. division
3. injury
4. epithelial

► FIBROUS CONNECTIVE TISSUE REPAIR

2-64

The healing mechanism called fibrous repair is basically a patchwork remedy that fills in defects after tissue necrosis and loss. In sharp contrast to regeneration, with fibrous repair there is no return of original _____(1). In some tissues there is little in the way of vital function to begin with. For example, the skin and all of the connective tissue that exists within the body provide their own function just by being present, by providing a covering and structural framework. If these tissues are repaired with fibrous connective tissue, there is little interference with the overall function of the body. The literature does not report any deaths due to scarring of the skin. Another name for fibrous connective tissue repair is the common term "scar tissue." An additional term used by health care professionals is fibrosis. The purpose of fibrous connective tissue repair is to provide a _____(2) remedy that fills _____(3) left after tissue loss. Two other terms for this type of healing are _____(4) and _____(5).

1. function
2. patchwork
3. defects
4. scar tissue
5. fibrosis

2-65

The significance of fibrosis is when this healing occurs in a vital organ. Two such organs that we said have great regenerative abilities are the _____(1) and _____(2). When the degree of injury overcomes even these organ's abilities to regenerate, then tissue loss is replaced with scar tissue. Scar tissue performs none of the work done by the original cells. Therefore the concern we have is how much healing in a vital organ will result in scar tissue or _____(3)? Again, this is determined by the amount or severity of injury. For example, if the damage to the liver is so severe that it results in 20 percent of the tissue being replaced by scarring, then 20 percent of liver function will be permanently lost. Fibrosis of the liver is called **cirrhosis,** and is due to long-term, continual damage generally from excessive alcohol intake. Eventually scar tissue predominates, there are not enough parenchymal cells remaining, and death results. (Referring back to Chap. 1, parenchymal means _____(4) _____(5) within an organ.) One vital organ you know that does not regenerate itself at all is the

1. liver or kidney
2. liver or kidney
3. fibrosis
4. functioning
5. cells

6. heart
7. scarring
8. prognosis
9. injury
10. regenerate
11. fibrosis or fibrous repair

_____(6). Following necrosis in the heart, fibrosis or _____(7) is the only mechanism of healing. The predicted future of the patient or the _____(8) then depends directly on the amount of _____(9). Another system previously mentioned is the central nervous system. A "stroke" causes necrosis in the brain. This tissue loss is not replaced by functioning cells, because neurons don't have the ability to reproduce themselves or _____(10). Healing in the brain is by _____(11).

2-66

1. wound
2. contraction
3. smaller
4. less
5. myofibroblasts
6. contraction

There are more events in fibrous repair than in the simpler cellular division of regeneration. The purpose of fibrosis is just to bridge the damaged area to provide continuity to the remaining tissue. A scar is a dense, tough mass of collagen, which is a ground substance consisting of supportive protein. The first step in repair is **wound contraction,** and this is visible in skin lacerations. Wound contraction is the process of shrinking the size of the defect to produce a smaller wound. The obvious purpose here is to leave less area to be repaired. The resulting scar would also be smaller, leaving less disruption to normal tissue. Myofibroblasts surround the wound and by nature of their movement, which is contraction, cause shrinkage. This is like drawing on a pouch string (Fig. 2–8). Contraction can be inhibited if the tissue is anchored tightly to underlying tissue (like the periosteum of a bone), so flexibility is a factor that influences this process. The shrinkage of a tissue defect is called _____(1) _____(2) and its purpose is to leave a _____(3) wound that needs _____(4) repair. It is accomplished mainly by cells called _____(5) that surround the wound and move by _____(6).

2-67

1. protein or cells
2. protein or cells
3. macrophage
4. demolition
5. granulation tissue
6. vessels or capillaries

After wound contraction comes the process of **granulation tissue** formation. Before and during contraction scavenger cells are removing necrotic tissue and debris left over from exudation. Remember, exudation is fluid release from vessels that contain _____(1) and _____(2). The scavenger cell responsible for most of the cleanup is the _____(3). This removal activity, which must come before healing, is called _____(4). After demolition, granulation tissue is formed, as shown in Figure 2–14. This delicate new tissue is a mixture of leftover fibrin from exudate, growth of tissue from surrounding areas, and myofibroblasts. Capillaries in the area produce buds of themselves that begin to grow across the defect. This will result in the necessary blood supply to nourish the area and support the repair process. This vascular network is reddish and very fragile, bleeding easily if disturbed. If you've ever prematurely removed a scab, or the dried clot covering the wound, then you've seen granulation tissue. (A scab that is allowed to fall off when ready reveals a mature scar.) The newly formed tiny vessels are thin and permeable so that the area is moist and nourishing fluid bathes the wound. The color and moisture of _____(5) is due to new _____(6) that bud across the wound from neighboring capillaries.

2-68

1. organization
2. granulation
3. collagen

Myofibroblasts infiltrate the wound along with the new vessels. In addition to contraction, these cells produce collagen fibrils (tiny fibers) that are laid down in the vascular bed. All of these elements will later mature and some will disappear. This initial stage is called **organization.** Organization results in the proper orientation or lining up of these elements before they mature. Also produced by fibroblasts are the compounds **proteoglycans** and **fibronectin,** which become part of the glue in this new ground substance. As the fibroblasts multiply, they lay down more and more collagen, which is the basis of the scar. The cells are nourished by the vascular bed that was formed for that purpose. With time, the number of cells and vessels decreases and the predominant substance that fills the defect is collagen, which condenses into a compact mass (Fig. 2–14). Remodeling occurs when organization and maturation are complete. The initial stage of vessel growth and myofibroblast migration into the wound is called _____(1). The red, moist, delicate new tissue that is formed during organization is _____(2) tissue. As part of organization, myofibroblasts produce _____(3) fibrils that later mature to dense collagen. Other

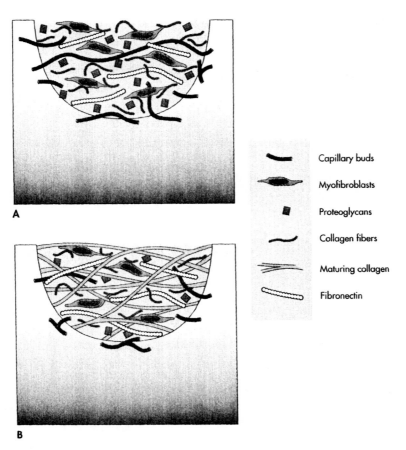

Figure 2–14. Fibrous connective tissue repair. **A.** Elements of granulation tissue. **B.** Maturation of granulation tissue (scar formation).

products from these cells include _____(4) and _____(5), which help make up the glue of the new matrix. The majority of the final mature tissue in a scar is _____(6).

4. proteoglycans or fibronectin
5. proteoglycans or fibronectin
6. collagen

2–69

On a final note, it is important to realize that both mechanisms of healing can occur simultaneously in the same tissue. Very few events in the body are isolated or occur in a vacuum. Even in regeneration there is some amount of fibrosis, which is necessary to replace the structural framework for the parenchymal cells. The following frames will illustrate how these mechanisms can be combined.

▶ REPAIR IN WOUNDS OF THE SKIN

2–70

In order to gain a better understanding of regeneration and fibrous repair, we can consider the example of healing in a skin defect. Skin wounds heal through a combination of regeneration by the outer epithelial layer, and fibrous connective tissue repair by the dermis or underlying connective tissue. Look at the example in Figure 2–15, which illustrates the tissue loss after a skin laceration. The immediate result is bleeding into the wound by the severed vessels. This blood will clot and begin to dry out and crust over, forming what we call a scab. Some of the elements of a clot are red blood cells, platelets (which are cell fragments important to the clotting process), and chemicals that cause clotting. Also of importance is the presence of fibrin. Recall that the structure of fibrin is _____-like (1) and that it weaves together to form a _____(2) or mesh that traps _____(3). This trapping of the solid elements forms the basis of the solid clot,

1. thread
2. net
3. cells and other particulate matter

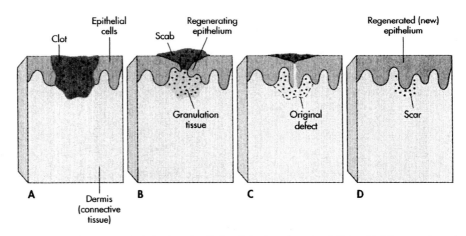

Figure 2–15. Healing in skin wounds. **A.** Clot formation. **B.** Granulation tissue formation. **C.** Early epithelial regeneration and maturation of granulation tissue. **D.** Regenerated epithelium and organized scar.

4. fibrinogen
5. blood
6. protein
7. fibrinous

especially as the liquid portion of blood begins to evaporate. The precursor to fibrin is _____(4), and it is normally found in the _____(5) stream. Fibrinogen is made of _____(6). The clot is not to be confused with the scaffold for phagocytosis formed by fibrin in exudate. Exudate that contains fibrin is called _____(7) exudate. Instead, the clot forms a protective barrier to prevent further injury or infection of the newly formed, fragile tissue (Figure 2–15A). The final scab will lie over the regenerating epithelial layer, which in turn lies over the granulation tissue of the fibrous repair of the dermis (Fig. 2–15B and C).

2–71

1. vascular
2. exudate
3. cellular
4. chemical
5. initiation
6. control
7. demolition
8. smaller
9. organization
10. granulation
11. scar

The wound then experiences the inflammatory reaction that consists of three main phases or responses you have learned:

1. The _____(1) response, which occurs early and produces the fluid rich in protein and cells called an _____(2).
2. The _____(3) response, which results in phagocytic cells arriving at the injury and destroying any invading agents such as bacteria.
3. The _____(4) response, which is responsible for the _____(5) and _____(6) of the whole process.

After the injury becomes stable, the process of healing can begin by cleaning up the dead cells, tissue, and debris in a phase called _____(7). Wound contraction occurs, which leaves a _____(8) wound to be repaired. A small amount of left-over exudate material mixes with ingrowing capillary buds and migrating myofibroblasts that secrete collagen fibrils. This all becomes oriented properly in the phase called _____(9). This freshly organized, red and moist tissue is called _____(10) tissue and will finally mature into a _____(11).

2–72

1. cell-to-cell
2. contact
3. inhibition
4. basal or germinal

After the injury is contained, regeneration of the epithelial layer begins. Loss of cell-to-cell contact is the signal that indicates tissue loss. This begins a migration of the epithelial cells from the edges of the wound toward the center. **Contact inhibition** occurs when the advancing sheets of cells meet each other, and is the signal for the migration to end. When they contact or touch each other, further movement is normally stopped or inhibited. Meanwhile the basal or germinal layer of cells is undergoing mitosis to produce new cells that mature into the epithelial cells of the upper layers. The signal for the movement of cells from the edges of the wound toward the center is loss of _____(1) contact. This is stopped when cells meet each other in what we call _____(2) _____(3). New cells are produced by the _____(4) layer by cell division or

_____(5). Because this method of healing produces functioning cells that are the same as the cells destroyed by the injury, this method is called _____(6). The advancing sheet of epithelial cells grows underneath the protective dried clot, which is commonly called a _____(7). When the scab detaches and falls off, it reveals regenerated epithelial tissue (Fig. 2–15D). This is provided so that the injury does not become infected, does not experience excessive inflammation, and does not lose the scab prematurely. Any of these events could destroy the regenerating cells and leave scarring as the method of tissue replacement.

5. mitosis
6. regeneration
7. scab

_2–73_

The healing mechanism of the dermis or underlying connective tissue is fibrous repair or _____(1). This tissue has the purpose of filling in the gap after injury or patching the defect. After exudation and phagocytosis, some fibrin may remain and mix with incoming myofibroblasts and loops of new capillary buds. These tiny vessels provide nutritional support for the myofibroblasts, which begin to secrete and weave collagen fibrils through the area. This early tissue with these components is called _____(2) tissue. These collagen fibrils mature to stronger fibers. After maturation, the vessels degenerate and disappear and the work of the myofibroblasts is complete. The fully matured repair tissue is commonly called a _____(3). The scar tissue generally does not contain hair follicles or glands, since these are structures that would require regeneration. The white color of the scar is due to the lack of melanocytes, which produce the skin pigment melanin. This method of healing that produces a scar is properly termed _____(4) or _____(5).

1. fibrosis
2. granulation
3. scar
4. fibrous repair or fibrosis
5. fibrous repair or fibrosis

_2–74_

Fibrotic tissue has a great amount of tensile strength and can therefore withstand tension placed upon it. It is this fact that allows patients to regain the former strength of the abdominal wall after a laparotomy incision. The final strength of the fibrotic tissue is directly proportional to the amount of collagen incorporated into the wound. This strength is not achieved until maturation is complete. We have already mentioned the fragility of granulation tissue; immature collagen is also weak. It is important during healing that strain on the new tissue be avoided. Constant straining, like coughing, could break down delicate strands of granulation tissue as it is formed. Rupture of an immature incisional scar could occur with any straining activity, and will be discussed under complications of healing. The strength of scar tissue depends on the amount of _____(1) in the wound. _____(2) must be complete to achieve full strength. It is important to avoid _____(3) of granulation tissue when it is new.

1. collagen
2. Maturation
3. strain

_2–75_

Healing of skin wounds has been divided into two categories that describe the wound more than the healing process itself. The process of repair is the same in both categories. The difference is the amount of work to be done, the time involved, and the size of the final scar. **Primary intention,** which is also known as **primary union,** occurs when the wound edges are brought closely together with sutures or tape, such as closing a surgical incision or getting "stitches" for a cut. Just as in natural wound contraction, the result is a smaller defect to bridge. The associated pressure also decreases the amount of continual bleeding and exudation, which means there is less demolition of the leftover material. The closely approximated edges result in smaller scar formation. Healing is neater and faster. Artificial wound contraction achieved by mechanically bringing the edges together is the feature of a wound in the category of _____(1) _____(2). This is also known as primary _____(3).

1. primary
2. intention
3. union

_2–76_

If a wound is left to gape open, or otherwise cannot be closed, this category is **secondary intention** or **secondary union.** In this case, oozing blood will leave a large clot, which holds apart the edges of the wound. More exudate is produced and contributes to the amount of necrotic debris that must be removed over a longer period of time. The distance to bridge is greater and the resulting scar will be larger than in the case of primary union. In addition to healing in from the sides, granulation activity also causes filling of the defect from the bot-

1. secondary
2. intention
3. union
4. greater
5. intention

tom upwards. In the past, healing in this manner was referred to as granulation, or it was said the wound would "granulate in." However, this is not an accurate description because granulation is a feature of both categories of skin wound repair. Figure 2–16 shows a wound that has healed by both primary and secondary intention. A wound that is not artificially reduced falls into the category of _____(1) _____(2) or secondary _____(3). In this case the size of the defect to repair, the amount of demolition needed, and the size of the scar will all be _____(4) compared to primary _____(5).

····· 2-77 ·····

1. stopped
2. debridement
3. demolition or cleanup
4. healing

In addition to primary union, another intervention in wound healing that speeds the process and leads to greater success is **debridement.** Debridement should be preceded by cleaning out the wound to remove dirt, any embedded objects, and bacteria. Thorough cleaning by flushing with copious (large) amounts of sterile saline is an important aspect of wound care. Debridement itself means removal of dead tissue and foreign material to where healthy tissue is exposed. The amount of necrosis that needs to be removed will depend on the severity of the injury, the age of the wound, and the presence of infection. So debridement is an intervention by health care professionals that mimics the cleanup function of the macrophages on a much larger scale. Techniques for debriding include surgical excision (cutting out), enzyme digestion of the tissue, and mechanical means. Remember, healing is initiated only when the injury has been contained or _____(1). In the face of relatively severe trauma or overwhelming infection, the body's ability to engage in successful demolition is overcome by the amount of material to be removed. Debridement is then necessary to allow the wound to heal. Intervention in a wound to remove necrotic tissue and other debris is called _____(2). This technique is like the macrophage function of _____(3) except on a macroscopic scale. Debridement may be required for _____(4) to begin.

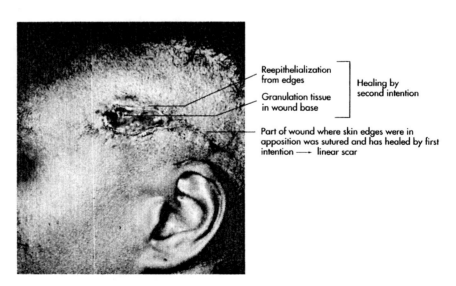

Figure 2–16. Ten-day-old laceration of the face. The posterior part of the wound was sutured and has healed by first intention. The anterior part, which had a large skin defect, was debrided and permitted to heal by second intention. Note the much greater time needed for healing by second intention and greater scar area. *(From Chandrasoma and Taylor,* Concise Pathology, *2nd ed., Appleton & Lange.)*

▶ COMPLICATIONS OF HEALING AND FACTORS INFLUENCING SUCCESS

2–78

Occasionally a side effect of healing may arise that has undesired consequences in either appearance or function. Some of these complications are illustrated in Figure 2–17. A **keloid** is an unsightly raised mass that occurs when the granulation tissue formation becomes excessive. The area becomes overgrown with capillary loops and collagen, and the mature scar is left raised above the plane of the original tissue. When any hollow organ of the body heals by fibrosis, **stenosis** or stricture is a possible result. After wound contraction and the production of relatively inelastic scar tissue, there may be an area that has become narrowed or cannot stretch. The effect is complete or partial blockage of the passage of material through the area. This blockage or closure is called an **occlusion.** Another common term would be obstruction. A stricture (a rigid narrow area) in an organ like the intestines can result in blockage as material tries to pass through. The urethra is a structure that often shows stenosis following surgery. A cosmetic side effect of excessive granulation tissue formation is a _____(1) and the mass is _____(2) above the original surface. Of more serious consequence is the formation of a rigid narrowed area called a _____(3) in an elastic hollow organ. This may cause blockage or _____(4) as material passes through.

1. keloid
2. raised
3. stenosis
4. occlusion

2–79

Some inflammatory processes can occur in a body cavity such as the abdomen. Peritonitis or inflammation of the lining of the abdomen (peritoneum) is an example. In this case, excessive scarring can occur in the form of **adhesions,** which are sticky rope-like structures running from one surface to another like a spider web. This is dangerous if mobile organs like the intestines become tangled in the stringy bands of adhesions. The intestines move in a wave-like fashion that propels material along their tracts. This movement is called peristalsis, and can cause the intestines to be caught in sticky rope-like scar tissue called _____(1). A section of intestine trapped in an adhesion can strangulate and necrose, which means the tissue _____(2). Strangulation and necrosis is a very serious consequence of _____(3) formation.

1. adhesions
2. dies
3. adhesion

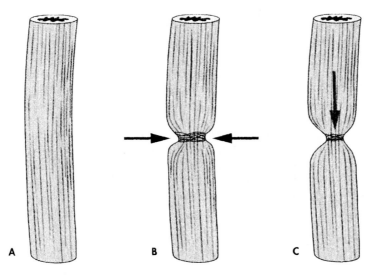

Figure 2–17. Complications of healing. **A.** Normal section of esophagus. **B.** Cicatrization of scar tissue following injury and inflammation. **C.** Resulting stenosis and occlusion.

2-80

1. inflammation
2. cicatrization
3. stenosis

Scar tissue generally contracts or shortens with time. Victims of severe burns or other extensive tissue loss may be left with deformities in areas. The term used to describe excessive deforming shortening is **cicatrization.** If the scarring involves a mobile area such as a joint, loss of function can occur if the joint becomes frozen from contracture. Chronic arthritis (which would mean _____(1) of a joint) can lead to loss of motion in the affected joints. Shortening of scar tissue over time leading to deformity or loss of function is called _____(2). This helps to also explain the narrowing of scarred hollow organs, which is called _____(3). This particular example is described as a cicatricial stenosis.

2-81

1. dehiscence
2. open
3. wound
4 dehiscence

Wound **dehiscence** is the rupture or bursting open of a wound, which can occur if too much tension is applied to the new tissue before it reaches the strength of maturity. This is especially serious in the case of postsurgical abdominal incisions. Actions producing too much strain on healing tissue may cause the wound to break open, which is called _____(1). Another example of a situation that may lead to dehiscence, or the bursting _____(2) of a _____(3), is if the attempted closure of the wound is over an area of normally high tension. For instance, if there was a large laceration with tissue loss on the inside of the lower leg, the sutures used to close the wound would be under a lot of strain. That is because there is not much excess tissue in that area and it is not very flexible. The tension produced by trying to bring the edges together might break the sutures and cause the wound to open or undergo _____(4).

2-82

1. virulence
2. numbers
3. contained

There are several factors that influence how well an individual may heal from injury or disease. This chapter has examined some of the agents of the body's defense, and there is much yet to be studied. With all of these defense mechanisms how does disease, such as infection, occur? One answer lies in the characteristic of the infectious agent, whether it is a bacterium or a virus. That characteristic is **virulence.** Virulence is the strength or potency of a microorganism in causing disease. A virulent or strong microorganism may be able to easily overcome our natural defenses and cause disease in spite of the response by the phagocytic cells. More will be said about this in Chapter 5 on pathogenic (disease-causing) microorganisms. Another characteristic is sheer numbers of invading organisms. This can overwhelm the cellular defenses if the body is not able to keep up with the demand for production of new defense cells. Two characteristics of invading organisms that can defeat body defenses and produce disease are _____(1) and _____(2) of organisms. This relates to healing ability, because, as you learned earlier, healing cannot take place until an injury has been stopped or _____(3). Degree of insult is a characteristic that can pertain to physical injury. The severity or amount of trauma, for example, may be such that the body could not possibly perform the amount of needed repair naturally. A ruptured spleen after a car accident is not a candidate for the body's healing abilities.

2-83

Another consideration in healing is **immune competence** on the part of the host or injured party. Chapter 4 on immunology will present this subject in more detail. For now, immune competence simply means that the antibodies and other agents of defense are present in normal amounts and that they are working effectively. If an individual is *not* immune competent, in other words if he or she is *immune suppressed,* even a relatively weak organism or small numbers can gain a foothold and cause disease that will not result in natural healing.

2-84

1. virulent
2. competent

Some cases of poor healing may occur even if invading organisms are not especially potent or _____(1), if the numbers are not overwhelming, or if the immune system is normal or _____(2). The following is a list of factors that can play a major role in the delay of healing:

1. Continued presence of the damaging agent, such as infection or foreign body.
2. Continued trauma or excessive movement, which destroys delicate granulation tissue.

3. Poor blood supply or circulation in a certain area, which can mean less vascular response and less nutritional support for granulation tissue. This can be due to vascular disease or simply that some areas of the body are naturally less perfused than others.
4. Advanced age of a patient may be associated with some other debilitating condition, so that healing is less than optimum.
5. Use of steroid medications, or diseases where natural steroid levels are high, interferes with immune competence and granulation tissue formation.
6. Poor nutrition, which results in a deficiency of materials, such as protein, necessary to form new tissue. Also, vitamin C is required for normal collagen production and capillary integrity.

2-85

Failure to contain or stabilize an injury will result in delayed healing. A few examples given above would be the continued _____(1) of the damaging agent or the continuation of _____(2). Destruction of delicate granulation tissue as it is formed by excessive _____(3) is another example. Certain medications, such as _____(4), interfere with immune function and wound healing. Delayed healing can occur if materials necessary for new tissue production are lacking in the diet, as is the case with poor _____(5). Two important nutrients are _____(6) and _____(7). A debilitating, or worn down condition can cause secondary problems with healing in a patient of advanced _____(8). Slow healing can be seen in some parts of the body that have less _____(9) supply or _____(10) than other parts.

1. presence
2. trauma
3. movement
4. steroids
5. nutrition
6. protein
7. vitamin C
8. age
9. blood
10. circulation

IV. REVIEW QUESTIONS

1. Which of the following processes result in scar formation as a method of healing? (choose all that are correct)
   a. fibrosis
   b. remodeling
   c. regeneration
   d. fibrous connective tissue repair
   e. granulation

2. The type of cells that most effectively heal through regeneration are a._____ cells. Some vital organs or systems like the b. _____ or c. _____ heal only through fibrosis.

3. Two vital organs that are vulnerable to injury and heal through regeneration are the a. _____ and b. _____.

4. The significance of healing by scar tissue in a vital organ is:
   a. it makes the organ larger than it originally was and increases function
   b. it results in permanent loss of function of the involved area
   c. the presence of scar tissue causes pressure necrosis of the surrounding area
   d. vital organs do not heal by scar tissue

5. Cells that are responsible for wound contraction are:
   a. myofibroblasts
   b. macrophages
   c. neutrophils
   d. lymphocytes

1. a–fibrosis; d–fibrous connective tissue repair

2. a–epithelial; b–heart or nervous system; c–heart or nervous system

3. a–liver or kidney; b–liver or kidney

4. b–it results in permanent loss of function of the involved area

5. a–myofibroblasts

6. d–new capillary buds and collagen fibrils from fibroblasts

7. true

8. d–contact inhibition

9. c–growth factors

10. primary

11. it takes longer because the defect is larger and there is more demolition needed. The final scar is larger.

12. 1. c–occlusion
    2. e–adhesion
    3. d–cicatrization
    4. a–stenosis
    5. b–keloid
    6. f–dehiscence

13. b–poor healing

14. d–debridement

6. Granulation tissue is primarily made of:
   a. debris and dead foreign agents
   b. necrotic tissue
   c. new capillary buds and collagen fibrils from macrophages
   d. new capillary buds and collagen fibrils from fibroblasts

7. True or false: The activity that precedes granulation tissue formation is demolition.

   _____

8. Sheets of growing epithelial cells in skin wounds stop growing due to:
   a. chemical mediators
   b. loss of cell-to-cell contact
   c. wound contraction
   d. contact inhibition

9. Proliferation of fibroblasts and epidermal cells as well as capillary growth in granulation tissue is stimulated by:
   a. chemotactic chemicals
   b. interleukin
   c. growth factors
   d. histamine

10. Artificial wound contraction describes wounds that are healing by _____ intention or union.

11. What is the result of healing in a wound that is allowed to heal by secondary intention?
    _____
    _____
    _____
    _____

12. Please match these complications of healing in the left column with their definitions in the right column:
    a. stenosis   1. ____ closing or blockage of a passageway
    b. keloid   2. ____ bands of scar tissue in a body cavity
    c. occlusion   3. ____ contraction of scar tissue
    d. cicatrization   4. ____ stricture or narrowing
    e. adhesion   5. ____ raised mass of granulation tissue
    f. dehiscence   6. ____ rupture of a sutured wound

13. Immunosuppression, poor diet, or poor blood supply can cause:
    a. inflammation
    b. poor healing
    c. excessive granulation tissue formation
    d. cicatrization

14. Intervention that removes excessive necrotic tissue is:
    a. primary intention
    b. secondary union
    c. wound contraction
    d. debridement

V. CHRONIC INFLAMMATION ◀ SECTION

The continued presence of a damaging agent, foreign body, trauma, or excessive movement leads to chronic inflammation. Length of duration is one difference between acute and chronic conditions. Complete healing cannot take place if an injury persists. The longer the agent is present, the longer the inflammatory response will continue to try and stop or eliminate the source of injury. The body enters the next stage, which is a response that is characteristic of chronic inflammation. Refer back to the list of factors causing delayed healing. The two factors most likely to lead to chronic inflammation are _____(1) and _____(2).

1. continued presence of damaging agent
2. continued trauma or excessive movement

Some cases do not involve acute inflammation leading to chronic inflammation. These situations involve mild injury that did not produce an acute response initially. The phases of response are the same as the acute condition, but the signs are much less intense. For example, there is less hyperemia and exudation. The difference between levels of response in acute and chronic inflammation can be compared to a fire burning initially, which later becomes a smoldering condition that is not extinguished. In pathology the term "chronic" can mean a specific cell pattern that produces a particular **histologic** picture. **Histology** is the study of tissues under the microscope. This pattern of cells is very helpful in diagnosing chronic inflammation. Often there is not a clear division between the stages of acute and chronic inflammation. As damage persists it produces more necrosis which causes another acute reaction. Necrosis causes inflammation because as dead tissue it is foreign material. Healing will be attempted and a chronic situation develops. Several phases and stages often occur together in a continuum. Chronic inflammation can mean either the length of _____(1) the condition has existed or a certain _____(2) pattern seen under the microscope. The phases are similar to the acute response, but the intensity of response is _____(3) than the acute. Both _____(4) and _____(5) inflammation can occur together.

1. duration
2. cellular
3. less
4. acute
5. chronic

▶ CAUSATIVE AGENTS

There are a variety of factors or agents that produce chronic inflammation. These include:

1. Some bacteria that are resistant to the acute response. Two examples are the bacillus that causes tuberculosis (TB) and the spirochete that causes syphilis.
2. A foreign body that is an insoluble object or particles that the cells cannot completely phagocytize or otherwise break down.
3. **Hypersensitivity,** which is an allergic response that can result in chronic inflammation due to the damage to normal tissue by the immune mechanism (Chap. 4). The damage continues as long as one is exposed to an allergen, which can be a long time. Hay fever is an example of allergic chronic inflammation.
4. Some viral infections that produce specific diseases of certain organs which we will discuss during this course. These diseases are classified as low grade chronic inflammation or "chronic inflammatory disease."
5. In the case of continued trauma or excessive movement, mechanical breakdown of the tissue prevents healing from occurring, and the reaction changes from acute to chronic.

Some viruses can infect organs in such a manner that the specific disease is classified as _____(1) grade _____(2) inflammatory disease. As an example of _____(3) chronic inflammation, hay fever may not have an _____(4) onset. There are some organisms that produce chronic inflammation because the acute phases do not destroy them. Examples given are organisms that cause _____(5) or _____(6). Chronic inflammation that develops after

1. low
2. chronic
3. allergic
4. acute
5. TB
6. syphilis

7. foreign body
8. trauma
9. movement

incomplete phagocytosis results from the presence of an insoluble irritant or _____(7). Chronic inflammation may also result in cases of ongoing _____(8) or too much _____(9) in an injured part.

▶ THE CELLULAR PATTERN OF CHRONIC INFLAMMATION

2–90

1. diagnosing
2. neutrophils
3. macrophages
4. monocytes
5. opsonin
6. opsonization

The predominant cells seen in the chronic response are different from the acute profile, and this is demonstrated microscopically as shown in Figure 2–18. Identifying these particular cells is very helpful in _____(1) chronic inflammation. Remember, the predominant early cells in acute responses are PMNs or _____(2) which are later replaced by _____(3). As macrophages remain in the area they become one of several cells to make up the chronic pattern. Macrophages are not multinucleated appearing cells like polymorphonuclear cells, so they are called **mononuclear.** Other mononuclear cells that are recruited to the chronic scene are **lymphocytes** and an offshoot of those, the **plasma cell.** Macrophages were previously _____(4) in the bloodstream, and plasma cells are derived from B-lymphocytes. Lymphs and plasma cells are the basis of the immune system. As was previously stated, chronic inflammation is a mixture of acute responses, demolition attempts, and healing attempts in the face of unresolved injury. Adding the presence of immune cells defines this condition. The hallmark for the diagnosis of chronic inflammation is few or no neutrophils, but primarily lymphs, plasma cells, and macrophages. Lymphocytes perform many functions such as secreting chemical mediators, one of which activates macrophages. Plasma cells produce antibodies. Antibodies attach to the foreign agents to make phagocytosis easier. Recall that a substance that facilitates (helps) phagocytosis is an _____(5), and the process is _____(6).

2–91

1. collagen

Another cell type very prominent and important in the definition of chronic inflammation is the fibroblast. Recall that fibroblasts (myofibroblasts) produce _____(1), which later matures into fibrous tissue. The large numbers of fibroblasts present and the amount of fibrous tissue is a good indicator of the duration of the condition. As fibrin is a signal of the acute response, immature fibrous tissue signals the chronic response. The production of large amounts of fibrous tissue is important, because it forms a barrier or wall around the source of the offending agent. The cells are usually incorporated into this wall. Even though cells

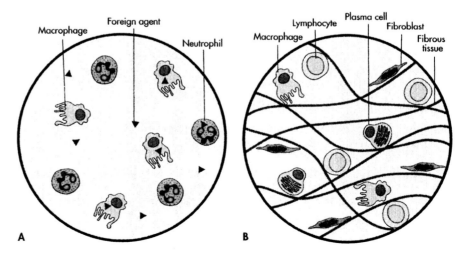

Figure 2–18. Differences in microscopic appearances between acute and chronic inflammation. **A.** Histology (tissue picture) of acute inflammation. **B.** Histology of chronic inflammation.

are heavily involved in the chronic response, it is not referred to as a cellular response as with the acute condition. The chronic reaction is better described as an immune reaction because the immune mechanisms of lymphocytes and plasma cells predominate. You will learn about these mechanisms in Chapter 4.

2–92

Two visible differences seen in chronic inflammation are the types of _____(1) present and the amount of _____(2) tissue. The general term that describes the nuclei of the predominant cells is _____(3). The system that these cells are associated with is the _____(4) system. The four cell types that are the hallmark of chronic inflammation are the _____(5), which is also part of the acute response, the _____(6) and its derivative the _____(7), and large numbers of _____(8). The large amounts of fibrous tissue form a _____(9) around the source of irritation. Compared to the cellular description of acute reactions, chronic inflammation is better described as an _____(10) reaction.

1. cells
2. fibrous
3. mononuclear
4. immune
5. macropahge
6. lymphocyte
7. plasma cell
8. fibroblasts
9. barrier or wall
10. immune

▶ CLASSIFICATIONS OF CHRONIC INFLAMMATION

2–93

There are a few variations seen in patterns of chronic inflammation, usually depending on the cause of irritation. **Chronic suppurative inflammation** is an example of the acute response that persists because pyogenic (pus-producing) bacteria such as staphylococcus are still present. [The term "suppurative" refers to the presence of _____(1).] These bacteria were able to resist destruction. Occasionally a large amount of pus itself incites the next stage of response due to the length of time it takes the macrophages to complete demolition. This is especially true of a localized, walled-off pocket of pus called an _____(2). The fibrotic, cellular wall is sometimes referred to as a **pyogenic membrane,** which is illustrated in Figure 2–19. The significance of this wall or _____(3) is that there are few things that can penetrate it, including vessels and cells. Any foreign body that may be in the center is protected from body defenses, even though the purpose of the wall is to barricade and protect the body from the foreign object. Also inside this festering mass is dead or _____(4) tissue. Necrotic tissue serves as an excellent medium or nutritional support for bacteria. Antibiotics are of little use in treatment of an abscess of chronic suppurative inflammation. The blood supply does not penetrate the wall or _____(5) membrane. The area must be surgically opened,

1. pus
2. abscess
3. pyogenic membrane
4. necrotic
5. pyogenic

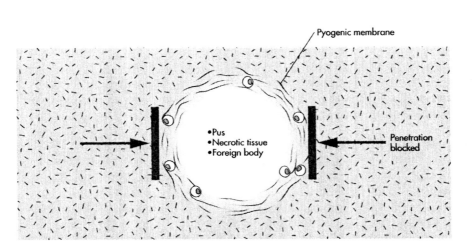

Figure 2–19. Chronic suppurative inflammation with a pyogenic membrane that is not penetrated by blood supply, cells, or other materials.

6. debridement
7. chronic suppurative
   inflammation

cleaned out or flushed, and necrotic tissue must be removed. This technique of artificial demolition is called _____(6). Long-standing inflammation associated with the presence of pus is called _____(7).

2-94

1. cheesy
2. granulomatous
3. granuloma
4. macrophage
5. tuberculoid
6. microscopic or histologic

Granulomatous inflammation is characterized by the appearance of a **granuloma** which means tumor-like swelling. The site is loaded with macrophage cells. The presence of T-lymphs recruits more macrophages to the area than normal. The necrosis associated with a granuloma is often the caseous type, which has a _____(1) consistency. TB is a classic cause of granulomatous inflammation, so the name **tuberculoid** is sometimes used to describe this condition. Today, fungal infections are more often the cause and may be seen in the immunosuppressed AIDS patient. A foreign body may sometimes produce a granuloma or _____(2) inflammation. In this case the foreign body can usually be seen in the center microscopically if a section of the granuloma is removed for examination. A histologic granuloma is a microscopic picture showing the presence of certain cell types and patterns. It is a diagnosis indicating that there is persistent irritation, and the cause, if not obvious, should be looked for. The foreign body can also be some type of organism such as a fungus or spirochete. The swollen site of granulomatous inflammation is called a _____(3) and it is packed with _____(4) cells. Another term used is _____(5), because TB is associated with this type of reaction. If a persistent foreign body is the cause of a granuloma, diagnosis by _____(6) examination can help in pinpointing the cause.

2-95

1. phagocytize
2. epithelioid
3. giant
4. nuclei
5. tuberculoid
6. foreign body
7. debris

The hallmark feature of a granuloma is two changes undergone by the macrophages. Refer to Figure 2–20, which demonstrates these changes. The first change is that they become **epithelioid,** or like epithelial cells. The cells enlarge, lose their ability to engulf or _____(1), and become packed tightly together in groups. Epithelioid cells are especially seen with the tuberculoid granuloma of classic TB. In the case of an insoluble foreign object or other remaining debris, **giant cells** are formed. The macrophages enlarge and fuse together to produce a very large cell with several nuclei that form a halo around the object or mass of debris. Again, histologic demonstration of epithelioid cells and giant cells can indicate this process and help put the pieces of the diagnostic puzzle together. Macrophages that enlarge and arrange themselves in close groups are called _____(2) cells. Enlargement followed by fusion or joining together produces a _____(3) cell that has several _____(4). Epithelioid cells are usually seen in a _____(5) granuloma. Giant cells form in the presence of a persistent _____(6) or remaining _____(7).

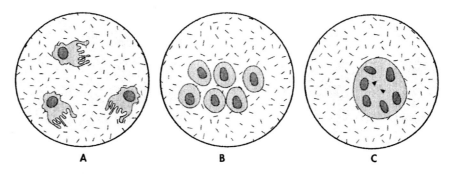

Figure 2–20. Changes in macrophages in chronic granulomatous inflammation. **A.** Normal macrophages. **B.** Epithelioid cells. **C.** Giant cell.

▶ EFFECTS OF CHRONIC INFLAMMATION

2-96

The effects of chronic inflammation can be localized or systemic. A local complication is excessive scarring. Remember that more fibrosis occurs in chronic situations. Recall also that excessive scar tissue can contract in a deforming manner in a process called _____(1). If this occurs in an organ of the body, serious complications can arise. Cicatrization can cause a narrowing or stricture of an area, called _____(2). A complication of stenosis is some degree of obstruction or _____(3). All result in disturbance of some body function.

1. cicatrization
2. stenosis
3. occlusion

2-97

Systemic effects include enlargement of regional lymph nodes and perhaps of the spleen as production of monocytic cells is increased. Higher or increased levels of antibodies from these cells are present, and this is an indicator of chronic inflammation. Specific antibody tests are very diagnostic for the causative agent. Because of the continued stress on the immune system, a strange protein substance called **amyloid** becomes deposited in various organs of the body. The mechanism for this is unclear. In severe cases the organs may become overloaded with amyloid and produce a condition called **amyloidosis.** Amyloidosis, by nature of infiltration, interferes with normal function and may even cause organ failure. Increased production of monocytic cells causes enlargement of _____(1) or of the _____(2). As more of these cells are present, levels of _____(3) increase because they are manufactured by these cells. A good indication of chronic inflammation is _____(4) levels of antibodies. An extreme consequence of chronic inflammation is organ failure due to infiltration by _____(5) in a condition called _____(6).

1. lymph nodes
2. spleen
3. antibodies
4. increased or high
5. amyloid
6. amyloidosis

V. REVIEW QUESTIONS

1. True or false: Chronic inflammation develops from unsuccessful acute inflammation or from particular causes of low-grade injury.

2. Chronic inflammation is often diagnosed by the presence of specific cells that form a certain _____ picture.

3. Individual causes of chronic inflammation include:
   a. certain viral infections
   b. allergy or hypersensitivity
   c. bacteria that resist acute inflammation
   d. all of the above

4. The predominant cell type in chronic inflammation is:
   a. mononuclear
   b. polymorphonuclear
   c. binuclear
   d. none of the above

5. Large numbers and amounts of the following cells and tissues are good indicators of the duration of a chronic condition:
   a. neutrophils and fibrin
   b. fibroblasts and fibrous tissue
   c. macrophages and fibrous tissue
   d. lymphocytes and necrotic tissue

1. true

2. histologic

3. d–all of the above

4. a–mononuclear

5. b–fibroblasts and fibrous tissue

6. a–suppurative; b–pyogenic; c–pus; d–pyogenic membrane; e–granulomatous; f–granuloma; g–macrophages

7. Epithelioid cells are macrophages that have enlarged and cluster themselves in groups. Giant cells are macrophages that have enlarged and fused together so that one very large cell has several nucleii. They usually encircle a foreign body.

8. false

6. Please complete the following sentences: Chronic a. _____ inflamation is a classification associated with b. _____ bacterial infections where an abscess or pocket of c. _____ has developed. The thick fibrotic wall surrounding the area is called a d. _____. Chronic inflammation characterized by a local swelling is called e. _____ inflammation and the swollen site is a f. _____. The swelling is due to large numbers of g. _____ that have infiltrated the area.

7. Briefly explain the difference between epithelioid cells and giant cells:
   _____
   _____

8. True or false: Amyloidosis is an infiltrative condition that can be seen in some organs as a result of acute inflammation. _____

CHAPTER ▶ SUMMARY

▶ SECTION I

Injury has its basis at the cellular level. Inflammation is a uniform reaction to injury that targets the agent of damage for destruction and leads to healing. Classic signs of inflammation as seen in skin are redness, swelling, heat, pain, and loss of function of some body parts. Irreversible injury causes death of individual cells. Necrosis is a sufficient number of dead cells that creates a visible area of tissue death. Several changes in the cell nucleus and various types of necrosis are described by terminology. Hypoxia is the most common cause of coagulation necrosis, while liquefaction necrosis is associated with bacterial infections containing pus. Necrosis itself causes inflammation, because dead tissue is foreign to the body. The stages or phases of acute inflammation are the response by local blood vessels (the vascular response), involvement by blood cells (the cellular response), and initiation and control of these responses by chemical mediators. The vascular response results in vasodilation and increased permeability, which produces the exudate, which is a mechanism to supply the injured area with agents of defense. In the cellular response neutrophils or PMNs act quickly to reach the site and begin the process of phagocytosis. They are followed by the slower macrophage, which will phagocytize even greater amounts of damaging agents, dead cells, and debris. Macrophages are also important in demolition. The fibroblast is a tissue cell that produces new tissue in the form of collagen in healing. Chemical mediators control these actions by acting as go-betweens to signal various cells to react in a specific manner. A successful result of inflammation is the halt of the damage, removal of the cause, and demolition of the aftermath so that healing may occur. In the case of excessive dead tissue and other debris, debridement greatly assists demolition so that healing can occur. Healing occurs in the form of regeneration, which returns function to the damaged area, or by fibrosis, which only fills the defect.

▶ SECTION II

Vasodilation, hyperemia, and stasis are terms that describe changes in vessels and blood flow that make up the vascular response. The increased flow to the area due to vasodilation slows down, which is helpful to the gathering forces in the vessels. Contracture of endothelial cells creates junctions through which the cellular elements may pass. Inside the vessels the WBCs line up or marginate along the endothelium in preparation for escape. Loss of fluid, cells, proteins, and other substances from the vessels creates an accumulation known as an exudate. A fibrinous exudate contains fibrinogen, which will become fibrin. A purulent exudate is associated with infections and also will contain dead neutrophils and bacteria in a collection known as pus. The fibrin in an exudate will form a network of fibers to wall off the damaging agents and provide support for phagocytosis. An exudate helps to dilute the area in the case of a chemical irritant, provides a means for the cells to reach the site, and gives the cells a place to anchor for phagocytosis. Signs of inflammation can be explained by vasodilation, hyperemia, and the buildup of exudate.

▶ SECTION III

The activities of the WBC are described by the terms phagocytossis, margination or pavementation, diapedesis, emigration, opsonization, and lysis. The order of the events of acute inflammation is vasodilation, margination, diapedesis, exudation, migration, opsonization, phagocytosis, and lysis. The neutrophil is the fastest cell to respond and is extremely active in engulfing and digesting particulate material, especially bacteria. The macrophage responds more slowly but performs more of the work of phagocytosis, engulfing dead cells and debris as well. The life span of the macrophage is much longer than that of the neutrophil. It is vital in the process of demolition. The mast cell is responsible for the production of histamine, an important mediator of vasodilation. The fibroblast is a tissue cell that produces collagen, a structural protein that is the basis of scar tissue. Chemical mediators begin (initiate) the inflammatory process, particularly when histamine is released by the mast cell. Most of the process is also controlled by these substances that carry messages to the tissues. The primary effects of chemical mediators are vasodilation, increased vascular permeability, and chemotaxis of white blood cells.

▶ SECTION IV

The two major mechanisms of healing are regeneration and fibrous connective tissue repair. Regeneration is very important, because it provides a mechanism to restore original function. Surviving cells of the injured tissue must have the ability to reproduce themselves through mitosis or cell division. Epithelial cells and organs made of those types of cells such as kidney and liver have very good powers of regeneration. Two vital tissues that have no such ability are the heart and central nervous system. Injury to them leaves fibrosis. Ability of other tissues falls somewhere in between these opposite examples. Fibrous repair or fibrosis has a much simpler purpose in that it fills in whatever tissue loss has been experienced, with no return of original function. It is a scar, which is a patching compound only. If a damage has been suffered in a vital organ with poor regeneration, then healing is by scar tissue, which leaves the organ permanently deficient in function. Enough scar tissue can result in death. Just before healing begins, the wound shrinks in size in a process called contraction as myofibroblasts surround the area and draw inward. This leaves a smaller wound, which takes less effort and time to repair as well as a smaller scar. The foundation of fibrosis is granulation tissue formation produced by the ingrowth of tiny new buds of vessels growing off local capillaries and the infiltration by myofibroblasts. Myofibroblasts weave new tissue by laying down collagen strands and cellular glue-like compounds. This material mixes together and matures into dense, tough scar tissue containing no cells or vessels. Healing can be assisted through primary intention, which is the closing of a wound by bringing the edges together. This results in faster, neater healing as opposed to the excessive granulation of an open wound in secondary intention. If there are great amounts of necrotic tissue or other debris in a wound, debridement replaces demolition more efficiently. Some problems associated with the production of scar tissue include stenosis, which can cause occlusion; adhesions, which can cause strangulation necrosis, cicatrization, which can prevent motion or result in stenosis, and dehiscence, in which the wound ruptures open. Success of healing is affected by both the nature of the injury and the condition of the host.

► **SECTION V**

Acute inflammation will lead to the chronic stage if the original injury cannot be stabilized or contained. This means that the presence of the agent persists or there is some ongoing injury that has not been stopped. Some conditions produce a chronic response at the start, which differs from the acute response in level of intensity. Microscopically, chronic inflammation is diagnosed by the different cell types as opposed to cells of acute inflammation. Mononuclear cells predominate such as the macrophage, lymphocyte, and plasma cell. These cell types are responsible for the immune description of the chronic condition. Numbers of fibroblasts and the amount of fibrosis is increased compared to acute responses. Chronic suppurative inflammation is defined by an unresolved infection where pus is present. An impenetrable pyogenic membrane surrounds the necrotic mass, which resists treatment by antibiotics. A granulomatous inflammation shows a swollen area caused by excessive numbers of macrophages. The site is called a granuloma. A granuloma can be specifically diagnosed if epithelioid cells and giant cells are present, both of which form from changes in macrophages. There are several systemic changes that can accompany chronic inflammation, including injury to organs by amyloid deposits during amyloidosis.

CHAPTER

....

Homeostasis and Associated Changes

▶ OBJECTIVES

SECTION II

Define all highlighted terms.

Specify the injury to cells as a result of hyperpyrexia.

Outline the events and chemicals involved in producing fever.

Differentiate between fever and hyperthermia, including origin of production and effect on the hypothalamic setpoint.

State the most common cause of fever.

Describe the three stages of fever, including the associated activities and their effect on body temperature.

Characterize the three syndromes of hyperthermia, including causes, circulatory changes, effects, and degree of severity.

Explain the different effects that fever, hyperthermia, and hypothermia have on the temperature-regulating mechanism.

State the primary cause of injury in hypothermia and relate this to the cause of death. Include also the consequences involving metabolism and respiratory depression.

SECTION III

Define all highlighted terms.

Identify the two main mechanisms that create dehydration and give examples of specific causes. Understand why these conditions create dehydration.

Explain how osmoreceptors stimulate polydipsia, including the relationship between solvent, solutes, and osmolarity.

List in order of occurrence the events of dehydration that are designed to maintain intravascular volume.

Relate dehydration to tissue hypoxia.

Differentiate between hypotonic fluid excess and isotonic fluid excess. State which is more common.

Relate two organ disorders to isotonic fluid excess.

Compare and contrast the effects of hypotonic versus isotonic fluid excess.

Differentiate between edema caused by increased hydrostatic pressure and edema caused by increased venous pressure. State what is the common outcome of each.

List specific causes of edema associated with abnormal distribution.

Explain the mechanism of hypoalbuminemia in producing abnormal distribution edema.

List both general causes of hypoalbuminemia and specific conditions.

Outline the adverse effects edema has on body functions.

State the primary deficiencies associated with diabetes insipidus.

State the role of antidiuretic hormone in water balance.

Explain how polyuria leads to polydipsia.

Differentiate between neurogenic and nephrogenic diabetes insipidus.

SECTION IV

Cite the two primary reasons for developing hyponatremia.

Describe the difference between an actual or true electrolyte imbalance and a relative imbalance. For example, what is meant by "dilutional hyponatremia"?

Explain the effects of aldosterone on sodium levels.

Outline the effects of abnormal sodium levels on cell size for both hypo- and hypernatremia.

State the body system most affected by abnormal cell size.

Cite the two primary reasons for developing hypernatremia.

State the most common reason for relative hypernatremia.

Given a specific cause for an imbalance in sodium, potassium, or calcium, classify the imbalance as true or relative.

Relate plasma potassium values to total body stores and give reasons why these two may actually differ.

List the effects of abnormal pH (acidosis or alkalosis) on the locations of potassium and extracellular fluid (ECF) levels.

State the most common reason for true hypokalemia.

For potassium and calcium, describe the effects of increased and decreased levels on the resting membrane potential of excitable tissue, the amount of stimulation needed to generate an action potential, and the overall effect on the excitability of the tissue.

State the two types of excitable tissue most affected by potassium and calcium imbalances.

State the usual causes of death in hypokalemia.

State the most common cause of true hyperkalemia.

Explain the effects of aldosterone on potassium levels.

State the most significant consequence of hyperkalemia and usual cause of death.

Relate the amounts of the ionized or active form of calcium to abnormal pH and the amounts of protein present.

Associate increased or decreased calcium with levels of parathyroid hormone and vitamin D. Explain how parathyroid hormone (PTH) affects plasma calcium levels.

Relate the presence of tetany and other effects to causes of death in hypocalcemia.

In addition to changes in the resting membrane potential (RMP), list other effects of hypercalcemia, including cause of death.

SECTION V

Define all highlighted terms.

Classify acid–base disturbances as to origin and abnormalities in pH.

Relate pH to functions of metabolism and respiration.

In defining the four imbalances, identify the primary defects for each (associate increases or decreases in bicarbonate or carbon dioxide with the correct classification).

Explain how amounts of carbon dioxide in the body relate to acid amounts and pH.

Relate pH to the ratio of base to acid rather then amounts of base or acid.

Compare and contrast the similarities and differences in correction and compensation.

Identify the organs of correction and compensation, compare response times and effectiveness between these two organs. State how each organ manipulates the acid–base pair to balance pH.

Relate acidosis or alkalosis to potassium and ionized calcium levels.

Classify the specific causes of metabolic acidosis.

Identify metabolic acidosis as the most common imbalance.

Relate hypoxia to lactic acidosis, and ketoacidosis to starvation or diabetes mellitus.

Describe how kidney disease or bacterial diarrhea produces metabolic acidosis.

For all four acid–base imbalances, relate the abnormality in number of H^+ ions (pH) to effects on body systems including nerve function, heart function, and potassium and calcium levels.

Given any of the acid–base imbalances, state the usual compensatory mechanism.

Identify the three major mechanisms that create metabolic alkalosis.

Characterize the relationship between hypercapnia and respiratory acidosis.

List the two main mechanisms for developing respiratory acidosis.

Characterize the relationship between hypocapnia and respiratory alkalosis.

Give examples of specific causes that produce excessive ventilation and respiratory alkalosis.

I. ANATOMY AND PHYSIOLOGY IN REVIEW ◄ SECTION

3-1

Homeostasis is defined as a tendency to uniformity or stability in normal body states or the internal environment. In other words, it is the process of maintaining a constant internal environment. The body has "settings" for what is normal and necessary for every parameter that makes up the whole health and function of the organism. Keeping internal conditions constant or steady provides cells and organs an environment in which to function properly. All body tissues contribute in some way to homeostasis. We do not have to consciously control things like heart rate and rate of respiration. In states of disease or imbalance, this automatic balance is interrupted. If one system becomes unable to contribute its part to maintaining the steady state, the rest of the body suffers. Disease can be thought of as a disturbance in homeostasis. All body processes are part of homeostasis. The heart, blood vessels, and hormones maintain a specific blood pressure. The lungs provide certain levels of oxygen. The kidneys regulate levels of ions. The aspects of homeostasis we will review and study in this chapter are temperature regulation, fluid balance, electrolyte balance, and acid–base balance.

3-2

Temperature regulation is vital to health. Our body's heat setting is in the range of 96.6 to 99.3°F, with normal temperature considered to be 98.6°F (37°C). All metabolic activities depend on this temperature, especially enzymes because they are heat sensitive. An area of the brain called the hypothalamus regulates this range by way of "temperature detectors" called thermal receptors found in various parts of the body. Normal temperature is a result of the balance between the production of heat and the loss of heat. Core tissues, such as the muscles and internal organs, produce most of the heat and are insulated by fat, subcutaneous tissue, and skin. Heat loss primarily involves the blood vessels and the skin.

3-3

The majority of heat production comes from normal metabolism, which is carried on in every cell of the body. Movement or exercise is another major contributor, since muscle contraction produces heat. When the body surface is in a cold environment, involuntary muscle contraction or **shivering** produces heat. Since no work is performed during the contractions of shivering, more energy is available for heat instead of ATP production. Since heat is made constantly in the body, there must be ways to release the excess or the core temperature would quickly climb to fatal levels. Loss of heat is primarily controlled by the blood vessels. As heat is produced by the inner core tissues, it is carried by the vessels to the surface for release. This release occurs through the skin to the environment. The skin is an important organ of heat regulation. Blood can be quickly passed to the surface as needed. Dilation of the superficial vessels of the skin allows heat loss that can occur in one or more of the following ways.

Radiation is the passage of heat from the body through the air in waves. This accounts for the majority of heat loss, usually about 60 percent. **Conduction** is the direct transfer of heat through surface contact, such as sitting in a chair. Heat travels from a warmer surface to the cooler surface. A cold rag placed on the forehead of a fevered patient conducts heat from the face. The layer of air immediately surrounding the body is also one of these surfaces so heat is actually conducted to that layer then radiates outward. **Convection** is the exchange of the warm layer of air next to the skin for a new, cooler layer. This constant replacement with cooler air causes faster heat loss. The wind does this, and hence, the reason for a "wind chill factor." Electric fans are another example of displacing the heat as soon as it is conducted to the surface air. **Evaporation** is very effective in heat loss. This is commonly called sweating. Sweat glands produce sweat from their secretions that contain water and sodium chloride (salt). This water on the skin surface is converted to vapor that then rises into the air. This conversion requires heat energy, so heat is used up in this process. Sweating accounts for about 22 percent of our heat loss. Figure 3–1 summarizes these mechanisms that create and maintain normal body temperature.

The heat created by the body can be conserved in several ways. In times when it is necessary to decrease the amount that is lost, the primary activity is **vasoconstriction.** This has the opposite effect of vasodilation, as the superficial vessels close down and shunt blood away from the skin. **Piloerection** is the contraction of muscles around the skin hairs that serves to decrease some of the surface area of the skin and provide less of an outlet of loss. The common term for this is "goose bumps." (This is actually more effective in animals

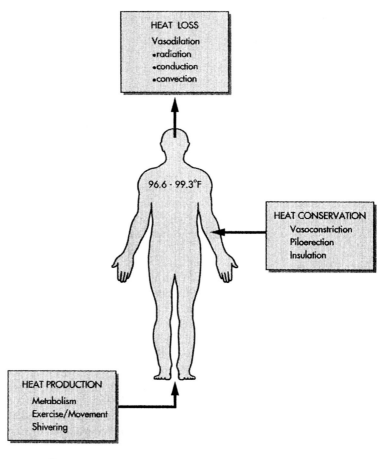

Figure 3–1. Mechanisms that create and maintain normal body temperature.

whose skin is covered with a haircoat.) The **insulation** provided by the skin, subcutaneous tissue, and especially, adipose tissue or fat, normally conserves heat.

Fluid balance is necessary for all metabolic processes. Water makes up about 60 to 70 percent of body weight. It provides a way of transportation for every substance in the body. Water aids in hydrolysis of foods and is vital in all the chemical reactions that occur. Normal metabolism would be impossible without water. The body's fluids are divided into two main compartments, the **intracellular fluid (ICF)** and the **extracellular fluid (ECF).** Fluid is found inside the cells in a particular environment. All other fluid is found outside of the cells. The ECF can be further divided into **intravascular** compartments (the plasma inside blood and lymph vessels), and **interstitial** compartments (in the matrix of tissues between vessels and cells). Figure 3–2 illustrates the major body fluid compartments.

Total body water is regulated by forces that direct intake (thirst) and control loss (the kidneys). Thirst is a sensation caused by the hypothalamus when detectors called **osmoreceptors** send a signal that means there is a decrease in the amount of body water. The receptors actually detect the osmolarity, or the numbers of dissolved particles in fluid, which you will learn more about later. Water loss is controlled by the kidneys which regulate both volume and osmolarity. An important hormone called **antidiuretic hormone** or **ADH** influences renal loss of water. This hormone controls and promotes reabsorption of water from the filtrate which will become urine as it moves through the kidneys. Because water reabsorption contributes to total blood volume and therefore pressure, this hormone is also called **vasopressin.** Increased ADH secretion causes more water to be retained by the kidneys.

Microcirculation is the exchange that occurs at the level of the capillary and provides the tissues with nutrients and removes wastes. Water and small molecules dissolved in plasma, such as oxygen and glucose, diffuse freely out of the capillaries on their way to the cells. Substances that are dissolved in fluid are called **solutes** and the fluid is called the **solvent.** Other solutes that are waste products of metabolism, such as lactic acid and carbon dioxide, diffuse back into the capillaries along with water. Between the ECF and ICF there is a constant exchange that produces the normal fluid balance or equilibrium between the compartments. The heart pumps and provides the pressure to force fluid and solutes out of the capillaries but how does fluid return? If capillary pressure is a force to expel fluid, then there must be an equal opposing force to draw it back into the vessels. This force is osmotic pressure.

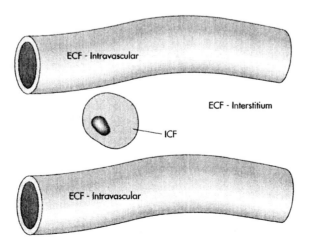

Figure 3–2. Major body fluid compartments, extracellular fluid (ECF), and intracellular fluid (ICF).

3–9

Osmotic pressure is the attraction of fluid back into capillaries by the presence of large molecules that cannot diffuse out. These molecules, that are confined to the capillaries, include the plasma proteins. **Albumin** is responsible for most of the osmotic pressure even though it is the smallest of the proteins. This is because osmotic pressure is related to the *number* of molecules present, not their size. Albumin is the most abundant plasma protein. Let us briefly review osmosis to understand osmotic pressure.

3–10

Osmosis, or the movement of water across different areas, is controlled by the number of solutes that are on one side or another of a membrane. Capillary membranes are **semipermeable** because they allow small molecules like water to pass through but prevent passage of larger molecules. In osmosis, water will move from an area of less solutes to the area that contains more solutes. This is also the same as saying that water moves from where water is more abundant to where there is less. When there is a difference in concentration or amount of a substance on two sides of a membrane, this is called a **concentration gradient.** The word *grade* is often used to describe the *steepness* of a hill or incline. Likewise, concentration gradient describes the *degree of difference between the two amounts.* The larger the gradient, the greater the force of attraction. Image letting a barrel roll down a hill. The steeper the hill, the faster the barrel will roll. Figures 3–3 and 3–4 illustrate the concepts of osmosis and concentration gradients.

3–11

Plasma in the capillaries changes in composition and pressure from the arterial end to the venous end so gradients are created. Look at Figure 3–5. Blood pressure is relatively high as it enters the capillary at the arterial end. This is because of the force of the heart's contraction. As blood leaves from the venous end, the pressure is much less because some of the force has dissipated and fluid has left the capillary. This allows osmotic pressure to be greater than blood pressure at the venous end and to exert the necessary force to draw fluid back inside the vessel. It is primarily albumin that is responsible for this attraction of fluid. Not all fluid is returned in this manner. Some is absorbed by vessels called lymphatics, which will be studied in Chapter 9.

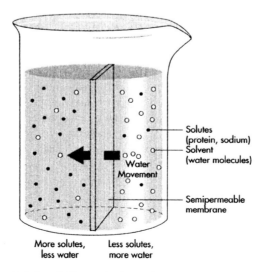

Solutes
(protein, sodium)
Solvent
(water molecules)

Water
Movement

Semipermeable
membrane

More solutes,   Less solutes,
less water   more water

Figure 3–3. Osmosis. Water molecules are drawn to the area of more solutes.

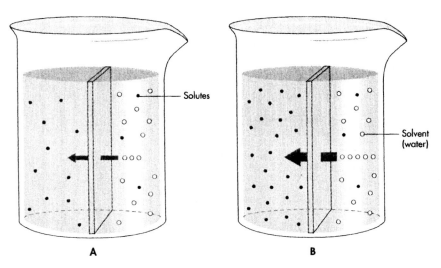

Figure 3–4. Concentration gradient (degree of difference in numbers of solutes on two sides of a membrane), which affects the force of attraction of solvent molecules. **A.** Force of attraction due to "X" number of solutes. **B.** Greater force of attraction due to "2X" number of solutes.

3–12

The concept of numbers of dissolved particles or solutes in a solution can be measured in terms of **osmolarity.** The body's osmolarity is a reflection of how concentrated the plasma is in terms of substances that are dissolved in it. Amounts of fluid or water would be opposite. In regulating amounts of total body water, the osmoreceptors interpret a rise in osmolarity to be a sign of less water since the plasma is now more concentrated. Osmolarity and relative changes in concentration are represented for you in Figure 3–6. Figure 3–6D represents dehydration, where the number of solutes is normal but water is less than normal. The effect is increased osmolarity that is detected by osmoreceptors. Thirst results to replace lost water. Figure 3–6E represents the opposite, or overhydration.

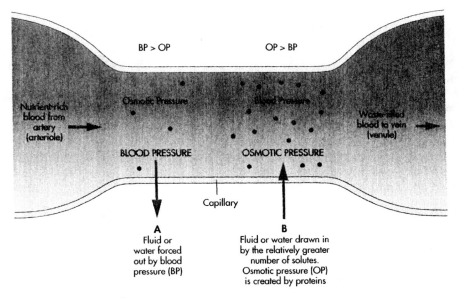

Figure 3–5. Control of fluid movement by blood pressure and osmotic pressure.

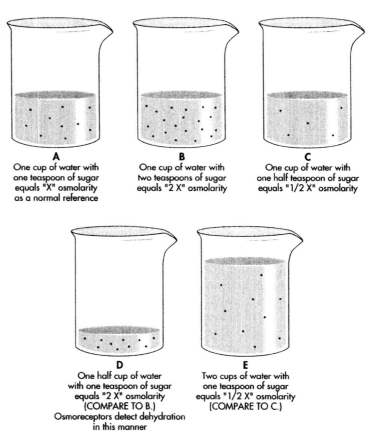

Figure 3–6. Osmolarity, the measure of the concentration of solutes dissolved in a solvent.

3–13

The last subject concerning fluid balance is that of **tonicity** (see Fig. 3–7). This is the effect of osmolarity on cell size due to the movement of water in and out of the cell. The cell is bathed in interstitial fluid. The interstitial fluid contains a certain number of solutes and inside the cell are solutes. Normally, the amounts on either side of the cell membrane are equal and so the interstitial fluid is **isotonic** in relation to inside the cell ("iso," meaning the same). Water moves in a normal fashion in and out of the cell. Following the principles of osmosis, if the interstitial fluid contains more solutes, it is **hypertonic** compared to intracellular fluid. Therefore, more water than normal will leave the cell, causing the cell to shrink or become **crenated.** Interstitial fluid with fewer solutes is **hypotonic,** causing excessive water to enter and swell the cell. Enough swelling will cause the cell membrane to rupture or **lyse.** The concentration of body fluid that causes it to be isotonic is created by sodium chloride in approximately a 0.9 percent solution. This concentration of sodium chloride is called **saline.** A 5 percent solution of glucose is also isotonic. This concept is important when administering intravenous fluids and when considering the effect of some disease states discussed later in this text.

3–14

Another important aspect of homeostasis is **electrolyte balance.** Molecules of some compounds have a natural tendency to dissociate into the individual particles that make up the molecule. You know from general chemistry that the force that creates compounds is the attraction and binding of the elements to each other. This is because of the difference in their net charge, either negative or positive. The molecules we call electrolytes have either a positive or negative charge associated with them once they have separated from the compound state. These charge particles are called **ions.** A positively charged ion is a **cation** and a neg-

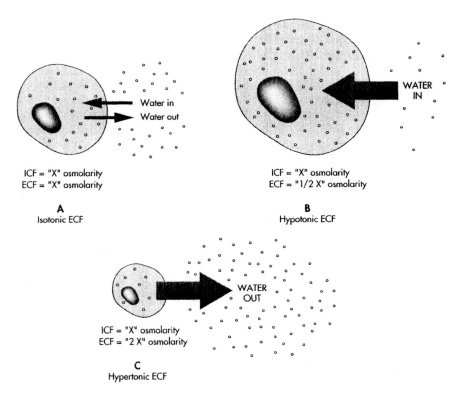

ICF = "X" osmolarity
ECF = "X" osmolarity

A
Isotonic ECF

ICF = "X" osmolarity
ECF = "1/2 X" osmolarity

B
Hypotonic ECF

ICF = "X" osmolarity
ECF = "2 X" osmolarity

C
Hypertonic ECF

Figure 3–7. The effect of fluid tonicity on cell size. **A.** Isotonic ECF. **B.** Hypotonic ECF = cellular swelling (rupture or lysis). **C.** Hypertonic ECF = cellular shrinking (crenation or dehydration).

ative ion is an **anion.** An example is sodium chloride. In plasma and other body fluids, it often exists as the cation sodium and the anion chloride. Electrolytes or ions are able to freely move among the different fluid compartments whenever there is a need to balance the charge in a particular area and cause it to be neutral. Electrolytes have many functions and are a vital part of homeostasis and health. They are important in regulating water balance, play a part in acid–base balance, maintain neutral body charges, assist many enzyme reactions, and are important in neuromuscular function. We will consider only the major electrolytes in the following frames.

3–15

The most numerous cation in the extracellular fluid is **sodium (Na$^+$).** It is responsible for most of the interstitial osmotic force that works with blood pressure to get fluid from the vessels, through the interstitium, and to the cells. The amount of sodium present determines most of the osmolarity of the ECF. This positive ion is the primary regulator of water balance among the compartments. Please note at this point that water balance and electrolyte levels, especially sodium, go hand in hand. Remember that "water follows sodium" under the guidelines of osmotic principles. Other functions of sodium include assisting the conduction of nerve impulses and acid–base balance. Sodium levels are controlled by a mineralocorticoid hormone from the adrenal cortex called **aldosterone.** The kidneys also contribute daily to sodium regulation through normal excretion and retention. When sodium levels drop, aldosterone stimulates the kidneys to retain or keep more sodium, while at the same time excreting more potassium. If blood volume or blood pressure should drop, such as in hemorrhage or shock, a hormonal "tag team" called the renal **renin–angiotensin system** will ultimately produce more aldosterone in the blood. This causes more sodium to remain in the body because of renal (kidney) retention. Since water follows sodium, more water is retained to contribute to blood volume and therefore pressure.

3-16

The major ECF anion is the counterpart to sodium, which is **chloride (Cl⁻).** Chloride participates in several functions along with sodium, but one function unique to chloride is the **chloride shift.** The chloride shift is an important event that occurs during the processes that create acid–base balance. Electroneutrality, or maintaining a neutral charged state, is vital for health of cells and tissues. In the course of hydrogen exchange during acid–base activities, the net charge of an area will be affected. Usually the ECF will contain too many negative charges. Therefore, the anion chloride moves or shifts into cells, usually red blood cells, and this restores the neutral charge.

3-17

Potassium (K⁺) is the predominant intracellular or ICF cation. The ECF contains much sodium but potassium is found mostly *inside cells.* What keeps most of the potassium inside the cells when it is small enough to diffuse out? And, incidently, what keeps most of the sodium out of the cells and in the ECF? The answer is the sodium–potassium pumps that are located in cell membranes. These pump systems use energy to perform the work of keeping sodium out and potassium in, so the process is called **active transport.** (Diffusion is passive transport because no work is done.) Potassium is responsible for most of the intracellular osmolarity. This ion is vital in maintaining membrane potentials for nerve impulses and muscle contraction, including skeletal and smooth muscle, as well as cardiac muscle. Potassium greatly affects heart function. It plays important roles in acid–base balance and in metabolic reactions.

3-18

Extracellular potassium levels are also regulated by aldosterone and the kidneys. The kidneys generally excrete potassium to keep plasma levels in a low normal range. If potassium increases, aldosterone stimulates the kidneys to excrete more potassium. However, if potassium is too low, the kidneys are not very effective in retaining this electrolyte. Plasma levels of potassium are greatly affected by changes in pH. In acidosis (low pH), potassium becomes elevated. In alkalosis (high pH), plasma potassium decreases. The reason for this is a shifting in and out of cells by both hydrogen ions and potassium ions to maintain electroneutrality. Since hydrogen is charged, abnormal amounts throw the ECF net charge out of balance so potassium movement in or out of cells restores balance. Levels of potassium have critical effects on heart function so disturbance in pH can affect heart function through potassium. Insulin also affects ECF potassium concentrations. Insulin stimulates movement of potassium into liver and muscle cells. This principle can be used to treat high levels of potassium. It can also cause a low potassium in a patient who was previously normal.

3-19

Calcium (Ca⁺) is a cation that is stored in bones, along with phosphate. Calcium provides bones and teeth their rigid structure necessary for normal function. It is part of the blood coagulation process. It is vital in nerve impulses and muscle contraction. This also includes heart contraction and automaticity. It also contributes to the stability of cell membranes. An interesting note about Ca⁺ levels is that they are *inversely proportional* to phosphate amounts. That is, when calcium is increased, phosphate decreases and vice versa. This is important because increases in both ions at the same time may result in precipitation of calcium phosphate salts in the tissues and injury to cells.

3-20

Calcium is regulated by **parathyroid hormone (PTH), calcitonin,** and **vitamin D.** PTH from the parathyroid glands increases plasma calcium by stimulating release from bone, increasing retention of Ca⁺ by the kidneys, and helping to activate vitamin D. Vitamin D passes through several steps, which include the liver and kidney, to become activated. This vitamin increases the amount of calcium that is absorbed from nutrients in the intestine. It also stimulates Ca⁺ release from bone. When calcium is too high, PTH causes increased excretion by the kidneys and calcitonin from the thyroid glands stimulates more deposit of calcium into the bones.

3–21

There are three forms of circulating calcium. The most important form, in terms of effects on body function, is the ionized form. The ionized form is the only *physiologically active* form. The others are bound to protein and other chemicals and so cannot diffuse out of the vessels. The ionized form is free to diffuse out of vessels to perform its functions. This ionized form is also affected by pH, just like potassium. Acidosis causes an increase in the ionized, or active form, while alkalosis produces a decrease. This is because the pH affects the amount of calcium that is bound to its carrier substances. Less binding means more ionized calcium and more effects on the body. And of course, the opposite is true. Table 3–1 summarizes the major mechanisms that control or effect electrolyte levels in the circulation.

3–22

Our last topic of review is acid–base balance. The presence of normal amounts of acid and base in the body is very important to homeostasis. You know from your chemistry studies that the description of an environment in terms of acid and base is called "pH." The close control of pH, or the regulation of the concentrations of hydrogen ions, is what acid–base balance is about. Slight changes from the normal pH greatly affects the rates of all chemical reactions, which form the basis for all metabolic processes. Some rates are accelerated, while others are severely depressed or stopped altogether. Another important consequence is that, as proteins, enzymes become denatured or lose their structural conformation. They are then deactivated. Therefore, the enzymes become useless to drive chemical reactions.

3–23

Before we begin discussion of acid–base balance, let us first review a few basic definitions. An **acid** is a molecule that can and does release hydrogen ions (H^+). An acid or base is strong or weak depending on the amount of this dissociation that takes place. Acids and bases in the body are generally weak. The predominant acid in our body is **carbonic acid** (H_2CO_3) which is produced from carbon dioxide (CO_2). A **base** is the opposite, or is a molecule that can and does accept H^+ from its environment. **Bicarbonate** (HCO_3^-) is the predominant base in the body and is produced from H_2CO_3. Acids and bases often occur as pairs, such as with H_2CO_3 and HCO_3^-. Think of them as two sides of the same coin. Whether the molecule is an acid or base at the time depends on the number of H^+ ions it contains. H_2CO_3 is able to donate a H^+ ion and become HCO_3^-, while HCO_3^- is "short" a H^+ ion and can accept one. Soon you will be asked to look at an equation that diagrams several relationships in acid–base balance, so this concept will become clearer. The **pH** is a measurement of the amount of free H^+ ions that are present and is *inversely proportional* to, or the *opposite* of, H^+ ion concentration. If an acid releases H^+, more will be present so the pH decreases. If a base takes on or removes H^+ from the environment, less will be present so the pH increases. So a lower pH is associated with **acidic** conditions and a higher pH is associated with basic or **alkaline** conditions.

TABLE 3–1. MECHANISMS THAT CONTROL OR AFFECT PLASMA LEVELS OF MAJOR ELECTROLYTES

	Sodium	Potassium	Total Calcium	Ionized Calcium
INCREASED BY	Aldosterone, by increasing retention by the kidneys	Acidosis, by movement out of cells	Parathyroid hormone, by bone resorption Vitamin D, by intestinal absorption	Acidosis, by decreasing binding to proteins
DECREASED BY	Increased excretion by the kidneys	Aldosterone, by increasing excretion by the kidneys Alkalosis, by movement into cells Insulin, by movement into cells	Calcitonin, by increasing bone deposition	Alkalosis, by increasing binding to proteins

3-24

The **Henderson–Hasselbalch equation** is a mathematical calculation that determines the normal pH in our bloodstream. This normal is determined by the *ratio* of our base and acid to each other (bicarbonate to carbonic acid). Please note it is the ratio of these chemicals to each other, not necessarily the actual amounts, that determines the pH. This will be important to understand when you learn about methods of compensating for abnormal pH. Because of this ratio concept, changes causing abnormal levels of H_2CO_3 or HCO_3^- can still lead to a pH in the normal range, if the ratio is normal. The ratio that produces a normal pH is 20 to 1, or 20 times as much HCO_3^- for every H_2CO_3. The Henderson–Hasselbalch equation is shown in Table 3–2.

3-25

The source of H^+ ions is largely through metabolism of glucose by cells that produce the waste product carbon dioxide (CO_2). CO_2 combines with water to form carbonic acid (H_2CO_3). This is catalyzed by the enzyme **carbonic anhydrase,** usually in the red blood cells. As an acid, H_2CO_3 dissociates into bicarbonate (HCO_3^-) and free H^+ ion. It is vital that this free H^+ be neutralized to maintain the pH at normal. Hemoglobin in red blood cells combines with the H^+ and carries it to the lungs. HCO_3^- diffuses out of the red blood cell, and since it is charged, another anion must move into the cell to maintain a neutral state. The anion that shifts into the cells is chloride and hence, the origin of the phrase **chloride shift.** The bicarbonate then combines with sodium and is transported by the circulation to the lungs as sodium bicarbonate. In the lungs, sodium leaves the bicarbonate and HCO_3^- combines back with the H^+ released from hemoglobin. This re-forms carbonic acid, again catalyzed by carbonic anhydrase, which splits into water and carbon dioxide. The carbon dioxide is expelled through exhalation by the lungs. Take a moment to study Figure 3–8 that shows these changes. These chemical changes are also given to you in the form of an equation in Figure 3–9. You may think of CO_2 as being "disassembled" in the tissues where it is formed, transported to the lungs, and "reassembled" back into CO_2 so it can be released into the atmosphere. This transport of CO_2 from tissues to lungs is primarily in the form of $NaHCO_3$ (70 percent), and as combined with hemoglobin ($HHbCO_2$, about 23 percent).

3-26

The next concept is that of **buffers.** A buffer is a chemical that will act as either an acid or a base, depending on the numbers of H^+ ions present. The purpose of acting both ways is that a buffer is able to donate H^+ to an environment that is too alkaline and able to absorb H^+ from an environment that is too acid. The net result of all this shifting around of H^+ is that the normal pH can be maintained and the body is not severely harmed. The buffers are what

TABLE 3–2. THE HENDERSON–HASSELBALCH EQUATION AND CHANGES IN ACID–BASE CONCENTRATIONS

A. Normal Amounts of Acid, Base, Ratio, and pH

pH = 6.1 + log base / acid

pH = 6.1 + log HCO_3^- / H_2CO_3

pH = 6.1 + log 20 / 1

pH = 6.1 + 1.3

pH = 7.4

B. Increased Amounts of Acid and Base, But a Normal Ratio and Therefore a Normal pH

pH = 6.1 + log 26 / 1.3

pH = 6.1 + 1.3 (26 / 1.3 = 20)

pH = 7.4

C. Decreased Amounts of Acid and Base, But a Normal Ratio and Therefore a Normal pH

pH = 6.1 + log 16 / .8

pH = 6.1 + 1.3 (16 / .8 = 20)

pH = 7.4

Venous
circulation
NaHCO3
HHb
HCO3−
HHb
H+
O2
H2CO3
HbO2−
CO2+ H2O
CO2
HbO2
Arterial
circulation
HHb
O2
H+
HbO2−
HCO3−
H2CO3
CO2 + H2O
CO2
TISSUES–
METABOLISM
PRODUCES CO2
LUNGS–
EXPIRE CO2

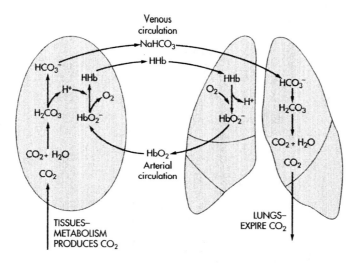

Figure 3–8. Generation, transport, and elimination of carbon dioxide.

keep the acid–base systems balanced and the pH compatible with life. Remember these facts about the need for buffers:

1. Free H^+ ions are constantly produced by the body and are generated from carbonic acid, which is formed from carbon dioxide.
2. Free H^+ ions determine the pH.
3. All metabolic processes are chemical reactions that depend on a specific pH to operate properly.
4. All chemical reactions depend on enzymes that are easily destroyed by abnormal pH. 3-27

With this in mind, let us consider the various buffer systems that help regulate pH. These buffers are found both inside and outside of the cell, or are intra- and extracellular. Their purpose is to act quickly in releasing or absorbing H^+ ions to prevent excessive changes in pH. This balancing act is meant to be a temporary measure. The true controllers of final pH are the lungs and kidneys. Buffers control local pH and transport H^+ to these sites of final release from the body. The first buffer system we have already mentioned and that is the carbonic acid–bicarbonate pair. H_2CO_3 is the acid and HCO_3^- is the base. The active sites for this pair are primarily the red blood cells, lungs, and kidneys. CO_2 diffuses into the red cells for the conversion we have already discussed (review Figures 3–8 and 3–9 if necessary). Once in the lungs, the reverse reaction occurs. The tubules of the kidneys are the site of H^+ release and HCO_3^- reabsorption. The H_2CO_3–HCO_3^- system works very quickly, converting to the different forms as needed in a fraction of a second.

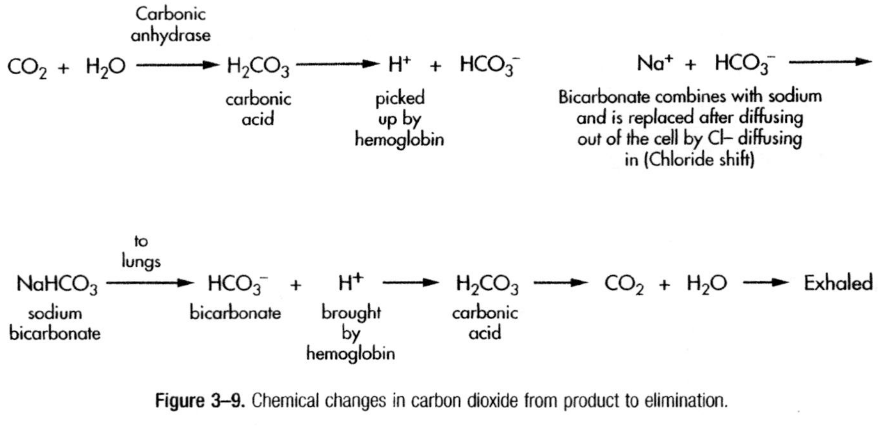

Carbonic
anhydrase
CO2 + H2O → H2CO3 → H+ + HCO3−
carbonic
acid
picked
up by
hemoglobin
Na+ + HCO3− →
Bicarbonate combines with sodium
and is replaced after diffusing
out of the cell by Cl− diffusing
in (Chloride shift)
to
lungs
NaHCO3 → HCO3− + H+ → H2CO3 → CO2 + H2O → Exhaled
sodium
bicarbonate
bicarbonate
brought
by
hemoglobin
carbonic
acid

Figure 3–9. Chemical changes in carbon dioxide from product to elimination.

3-28

Phosphate is another buffer pair, in the form of $H_2PO_4^-$ and HPO_4^-. The phosphates are found in the cells and are especially concentrated in the tubules of the kidneys because phosphate is eliminated in the urine. Because of the high amounts of phosphate in the tubules, this results in the very important function of buffering the filtrate itself as it passes through the nephron. During the process of readying H^+ for elimination, it would be possible for very strong acids to be formed in the filtrate and cause lethal injury to the kidney cells. The presence of phosphate helps to prevent this from happening by absorbing H^+ and forming the weak acid $H_2PO_4^-$.

3-29

Proteins are another important pH regulator. The amino group that is part of an amino acid is responsible for its ability to act as a buffer. The amino group buffer system consists of NH_2^- (accepts H^+) and NH_3 (donates H^+). A specific kind of protein-based molecule is **hemoglobin** (Hb) that binds oxygen for transport by the red blood cells. We mentioned the transport of H^+ by hemoglobin to the lungs. Oxyhemoglobin (oxygen and Hb) travels to the tissues from the lungs through the blood. There the oxygen is released and Hb accepts the H^+ which has just split off from H_2CO_3. This is deoxyhemoglobin or HHb. HHb makes its way back to the lungs, releases the H^+, picks up oxygen, and the process repeats. The released H^+ now recombines with the HCO_3^- that traveled to the lungs attached to sodium. The resulting H_2CO_3 is catalyzed by carbonic anhydrase back to water and CO_2. Refer to Tables 3–8 and 3–9 again to understand these processes.

3-30

The lungs are a vital part of pH balance because they ultimately rid the body of CO_2 and therefore H^+ ions through the process of expiration. This elimination of CO_2 occurs continuously but, when levels of CO_2 increase beyond normal, this directly stimulates the respiratory center in the brain. Autonomic nerve impulses cause an increase in ventilation so that the body can literally "blow off" extra carbon dioxide. This hyperventilation is a relatively fast response toward normalizing the pH (about 3 to 12 minutes). However this rate of ventilation is short lived. The body cannot sustain this type of respiration and remain healthy. So even though the lungs play an important and fast role in pH regulation, they cannot completely return the pH to normal. They begin the job that the kidneys ultimately finish. The effectiveness of increased respiration is to normalize the system until the kidneys can finish the task.

3-31

The kidneys eliminate H^+ ions through the urine and conserve HCO_3^- in the body. That is why urine is more acidic than blood. If CO_2 levels increase, this speeds up the secretion of H^+. The resulting urine will be more acidic. The opposite is also true if pH decreases, that is, the kidneys will conserve more H^+ ions and secrete more HCO_3^-, making the urine alkaline. Buffering of the urine by phosphate and ammonia is the key element in the ability to adjust the urine pH without damaging the kidneys. The urine itself does not become so acidic or alkaline that it destroys the tubules. The action of these buffers allows more H^+ to be secreted before any damage to the kidneys occurs. The kidneys are the slowest of the regulators to respond, often taking hours to even days to full effectiveness. However this is the most effective organ in correcting acid–base imbalances. The response may be slower but it is capable of being sustained, unlike the respiratory response. Changes in urine composition by the kidneys will continue until the pH is actually returned to normal, not just brought closer to normal. The exceptions to this are if the kidneys are diseased or if the cause of the original imbalance continues. Table 3–3 summarizes some of the mechanisms that produce the normal balance between acid and base and therefore the normal pH.

3-32

Before we leave the subject of acid–base balance, only two points remain. First, while the majority of H^+ ion concentrations are from glycolysis, there are certainly other sources of acid production. Lactic acid is a waste product generated from muscle activity while protein and fat metabolism form additional acids. Sometimes imbalances stem from these sources. (The kidneys still control pH through processing these additional acids as well.) Second is the effect of pH on electrolytes and vice versa. Remember cations and anions will shift from one compartment to another to maintain electroneutrality. Na^+, K^+, Cl^-, HCO_3^-, and H^+ ions are mainly involved in these shifts. The net effect of these exchanges is a deviation from

TABLE 3–3. MECHANISM OF CONTROL OF ACID–BASE BALANCE

	Mechanism	Rate of Action

Buffer pairs
  Carbonic acid / bicarbonate (H_2CO_3/HCO_3^-)
  Proteins and hemoglobin (Hb/HHb)
  Phosphate (HPO_4^-)
	Release or absorb hydrogen ions	Immediate

Kidneys	Retain or eliminate HCO_3^- or H^+ as needed, phosphate and ammonia buffering	Hours to days
Lungs	Retain or eliminate CO_2 (H_2CO_3)	Minutes to hours
Movement of electrolytes in and out of cells	Exchanges Na^+ and/or K^+ for H^+ in the ECF	Minutes to hours

normal in plasma potassium levels. The relationship of H^+ and K^+ ion movements is an important aspect of pH.

II. DISORDERS IN TEMPERATURE REGULATION ◀ SECTION

Increased body temperature is the first disorder we will consider. Before specific syndromes are covered, there are some points to be made about increased temperature. It is one of the most frequent physiologic responses to be seen in several kinds of disease. The body temperature is an excellent indicator of general health status, particularly in infectious conditions. A high temperature is generally not harmful until it exceeds about 104°F. Levels higher than that will cause severe nerve damage and cause cell proteins to coagulate and be destroyed. The cooking of an egg, causing the white part to solidify and be permanently changed, is the classic example of protein coagulation by heat. An easy way to gauge the degree of sickness in an individual with an infection is taking the _____(1). As long as levels do not go above _____(2), there is no real danger. However, beyond that is the possibility that cell proteins will _____(3) and there will be _____(4) damage.

1. temperature
2. 104°F
3. coagulate
4. nerve

▶ FEVER

Another term for fever is **pyrexia.** Pyrexia is an increase in body temperature that follows a change in the regulating mechanism. Fever is caused by endogenous factors, which means the disturbance is coming from _____(1) the body. (Shortly we will contrast this with hyperthermia.) Temperature greater than 104°F is called **hyperpyrexia.** Hyperpyrexia is the range in which the regulating mechanism is in danger of being lost, which means the temperature could then climb to fatal levels. Also, even if the regulation were to remain effective, temperatures higher than 106°F can mean that some additional activity is occurring that is overriding the body's efforts to lose enough heat. A **pyrogen** is a chemical that will cause a fever. Most pyrogens come from bacteria and are therefore called exogenous pyrogens. Exogenous pyrogens affect white blood cells and cause them to secrete their own fever producing chemical. This *endogenous* pyrogen is **interleukin-1.** Interleukin-1 increases the production of **prostaglandin** which directly affects the hypothalamus. The result is that the setpoint of the hypothalamus is changed to a higher setting. This higher setting causes more heat producing activity until the new temperature is reached. Fever is properly termed _____(2) and is called _____(3) if it reaches greater than _____(4). A chemical that stimulates a fever is a _____(5). Interleukin-1 is an _____(6) pyrogen and comes from stimulated _____(7) cells. Interleukin-1 causes production of _____(8),

1. inside or from within
2. pyrexia
3. hyperpyrexia
4. 104°F
5. pyrogen
6. endogenous
7. white blood
8. prostaglandin

9. hypothalamus
10. setpoint

which acts directly on the _____(9). The hypothalamic _____(10) is increased so the body acts accordingly to increase the temperature.

------- 3-35 -------

1. conservation
2. production
3. loss
4. cold
5. conserved
6. produced
7. vasoconstriction
8. shivering
9. production
10. loss
11. hot
12. sweating

The most common cause of fever is infection. This kind of temperature increase can be composed of three distinct stages. The **cold stage** is the group of activities that responds to the higher setpoint of the hypothalamus. Just like turning up the thermostat of a room, the furnace will "kick on" and run until the new temperature is reached, and then shut off. Cold stage activities are primarily vasoconstriction and shivering, which you know to be effective methods of heat _____(1) and _____(2) respectively. Because the vessels close down, people feel colder and start to shiver. Between these small muscle contractions that generate heat, and prevention of heat loss through vasoconstriction, the new temperature is reached. When this happens, this begins the next stage which is the **hot stage.** The patient feels overwarm and shivering stops. Vessels return to normal so the effect is that heat production and loss are once again balanced and the new temperature maintained. A properly working thermoregulation system will not allow the temperature to exceed dangerous levels (104 to 106°F). The end of pyrexia is signaled by the **sweating stage.** You know that sweat is a very effective means of heat _____(3). The patient feels hot and heat loss behavior accompanies sweating. These stages are illustrated for you in Figure 3–10. Turning up a furnace thermostat is very like the _____(4) stage of a fever. Various activities will cause heat to be _____(5) and _____(6) until the new temperature is reached. These activities are _____(7) and _____(8). The balance between heat _____(9) and _____(10) maintain the new temperature in the _____(11) stage. Cooling back down to normal is the function of the _____(12) stage.

------- 3-36 -------

Less common causes of fever include tissue injury such as in infarction, thrombosis, or hemorrhage. Catabolism (breakdown) of the dead or injured tissue involves the phagocytic macrophages that also release interleukin. The fever in these cases is mild. Tumors produce slightly higher temperatures and this is thought to be due to a pyrogen called **tumor necrosis factor.** Some cases of pyrexia cannot be traced to any cause and are classified as a **fever of unknown origin** or **FUO.** Since cancer can be occult or hidden until it is advanced, an

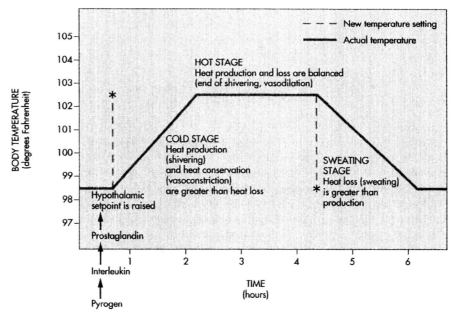

Figure 3–10. Stages of fever.

undiagnosed FUO should alert the health care professional to the possibility of cancer. The pyrogen from tumors is _____(1). Because tumors can cause fever, they should be suspected as the cause in a case of a fever of _____(2). The purpose of fever and what good it may serve is not clearly known and theories vary among authorities. It is assumed to be part of our basic defense mechanism against disease since research has shown some parts of the immune response to be enhanced by higher temperatures. Also some bacteria do not grow well or are even destroyed at higher temperatures so this may be another function.

1. tumor necrosis factor
2. unknown origin

▶ HYPERTHERMIA

3-37

The literal meaning of **hyperthermia** is an increased or higher than normal body temperature. So what then is the difference between fever and hyperthermia? The answer is from where the inciting cause is originating, and if there is any effect on the hypothalamic setpoint. Fever is of endogenous/exogenous (choose one) _____(1) origin and the temperature setting is turned up. In hyperthermia the origin is *external* or is endogenous/exogenous (choose one) _____(2). This means the disturbance is coming from the environment in the form of heat and humidity. Also there is no resetting of the body's temperature level. Rather, hyperthermia damages the body by overcoming the body's ability to maintain normal temperature. Mechanisms for balancing heat production and heat loss become overwhelmed. Often hyperthermia is a combination of increased production and decreased loss of heat. An example of this is heavy work or exercise in a hot, humid environment. Muscle exertion produces quite a lot of heat, and humid air greatly decreases heat loss through evaporation. The challenge to regulate temperature in these conditions becomes greater than the ability to keep the temperature in normal ranges. The difference between fever and hyperthermia is that in hyperthermia, the causes are _____(3) or _____(4) and this is due to an environment that is _____(5) and _____(6). There is no change in the hypothalamic _____(7) of what the temperature should be. Instead, the conditions of hyperthermia overwhelm homeostatic efforts to keep the temperature _____(8).

1. endogenous
2. exogenous
3. external
4. exogenous
5. hot
6. humid
7. setpoint
8. normal

3-38

There are three recognized syndromes of hyperthermia. The first is **heat cramps** and this is the least severe problem. This is probably because heat cramps are a localized problem involving only some muscle groups. If a group of muscles are sorely taxed beyond their limits by exertion and exercise, spasms usually result. These painful bursts of involuntary rigidity are thought to be due to exhausted aerobic metabolism and loss of sodium and water through excessive sweating. (In physiology you would have learned the difference between aerobic metabolism that is fueled by oxygen and anaerobic, an alternate pathway during low oxygen. The waste product lactic acid is then formed in excess.) While local temperature is increased, body temperature overall is normal. Recall that sodium has a role in assisting nerve impulses. Local electrolyte depletion combined with local dehydration and lactic acid production create heat cramps. The least severe heat syndrome is _____(1). This is a generalized/localized (choose one) _____(2) condition involving loss of _____(3) and _____(4) through excessive sweating. The area affected is overworked _____(5) groups. Generally body temperature is _____(6).

1. heat cramps
2. localized
3. water
4. sodium or electrolytes
5. muscle
6. normal

3-39

A condition of moderate severity is **heat exhaustion.** This is somewhat like heat cramps except it is a generalized effect of severe water and electrolyte loss. Affected individuals are weak, have headaches and dizziness, and are nauseated. Brief collapse is possible. Because of generalized increase in heat, intense peripheral vasodilation occurs and this results in blood volume being removed from effective cardiac output. Both cardiac output and blood pressure decrease (hypotension), directly causing the signs and symptoms of heat exhaustion. It is unusual to have a high body temperature because the vasodilation compensates

1. water
2. electrolytes
3. dilation
4. signs and symptoms
5. cardiac output
6. blood pressure
7. normal
8. do

well for the heat. Loss of water and electrolytes through excessive sweating compound the effects of changes in how the blood volume is distributed. If the individual is removed from the environment, allowed to rest, and receives replacement fluids, heat exhaustion becomes self-limiting. The body's homeostatic mechanisms of temperature regulation will restore balance because there has been no true damage. Heat exhaustion is generally characterized by loss of _____(1) and _____(2), as well as vaso _____(3). Vascular changes that attempt to compensate for increased heat are responsible for the _____(4) seen in the individual. These signs and symptoms are the direct result of decreased _____(5) and _____(6). Overall body temperature is generally _____(7) and individuals usually do/do not (choose one) _____(8) recover.

3-40

1. 104°F
2. heat stroke
3. thermoregulation
4. hyperpyrexia
5. circulatory failure
6. shock
7. ischemic necrosis
8. treatment

Heat stroke, sometimes called **sunstroke,** is the most severe ailment and is life threatening. This condition is most true to the definition of hyperthermia in that heat stroke represents the failure of thermoregulation. Heat stroke is caused by heat exposure. The body's attempts to normalize temperature are overwhelmed, or there may be insufficient response. A healthy adult in extreme enough conditions will succumb and the elderly are especially susceptible because of suppressed function of normal body activities. Persons already compromised with chronic disease are also candidates for failed temperature regulation. There *is* increased body temperature into the range of hyperpyrexia, which means the temperature is at least _____(1). In heat stroke the same blood volume changes of heat exhaustion exist, but they are intensified to the point of circulatory failure and shock. The heart and kidney are especially susceptible to ischemic necrosis caused by lack of adequate circulation and blood pressure. Death will occur without aggressive treatment. The most dangerous and life threatening of the heat syndromes is _____(2). The basic mechanism of injury is failure of _____(3). Body temperatures reaches 104°F or greater, which is called _____(4). Extreme blood volume changes occur which cause _____(5) and _____(6). Vital organs such as the heart and kidney will undergo _____(7) and death is imminent without _____(8). Table 3–4 compares the three syndromes of hyperthermia.

▶ HYPOTHERMIA

3-41

1. vasoconstriction
2. hypothermia
3. normal, intact, etc.
4. temperature
5. vasoconstriction
6. ischemic

Hypothermia is a core body temperature of less than 95°F. Most causes of hypothermia are accidental exposure to extreme cold for long periods of time or immersion in cold water. Many factors determine survival of hypothermia, including the severity of temperature drop, the duration, immersion in water, and the age and condition of the individual. Temperature regulation becomes overwhelmed as the severity of external conditions are greater than regulation ability. Mechanisms for heat conservation are called upon. The vascular reaction that conserves heat is _____(1). When this reaction is very intense, such as in hypothermia, the vasoconstriction greatly decreases the amount of blood and therefore oxygen available to the tissues. Ischemic injury and necrosis, especially of sensitive vital organs, play a major role in the cause of death. Other effects of hypothermia include increased heart rate and blood pressure at first to try to perfuse vital tissues. Heart rate and blood pressure then falls, and metabolism is greatly reduced. When this occurs, it sets a cycle of depression into motion. Decreased metabolism uses less oxygen. Less carbon dioxide is produced. Carbon dioxide levels are a direct stimulant to the respiratory center of the brain. Therefore breathing becomes depressed and even less oxygen is introduced into the system. This compounds the effects of extreme vasoconstriction and resulting ischemic necrosis. The individual feels very sleepy due to lack of oxygen to the brain. This leads to loss of consciousness and death. A core body temperature less than 95°F is the definition of _____(2). Temperature regulation is usually _____(3) but conditions overcome the ability to maintain normal body _____(4). The heat conservation mechanism of _____(5) causes _____(6) damage to tis-

TABLE 3–4. HYPERTHERMIA SYNDROMES

Syndrome	Cause	Effect
Heat cramps	Muscle exertion, local depletion of sodium and water, anaerobic metabolism causing increased lactic acid production	Local spasms, pain, normal temperature
Heat exhaustion	High environmental temperature and humidity, generalized sodium and water depletion (dehydration) due to excessive activity	Weakness, headache, dizziness, collapse due to hypotension caused by vasodilation to dissipate heat. Normal body temperature
Heat stroke	Extreme environmental temperature and humidity, severe dehydration and electrolyte loss due to excessive activity Poor temperature regulation in susceptible individuals (elderly, infants)	Vascular and blood volume changes producing shock, ischemic injury to vital organs, hyperpyrexia and death

sues because of lack of _____(7) and _____(8). A cycle of depression begins when _____(9) is reduced by the cold temperature. The result is less _____(10) in the blood to stimulate respiration and _____(11) is depressed to the point of death.

7. blood supply
8. oxygen
9. metabolism
10. carbon dioxide
11. breathing

Frostbite is localized hypothermia that causes direct damage to tissues, and perhaps even necrosis depending on the extent. Tissues most susceptible include the fingers, toes, ears, and nose because these tissues have a high surface area to mass ratio. They are largely "skin and bones" with little muscle for heat production and fat for insulation. Destruction of capillaries and vessel obstruction cause ischemic injury and necrosis. Tissues that are susceptible to local hypothermia or _____(1) have a high _____(2) ratio that makes them more prone to cold injury.

1. frostbite
2. surface area to mass

II. REVIEW QUESTIONS

1. Another term for fever is _____.

2. Circle the correct responses:
   Fever is caused by (endogenous/exogenous) sources and (does/does not) result in a change in the hypothalamic setpoint. Hyperthermia is caused by (endogenous/exogenous) sources and (does/does not) result in a change in the hypothalamic setpoint.

3. A pyrogen is:
   a. a chemical that lowers body temperature
   b. a white blood cell that increases body temperature
   c. a chemical that produces fever
   d. a chemical that directly affects the hypothalamus

4. The endogenous pyrogen is:
   a. interleukin-1
   b. prostaglandin
   c. from bacteria
   d. white blood cells

1. pyrexia

2. endogenous; does; exogenous; does not

3. c–a chemical that produces fever

4. a–interleukin-1

5. b–infection

6. a–temperature is increased;
   b–new temperature is
   maintained; c–temperature
   returns to normal

7. tumor

8. b–hyperthermia

9. 1. b–heat exhaustion; 2.
   a–heat cramps; 3. c–heat
   stroke; 4. b–heat exhaustion; 5. c–heat stroke; 6.
   a–heat cramps; 7. c–heat
   stroke; 8. b–heat exhaustion; 9. c–heat stroke

10. d–vasoconstriction and
    ischemic necrosis

11. a–hypothermia

12. d–muscle and fat

5. The most common cause of fever is:
   a. a tumor
   b. infection
   c. tissue injury
   d. endogenous pyrogen from macrophages

6. Please match these stages of fever with their activities:
   a. cold stage   _____ new temperature is maintained
   b. hot stage   _____ temperature returns to normal
   c. sweating stage   _____ temperature is increased

7. Fever of unknown origin may be a sign of hidden _____.

8. Increased production of heat combined with decreased heat loss most describes:
   a. fever
   b. hyperthermia
   c. hypothermia
   d. hyperpyrexia

9. Please match these heat syndromes with their characteristics:
   a. heat cramps   1. _____ peripheral vasodilation and hypotension
   b. heat exhaustion 2. _____ least severe
   c. heat stroke   3. _____ hyperpyrexia
                       4. _____ self-limiting with rest and fluids
                       5. _____ life-threatening
                       6. _____ involves muscle groups
                       7. _____ circulatory failure and shock
                       8. _____ generalized water and electrolyte loss
                       9. _____ ischemic necrosis of vital organs

10. The mechanism of damage to the body in hypothermia is:
    a. vasodilation and ischemic injury
    b. decreased cardiac output
    c. vasoconstriction and hypotension
    d. vasoconstriction and ischemic necrosis

11. Slowed metabolism, decreased carbon dioxide, and depressed respiratory stimulation
    occurs in:
    a. hypothermia
    b. frostbite
    c. fever
    d. hyperthermia

12. Body parts that are sensitive to frostbite have less:
    a. skin and bones
    b. muscle and bones
    c. skin and fat
    d. muscle and fat

<h1>III. DISORDERS IN FLUID BALANCE ◀ SECTION</h1>

▶ **DEFICIENCY IN FLUID VOLUME**

3-43

A deficit in water volume, or a negative water balance, is called **dehydration.** There are two mechanisms that produce this condition as outlined in Table 3–5. The first is water intake which is less than normal output. Output includes **sensible** loss, or that which is noticeable, such as through urine production. It also includes **insensible** loss, or that which is less noticeable and therefore difficult to measure. Insensible losses occur through sweat, in the feces, and as a part of respiration. Insufficient intake can be a result of lack of access to water or by being unconscious or otherwise unable to communicate the need for water. Impaired thirst or **hypodipsia** and difficulty in swallowing (**dysphagia**) are other reasons for insufficient intake. The other category of cause of dehydration is when water output is greater than normal intake. There are several examples of this. The diarrhea that accompanies cholera is extreme, and death due to dehydration can occur in one or two days in untreated cases. The amount of water secreted into the intestines is excessive and the amount that would normally be absorbed is greatly decreased. Kidney disease can produce large volumes of urine (**polyuria**) that is dilute because the kidneys have lost their ability to concentrate urine. The more dilute the urine, the greater the water content. In diabetes mellitus (high blood sugar) the principle of osmosis leads to greater water loss through the urine because as glucose spills over into the urine, water will follow glucose. This is called **osmotic diuresis. Diuresis** refers to a condition or a drug (**diuretic**) that increases the volume of urine being produced. Another condition relating to loss through the urine is diabetes insipidus, which is discussed later in this chapter. In this disease, water conservation mechanisms are not working properly. Exorbitant sweating is a mechanism of loss through the skin, as is widespread burns. This is because water evaporation cannot be prevented if large areas of the skin are destroyed. It is also possible to have **third space** loss, meaning water is sequestered where it is of no use to the fluid compartments that are responsible for fluid balance (the ECF and ICF). An example would be in the intestines or in the peritoneal space (abdominal cavity). Less than normal amounts of body water are called _____(1). This can develop in one of two ways. The first way is when _____(2) is less than output. The second is when _____(3) is greater than intake. Lack of access, unconsciousness, hypodipsia, or dysphagia are causes of insufficient _____(4). Polyuria, osmotic _____(5), and burns are causes of too much _____(6).

1. dehydration
2. intake
3. output
4. intake
5. diuresis
6. output

TABLE 3–5. CAUSES OF DEHYDRATION

Fluid Intake Less Than Output	Fluid Output Greater Than Intake
Hypodipsia	Diarrhea
Dysphagia	Kidney disease—polyuric phase
Inability to communicate	Osmotic diuresis of diabetes mellitus
Restricted access	Diabetes insipidus
	Excessive sweating
	Widespread burns
	Third space loss

3–44

1. sodium
2. retain or keep
3. water

Since sodium and water balance are intimately related, conditions of low sodium will decrease the body's ability to retain normal amounts of water. Remember that water follows sodium through the principle of osmosis. In circumstances such as vomiting and diarrhea, or the heavy sweating of heat exhaustion, both water and sodium are lost. This makes it more difficult to regulate the remaining amounts of water. In Addison's disease (see Chap. 16) aldosterone levels are subnormal. You know that aldosterone is the hormone that controls levels of _____(1) by causing the kidneys to _____(2) this electrolyte. Less aldosterone means that more sodium is lost in the urine and therefore, _____(3) also.

3–45

1. hyper
2. shrink or crenate
3. intravascular
4. pressure
5. shock
6. interstitial
7. hypertonic
8. ICF
9. osmosis
10. lethal

An effect of dehydration is reduced intravascular volume. The amount of fluid inside vessels, or the volume, contributes a great deal to the blood pressure. A certain blood pressure is required to be able to perfuse or supply the tissues with blood, and therefore, oxygen. Lack of sufficient volume and pressure can lead to **hypovolemic shock** (see Chap. 9) and death. The body takes immediate steps to prevent shock and correct the situation. The heart rate climbs to pump blood faster. More importantly, fluid is drawn from the interstitial tissues into the vessels to make up for the deficit. The number of solutes remaining in the interstitium stays the same. However, with less water, the interstitium becomes _____(1) tonic in relation to the intracellular volume concentrations. The hypertonicity of the interstitium draws water from the cells through osmosis. The effect of hypertonicity on cells is that they _____(2). This is lethal to cellular enzymes and metabolism. Nerve cells and the brain are especially affected. Death occurs when water loss is about 15 percent of body weight, although signs of severe dehydration are apparent much sooner. The precipitating event that sets the cycle of injury in motion in dehydration is decreased _____(3) volume. This creates decreased blood _____(4) and the danger of hypovolemic _____(5). To prevent this, fluid is taken from the _____(6) tissues. This makes the interstitium _____(7) in relation to the _____(8). This causes water to leave the cells through the principle of _____(9). Hypertonicity causes cell crenation or intracellular dehydration that is _____(10) to cell metabolism. The order of these events is shown to you in Figure 3–11. The signs of dehydration include an acute decrease in body weight. This is a convenient way to monitor fluid status in babies. Extreme thirst is present but cannot be expressed in babies. If the kidneys are healthy and there is no

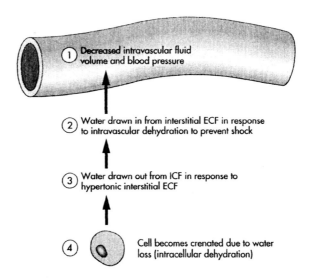

Figure 3–11. Effects of dehydration on ECF and ICF water distribution. (1 to 4 = order of events.)

underlying disease, the urine becomes scant and very concentrated. Loss of tissue turgor causes the eyes to have a sunken appearance. Dehydration is another cause of mild fever.

► EXCESS IN FLUID VOLUME

3-46

Excessive amounts of fluid in the body is classified as either too much water and sodium or too much water alone. The retention of both sodium and water does not change tonicity so the ECF is still considered isotonic. There is not a direct effect on cell size. Increased water over normal sodium levels does produce an ECF that is hypotonic so the danger of cellular swelling does exist. A primary cause of hypotonic fluid excess, which is termed **water intoxication,** is psychogenic compulsive water drinking. This is a psychiatric disorder. The patient is driven to consume water far in excess of what the kidneys can excrete and death will occur unless the practice is stopped or aggressively treated. More common is isotonic fluid excess and this has several causes. Increased intake greater than normal excretion often has **iatrogenic** causes, meaning a treatment is responsible for the imbalance. This is described as **circulatory overload.** It occurs during IV infusion of either high volumes of fluids in some patients or during infusion of normal amounts in patients susceptible to fluid excess, such as in heart disease or in the elderly. More common are conditions of decreased excretion of water and electrolytes that are less than normal intake. In congestive heart failure, blood pressure is not sufficient for the kidneys to produce normal amounts of urine, which contains unneeded water, electrolytes, and wastes. Blood must be filtered through the functional units of the kidneys (nephrons) with enough pressure to form the filtrate that is a precursor of urine. In kidney disease urine production may be greatly decreased (**oliguria**) or stop all together (**anuria**). Fluid excess may be isotonic which means there is an increase in both _____(1) and _____(2). Water increase alone is _____(3) fluid excess. Hypotonic fluid excess is also called water _____(4) and its usual cause is compulsive _____(5). Isotonic fluid excess may be iatrogenic in origin and it is described as _____(6). Usually, increased fluid volumes are due to decreased _____(7) that is less than normal intake. Two organs whose disease or failure can cause this are the _____(8) and _____(9).

1. water
2. sodium
3. hypotonic
4. intoxication
5. water drinking
6. circulatory overload
7. excretion
8. heart
9. kidney

3-47

The effects of pure water intoxication are as follows. In the presence of a hypotonic solution, cells _____(1) and may actually _____(2). The most dramatic signs of what is happening at the cellular level are seen through neurological signs caused by swelling of brain cells. Patients show confusion and dementia followed by stupor, seizures, and finally coma and death. Retention of both sodium and water naturally affects the body differently since the ECF is primarily isotonic. As in dehydration, body weight is a good indicator and weight increases. The pulse is described as pounding since intravascular volumes are increased. Edema is often seen and this imbalance is described in frame 3–60. This abnormal fluid in the interstitium may be generalized (widespread) or seen in "dependent" areas that are affected by gravity. Edema in the lungs, or pulmonary edema, produces signs of respiratory distress, and this is the most serious consequence. Water _____(3) causes cellular swelling, and death results because of the effects this has on the _____(4). A good sign of isotonic fluid retention is _____(5) body weight. Edema is generally present and can prove dangerous if the fluid accumulation is in the _____(6).

1. swell
2. lyse
3. intoxication
4. brain
5. increased
6. lungs

▶ POLYDIPSIA, EDEMA, AND DIABETES INSIPIDUS

3–48

1. polydipsia
2. consumption or drinking
3. dehydration
4. osmoreceptors
5. osmolarity
6. tissues

Polydipsia means excessive thirst. Some confuse this definition with excessive *drinking*, but increased fluid consumption is a result of being abnormally thirsty. Polydipsia is a *sign* of some imbalance. If a person is dehydrated, the normal mechanism to correct this is polydipsia. Recall that dehydration, and therefore polydipsia, will develop if intake is less than output. Also it results from increased loss such as vomiting and diarrhea, osmotic diuresis of diabetes mellitus, or from diabetes insipidus. A false type of polydipsia can accompany kidney and heart failure. The person isn't really dehydrated but large amounts of fluid can be trapped as edema in the tissues. The osmolarity of the plasma is increased as a result (less water in vessels, so more solutes). Osmoreceptors sense this and interpret it as dehydration, stimulating thirst through the hypothalamus. Finally there is polydipsia that can be associated with psychogenic compulsive water drinking. The term for excessive thirst is _____(1). This is seen as increased _____(2) of fluids. True polydipsia is a result of _____(3), which has several causes. False polydipsia is triggered by _____(4) that detect a rise in plasma _____(5). This rise is the result of fluid trapped in the _____(6) as edema.

3–49

1. fluid
2. interstitial
3. tissue
4. pitting edema
5. lungs
6. breathing or gas exchange
7. fluid
8. distribution

Another sign of a fluid imbalance is **edema.** This is an abnormal collection of fluid outside of the vessels and cells, in the interstitial or tissue spaces. Edema in the extremities can be demonstrated by pressing on the area, and when the pressure is released, seeing an indentation in the tissues. This is called **pitting edema.** This is like the impression that is seen after pressing on a piece of ripe fruit. Edema can be localized if there is a blockage in the venous or lymphatic drainage in that area. It can also be generalized in systemic causes such as congestive heart failure. Often this is seen as swelling of **dependent** areas, or body parts that are affected by gravity, such as the lower legs and ankles. **Pulmonary edema** (see Chap. 11) is fluid accumulation in the lungs. This develops in cases of left sided heart failure. Since the presence of fluid interferes with gas exchange, or the ability to breathe, this can deteriorate into an emergency condition. Overall fluid excess can be the reason for edema. However there may just be a problem with *distribution* of fluid when total body water is normal. Edema is too much _____(1) present in the _____(2) or _____(3) spaces. Visible denting of tissues after digital pressure is called _____(4). The most life-threatening consequence is edema in the _____(5) because _____(6) is compromised. Edema can be an indication of excessive _____(7) volume or may be an imbalance in fluid _____(8).

3–50

The first cause of edema is related to increased body fluids that develop during kidney disease. Loss of the ability to excrete normal amounts of sodium leads to sodium and therefore water retention. This causes an increased **hydrostatic pressure** because of increased fluid volume in the vessels. The increased pressure results in greater filtration force that normally pushes fluid out of the vessels. Fluid reabsorption requires osmotic pressure to be greater at the venous end of the capillary than blood pressure. Increased hydrostatic pressure interferes with normal return of fluid back into the vessels because blood pressure is not decreased enough. So we have two mechanisms at work. Related to this cause is increased **venous pressure** when there is right sided congestive heart failure. The pressure is increased because there is resistance to outflow at the venous end of the capillary. A failing right ventricle leads to backup of blood supply which is the resistance encountered in the capillary. Again, the difference between osmotic and blood pressure may not be great enough and this interferes with the ability of osmotic pressure to return fluid to the vessel. Any occlusion (blockage) of the large veins in the body will increase resistance and therefore pressure and create edema. Both of these mechanisms are illustrated in Figure 3–12. (Compare this to the normal state of events in Figure 3–5.) The fluid that accumulates in the tissues is called a **transudate** because it does not contain large amounts of proteins or cells. As you learned in Chapter 2, extravascular fluid from inflammation may contain proteins and cells and there-

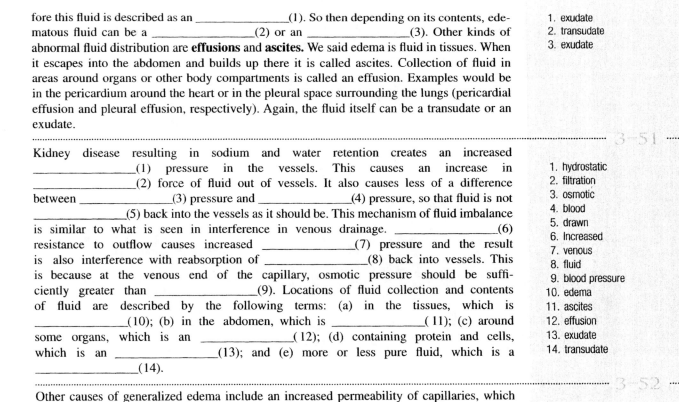

Figure 3–12. Edema due to increased fluid pressure (blood pressure greater than osmotic pressure).

fore this fluid is described as an _____(1). So then depending on its contents, edematous fluid can be a _____(2) or an _____(3). Other kinds of abnormal fluid distribution are **effusions** and **ascites.** We said edema is fluid in tissues. When it escapes into the abdomen and builds up there it is called ascites. Collection of fluid in areas around organs or other body compartments is called an effusion. Examples would be in the pericardium around the heart or in the pleural space surrounding the lungs (pericardial effusion and pleural effusion, respectively). Again, the fluid itself can be a transudate or an exudate.

1. exudate
2. transudate
3. exudate

3–51

Kidney disease resulting in sodium and water retention creates an increased _____(1) pressure in the vessels. This causes an increase in _____(2) force of fluid out of vessels. It also causes less of a difference between _____(3) pressure and _____(4) pressure, so that fluid is not _____(5) back into the vessels as it should be. This mechanism of fluid imbalance is similar to what is seen in interference in venous drainage. _____(6) resistance to outflow causes increased _____(7) pressure and the result is also interference with reabsorption of _____(8) back into vessels. This is because at the venous end of the capillary, osmotic pressure should be sufficiently greater than _____(9). Locations of fluid collection and contents of fluid are described by the following terms: (a) in the tissues, which is _____(10); (b) in the abdomen, which is _____(11); (c) around some organs, which is an _____(12); (d) containing protein and cells, which is an _____(13); and (e) more or less pure fluid, which is a _____(14).

1. hydrostatic
2. filtration
3. osmotic
4. blood
5. drawn
6. Increased
7. venous
8. fluid
9. blood pressure
10. edema
11. ascites
12. effusion
13. exudate
14. transudate

3–52

Other causes of generalized edema include an increased permeability of capillaries, which could also be described as the loss of selective permeability. In several conditions such as shock, anoxia, or anaphylaxis (life-threatening allergic response), capillaries become damaged on a wide scale basis and lose selective permeability. The loss of proteins into the interstitium, along with fluid, means much less osmotic pressure to draw fluid back in, as well as attracting even more fluid out of the vessels. We will be studying several disease states that

1. selective
2. permeability
3. proteins
4. osmotic
5. osmotic
6. attraction or draw
7. vessels

3-53

1. proteins
2. albumin
3. osmotic
4. albumin
5. hypoalbuminemia
6. kidneys
7. glomerulus
8. protein-losing
   enteropathy
9. liver
10. edema
11. ascites

damage capillaries in this manner. Loss of _____(1) _____(2) of the capillaries allows _____(3) to escape into the tissues. This creates more _____(4) pressure in the tissues that pulls more fluid there. It also leaves less _____(5) pressure in the vessel. This decreases fluid _____(6) back into the _____(7).

The last reason for edema production is decreased osmotic pressure that would lessen the attraction of water back into the capillary, as shown in Figure 3–13. The substances most responsible for osmotic pressure are plasma _____(1). Of these substances, the specific molecule responsible for most of the osmotic pressure in capillaries is _____(2). The condition in which there is less than normal amounts of albumin in the blood is called **hypoalbuminemia.** It makes sense that less albumin means less osmotic pressure and therefore retention of fluid in the tissues. There are two reasons for hypoalbuminemia, loss of albumin from the body at greater than production rates and less production of albumin. Loss of albumin into the urine is a feature of some kidney diseases, most notably, glomerulonephritis. This is an inflammatory condition of the glomerulus in which albumin escapes through the loosened capillary endothelial junctions. In hypoalbuminemia due to kidney disease, there will be albumin present in the urine. Albumin in the urine is called **albuminuria.** (The suffix **"emia"** means blood or plasma and the suffix **"uria"** means urine). Other routes of loss of protein include specific intestinal diseases that are collectively called **protein-losing enteropathy.** Literal interpretation of this phrase reads as "disease of the intestines in which protein is lost." Less production of albumin is due to liver disease since the liver is the organ responsible for manufacturing albumin from dietary protein. Signs of significant liver disease include edema and ascites as a direct result of the hypoalbuminemia. Starvation has the same effect, since amino acids for making albumin are not available. Another cause of edema formation is decreased _____(3) pressure because of decreased amounts of the specific protein _____(4). The term for this is _____(5). Loss of albumin can occur through the _____(6) when there is inflammatory disease of the _____(7). Another route of loss is through the intestines in a condition known as _____(8). Decreased production of albumin can be a result of _____(9) disease, since this organ makes albumin. Two fluid imbalances seen as signs of liver disease are _____(10) and _____(11).

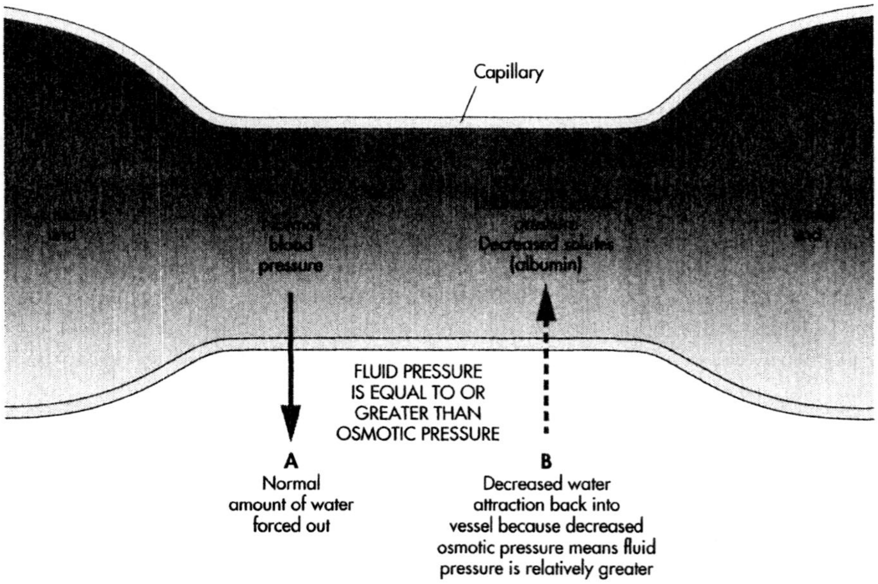

FLUID PRESSURE IS EQUAL TO OR GREATER THAN OSMOTIC PRESSURE

A
Normal amount of water forced out

B
Decreased water attraction back into vessel because decreased osmotic pressure means fluid pressure is relatively greater

Figure 3–13. Edema due to decreased osmotic pressure (blood pressure equal to or greater than osmotic pressure).

Table 3–6 outlines the causes of edema that you have just learned. Visible signs of edema include swelling or puffiness of extremities or other affected parts such as the eyelids. Pulmonary edema is not visible without an x-ray but respiratory signs are apparent. If edema is a result of fluid excess there will be weight gain. Generally the specific cause of this imbalance will produce its own signs and symptoms. The detrimental effects of edema include interference with passage of oxygen and nutrients through the fluid filled interstitial space to the cells, and elimination of wastes. The presence of edema also increases the pressure in the tissues, making it more difficult for normal capillary blood flow. Therefore ischemia may develop. As you learned in Chapter 1, ischemia is decreased _____(1) to an area. Life-threatening effects occur when edema is in the lungs, surrounding the larynx in the throat, and when brain cells are compressed by fluid inside the skull. Sequestering of fluid in third spaces, or effusions of a large nature, can produce functional dehydration. Interference in body function by edema is due to difficulty in the passage of _____(2) and _____(3) to the cells and _____(4) from them. Dehydration can result if large amounts of fluid are trapped in _____(5). The organs most severely affected by edema are the _____(6), _____(7), and _____(8).

3–54

1. blood supply
2. oxygen
3. nutrients
4. waste
5. third spaces
6. lungs
7. larynx
8. brain

The last fluid imbalance we will consider is **diabetes insipidus.** Unlike polydipsia and edema, which are *signs* of imbalance, this is a disease itself. Don't be confused by using the term "diabetes," which most people think of to mean high blood sugar. The word diabetes comes from the Greek and literally means "running through." In this case what is running through is fluids, or urine, from the body. In cases of high urine losses, this is a stimulant for polydipsia as people become thirsty and drink to replace lost water. This was seen by the Greek physicians as a lot of water in and a lot of water out. The word insipidus means "tasteless" to distinguish it from the sugar-laden or sweet-tasting urine of a diabetic. Earlier we mentioned that antidiuretic hormone (ADH) and the thirst mechanism were vital parts of normal water balance. If a diuretic is an agent that promotes urine production and water loss, then the term *anti*diuretic is an agent that *inhibits* water loss. That is precisely what ADH does. It closely governs the water content of urine, helping the kidneys to produce normally concentrated urine. What causes diabetes insipidus is lack of ADH, less than normal amounts of this hormone, or decreased response by diseased kidneys. Loss of control of water content of urine, or decreased concentrating ability, produces a dilute urine with high volume. Too much water is lost from the body. This increased urine production is called **polyuria.** Polyuria creates dehydration and an increase in plasma osmolarity that stimulates the hypothalamus and causes polydipsia. Diabetes literally means _____(1),

3–55

1. running through

TABLE 3–6. CAUSES OF EDEMA

Localized	Generalized
Obstructed drainage	Fluid excess
Veins	Kidney disease
Lymph vessels	Overhydration
Left-sided congestive heart failure	Abnormal distribution
Pulmonary edema	Increased resistance to flow—right-sided
	congestive heart failure
	Decreased osmotic pressure—hypoalbuminemia
	Decreased liver production
	Increased kidney or
	intestinal loss
	Increased capillary permeability
	Inflammation
	Shock
	Anoxia
	Anaphylaxis

2. polyuria
3. polydipsia
4. antidiuretic hormone
5. water

········ 3-56 ········

1. production
2. release
3. hypothalamic
4. posterior pituitary
5. Nephrogenic
6. kidneys
7. response
8. concentration
9. conservation
10. polyuria

1. dehydration

2. a–1. fluid intake less than output; b–2. fluid output greater than intake; c–2. fluid output greater than intake; d–2. fluid output greater than intake; e–1. fluid intake less than output; f–2. fluid output greater than intake; g–1. fluid intake less than output; h–2. fluid output greater than intake

3. true

4. c–dehydration

and this description comes from signs of increased urine production, called _____(2), and increased fluid consumption, called _____(3). Diabetes insipidus is a result of a deficiency of _____(4), which controls the amount of _____(5) lost through the urine.

Neurogenic diabetes insipidus implies that the reason for deficient ADH lies in the central nervous system. It is in the region or gland responsible for normal production and release. The hypothalamus produces ADH so damage or disease of this region could lead to low ADH levels. The posterior pituitary gland releases ADH from its storage place there so a defect in this process would produce the same results. **Nephrogenic** diabetes insipidus refers to difficulty in kidney function, since the nephron is the functional unit responsible for urine production. The particular difficulty is poor response by the kidney cells to normal amounts of ADH because the cells are damaged through some disease process. Hormones are like the chemical mediators of Chapter 2 because they send messages and tell cells what to do. In this case, the cells aren't getting the message. The message is to concentrate urine and conserve water so the result is polyuria because these actions don't occur. Neurogenic diabetes insipidus is a result of a disorder in either _____(1) or _____(2) of ADH. Decreased or lack of production is related to _____(3) disease while impaired release is the fault of the _____(4). _____(5) diabetes insipidus indicates that the problem lies with the _____(6). The specific disorder is lack of _____(7) to ADH by kidney cells. Therefore the message of urine _____(8) and water _____(9) is not received and the sign of this is _____(10).

III. REVIEW QUESTIONS

1. A deficiency in total body fluid is called _____.

2. Please match these categories of dehydration with their related conditions:
   1. fluid intake less than output
   2. fluid output greater than intake

   a. _____ restricted access to fluid
   b. _____ polyuria in kidney disease
   c. _____ diarrhea
   d. _____ osmotic diuresis
   e. _____ hypodipsia
   f. _____ diabetes insipidus
   g. _____ unconsciousness
   h. _____ excessive sweating

3. True or false: Third space sequestering of fluid can cause functional dehydration because the fluid is not available to the ECF and ICF for proper balance.

   _____

4. Reduced intravascular volume, and therefore reduced blood pressure, can produce hypovolemic shock. To avoid this, the body draws fluid from the interstitial spaces, making them hypertonic in relation to the ICF. This causes water to flow from the cells through osmosis. The cells shrink and the resulting crenation can be lethal to cell processes. This pathogenesis best describes the effects of:
   a. water intoxication
   b. circulatory overload
   c. dehydration
   d. edema

5. Sunken eyes, loss of body weight, little urine, and polydipsia are signs of:
   a. edema
   b. dehydration
   c. circulatory overload
   d. water intoxication

6. In cases of fluid excess, the imbalance that does NOT cause swelling of the cells is (choose all that apply):
   a. water excess
   b. isotonic increase in fluid
   c. water and sodium excess
   d. hypotonic increase in fluid

7. Heart failure and kidney disease can produce fluid excess because of decreased excretion. This is best described as (choose all that apply):
   a. water excess
   b. isotonic increase in fluid
   c. water and sodium excess
   d. hypotonic increase in fluid

8. The effects of fluid volume excess depend on whether it is water intoxication or isotonic (sodium and water) excess. Lethal effects of water intoxication affect the _____ and isotonic excess causes pulmonary edema, which is seen as _____.
   a. heart; respiratory distress
   b. brain; kidney failure
   c. lungs; weight increase
   d. brain; respiratory distress

9. Extreme thirst is called _____.

10. Dehydration, severe edema, vomiting, and diarrhea can cause the sign:
    a. polydipsia
    b. polyuria
    c. ascites
    d. effusion

11. Fluid collection in the tissues of the extremities that can be demonstrated by leaving an indentation after applying pressure is called _____.

12. Edema is too much fluid in the:
    a. vessels
    b. interstitium
    c. cells
    d. any of the above

5. b–dehydration

6. b–isotonic increase in fluid; c–water and sodium excess

7. b–isotonic increase in fluid; c–water and sodium excess

8. d–brain; respiratory distress

9. polydipsia

10. a–polydipsia

11. pitting edema

12. b–interstitium

13. a–sodium; b–resistance; c–hydrostatic; d–venous; e–filtration; f–osmotic; g–fluid

14. b–increased capillary permeability; c–hypoalbuminemia; e–decreased osmotic pressure

15. b–inflammatory kidney disease; e–specific intestinal disease; f–liver disease

16. 1. b–inflammatory kidney disease; 2. e–specific intestinal disease; 3. f–liver disease

17. d–edema

18. a–diabetes insipidus

19. a–antidiuretic hormone; b–concentrate; c–conserve

20. a–Neurogenic; b–Nephrogenic

13. Please complete these sentences using the terms listed below:
Causes of edema include retention of a. _____ by the kidneys and increased b. _____ to outflow from the veins. The kidney condition leads to increased c. _____ pressure and the venous drainage problem causes increased d. _____ pressure. Both lead to greater e. _____ force of fluid out of the vessels and blood pressure that may be greater than f. _____ pressure, which interferes with drawing g. _____ back into the vessels.

osmotic	potassium	venous	sodium
resistance	dilation	hydrostatic	cells
fluid	filtration	diuretic	gravitational

14. Other causes of edema include (choose all that apply):
a. hyperalbuminemia
b. increased capillary permeability
c. hypoalbuminemia
d. decreased capillary permeability
e. decreased osmotic pressure
f. increased osmotic pressure

15. Conditions that can produce hypoalbuminemia are (choose all that apply):
a. excessive sweating
b. inflammatory kidney disease
c. vomiting and diarrhea
d. diabetes insipidus
e. specific intestinal diseases
f. liver disease
g. dehydration

16. Look at the choice of answers in question 15. The two routes of loss of albumin are 1. _____ and 2._____. Decreased production is seen in 3. _____.

17. Interference in passage of substances through the tissues, ischemia, and respiratory distress are some of the effects of:
a. diabetes insipidus
b. dehydration
c. water intoxication
d. edema

18. Polyuria and polydipsia are signs of:
a. diabetes insipidus
b. dehydration
c. edema
d. circulatory overload

19. The hormone responsible for diabetes insipidus is a. _____. This hormone normally tells the kidneys to b. _____ urine and therefore c. _____ water.

20. a. _____ diabetes insipidus is impaired production or release of ADH.
b. _____ diabetes insipidus is little response to ADH by kidney cells.

IV. DISORDERS IN ELECTROLYTE BALANCE ◀ SECTION

▸ HYPONATREMIA

3-57

When we talk about electrolyte levels in blood, plasma, or serum it is understood to represent about the same concentration in the ECF. Remember the ECF is both intravascular and interstitial fluid but we do not measure interstitial fluid. It is these measured blood levels that affect body function. A blood level of sodium that is lower than normal is called **hyponatremia.** There are two primary reasons for developing hyponatremia. First is loss of sodium from the body and the second is water retention. Increased amounts of total body water causes a *relative* decrease in sodium even if total sodium is actually normal. This is a dilution of sodium by excess water. The result is still the same because tissues respond to blood levels for any electrolyte that we discuss. Also keep in mind the very close relationship between sodium and water balance. Upsets in sodium affects water balance as well. One cause of true sodium loss is a condition called Addison's disease, a deficiency in hormones from the adrenal cortex. One important hormone we already introduced is aldosterone. Write here the two main functions of aldosterone: a. retention of _____(1); b. excretion of _____(2). If aldosterone is decreased then the effect is loss of these functions. Therefore, in Addison's disease, _____(3) would be lost in abnormal amounts, along with water, and _____(4) would be kept in abnormal amounts. So this adrenal insufficiency leads to unregulated loss of total body sodium. Sodium level that is less than normal is called _____(5). Hyponatremia can be due to actual sodium loss or to _____(6) of normal sodium by excess water.

1. sodium
2. potassium
3. sodium
4. potassium
5. hyponatremia
6. dilution

Other causes of sodium depletion are heavy sweating, vomiting, and diarrhea. Both water and sodium are lost, so hyponatremia and dehydration can exist together. A dilutional hyponatremia can develop if fluid replacement is pure water, and not an electrolyte drink. It is more likely to occur in kidney dysfunction where water is retained or in cases of increased amounts of ADH. Increased amounts of ADH would cause retention of _____(1). Overzealous use of water enemas, low sodium IV infusions, and diuretics are iatrogenic causes of hyponatremia. Pure water replacement after excessive sweating, vomiting, and diarrhea can lead to hyponatremia because of _____(2) of sodium. Disease of the _____(3) or an increase in _____(4) may cause dilutional hyponatremia because of _____(5) retention.

1. water
2. dilution
3. kidney
4. antidiuretic hormone (ADH)
5. water

Less sodium in the ECF means that the fluid there is _____(1) tonic in relation to the ICF or inside the cells. Therefore, _____(2) will move into the cells according to the principle of _____(3). When sodium levels are low, muscles will cramp and become weak from cellular swelling. The brain and nervous system is most seriously and obviously affected by this. Swelling of the brain produces the neurologic signs of confusion. Convulsions and coma develop at very low levels. One of the many injurious effects of neuron swelling is the decreased ability to depolarize and repolarize normally, so nerve impulse transmission is seriously impaired. Dilutional hyponatremia is accompanied by the signs of water excess, such as increased weight and edema. The primary mechanism of injury in hyponatremia is hypotonicity of the _____(4) that causes water to move _____(5) the cells. The resulting _____(6) of the cells most seriously affects the _____(7) and _____(8). There is grave impairment of nerve impulse _____(9). Table 3–7 summarizes the causes of hyponatremia.

1. hypo
2. water
3. osmosis
4. ECF or extracellular fluid
5. into
6. swelling
7. brain
8. nervous system
9. transmission

TABLE 3–7. CAUSES OF HYPONATREMIA

True	Relative
Sodium Loss	Increased Body Water
Addison's disease	Water replacement following sodium loss
Decreased aldosterone	Water intoxication
Heavy sweating	Kidney disease—oliguric or anuric phases
Vomiting	Increased antidiuretic hormone
Diarrhea	Iatrogenic (fluid administration)
Iatrogenic (diuretic drugs)	

▶ HYPERNATREMIA

┉ 3–60 ┉

1. sodium
2. normal
3. retention
4. water
5. loss
6. water
7. sodium
8. water

Hypernatremia is sodium concentrations greater than normal in the blood. This can be due to a rise in the intake of sodium or a relative increase compared to water concentration. Decreased water intake or increased loss of water from the body (dehydration) leads to a relative increase in sodium because it is now more concentrated in less water. Any state of dehydration creates *relative hypernatremia*. The most common reason for hypernatremia is loss of both sodium and water, but water losses are greater so this is a relative increase in sodium. Conditions where this occurs are diabetes insipidus and watery diarrhea. *True hypernatremia* may develop in Cushing's disease. Cushing's disease is excessive hormones from the adrenal cortex. It is the opposite of Addison's disease. High levels of cortisol, a natural steroid, in Cushing's disease amplifies sodium retention. At the same time, increased aldosterone, also from the adrenal cortex, retains more sodium. Hypernatremia is a _____(1) level above _____(2). True hypernatremia results from excessive _____(3) of sodium because of increased cortisol and aldosterone. Relative hypernatremia results from decreased _____(4) intake or too much _____(5) of water from the body. Diabetes insipidus and diarrhea are examples of loss of both _____(6) and _____(7), but with more loss of _____(8). When you look at Table 3–8, which lists causes of hypernatremia, you may be confused by the fact that diarrhea is listed as a cause for both hyponatremia (see Table 3–7) and hypernatremia. Please realize, as with many pathophysiology concepts, there are more shades of gray than there are black and white. Sodium may be lost excessively during diarrhea, causing hyponatremia. However, if the water content is very high in the stool, water losses can exceed sodium loss and cause a relative hypernatremia.

TABLE 3–8. CAUSES OF HYPERNATREMIA

True	Relative
Excess Sodium	Decreased Body Water
Cushing's disease	Decreased intake of fluids
Increased aldosterone	Increased loss
Increased cortisol	Very watery diarrhea
Salt water ingestion	Diabetes insipidus
Iatrogenic (administration of	Decreased antidiuretic hormone
sodium-containing drugs)	or response to ADH
	Kidney disease—diuretic phase

The effects on the body of hypernatremia are related to changes in tonicity of the ECF. In this case the increased sodium would make the ECF _____(1) tonic compared to intracellular fluid. This would draw _____(2) out of the cells, causing intracellular dehydration. If the hypernatremia is caused by water loss, then the events of dehydration (decreased intravascular volume and blood pressure) come into play. Truly excessive sodium causes the same intracellular dehydration, but water content of the ECF, which was normal, now becomes overloaded from cellular fluid. Circulatory overload is a concern in predisposed patients. As in true dehydration, shrinking, or crenation of cells, most dramatically affects cells of the brain and central nervous system, leading to convulsions and coma. The effects of abnormal sodium levels on cells is shown to you in Figure 3–14. The result of hypernatremia is dehydration of _____(3) because _____(4) is pulled out of them. Depending on the cause of increased sodium, the extracellular fluid space will have _____(5) fluid than normal (dehydration) or will end up having _____(6) fluid than normal. Either way, the same effect is seen on cells of the _____(7) and _____(8), with visible signs being _____(9) and _____(10) if the condition is not corrected.

1. hyper
2. water
3. cells
4. water
5. less
6. more
7. brain
8. central nervous system
9. convulsions
10. coma

▶ HYPOKALEMIA

When the concentration of potassium in the circulation is less than normal, this is **hypokalemia.** It is important to realize that because of the shifting of potassium between the ECF and ICF in various conditions, the *plasma* level may not accurately reflect *total* body stores. So hypokalemia may mean decreased potassium in the body or it may mean uptake of potassium into the cells. But again, the ECF levels of electrolytes are what affect body function, so excessive sequestering of potassium in the ICF has the same result as true depletion. A small change in extracellular potassium, for whatever reason, can have serious consequences. Unfortunately, preservation of potassium is *not* one of the homeostatic mechanisms of the body that works very well. The kidneys do a poor job of conserving potassium even in situations of great need so urinary loss continues in spite of true deficits. Because of this hypokalemia can develop very quickly. However the signs of deficiency can be gradual in onset and may go undetected until quite late. This is because as the body continues to lose potassium and blood levels drop, more potassium shifts out of the cells to maintain normal levels. It is when intracellular amounts become so depleted that the extracellular amounts

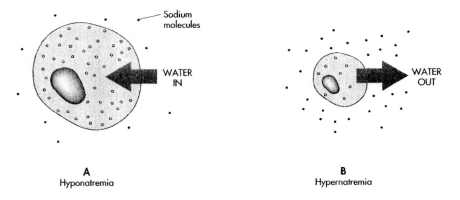

A
Hyponatremia

B
Hypernatremia

Figure 3–14. Effects of abnormal sodium levels on cells. **A.** Hyponatremia. Hypotonic ECF with swelling and rupture or lysis of cells. **B.** Hypernatremia. Hypertonic ECF with shrinking and crenation or dehydration.

1. potassium
2. cells or ICF
3. plasma or blood
4. poorly
5. late
6. potassium
7. cells or ICF
8. extracellular fluid or ECF

3–63

1. excrete or lose
2. intake
3. loss or excretion
4. vomiting
5. diarrhea
6. sodium
7. water
8. loss or excretion
9. aldosterone
10. hypokalemia
11. Alkalosis

can't be preserved that signs may be detected. Hypokalemia can be due to decreased total _____(1) in the body or it may mean that more potassium is entering the _____(2). Therefore _____(3) levels may not truly reflect body stores. Homeostatic conservation of potassium works _____(4) well / poorly (choose one) in time of increased loss. Signs of hypokalemia can be seen _____(5) early / late (choose one) in the course of this condition because of movement of _____(6) from the _____(7) to the _____(8) to keep blood levels normal.

Poor nutrition or decreased intake can cause hypokalemia but this is a greater problem in the elderly than most people. Limited income and imbalanced diet contribute to the problem. Excessive loss is the more common reason for hypokalemia. As with sodium, vomiting and diarrhea can deplete levels and this also stimulates aldosterone because of the sodium loss. Aldosterone works to _____(1) potassium from the body through the kidneys, so the intestinal loss is compounded. Other reasons for increased aldosterone production are sodium and water loss because of diuresis in kidney disease, and Cushing's disease, which produces too much aldosterone. Kidney disease that is in the **diuretic phase,** which is excessive production of urine, is a mechanism of true loss of potassium. Drugs that produce diuresis to treat other conditions, such as congestive heart failure, increase potassium losses through the urine. Diabetic acidosis causes an ICF to ECF shift in potassium. The acid ECF has too many H^+ ions so some of them move inside the cell and the K^+ ion moves out. This causes a temporary *hyperkalemia* until the kidneys rid the excess. But if the conditions remain the same, the result is depletion of total potassium stores. This is an example of normal plasma levels that because of shifting do not indicate an abnormality. When insulin is administered to treat the diabetes, hypokalemia will become evident because insulin draws potassium back into the cells. In addition to acidosis and insulin, alkalosis causes shifting of potassium, but it is *not* a true depletion of body stores. However, the result is ECF hypokalemia. When there are not enough H^+ ions in the ECF (alkalosis), H^+ inside the cell passes out into the ECF and K^+ moves inside to balance the charges. Decreased _____(2) of potassium can cause hypokalemia but more common is increased _____(3) from the body. This can take place from the stomach and intestines in the form of _____(4) and _____(5). Aldosterone can be stimulated by loss of _____(6) and _____(7) through the GI tract or by kidney disease. Aldosterone causes _____(8) of potassium. Cushing's disease results in too much _____(9) and other hormones so this is another stimulus for loss of potassium. Acidosis causes true _____(10) because potassium that should be inside cells is being excreted. _____(11) causes a relative hypokalemia because potassium that should be outside cells has shifted inside.

3–64

Hypokalemia affects kidney function and the GI tract but we will focus on muscle and nerve function as the major consequences. You know from physiology that nerve impulses and muscle contraction depend on electrical activity of cell membranes. The **resting membrane potential** or RMP is the state of normal negative electrical fields that lead to proper response by the cells. In hypokalemia, the RMP becomes more negative because of fewer positive K^+ ions. At low levels, there is decreased response at the neuromuscular junctions so that greater stimulation is required to generate normal contractions. Figure 3–15 compares the normal RMP and action potential (AP) to several electrolyte imbalances. Take a moment to see the effect of hypokalemia. Hypokalemia also interferes with glycogen metabolism and other cell activities. Muscles cramp, become weak, and paralysis is possible. If this happens to the diaphragm, respiratory arrest can occur and the patient stops breathing. If hypokalemia is not severe but is chronic or present for a long time, muscle atrophy may develop. This interference with electrical activity and metabolism also affects the heart. An **electrocardiogram** or ECG will show abnormal tracings of heart activity. These abnormal electrical impulses, and therefore abnormal contractions in response, make up the condition of cardiac **arrhythmia.** Arrhythmia is loss of the coordination between different parts of the heart that is necessary for effective contractions. Severe arrhythmias prevent the heart from pumping blood nor-

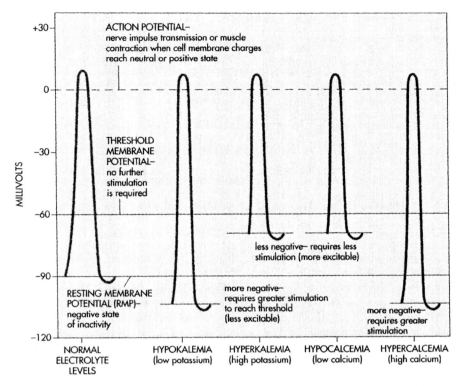

Figure 3–15. Effects of abnormal potassium and calcium levels on the resting membrane potential of excitable tissue (nerve and muscle).

mally. One example is a **fibrillation.** Instead of a squeezing contraction that pumps blood, the heart quivers and is completely ineffective in forcing blood out to the rest of the body. This severely compromised cardiac output produces hypovolemic shock and death. Since nerve function is impaired, hypokalemia also causes depression of the brain and nervous system. Hypokalemia adversely affects the _____(1) of cell membranes, causing abnormal nerve _____(2) and muscle _____(3). Because of the increased negativity of the RMP, more _____(4) is required to generate normal _____(5). If muscles become paralyzed and this affects the diaphragm, the patient will experience _____(6). The effect of hypokalemia on the heart is abnormal _____(7) impulses and abnormal _____(8). This loss of coordinated and effective contractions is called _____(9). A fatal consequence of one type of severe arrhythmia is loss of output from the heart and this can happen during _____(10). Hypokalemia also impairs the _____(11) and _____(12) function. Table 3–9 summarizes the causes of hypokalemia.

1. resting membrane potential or RMP
2. impulses
3. contractions
4. stimulation
5. contractions or response
6. respiratory arrest
7. electrical
8. contractions
9. arrhythmia
10. fibrillation
11. brain
12. nervous system

▶ HYPERKALEMIA

Plasma potassium values greater than normal define **hyperkalemia.** Generally, homeostatic mechanisms of renal loss of potassium and ICF shifting or uptake of potassium by cells work very well in preventing hyperkalemia. The only time this would not be true is if intake exceeds the body's ability to handle the extra load. This is unusual except in people with kidney disease who have extra potassium in their diet. For example, salt substitutes use potassium instead of sodium. The most common cause of high potassium is kidney failure. Remember kidneys normally save _____(1) and get rid of _____(2). So when there is failure of these normal functions, potassium would naturally become elevated. This especially occurs during **oliguria,** which is greatly

1. sodium
2. potassium

TABLE 3–9. CAUSES OF HYPOKALEMIA

True	Relative
Potassium Loss or Deficiency	*Cellular Uptake*
Inadequate diet	Insulin treatment following acidosis
Vomiting	Alkalosis
Diarrhea	
Increased aldosterone	
Stimulated by sodium loss	
Diarrhea	
Kidney disease—diuretic phase	
Cushing's disease	
Diuretic drugs	

3. aldosterone
4. potassium
5. homeostatic
6. kidney failure
7. oliguria
8. aldosterone
9. response

decreased urine formation and output. The hormone you have learned about that regulates this sodium retention and potassium loss of the kidneys is _____(3). In Addison's disease, a deficiency of aldosterone, the result is loss of more sodium and retention of more potassium so this is another mechanism of hyperkalemia. Hyperkalemia is an elevated level of _____(4) in the blood or plasma. Normally _____(5) mechanisms prevent hyperkalemia. The most common cause of this electrolyte imbalance is _____(6). The type of urine production where this is most likely to happen is during _____(7). Deficiency of the hormone _____(8) also leads to hyperkalemia, as does decreased _____(9) to this hormone by the kidneys.

3-66

1. inside
2. distribution
3. potassium
4. acidosis
5. electrical neutrality

•

Another reason for development of hyperkalemia is *not a true increase* in total body amounts, but a *change in distribution* of potassium. Remember potassium is one of those simple compounds that can pass through cell membranes. Several conditions cause shifting of potassium out of cells. The majority of potassium in the body is found _____(1) the cells and the ECF contains very little. Just a small amount of shifting from cells causes relatively large changes in ECF potassium and noticeable effects on the body. Shifting is caused by acidosis, in which excessive H^+ ions want to move inside the cells to raise the ECF pH. To maintain electrical neutrality, K^+ moves out into the ECF. Also, in **diabetic ketoacidosis,** which you will learn about in Chapter 8, in addition to the acid environment there is decreased insulin. Insulin promotes movement of potassium into cells so there is a lack in this mechanism to lower ECF potassium. Shifting of potassium, or a change in _____(2), produces hyperkalemia that is not due to increase in total body amounts. The abnormal ECF pH which draws _____(3) out of cells is _____(4). This is a balancing act with positive ions that helps maintain _____(5).

3-67

1. neuromuscular
2. muscles
3. heart
4. bradycardia
5. arrest

Hyperkalemia causes changes in neuromuscular function, as in hypokalemia, but the RMP in this case is less negative and therefore closer to the AP state. This causes increased responsiveness to nerve impulses or overexcitability. Refer again to Figure 3–15. Besides general gastrointestinal (GI) discomfort, such as nausea and diarrhea, skeletal muscles cramp, become weak and may be paralyzed. The most significant consequence of high potassium is its action on the heart. Cardiac muscle is also abnormally responsive to nerve impulses and the heart rate slows alarmingly. This is because the electrical impulses are so abnormal it is impossible to produce a normal rate of contraction. A slow heart rate is called **bradycardia.** If not treated, bradycardia leads to cardiac arrest. The common result of hypo- and hyperkalemia is a change in _____(1) function. Skeletal _____(2) do not function normally and the most serious repercussion is abnormal function of the _____(3). In this case, the heart slows down and this is known as _____(4). If hyperkalemia continues, it will lead to cardiac _____(5). Table 3–10 summarizes the causes of hyperkalemia.

TABLE 3–10. CAUSES OF HYPERKALEMIA

True	Relative
Excess Potassium	*Cellular Release or Decreased Uptake*
Potassium-rich diet in patient with renal dysfunction	Trauma or injury to potassium-rich tissue such as muscle
Kidney failure—oliguric or anuric phases	Acidosis
Addison's disease Decreased aldosterone	Insulin deficiency
Iatrogenic (potassium administration)	

▶ HYPOCALCEMIA

Hypocalcemia is less than the normal amount of calcium in the blood. Refer back to Frame 3–21 on the different circulating forms of total body calcium. The form that is active, or affects body function, is the _____(1) form. Because of this, total calcium measurements may not accurately reflect what is available for action. Calcium, which is bound to proteins such as albumin and other substances, is not the ionized or active form. Therefore changes in concentrations of these binding substances change the amount of ionized calcium. Therefore hypocalcemia may be relative instead of a true decrease. Causes of relative hypocalcemia include increased binding with extra protein in the system. Alkalosis causes increased binding of calcium to normal amounts of protein. In a disease called acute pancreatitis, the fat-digesting enzyme **lipase** frees fatty acids from tissues and the fatty acids promote calcium binding to those acids.

Serum levels of phosphate and calcium are inverse, or the opposite of each other, in states of imbalance. Therefore in kidney disease, where there is retention of phosphate, more calcium will be lost in the urine to maintain this relationship. This is true hypocalcemia because this ion is lost from the body instead of experiencing a change in form. Other conditions leading to true hypocalcemia are **hypoparathyroidism** and decreased gastrointestinal absorption. Parathyroid hormone (PTH) is a major calcium regulator whose function is to maintain normal levels by providing calcium to the circulation from bone stores. In hypoparathyroidism, it follows that this calcium mobilization, or release from the bones, is decreased. While calcium is not actually lost from the body, it is sequestered in bones as an unavailable substance. The parathyroid glands, located with the thyroids in the neck, may not be functioning properly and not releasing PTH. Or the glands may be damaged or removed during removal of the thyroid gland or other surgeries involving the neck. Decreased GI absorption of calcium is usually related to problems with vitamin D. Vitamin D is required to absorb calcium. Dietary insufficiency may exist, or there may be a state of malabsorption affecting not only vitamin D and calcium but other nutrients as well. In addition, vitamin D must go through several stages in both the liver and kidney to become activated and facilitate calcium absorption. Therefore, disease of either of these organs could lead to inadequate amounts of this vitamin and subsequent hypocalcemia. Increases in substances that bind to calcium can produce a relative _____(1) because there is a decrease in the _____(2) form of this electrolyte. Kidney disease can produce hypocalcemia two ways. First, when _____(3) is retained in abnormal amounts, _____(4) is lost to keep the levels of these two ions inverse. Second, the kidney is necessary to activate _____(5), which is required to absorb _____(6) in the gut. Release of calcium from the _____(7) requires the hormone _____(8). Therefore deficiency of this hormone, or _____(9), can cause hypocalcemia. Liver disease, malabsorption, and poor nutrition can lead to deficiency of vitamin _____(10) and therefore to the electrolyte deficiency _____(11).

3–68

1. ionized

3–69

1. hypocalcemia
2. ionized or active
3. phosphate
4. calcium
5. vitamin D
6. calcium
7. bones
8. parathyroid hormone
9. hypoparathyroidism
10. D
11. hypocalcemia

3-70

1. nerve
2. increase
3. muscles
4. tetany
5. larynx
6. diaphragm
7. heart

Calcium is essential to normal electrical activity involving nerve impulses. Low calcium leads to an increase in nerve excitability (see Fig. 3–15). If the nerves are overactive and spastically sending impulses, the muscles will try to respond by contracting according to the orders received from the nervous system. Clinically, this is seen as **tetany,** a state of paralysis that is rigid or stiff, not limp. This is because the muscles contract so fast and hard without rest that they produce spasms and do not move normally or voluntarily. The danger to the patient is spasm of the laryngeal muscles in the throat that would cut off air supply or spasm of the diaphragm causing respiratory arrest. The heart muscle is also abnormal in its contractions, producing arrhythmias and perhaps insufficient cardiac output. Hypocalcemia of a severe nature leads to seizures and death. The primary adverse effect of hypocalcemia involves _____(1) function. There is an _____(2) in nerve excitability. Because of this, the secondary effect is on the _____(3), which respond to this excessive stimulation. The rigidity and inability to move is described as _____(4). Spasms of the muscles of the _____(5) or _____(6) can result in death. Seizures are not uncommon and arrhythmias of the _____(7) are also a concern. Table 3–11 summarizes the causes of hypocalcemia.

▶ HYPERCALCEMIA

3-71

1. hypercalcemia

You should know that a calcium level greater than normal in the blood is called _____(1). The causes of this excess are opposite of some of the causes of hypocalcemia. The most common reason for *true hypercalcemia* is an increase in the resorption of calcium from the bone. This can be due to too much PTH, as in **hyperparathyroidism.** Tumors of the parathyroid gland can release too much PTH. Immobility of bone, such as during multiple fracture healing, causes atrophy of bone as it does other tissues like muscle. This atrophy contributes to increased dissolving of bone. A common reason for destruction of bone and calcium release is **neoplasia,** or cancer. **Primary bone cancer,** or cancer of the bone itself, can produce this. Also any cancer that originated elsewhere that spread to the bone causes the same destruction. This spread, or **metastasis,** is **secondary bone cancer.** An interesting phenomenon is that some tumors produce a compound that acts like PTH, therefore increasing calcium release. The finding of hypercalcemia on a blood test may suggest to the physician the need to look for cancer if there are no other reasons for the increased calcium. *Relative hypercalcemia* is an increase in the ionized form of calcium. This occurs in hypoalbuminemia because there is less protein to bind free calcium. Another relative increase is in acidosis, which decreases the binding of free calcium to normal amounts of protein. The most common reason for true hypercalcemia is an

TABLE 3–11. CAUSES OF HYPOCALCEMIA

True	Relative
Decreased Total Calcium	*Decreased Ionized Form*
Increased phosphate retention Kidney disease	Increased binding to increased proteins

Hypoparathyroidism
   Decreased parathyroid hormone
	Increased binding to normal protein
	   Alkalosis

Decreased GI absorption
   Decreased vitamin D
     Dietary insufficiency
     Kidney disease
     Liver disease
	Increased binding to fatty acids
	   Pancreatitis

_____(2) in resorption of calcium from bone stores. Hyperparathyroidism causes hypercalcemia because there is too much _____(3) in the circulation. The function of this hormone is to release _____(4) from the _____(5). Bone destruction due to _____(6) may cause hypercalcemia. This can originate in the bone, or be _____(7) cancer, or spread there and be _____(8) cancer. Relative hypercalcemia can occur if there is less _____(9) to bind calcium, which leads to an increase in the _____(10) form. The decreased protein is usually because of a state called hypo_____(11). Acidosis can also interfere with the binding of calcium to _____(12), causing relative hypercalcemia.

2. increase
3. PTH
4. calcium
5. bones
6. neoplasia or cancer
7. primary
8. secondary
9. protein
10. ionized
11. albuminemia
12. proteins

3–72

Hypercalcemia depresses neuromuscular activity, making the membranes less excitable or responsive (see Fig. 3–15). Muscles become weak and there may be cardiac arrhythmias. Severe hypercalcemia causes cardiac arrest. Effects on the nervous system include stupor and coma. It is interesting to note that hypercalcemia also produces behavioral or mental changes in the form of an **acute psychosis.** Since calcium gives bone its strength, too much loss will weaken bones and make them susceptible to **pathologic fractures.** This means bones break not because of trauma, but because disease has weakened them. Pathologic fractures are generally painful, hairline breaks that happen during the course of normal activity. This is another indication of the possibility of a cancerous process in the bone. **Calculi,** or stones made of calcium, can precipitate in the kidneys causing damage to that tissue. Severe hypercalcemia leads to **hypercalcemic crisis.** The prognosis is poor because of cardiac arrest. The effect of hypercalcemia on neuromuscular function is to _____(1) it. The most serious loss of response is cardiac _____(2). Nervous system depression may make the patient slip into a _____(3) or show signs of acute _____(4). Breaks in bone during normal use are _____(5) fractures because _____(6) has weakened them. In this case, the disease is excessive resorption of _____(7) from the bones. A hypercalcemic crisis has a _____(8) prognosis because of _____(9). Table 3–12 summarizes the causes of hypercalcemia.

1. depress
2. arrest
3. coma
4. psychosis
5. pathologic
6. disease
7. calcium
8. poor
9. cardiac arrest

3–73

If you are confused about some imbalances of homeostasis at this point, do not be discouraged. Traditionally the subjects of fluid, electrolyte, and acid–base imbalances have been challenging. If you pay close attention to the following, and understand this information, you should have a good grasp of the concepts:

1. Figures and tables that visually present fluid, electrolyte, and acid–base balance and imbalances.
2. The review questions.
3. The chapter summary.

TABLE 3–12. CAUSES OF HYPERCALCEMIA

True	Relative
Increased Total Calcium	*Increased Ionized Form*

Hyperparathyroidism
  Increased parathyroid hormone
	Decreased binding to decreased protein
	  Hypoalbuminemia

Bone atrophy	Decreased binding to normal protein Acidosis
Bone cancer—primary	
Bone cancer—secondary or metastatic	
Milk–alkali syndrome	

IV. REVIEW QUESTIONS

1. c–loss of water from the body produces hyponatremia

2. a–2. relative hyponatremia; b–1. true hyponatremia; c–2. relative hyponatremia; d–1. true hyponatremia

3. a–the ECF is hypotonic and causes water movement into the cells

4. d–cellular swelling

5. b–hypernatremia only develops because of excessive salt intake

6. c–the ECF is hypertonic and draws water out of the cells

7. c–crenation; central nervous system

8. a–potassium can move between the ICF and ECF in response to varying conditions

1. Please select the INCORRECT statement:
   a. Effects on the body by electrolytes depend on the blood concentrations rather than on total levels of the electrolyte
   b. Loss of sodium from the body produces hyponatremia
   c. Loss of water from the body produces hyponatremia
   d. Serum sodium concentration affects water balance

2. Please match these causes of hyponatremia according to true loss or relative decrease:
   1. true hyponatremia
   2. relative hyponatremia
   a. _____ increased antidiuretic hormone
   b. _____ vomiting or diarrhea
   c. _____ water replacement following sodium loss
   d. _____ Addison's disease (decreased aldosterone)

3. Hyponatremia causes swelling of cells because:
   a. the ECF is hypotonic and causes water movement into the cells
   b. the ICF is hypotonic and causes water movement into the cells
   c. the ECF is hypertonic and causes sodium movement into the cells
   d. the ICF is hypertonic and causes sodium movement into the cells

4. Impaired nerve transmission and neurologic signs in hyponatremia are primarily due to:
   a. changes in RMP or electrical activity of cell membranes
   b. cellular dehydration
   c. increased cell membrane permeability
   d. cellular swelling

5. Please choose the INCORRECT statement:
   a. Thirst develops in hypernatremia to lower sodium concentration and maintain homeostasis
   b. Hypernatremia only develops because of excessive salt intake
   c. Increased aldosterone and cortisol in Cushing's disease causes sodium retention and hypernatremia
   d. Water losses greater than sodium losses produces hypernatremia

6. Hypernatremia causes cellular dehydration because:
   a. the ECF is hypotonic and draws water out of cells
   b. the ICF is hypotonic and draws sodium into cells
   c. the ECF is hypertonic and draws water out of cells
   d. the ICF is hypertonic and draws sodium into cells

7. Cellular dehydration causes _____ of cells and most obviously affects cells of the _____.
   a. lysis; heart
   b. crenation; kidney;
   c. crenation; central nervous system
   d. lysis; central nervous system

8. Total body stores of potassium may not be represented accurately by serum levels because:
   a. potassium can move between the ICF and ECF in response to varying conditions
   b. potassium can be sequestered as a third space loss in effusions
   c. potassium can move between the vascular fluid and interstitial fluid in response to varying conditions
   d. potassium is conserved by the kidneys and stored in kidney cell ICF in times of need

9. One aspect of homeostasis that works poorly is preserving levels of:
   a. water
   b. sodium
   c. calcium
   d. potassium

10. The most common reason for hypokalemia is:
    a. shifting among fluid compartments
    b. increased loss
    c. decreased aldosterone
    d. decreased intake

11. Signs of hypokalemia become noticeable when:
    a. potassium is first lost excessively in the urine
    b. so much ECF potassium has shifted into cells the ECF becomes depleted
    c. potassium is first lost excessively through the GI tract
    d. so much ICF potassium has shifted out of the cells the ICF becomes depleted

12. Please complete these statements using the terms listed below: Decreased ECF potassium may be caused by loss through the urine due to increases in the hormone a. _____. One disease of the adrenal glands that causes this increased hormone is b. _____. The c. _____ phase of kidney disease loses too much potassium. Both the acid–base imbalances called d. _____ and e. _____ cause f. _____ of potassium in and out of cells to produce ECF hypokalemia. Another hormone used to treat diabetes also causes potassium shifting into cells and this is g. _____.

acidosis	nutrition	diuretic	aldosterone
alkalosis	oliguria	ADH	cortisol
movement	insulin	Cushing's	Addison's

13. Please mark these results of hypokalemia as true or false:
    a. _____ Decrease in cell membrane permeability causes changes in RMP
    b. _____ A more negative RMP causes decreased response to normal stimuli that produces muscle contractions
    c. _____ Hypokalemia causes cardiac arrhythmias, which is a heart rate that is too fast
    d. _____ Death can occur from decreased cardiac output and shock as a result of cardiac fibrillation

14. The most common reason for hyperkalemia is:
    a. diuretic phase of kidney disease
    b. kidney failure
    c. excessive aldosterone
    d. decreased aldosterone

15. A change in potassium distribution that causes ECF hyperkalemia can be caused by (choose all that apply):
    a. acidosis
    b. alkalosis
    c. increased insulin
    d. decreased insulin

16. The most significant result of hyperkalemia is:
    a. bradycardia and cardiac arrest
    b. arrhythmia and fibrillation
    c. bradycardia and arrhythmia
    d. fibrillation and cardiac arrest

9. d–potassium

10. b–increased loss

11. d–so much ICF potassium has shifted out of cells the ICF becomes depleted

12. a–aldosterone; b–Cushing's; c–diuretic; d–acidosis; e–alkalosis; f–movement; g–insulin

13. a–false; b–true; c–false; d–true

14. b–kidney failure

15. a–acidosis; d–decreased insulin

16. a–bradycardia and cardiac arrest

17. true

18. c–decreased protein binding; d–hypoalbuminemia

19. b–decreased PTH

20. d–any of the above

21. false

22. d–an increase in nerve excitability leads to increased impulses to the muscles and a rigid paralysis

23. a–increased calcium release from the bone

24. d–cancer

25. a–pathologic fractures; c–cardiac arrest; f–mental disturbances; g–hypovolemic shock

17. True or false: Total calcium levels may not accurately represent calcium activity because there may be abnormalities only in the ionized form of calcium.

_____

18. Causes of *normal total* calcium but *increased active* calcium include (choose all that apply):
    a. increased protein binding
    b. hyperalbuminemia
    c. decreased protein binding
    d. hypoalbuminemia

19. The mechanism of hypocalcemia in hypoparathyroidism is:
    a. increased GI absorption
    b. decreased PTH
    c. decreased GI absorption
    d. increased PTH

20. Hypocalcemia can result from:
    a. disease of the liver or kidney
    b. malabsorption
    c. decreased vitamin D
    d. any of the above
    e. none of the above

21. True or false: Hypocalcemia primarily affects muscle function so that muscles do not respond properly to normal nerve impulses. _____

22. Tetany develops in hypocalcemia because:
    a. there is interference in ATP production and muscles become paralyzed from lack of energy
    b. a decrease in nerve excitability leads to decreased impulses to the muscles and a limp paralysis
    c. laryngeal spasm cuts off oxygen supply to the muscles and they become paralyzed
    d. an increase in nerve excitability leads to increased impulses to the muscles and a rigid paralysis

23. Hypercalcemia is most often a result of:
    a. increased calcium release from the bone
    b. increased GI absorption of calcium
    c. increased calcium deposits into the bone
    d. decreased calcium loss through the urine

24. A hidden cause of hypercalcemia can be:
    a. renal failure
    b. hyperparathyroidism
    c. bone atrophy
    d. cancer

25. The effects of hypercalcemia include (choose all that apply):
    a. pathologic fractures   e. tetany
    b. cellular swelling   f. mental disturbances
    c. cardiac arrest   g. hypovolemic shock
    d. bradycardia   h. cellular dehydration

V. DISORDERS IN ACID–BASE BALANCE ◀ SECTION

▶ METABOLIC AND RESPIRATORY ORIGIN OF ACID–BASE IMBALANCE

.... 3–74 ......

Acid–base imbalances are classified as either **metabolic** or **respiratory,** and either **acidosis** or **alkalosis.** Acidosis is defined as a decrease in pH due to an increase in H^+ ions, or a decrease in the bicarbonate base. Alkalosis is the opposite or increased pH (which is a deficiency of H^+ ions) or an excess of base. Metabolic origin of imbalance means that the primary problem is with amounts of bicarbonate of HCO_3^-. From the review in Section I, you should know that an increase in bicarbonate, or the base, causes the pH to be _____(1) than normal. This produces the clinical condition of metabolic acidosis / alkalosis (choose one) _____(2). When there is a deficiency of bicarbonate, the pH will be _____(3) than normal, and the condition is called metabolic acidosis / alkalosis (choose one) _____(4). The respiratory origin of imbalance means that the primary problem is with amounts of carbon dioxide. It is related to pulmonary, or lung function, and is usually due to a change in the rate of ventilation. Remember that the lungs rid the body of CO_2. Carbon dioxide (CO_2) is the acid component since it combines with water to form carbonic acid (H_2CO_3). So when there is a change in the amount of CO_2 in the body there is a change in the amount of H_2CO_3 or acid. (Even though CO_2 is generated through metabolism, the term respiratory helps to classify the imbalance and distinguish it from abnormal base levels.) Since acid and base balances to produce normal pH, too much base results in the same conditions as not enough acid. Conversely, not enough base is like too much acid. Table 3–13 shows the relationships of base to acid as a function of metabolism and respiration.

1. greater or higher
2. alkalosis
3. less or lower
4. acidosis

.... 3–75 ......

Decreased ventilation, or breathing, would allow a buildup of _____(1), or the acid component. The pH would then be _____(2) than normal and the clinical condition is called _____(3). Increased rate of ventilation causes excessive loss of _____(4), or the _____(5) component. The pH would then be _____(6) than normal and the clinical condition is called _____(7).

1. CO_2
2. lower or less
3. respiratory acidosis
4. CO_2
5. acid
6. higher or greater
7. respiratory alkalosis

.... 3–76 ......

Frame 3–24 explained that the normal pH depended on a ratio of base to acid as calculated by the _____(1) equation. While strict definitions of imbalance are related to changes in H^+ ion concentration, it is important to remember that an upset in the *ratio* of 20 to 1 produces an abnormal pH. Homeostasis takes advantage of this relationship because while the primary upset may still exist (changes in H^+ concentration), the pH can be normalized if this ratio can be adjusted accordingly. Regardless of actual amounts of base and acid, 20 times more base than acid normalizes pH. We will come back to this when we study the concept of compensation. The pH approaches normal when the ratio of _____(2) is maintained and there is 20 times more _____(3) compared to amounts of _____(4).

1. Henderson–Hasselbalch
2. 20 to 1
3. base
4. acid

TABLE 3–13. pH AS A FUNCTION OF METABOLISM AND RESPIRATION

$$pH = \frac{\text{Base—bicarbonate } (HCO_3^-)}{\text{Acid—carbonic acid or carbon dioxide } (H_2CO_3 \text{ or } CO_2)}$$

$$pH = \frac{\text{Metabolic function}}{\text{Respiratory function}}$$

$$pH = \frac{\text{Renal control}}{\text{Pulmonary control}}$$

► CORRECTION AND COMPENSATION

Correction of acid–base imbalance is a straightforward process. The abnormal component of the ratio equation is returned to normal. The actual values of the buffer pair measure as normal. Excessive acid or H^+ ions are consumed by buffers or lost from the body. Excessive base is secreted in greater amounts into the urine. Correction is the mechanism of choice if it is possible. It may not always be possible because of underlying disease. Also, there may be other factors, such as time, that call for another mechanism of normalizing pH. (Remember, it is *pH* that affects body function, not absolute amounts of base and acid.) When correction cannot occur right away, compensation is the interim, or temporary measure, for survival. Think of the term "compensation" as meaning "making up for." In this case, it is making up for the acid–base imbalance. The true definition of **compensation** is reacting to abnormal conditions to *maintain a normal pH without* correcting or repairing the abnormality. How is this done if the abnormality still exists? By changing the other component of the ratio formula. Table 3–14 demonstrates this principle. As long as the ratio is normal, regardless of actual amounts of the buffer pair, the pH will approach normal. If the abnormal acid or base concentration can directly be returned to normal, this describes the process of _____(1). Changes in the acid–base _____(2) formula occur in the process of _____(3) and the effect is to maintain the normal _____(4).

The two organs primarily involved in correction and compensation are the kidneys and lungs. The kidneys can retain more or secrete more H^+ and HCO_3^- as needed. The lungs, through changes in ventilation, can lose more or keep more CO_2. In disease of either of these two organs, only the opposite organ can compensate for imbalances. In lung disease, the kidneys compensate by H^+ loss or retention. In kidney disease, the lungs compensate through CO_2 loss or retention. In states of disease and compensation, it important to note that while homeostasis works diligently to maintain pH, it may not quite reach the state of healthy balance. Also, some conditions can only be compensated for a limited time before mechanisms fail. However, compensation is a vital stop gap to ensure immediate survival. The timing and effectiveness between these two organs are different in that the lungs respond rapidly, are only a temporary measure, and are less effective because the pH is only improved towards normal. While the kidneys are relatively slow to respond, they continue in compensation efforts. Changes in urine components are much easier to maintain than an abnormal breathing pattern. The kidneys are also more effective because they may be able to return pH to normal, if other conditions allow. The two organs responsible for correction and _____(1) of acid–base imbalances are the _____(2) and _____(3). The kidneys process _____(4) and _____(5) while the lungs are responsible for handling _____(6) levels. A quick, short-lived response is a typical reaction of the _____(7). Delayed, but long-term and effective measures are performed by the _____(8).

TABLE 3–14. A COMPARISON BETWEEN CORRECTION AND COMPENSATION

	pCO$_2$ Levels	HCO$_3^-$ Levels	pH
Respiratory malfunction (hypoventilation)	↑	Normal	↓
Correction (hyperventilation)	↓ to normal	Normal	Normal
Compensation (renal retention of HCO$_3^-$)	↑	↑	Normal

▶ METABOLIC ACIDOSIS

Metabolic acidosis is a deficiency in the base, or bicarbonate, of the buffer pair. It can be a true deficit, or a relative decrease because of increased acid in the body. Metabolic acidosis is the most common of the acid–base imbalances. There are three major mechanisms that lead to metabolic acidosis. The first is an increase in acid production and the second is retention of acid by the kidneys. These represent a relative decrease in bicarbonate, simply because there is more acid present than normal. The third is a true deficiency of base that occurs when too much bicarbonate is lost through the urine. Look at Table 3–15, which compares the true and relative defects in the four acid–base imbalances. Refer to this table for each of the imbalances. In metabolic acidosis the primary abnormality is too little _____(1) in the body compared to amounts of _____(2). This can be an actual decrease or a _____(3) decrease depending on which mechanism is responsible. The most common acid–base imbalance is _____(4). Acid levels may be increased if there is too much _____(5) of acid, or if there is too much _____(6) by the kidneys. True base deficiency occurs when too much _____(7) is lost by the kidneys.

3-79

1. bicarbonate or base
2. acid
3. relative
4. metabolic acidosis
5. production
6. retention
7. bicarbonate

Acid production is increased during times of increased lactic acid formation. Lactate, or lactic acid, is part of normal metabolism but when amounts of oxygen are sufficient, **aerobic metabolism** does not lead to excessive lactic acid. When oxygen is insufficient **anaerobic metabolism** is the alternate pathway and leads to more lactate production. Any state of hypoxia, which means decreased _____(1) to the tissues, can cause increased lactic acid levels. Poor perfusion of the tissues by blood and the resulting hypoxia develop during shock, insufficient cardiac output, or cardiac arrest. Since the liver is also poorly perfused, this worsens the problem because the liver is responsible for clearing lactic acid from the circulation. Metabolic acidosis that develops due to this reason has a high mortality rate because the underlying cause is very serious. Increased formation of lactic acid causes metabolic _____(2). This occurs during times of _____(3), or decreased oxygen to the _____(4). The alternate state of metabolism during hypoxia is _____(5) and an end product is _____(6).

3-80

1. oxygen
2. acidosis
3. hypoxia
4. tissues
5. anaerobic metabolism
6. lactic acid or lactate

Ketoacidosis is another condition of elevated levels of acidic compounds. Fat in our body can be used as a fuel source when carbohydrate stores are low. Fat is broken down to fatty acids that enter the Krebs's cycle to produce energy. The liver turns some of these fatty acids into compounds called **ketones.** Ketones are acid compounds by nature. Starvation is one way ketoacidosis can develop. Carbohydrates are not available so the body increases fat breakdown and the result is higher levels of ketones. A more common reason for ketoacidosis is uncontrolled diabetes mellitus. In diabetes, insulin is insufficient. Insulin is required for the cells to use carbohydrates because this hormone activates the transport of carbohydrates across the cell membrane to the inside for use. It doesn't matter what the blood levels of

3-81

TABLE 3–15. DEFECTS IN ACID-BASE BALANCE

	True	Relative
Metabolic acidosis	Decreased bicarbonate through loss (HCO_3^- deficit)	Decreased bicarbonate through buffering or consumption (acid excess)
Metabolic alkalosis	Increased bicarbonate (HCO_3^- excess)	Increased bicarbonate through decreased buffering (acid deficit)
Respiratory acidosis	Increased carbonic acid (H_2CO_3 or CO_2 excess)	
Respiratory alkalosis	Decreased carbonic acid (H_2CO_3 or CO_2 deficit)	

1. fat
2. carbohydrates
3. starvation
4. diabetes
5. insulin
6. ketones

carbohydrates are; in fact, blood glucose is very elevated in uncontrolled diabetes. The end result is that the cells begin to starve because glucose cannot enter so the body reacts to this "starvation" through fat breakdown. Therefore ketone formation is abnormally high. The main mechanism of increased acidic ketone formation is increased _____(1) breakdown that occurs when enough _____(2) are not available. This can be a true lack of carbohydrates such as in _____(3) or it may be associated with the disease _____(4). In this disease, there is not enough _____(5) so cells do not receive necessary amounts of glucose. The body begins to break down more fat in this case so there are more _____(6) produced.

----- 3-82 -----

1. kidneys
2. metabolic
3. hydrogen

In kidney disease, "uremic acidosis" or "retention acidosis" develops through decreased elimination of acid from the body. The kidneys normally retain bicarbonate and eliminate H^+ ions. More H^+ is retained by kidneys that are not working properly. One specific condition that causes this is **renal tubular acidosis,** which is explained in Chapter 14. Metabolic acidosis due to kidney disease is chronic in nature. Dysfunction that approaches kidney failure especially causes metabolic acidosis. Dysfunction of the _____(1) can cause _____(2) acidosis because there is an increase in the amount of _____(3) ions that are kept in the body.

----- 3-83 -----

1. fluids
2. kidneys
3. chloride
4. bicarbonate

Another mechanism for metabolic acidosis is loss of bicarbonate. Loss of body fluids, such as in severe diarrhea, is a common reason for this. This is especially true in diarrhea due to pathogenic or disease-causing bacteria in the intestines. In addition to loss of bicarbonate in intestinal secretions, more bicarbonate than usual is secreted into the intestines to neutralize acids produced by the bacteria. Bacterial diarrhea in children especially can lead to acidosis. Another cause of excessive loss of bicarbonate is kidney failure and renal tubular acidosis. Just as H^+ is abnormally retained, bicarbonate is abnormally lost. These causes of metabolic acidosis are summarized in Table 3–16. Chloride is also excessively conserved in severe kidney disease. As the ECF chloride levels increase the body tries to maintain electrical neutrality. Remember chloride is an anion. Since bicarbonate is also an anion, this negative ion shifts inside cells to compensate for the increased chloride. This has the effect of decreased bicarbonate. Bicarbonate can be lost from the body through _____(1), such as occurs in severe bacterial diarrhea. Severe disease of _____(2) is another route of bicarbonate loss. A relative decrease in bicarbonate develops when levels of _____(3) increase. This is because _____(4) moves into the cells to make up for increased negative charges that accompany increased chloride.

TABLE 3–16. CAUSES OF METABOLIC ACIDOSIS

True	Relative	Relative
Bicarbonate Loss	*Increased Acid Production*	*Increased Acid Retention by Kidneys*
Diarrhea	Lactic acid through anaerobic metabolism	Uremic or retention acidosis
Bacterial infection	Hypoxia	Severe kidney disease
Severe kidney disease	Ketoacidosis	Renal tubular acidosis
Renal tubular acidosis	Diabetes mellitus	
	Starvation	
	Acute alcohol abuse	
	Acidic poisoning	
	Methanol	
	Ethylene glycol (antifreeze)	
	Salicylate (aspirin)	

TABLE 3–17. PRIMARY EFFECTS OF ABNORMAL pH DUE TO ACID–BASE IMBALANCE

Acidosis (acidemia)	Decreased nerve function, decreased excitability—central nervous system depression, stupor, coma, cardiac arrhythmias Hyperkalemia Hypercalcemia
Alkalosis (alkalemia)	Increased nerve function, increased excitability—central nervous system overstimulation, stupor, coma, cardiac arrhythmias Hypokalemia Hypocalcemia

······· 3–84 ·······

Decreased bicarbonate is either a true loss or it is consumed by buffering excess acids. The pH drops because there are insufficient amounts of base in relation to acids. Almost always, metabolic acidosis is a secondary problem due to disease such as diabetes or kidney failure. The acid pH causes generalized signs and symptoms such as anorexia (loss of appetite), nausea, vomiting, and lethargy. More specifically, acid pH causes a decrease in nerve function. Increased H^+ ions cause a decrease in the excitability of nerve cell membranes and other excitable tissue such as muscle. Severe depression of central nervous system function can lead to stupor and to coma. Significant acidosis is fatal if not corrected. Heart muscle is also affected and cardiac arrhythmias contribute to mortality. As levels of the cation H^+ increase, the body attempts to normalize ECF pH by shifting H^+ inside cells. To balance charges, potassium moves out. This creates hyperkalemia and its harmful effects. Acidosis also causes an increase in the ionized form of calcium and so may create the effects of hypercalcemia. Table 3–17 lists the effects of abnormal pH that are seen in all four of the acid–base imbalances. Tissues that are adversely affected by low pH include the _____(1) and _____(2). The pH is low because there is not enough _____(3) in the body compared to _____(4). Decreased levels of _____(5) classify this disorder as metabolic acidosis. Excessive H^+ ions depress _____(6) of membranes. The _____(7) system and the _____(8) can be depressed to the point of death. Because of ion shifting and changes in electrolyte binding, the electrolyte imbalances _____(9) and _____(10) also contribute to the harmful effects.

1. nerves
2. muscles
3. bicarbonate
4. acids
5. bicarbonate
6. excitability
7. central nervous
8. heart
9. hyperkalemia
10. hypercalcemia

······· 3–85 ·······

Decreased pH is a direct stimulus for increasing ventilation, so the lungs will compensate for the acidosis to some degree, and for a limited time, through hyperventilation. By increasing the rate and depth of breathing, the lungs are able to release more carbon dioxide, the acid component of the buffer pair. In diabetes, this breathing pattern is called **Kussmaul's breathing.** Table 3–18 outlines the compensatory mechanisms for acid–base imbalances. Study this table carefully for each condition we discuss.

TABLE 3–18. ACID–BASE IMBALANCES AND COMPENSATORY MECHANISMS

	Primary Imbalance			Compensatory Change		
	pH	pCO₂	HCO₃⁻	pH	pCO₂	HCO₃⁻
Metabolic acidosis	↓	N	*↓	↑ Toward N	↓* (Lungs—hyperventilation)	↓
Metabolic alkalosis	↑	N	*↑	↓ Toward N	↑* (Lungs—hypoventilation)	↑
Respiratory acidosis	↓	*↑	N	↑ Toward N	↑	↑* (Renal retention and H⁺ elimination)
Respiratory alkalosis	↑	*↓	N	↓ Toward N	↓	↓* (Renal elimination)

On the 1° imbalance side, the initial abnormality is marked by *. On the compensatory change side, the parameter that changes to make up for the 1° problem is marked by **.

▶ METABOLIC ALKALOSIS

1. hypokalemia
2. hydrogen

In **metabolic alkalosis** the primary upset is an increase in the base bicarbonate that is either real or in relation to decreased acid. This condition does not occur as frequently as metabolic acidosis. The three major mechanisms that create metabolic alkalosis are an abnormal loss of hydrogen ions, an increase in bicarbonate levels, and less extracellular fluid or volume contraction. Excessive loss of H^+ ions develops during times of continued vomiting. Stomach or "gastric contents" include hydrochloric acid or "HCl." As this acid is lost, a H^+ deficit occurs. Since chloride is also lost, this anion is replaced in the ECF with HCO_3^-, or bicarbonate, by cellular shifting to maintain neutrality. So this contributes to an alkaline ECF. In **bulimia,** the eating disorder characterized by food binges and self-induced vomiting, metabolic alkalosis is often a finding. Decreased levels of potassium, which is called _____(1), is another contributing factor of this imbalance. You know that if ECF K^+ decreases, potassium will leave cells to make up this deficit. Since charges must be balanced inside and outside cells, the cation _____(2) will move inside the cell. So more H^+ is lost from the ECF in this manner. Hypokalemia can develop in several ways. First, during vomiting, potassium chloride is also part of gastric contents that are lost. Several diuretic drugs that promote urine excretion typically increase loss of potassium as well. In Cushing's disease increased aldosterone, which normally promotes potassium loss, causes even greater excretion of this electrolyte, as well as greater excretion of H^+ ions. This hydrogen loss is an attempt by the kidneys to maintain electrical balance. Even though overall loss of potassium is greater than the amounts that are retained, the kidneys will still try to conserve what they can. For every K^+ that is kept, a H^+ is lost to even the charge differences.

1. bicarbonate
2. acid
3. hydrogen
4. bicarbonate
5. extracellular fluid
6. vomiting
7. extracellular
8. shifting
9. into
10. kidneys
11. electrical charges

In metabolic alkalosis there is either too much of the base _____(1) or not enough H^+ ions or _____(2). Three ways this develops is loss of too much _____(3), retaining too much _____(4), or decreased _____(5). Loss of too much H^+ follows continued _____(6) because of the HCl contents in the stomach. Hypokalemia causes decreased hydrogen in two ways. The first is a relative decrease of H^+ in the _____(7) fluid because of cellular _____(8). Hydrogen moves _____(9) the cell. The second is actual loss of H^+ by the _____(10) as these organs try to retain potassium during diuretic use or Cushing's disease. The exchange of H^+ for K^+ by the kidneys is a way to balance _____(11).

1. intake
2. kidneys
3. pressure
4. volume contraction

Excessive hydrogen loss causes blood tests to show elevated bicarbonate levels because there is not enough H^+ for this base to buffer. Therefore, there is more free bicarbonate to be measured. Actual increases in bicarbonate are less common. HCO_3^- is normally conserved by the kidneys and there are no mechanisms to cause the kidneys to increase this conservation. However, excessive ingestion of bicarbonate compounds can produce an excess. People with gastric or duodenal ulcers who self-medicate tend to consume a lot of antacids that are some form of bicarbonate. Dehydration can be described as **volume contraction** because the volume or amount of ECF fluid has "shrunk" or contracted and is now less. Filtration of blood by the kidneys is very dependent on blood pressure and blood pressure depends in part on blood volume. Volume contraction decreases filtering pressure for the kidneys. Therefore, several urine components end up being retained in the body, one of which is bicarbonate. Actual increases in bicarbonate levels can develop in one of two ways. One is by excessive _____(1) of bicarbonate. The other is by retention of bicarbonate by the _____(2) during times of decreased filtering _____(3). This decreased pressure can develop from dehydration, which is described as _____(4). Table 3–19 summarizes the causes of metabolic alkalosis.

TABLE 3–19. CAUSES OF METABOLIC ALKALOSIS

True	Relative
Increased Base Levels	*Increased Acid Loss*
Ingestion of bicarbonate compounds	Vomiting
Decreased ECF (dehydration)	H^+ ion loss
Decreased glomerular filtration rate	Cellular release of HCO_3^- to replace Cl^- loss
Retention of bicarbonate	Hypokalemia
Iatrogenic (bicarbonate administration)	Cellular release of K^+ shifts H^+ inside
	Increased excretion of H^+ by kidneys
	Cushing's disease

3–89

The signs of metabolic alkalosis are generally shadowed by signs of the cause, such as dehydration, vomiting, or hypokalemia. When the pH rises to a severe alkalosis, neurologic signs develop. Instead of depression of excitability as in acidosis, alkalosis causes overexcitability. The end result is still the same, with cardiac arrhythmias and coma leading to death. While neurologic and muscular effects are occurring, an alkalotic pH also causes a decrease in the amounts of ionized calcium because it increases calcium binding to proteins. The result is ECF hypocalcemia, which if severe enough, leads to tetany. In these cases, respiratory failure can happen if the diaphragm becomes paralyzed. Signs of mild to moderate metabolic alkalosis are usually seen as signs of the _____(1) of the imbalance such as dehydration, _____(2), or _____(3). Severe alkalosis causes _____(4) signs. The primary effect on excitable tissue is _____(5). The electrolyte imbalance known as _____(6) can develop as the pH affects active levels of this electrolyte. The rigid muscular paralysis known as _____(7) can cause _____(8) failure if it affects the diaphragm.

1. cause
2. vomiting
3. hypokalemia
4. neurologic
5. overexcitability
6. hypocalcemia
7. tetany
8. respiratory

3–90

The compensatory reaction by the lungs in metabolic alkalosis is hypoventilation, or a decrease in the rate of breathing. In this manner more CO_2, the acid component of the buffer pair, is retained. This helps to bring the HCO_3^- to H_2CO_3 ratio toward normal. If the ratio can be improved, the _____(1) approaches normal because this ratio determines the _____(2). This is only a temporary measure because hypoventilation cannot continue without ill effects.

1. pH
2. pH

▶ RESPIRATORY ACIDOSIS

3–91

The origin of this acidosis is the lungs where ventilation abnormalities lead to retention of CO_2 and therefore H_2CO_3. **Respiratory acidosis** has as its primary abnormality increased levels of CO_2, which is called **hypercapnia.** If the lungs are the origin of the imbalance then the compensating organs would have to be the _____(1) as shown in Table 3–18. You know that compensation by the kidneys is relatively slow, taking a day or two. Therefore acute respiratory acidosis can develop rather quickly because there is not an immediate compensatory response. There are two main mechanisms for development of this acid–base imbalance, which are presented in Table 3–20. The first is *impaired ventilation,* which is the physical act of inhalation and exhalation. Depression of the respiratory center of the brain by certain drugs such as barbiturates causes decreased rate of breathing. Head injury that affects this area of the brain interferes with messages to nerves and muscles responsible for breathing. Problems with the chest wall or respiratory muscles such as injuries. paralysis, or congenital deformities can interfere with the ability to expand the lungs and take in air. The second mechanism is disease of the lungs themselves that interferes with

1. kidneys

2. carbon dioxide
3. hypercapnia
4. lungs
5. ventilation
6. gas
7. carbon dioxide
8. acidic

normal *gas exchange.* Air may be able to reach the alveoli (air sacs) normally, but diseased tissue interferes with the ability of oxygen to pass into the capillaries and for carbon dioxide to be released. Examples of diseases of the lung parenchyma are emphysema, pneumonia, and pulmonary edema. Diseases of the airways, such as chronic bronchitis or asthma, also decrease gas exchange and lead to CO_2 retention. Chronic respiratory acidosis usually accompanies these **chronic obstructive pulmonary diseases** or **COPD.** In respiratory acidosis, the primary abnormality is increased _____(2) in the blood, which is called _____(3). The organs responsible for this imbalance are the _____(4). Two ways this condition develops is impaired _____(5), or physical breathing, and interference with normal _____(6) exchange. The results of these two abnormal lung functions is that more _____(7) is retained by the body so the pH becomes more _____(8).

3–92

1. central nervous
2. heart
3. depress

In respiratory acidosis, because ventilation or gas exchange is impaired, levels of oxygen may be below normal. Chronic conditions of lung disease will usually result in signs of low oxygen in the blood, or hypoxemia. Severe respiratory acidosis has the same effects we discussed in metabolic acidosis because it is the concentration of H^+ ions, or the pH, which alters function of excitable cell membranes. Looking back to Frame 3–84, you can see that acidosis can cause death because of its impact on the _____(1) system and the _____(2). The effect of too many H^+ ions is to _____(3) the excitability of cell membranes.

3–93

1. hydrogen
2. bicarbonate
3. healthy or working
   normally

Once the kidneys begin to compensate for the acidosis, excess H^+ is eliminated in the urine making it more acidic. As indicated earlier, the kidneys are very effective in normalizing the buffer pair ratio and returning the pH to near normal. They are able to continue this compensation indefinitely. If the kidneys are also diseased, then respiratory acidosis can become severe. Another consideration in normalizing conditions is maintaining adequate levels of oxygen. Carbon dioxide is the usual stimulant for changing respiratory patterns. If CO_2 becomes chronically increased the respiratory center of the brain adapts to this and CO_2 is no longer as strong a stimulant. Oxygen levels become the stimulus so it is important to maintain as normal a level as possible with treatment. The kidneys compensate for respiratory acidosis by eliminating as much _____(1) as possible and keeping more _____(2) in the body. If respiratory acidosis is to be effectively compensated for the kidneys must be _____(3). Table 3–20 summarizes the causes of respiratory acidosis.

TABLE 3–20. CAUSES OF RESPIRATORY ACIDOSIS

Impaired Ventilation	Impaired Gas Exchange
Impaired respiratory center	Pulmonary disease
Drug depression	Emphysema
Injury to respiratory center	Pneumonia
Impaired chest expansion	Pulmonary edema
Injuries to chest wall	Airway disease (COPD)
Paralysis of respiratory muscles	Bronchitis
Congenital defect of thorax	Asthma

TABLE 3–21. CAUSES OF RESPIRATORY ALKALOSIS

Excessive Ventilation

Increased metabolism
  Fever
  Hyperthyroidism
Stimulation of respiratory center
  Increased ammonia in liver disease
Hypoxia
Pyschogenic
  Extreme fear
Iatrogenic (overventilation)

▶ RESPIRATORY ALKALOSIS

Decreased carbon dioxide in the blood or **hypocapnia** is the origin of **respiratory alkalosis.**
As in the other alkalosis imbalance, a decrease in the acid component leads to a higher pH.
If hypoventilation retains too much CO_2 and causes acidosis then _____(1)
ventilation loses too much CO_2 and causes _____(2). There are metabolic reasons for hyperventilation such as fever and hyperthyroidism. These are states of hyperme-
tabolism (increased rates of metabolism) so ventilation also increases. Liver disease, which
allows levels of ammonia to build up in the blood, produces stimulation of the respiratory
center by the ammonia. Conditions that cause decreased oxygen in the blood, such as high
altitudes or congestive heart failure, will cause respiration to increase to bring in more oxygen. Persons on mechanical breathing devices can be overventilated, producing an iatrogenic
respiratory alkalosis. A commonly recognized condition called "hyperventilation syndrome"
is a situation of overbreathing due to anxiety, fear, or hysteria. These are considered psychogenic causes of respiratory alkalosis. The primary abnormality in respiratory alkalosis is
decreased _____(3), which is called _____(4). This develops
when the rate of breathing _____(5) as a result of certain disease states or
extreme fear.

3–94

1. hyper
2. alkalosis
3. carbon dioxide
4. hypocapnia
5. increases

In respiratory alkalosis, **apnea,** the cessation of breathing, can occur if carbon dioxide falls
too low because CO_2 is the stimulus for breathing. The dangers of alkalosis are a consideration if the pH becomes too high. Again, hyperexcitability of cell membranes and overstimulation of nervous and muscular tissue is the mechanism of damage. Tetany, respiratory failure, and coma are possibilities. Based on what you have learned about compensation to this
point, you know that the _____(1) would retain more _____(2)
ions, or acid, and lose more _____(3), or base. Table 3–21 summarizes the
causes of respiratory alkalosis.

3–95

1. kidneys
2. hydrogen
3. bicarbonate

V. REVIEW QUESTIONS

1. Acid–base disturbances are classified according to (choose all that apply):
   a. changes in pH
   b. changes in the buffer pair ratio
   c. the organs responsible for the imbalance
   d. abnormal levels of bicarbonate and carbon dioxide

1. a–changes in pH; d–abnormal
   levels of bicarbonate and carbon dioxide

2. 1b–metabolic alkalosis;
   2c–respiratory acidosis;
   3d–respiratory alkalosis;
   4a–metabolic acidosis

3. 1–hydrogen 2–ratio

4. c–normalize the ratio of the
   buffer pair

5. 1a–lungs; 2b–kidneys;
   3b–kidneys; 4a–lungs;
   5a–lungs; 6b–kidneys

6. a–metabolic acidosis

7. a–acid; b–hydrogen;
   c–bicarbonate

8. d–ketones and lactic acid

9. 1–anaerobic 2–hypoxia
   3–fat 4–starvation 5–diabetes

10. d–bacterial diarrhea and
    kidney failure

2. Please match these acid–base disturbances with their definitions:
   a. metabolic acidosis   1. _____ pH greater than normal, increased bicarbonate
   b. metabolic alkalosis   2. _____ pH less than normal, increased carbon dioxide
   c. respiratory acidosis   3. _____ pH greater than normal, decreased carbon dioxide
   d. respiratory alkalosis   4. _____ pH less than normal, decreased bicarbonate

3. Please complete: Changes in pH are a direct reflection of the concentration of
   _____(1) ions, and this is mathematically determined by changes in the
   HCO_3^- to H_2CO_3 _____(2).

4. In compensation measures during acid-base imbalance, the pH can be improved by:
   a. normalizing the component of the buffer pair that is abnormal
   b. intervening with medical treatment
   c. normalizing the ratio of the buffer pair
   d. producing more acid or base as needed

5. Please match these organs of compensation with the characteristic response:
   a. lungs   1. ____ very fast response
   b. kidneys   2. ____ long-term ability to respond
                    3. ____ slower response
                    4. ____ less efficient in normalizing pH
                    5. ____ short-term ability to respond
                    6. ____ most efficient in normalizing pH

6. The most common acid–base imbalance is:
   a. metabolic acidosis
   b. metabolic alkalosis
   c. respiratory acidosis
   d. respiratory alkalosis

7. The three mechanisms that produce metabolic acidosis are
   a. increased _____ production
   b. kidney retention of _____ ions
   c. loss of _____ from the body

8. Two common acids that can be formed in excess in metabolic acidosis are:
   a. lactic acid and carbonic acid (from CO_2)
   b. salicylates and ketones
   c. fatty acids and lactic acid
   d. ketones and lactic acid

9. Please complete these sentences using the terms below: The mechanism of increased
   lactic acid production is _____(1) metabolism, such as occurs during low
   oxygen or _____(2). Ketones are formed from increased
   _____(3) breakdown, such as occurs during _____(4). The
   disease that mimics starvation to cells is _____(5).

fat	hydrogen ions	hypoxia
diabetes	anaerobic	carbohydrate
aerobic	ischemia	starvation

10. Metabolic acidosis due to increased bicarbonate loss is commonly associated with:
    a. continued vomiting and kidney failure
    b. hyperventilation and bacterial diarrhea
    c. continued vomiting and bacterial diarrhea
    d. bacterial diarrhea and kidney failure

11. In general, acidosis causes _____(1) of nerve cell membrane function while alkalosis causes _____(2) of nerve cell membrane functions. Either condition, if severe enough, can result in _____(3).

12. In metabolic acidosis compensation occurs through the:
    a. lungs and hyperventilation
    b. lungs and hypoventilation
    c. kidneys and hydrogen retention
    d. kidneys and bicarbonate loss

13. Three mechanisms that cause metabolic alkalosis are:
    a. excessive loss of _____ ions
    b. fluid volume _____
    c. excessive intake of _____

14. Metabolic alkalosis due to increased hydrogen loss is commonly associated with (choose all that apply):
    a. continued vomiting
    b. shifting of bicarbonate out of cells to replace chloride loss
    c. severe diarrhea
    d. shifting of bicarbonate out of cells to replace potassium loss

15. Metabolic alkalosis can be produced by, or worsened by, this electrolyte imbalance:
    a. hyperkalemia
    b. hypocapnia
    c. hypokalemia
    d. hypercapnia

16. Retention of bicarbonate and other compounds can develop from (choose all that apply):
    a. ECF volume contraction
    b. decreased blood volume
    c. decreased blood pressure
    d. decreased kidney filtering pressure

17. In addition to overexcitability of nerve cell membranes, metabolic alkalosis causes an electrolyte imbalance that results in tetany and this is:
    a. hypocalcemia
    b. hypokalemia
    c. hypercalcemia
    d. hyperkalemia

18. In respiratory acidosis the primary abnormality is:
    a. base excess
    b. base deficit
    c. hypocapnia
    d. hypercapnia

19. Choose the two mechanisms of developing respiratory acidosis:
    a. diaphragm paralysis during tetany
    b. impaired ventilation
    c. excessive gas exchange
    d. impaired gas exchange

20. In respiratory alkalosis the primary abnormality is hypercapnia/hypocapnia (choose one) _____(1) and this is caused by hyperventilation/hypoventilation (choose one) _____(2) .

11. 1–depression; 2–overexcitability; 3–death

12. a–lungs and hyperventilation

13. a–hydrogen; b–contraction; c–bicarbonate;

14. a–continued vomiting; b–shifting of bicarbonate out of cells to replace chloride loss

15. c–hypokalemia

16. a–ECF volume contraction; b–decreased blood volume; c–decreased blood pressure; d–decreased kidney filtering pressure

17. a–hypocalcemia

18. d–hypercapnia

19. b–impaired ventilation; d–impaired gas exchange

20. 1–hypocapnia; 2–hyperventilation

CHAPTER ▶ SUMMARY

▶ SECTION II

Elevated body temperature can be either fever (of an endogenous or internal source) or it can be hyperthermia (of an exogenous of external source). Hyperpyrexia is temperature greater than 104°F. The danger of hyperpyrexia is that it destroys cells by coagulating their proteins. Fever is also termed pyrexia. Pyrexia is due to a change in the setpoint of the hypothalamus, which determines body temperature. This alteration is caused by a chain of chemical events that begins with a pyrogen. Infections are the most common cause of fever. In fever, the cold stage increases temperature to the new setting by producing heat in greater amounts than heat is lost. The activities are shivering, which produces heat, and vasoconstriction, which conserves heat. The hot stage maintains the new temperature through balancing heat production and heat loss. The sweating stage lowers temperature by heat loss that is greater than production. Hyperthermia is increased temperature that is NOT caused by a change in the setpoint. Intense activity in a hot, humid environment can cause hyperthermia. Heat production from exercising muscles and decreased loss to the environment may overwhelm the body's heat regulating abilities. The three syndromes of hyperthermia are:

1. Heat cramps—localized muscle spasms resulting from lactic acid production and water and electrolyte loss.
2. Heat exhaustion—generalized loss of water and electrolytes with intense vasodilation that causes hypotension.
3. Heat stroke (sun stroke)—life-threatening hyperthermia that leads to intense circulatory changes preceding shock, ischemic organ injury, and death.

Hypothermia is core body temperature less than 95°F. External conditions overcome thermoregulation. The primary injury is extreme vasoconstriction in an attempt to conserve heat. This causes ischemic injury to vital organs and tissues. Respiration is depressed to the point of death due to greatly slowed metabolism and decreased carbon dioxide production. Frostbite is local hypothermia of susceptible body parts that can produce necrosis or tissue death of those parts.

▶ SECTION III

Dehydration develops when fluid intake is less than fluid loss, or if losses are greater than intake. Causes of excessive loss include severe diarrhea, polyuria in kidney disease, osmotic diuresis in diabetes mellitus, diabetes insipidus, excessive sweating, severe burns, and third space sequestering of fluid. Hyponatremia contributes to dehydration since sodium is necessary to draw water back into the body from pre-urine filtrate. Dehydrate causes decreased intravenous blood volume and blood pressure. Perfusion of tissues with blood and oxygen decreases. Severe cases result in hypovolemic shock. To prevent this, water is shifted from the interstitial ECF to the intravascular ECF. The now hypertonic interstitial ECF draws water from cells and causes crenation of the cells and can lead to death. Polydipsia, or increased thirst, is a feature of dehydration. Osmoreceptors sense the increase in osmolarity (less solvent equals relative increase in number of solutes) and stimulate the hypothalamus to initiate thirst. Pure water increases, usually seen as psychogenic water intoxication, is hypotonic, and causes swelling of cells. Fluid excess that is also accompanied by sodium increase is isotonic and does not adversely affect cell size. This is more commonly seen. Usually, isotonic fluid excess is seen in cases of congestive heart failure where blood pressure is insufficient to produce normal amounts of urine. Kidney disease that does not produce enough urine is another cause of fluid excess. The cellular swelling of hypotonic fluid excess most obviously impairs brain function while isotonic fluid excess shows less intense signs, except in the case of pulmonary edema. Edema is increased ECF interstitial fluid and can be seen as "pitting" in the extremities. Edema can be localized or generalized. Left-sided congestive heart failure is one cause of generalized edema that can lead to pulmonary edema or fluid in the lungs. Edema due to true body fluid increase is caused by retention of sodium and water by diseased kidneys. The mechanism for edema production in this case is increased hydrostatic pressure. Other causes of edema can be described as normal body fluid levels but with a change in the normal distribution of that fluid. One of these is right-sided congestive heart failure, which causes increased venous pressure. Both of these pressure increases make the blood pressure too high at the venous end of the capillary. Therefore osmotic pressure is not greater than blood pressure and enough fluid is not drawn into the vessel. Transudate, exudate, effusion, and ascites are terms that describe fluid contents and locations. Shock and inflammation are events that cause capillaries to become leaky and allow edema to develop. Decreased osmotic pressure is the cause of distribution edema when hypoalbuminemia exists. Albumin creates the majority of osmotic pressure. Albumin can be lost from the body in inflammatory disorders of the kidneys and will be found in the urine. Protein-losing enteropathy is another reason for albumin loss, while liver failure and starvation mean enough albumin is not being synthesized. The primary mechanism of injury in edema is decreased ability to pass oxygen, nutrients, and wastes to and from the cells. Mechanical pressure on small vessels can produce ischemia if blood has a difficult time flowing through the area. The brain, larynx, and lungs are susceptible to immediate life-threatening effects. Neurogenic diabetes insipidus is insufficient antidiuretic hormone, while nephrogenic is the form caused by lack of response to ADH by the kidneys. ADH prevents abnormal water loss so in diabetes insipidus urine output is excessive and dilute (polyuria). Neurogenic diabetes insipidus arises from problems in the hypothalamus or posterior pituitary gland. In the nephrogenic form diseased kidney cells turn a "deaf ear" to the water conservation message from ADH. Polyuria and polydipsia are obvious clinical signs.

▶ SECTION IV

Levels of electrolytes are measured in terms of amounts in the circulation. Electrolyte levels in the circulation are what affect body function even if those levels are not a true picture of total body levels. Hyponatremia is decreased sodium in the circulation. True hyponatremia is sodium loss due to decreased aldosterone in Addison's disease or loss of body fluids (sweating, vomiting, or diarrhea). Relative hyponatremia is due to increased body water that dilutes normal sodium amounts. Sodium and water balance is closely related. Relative hyponatremia can be due to water intoxication, retention of water by increased levels of ADH, or diseased kidneys. Hyponatremia creates a hypotonic ECF that leads to cellular swelling and possible lysis. The most visible signs of this are abnormalities in central nervous system function. Hypernatremia is increased sodium in the circulation. True elevated sodium can be due to elevated aldosterone and cortisol in Cushing's disease, or ingestion of sodium. Relative hypernatremia occurs with decreased body water or dehydration. This can be because of decreased intake of water, increased loss of water seen in watery diarrhea, diabetes insipidus, or kidney disease. Hypernatremia creates a hypertonic ECF that leads to cellular shrinking or crenation. Dehydration compounds the problem as fluid is redistributed from the interstitium and cells to maintain intravascular volumes. The function of CNS cells is most obviously affected. Hypokalemia is decreased potassium in the circulation. Potassium is one electrolyte that may not be truly represented by blood tests because of the movement of potassium among fluid compartments. However blood levels are what influence body function. Hypokalemia is a unique imbalance owing to poor conservation by the kidneys in time of need. Because of cellular shifting out to the ECF and resulting cellular depletion, serious signs of hypokalemia usually mean the condition has existed for some time and now has reached a critical point. True hypokalemia due to deficiency can be seen as a result of insufficient intake, direct loss (vomiting, diarrhea, diuretics), or loss due to increased aldosterone in Cushing's disease. Aldosterone is also stimulated by sodium loss so hyponatremia can contribute to hypokalemia. Relative hypokalemia is usually the result of cellular shifting into the ICF or cellular uptake. This can be because of diabetic acidosis, which is treated with insulin or alkalosis. Hypokalemia creates a more negative RMP that is less excitable, or needs more stimulation to reach the threshold and action potentials. This is because the RMP is now farther from the threshold. Nerve transmission and muscle contraction is depressed. An ECG reveals abnormal cardiac muscle activity called arrhythmia.

Severe arrhythmia, such as fibrillation, can halt cardiac output causing shock and death. Hyperkalemia is increased potassium in the circulation. This condition generally develops during kidney failure because otherwise homeostatic mechanisms work efficiently to prevent it. True hyperkalemia can be due to kidney failure, increased intake of potassium concurrent with kidney disease, or decreased aldosterone in Addison's disease. Relative hyperkalemia is generally a development of cellular shifting in the form of increased release from cells or decreased uptake. Causes of this include acidosis and lack of insulin. Opposite effects on the RMP are seen in hyperkalemia, with more excitability of tissues and less required stimulation. This is because the RMP is less negative, or closer to the threshold. One excitable tissue that is profoundly affected is the heart. Slowed heart rate or bradycardia can turn into cardiac arrest. Hypocalcemia is decreased calcium in the circulation. Amounts of the free, or ionized form, are extremely important because it is only this form that is active in the body. This is another electrolyte for which levels in the circulation may not represent total body stores. True hypocalcemia can be caused by kidney disease where phosphate is retained, decreased PTH in hypoparathyroidism, and decreased vitamin D, which causes decreased calcium absorption from the intestines. Relative hypocalcemia is actually a decrease in the active or ionized form of calcium. This occurs with increased protein, which binds more calcium, and alkalosis, which increases binding to proteins and increased binding to other substances. Hypocalcemia causes an increase in the excitability of nerves and muscles and clinically produces the sign tetany, a rigid paralysis. Respiratory arrest due to tetany of the diaphragm or laryngeal spasm can cause death. Cardiac output can be severely impaired by arrhythmias, and CNS abnormalities are seen as seizures. Hypercalcemia is increased calcium in the circulation. True hypercalcemia is seen with increased PTH in hyperparathyroidism and abnormalities of bone, such as atrophy or cancer, that causes greater release of calcium from bone. Relative hypercalcemia is an increase in the ionized form in cases of hypoalbuminemia, where there is less protein available for binding, and acidosis, which inhibits binding to protein. Hypercalcemia causes a decrease in the excitability of nerves and muscle. In addition to the typical problems of cardiac arrhythmias, arrest, and possible coma, behavior changes are seen as an acute psychosis. Pathologic fractures can also develop if calcium stores in bone are depleted because of bone disease. Increased calcium causes decreased response to ADH by kidney cells leading to less concentration of the urine and more water and sodium loss. Precipitation of calcium crystals in the kidneys, or calculi, damages that organ. All of these signs can culminate in a hypercalcemic crisis.

▶ SECTION V

Acid–base imbalances are classified according to the origin of disturbance (metabolic or respiratory) and pH abnormality (acid or alkaline). Changes in bicarbonate are metabolic disturbances, while changes in carbonic acid (carbon dioxide) are respiratory disturbances. Abnormal pH is directly related to the ratio of base to acid rather than actual amounts. The mechanism of compensation uses this relationship to help normalize pH. In correcting acid–base imbalances, the body is able to adjust the abnormal value directly and return the pH to near normal. In compensating, the opposite member of the ratio is adjusted to help normalize the ratio and therefore, the pH. In compensation, the original abnormality still exists. The kidneys and the lungs provide these two functions of correction and compensation. The kidneys are slow but more effective in the long run while the lungs are quick but short lived in their effect. Metabolic acidosis is decreased pH due to increased acid or decreased base. Lowered bicarbonate may be a true deficit because of loss, or a relative one because more acid uses up base during buffering. Metabolic acidosis is the most common imbalance. The mechanisms of metabolic acidosis in relative bicarbonate decreases include increased acid formation (lactic acid during anaerobic metabolism) and ketoacidosis (uncontrolled diabetes or starvation). Retention of more acid by the kidneys occurs in renal tubular acidosis in kidney disease. Metabolic acidosis caused by true bicarbonate loss is seen in severe diarrhea of bacterial infections and renal tubular acidosis. The effect of metabolic acidosis is the same as respiratory acidosis, increased H^+ ions (decreased pH) depresses nerve function and excitability causing CNS depression and cardiac arrhythmias. It also increases levels of potassium and calcium. The lungs attempt to compensate through hyperventilation to decrease CO_2 or H_2CO_3. Metabolic alkalosis is increased pH due to decreased acid or an increase in bicarbonate. The mechanism of metabolic alkalosis during relative bicarbonate excess is acid deficit found in vomiting (which loses H^+ ions), hypokalemia (which moves H^+ inside cells), and Cushing's disease (increased aldosterone and cortisol), which increases H^+ and K^+ excretion by the kidneys. True bicarbonate excess is because of ingestion of basic compounds and retention of bicarbonate during reduced kidney filtering caused by volume contraction (dehydration). The effect of metabolic alkalosis is the same as respiratory alkalosis, decreased H^+ ions (increased pH) overexcites nerve function causing CNS overstimulation and cardiac arrhythmias. It also lowers levels of potassium and calcium. The lungs attempt to compensate through hypoventilation to retain more carbon dioxide (CO_2) that is derived from carbonic acid (H_2CO_3). Respiratory acidosis is decreased pH because of increased H_2CO_3 or CO_2, which is called hypercapnia. This develops when there are problems in ventilation or in gas exchange. Hypoxia may exist. Respiratory acidosis caused by ventilation difficulty is seen in depression or injury to the respiratory center of the brain and difficulty in expanding the chest because of injury, paralysis, or birth defects. Respiratory acidosis associated with poor gas exchange is seen in disorders of the lung tissue (emphysema, pneumonia, or edema) and disorders of the airways (COPD in bronchitis or asthma). Compensation for respiratory acidosis by the kidneys is slow so respiratory acidosis may persist in its initial effects. The kidneys eliminate more H^+ ions to raise the pH. Respiratory alkalosis is increased pH due to decreased H_2CO_3 or CO_2, which is called hypocapnia. Hyperventilation is the cause and is associated with fever, hyperthyroidism, liver disease, hypoxia, and anxiety or fear. Apnea may develop because severe hypocapnia leads to little or no stimulation of the respiratory center. The kidneys compensate by retaining more H^+ ions and losing more bicarbonate.

The Immune System

▶ OBJECTIVES

SECTION II

Define all highlighted terms.

Explain the difference between a normal immune response, hypersensitivity, and allergy.

List the classifications of hypersensitivity and state common titles of each class.

For each type of hypersensitivity, relate how antigens are destroyed, what antigens are targeted, and how this destruction may injure the body.

Identify the difference between atopy and anaphylaxis in type I hypersensitivity.

State the most common atopic condition.

Explain the pathogenesis and effects of anaphylaxis.

State the secondary effect of type II antigen destruction and the most common cells involved.

Give examples of antibody-dependent cell-mediated cytotoxic diseases.

List secondary effects of type III acute vasculitis.

Identify the difference in mechanism between delayed cell-mediated hypersensitivity and types I, II, and III.

Describe the kind of inflammation present in type IV hypersensitivity.

Classify specific disease examples or conditions according to the type of hypersensitivity mechanism.

Name a broad category of type IV hypersensitivity reactions.

SECTION III

Define all highlighted terms.

Explain the concept of immunodeficiency and related terms.

List causes of nonspecific immunosuppression.

Explain the pathogenesis of inherited immunosuppression.

Describe the original findings in AIDS epidemiology, including geographic location, populations identified, presenting signs, and specific diseases.

Define the acronyms HIV and AIDS.

Explain the difference between HIV infection and AIDS.

Equate some of the signs and conditions in AIDS with specific causes. For example, behavior abnormalities due to AIDS dementia complex.

List substances infectious for HIV and routes of infection.

Describe the pathogenesis of HIV, including specific target cells and secondary results.

Explain the typical CD4 to CD8 ratio in AIDS and its significance.

Relate the stages of HIV infection to events in the patient.

List infections or conditions that are relatively common to AIDS.

SECTION IV

Define all highlighted terms.

Describe the concept of autoimmunity and autoantibodies.

Relate autoimmunity to hypersensitivity.

List criteria for classifying a disease as autoimmune.

Explain how autoimmune disease causes injury to body tissues.

For each example of autoimmune disease (if applicable), list specific diseases, identify the antigens, and state the tissue injuries.

Explain why systematic lupus erythematosus (SLE) is called diffuse collagen vascular disease and identify primary targeted tissues.

List assumed antigens in SLE.

State a classic superficial sign of SLE, as well as systemic signs common to SLE, and relate them to the pathogenesis of this disease.

State the effects of SLE most responsible for death.

SECTION ▶ 1. ANATOMY AND PHYSIOLOGY IN REVIEW

4–1

Immunology is the study of the immune system. Before you learn about the immune system there are other types of defenses to consider. There are two classes of defense. One is the immune system that is a **specific** defense. This is an attack or an offensive launched against particular disease agents through complicated mechanisms. The second class is a **nonspecific** or sometimes called an **innate** defense. Innate means present at birth or "inborn" and does not require activation by disease agents. It is called nonspecific because it is made of general barriers that react to all invaders the same way. A critical difference between specific and nonspecific defense is the development of future protection. Only the specific response by the immune system causes future protection (immunity).

4–2

The innate, or nonspecific, guards against disease are listed and explained in this frame.

1. Barrier epithelial cells. These are the skin and mucous membranes of the gastrointestinal tract, respiratory tract, and genitourinary tracts. The covering and lining formed by joined epithelial cells is a physical barrier that prevents microorganisms from entering body tissue. A breakdown in this sheet of cells, such as a cut, can lead to infection of the underlying tissue.

2. Secretions. Several body fluids such as tears, saliva, and mucous membrane secretions contain chemicals that are harmful to microorganisms. One example is **lysozyme,** which will lyse, or rupture, cells.

3. Physical body properties. These include temperature, a very acid stomach pH, digestive enzymes, populations of harmless bacteria (normal flora) that prevent pathogens from gaining hold, cilia of the respiratory tract, and the sneeze and cough reflex.

4. Inflammation and phagocytosis. Chapter 2 centered on these concepts of the "search and destroy" function of inflammation and phagocytosis.

5. The complement system. This series of reactions will be covered later.

4–3

Immunity or protection against disease can be either natural or acquired. **Natural immunity** means that only a particular host can develop disease. This is a species specific concept and an example is that humans are not susceptible to many animal diseases. **Acquired immunity** is being a host for a disease agent and successfully fighting against it. This contact and resulting fight is the **immune response.** The immune response is divided into two types. The first is **humoral immunity.** It is especially effective against bacteria. A type of white blood cell called a **lymphocyte** takes part in humoral immunity. This is further broken down to a particular kind of lymphocyte called a **B lymphocyte.** B lymphocytes secrete proteins called **antibodies** that attack foreign substances **(antigens).** In this way, B cells act indirectly on antigens. After the attack, the antigen is more easily phagocytized. Do you remember the term used in Chapter 2 to describe the process in which a substance was made easier to phagocytize? It is called _____(1). In addition to phagocytosis these activities stimulate the complement system that further destroys antigens.

1. opsonization

4–4

The second type of immune response is called **cell-mediated immunity.** It acts against viruses, fungi, parasites, tumor cells, and some bacteria. It is also created by a special kind of lymphocyte, the **T lymphocyte.** The T cell does not produce antibodies but instead attacks the invader itself. So T cells act directly on antigens. There are several kinds of T cells that you will learn about shortly. These "killer Ts" prevent the antigens from spreading and phagocytize them extremely well. An important note here is this particular cell activity is capable of causing damage to normal tissue. This destruction may be referred to later when discussing some diseases. This is another example of protective measures that can cause harm, especially if the activity is intense.

4–5

An antigen is any substance that is not a natural part of an individual. It is necessary to say "individual" because substances that are natural to the human body in general still are not the same from one person to the next. An antigen is a substance that the immune system recognizes as foreign, or not belonging in the individual's body. It is usually a protein or some other large molecule. Pathogens or microorganisms that cause disease are antigens. On the surface of antigens are sites that cause recognition by the immune system. These sites are called **antigenic determinants** or **epitopes.** A **hapten** is a foreign substance that is too small to cause immune recognition. When a hapten is joined to a larger molecule an immune response can take place. This larger molecule is called a **carrier.** An example is an allergic response to penicillin. An antibody is a specialized protein made by B cells whose only function is to destroy a particular antigen. It is important to understand the specificity that is involved here. The example of a lock and key is often used to explain this interaction between an antibody and its target antigen. Only keys made to fit a particular lock will turn the barrels.

4–6

Immunologic tolerance is the concept of "self" versus "non-self." Substances are recognized as either belonging in the individual (self) or not belonging (non-self). If it doesn't belong it is foreign. There are "markers" on body tissues that are interpreted by lymphocytes as self. A major marker system is the major histocompatibility complex (MHC) that is presented in later frames. The MHC from another person is considered just as foreign as any virus or bacteria and is targeted for destruction. A failure in this mechanism to recognize your own tissue is one of the three categories of immune system disorders. The first one we will consider later in this chapter is "over response." This is **hypersensitivity.** The second category is "under response" or **immunodeficiency.** The failure to recognize self is the category of **autoimmune disease** or "misdirected response."

4–7

Immunity is a result of the immune response in which you are no longer susceptible to a particular disease agent. A person who is immune to chickenpox mounted a successful defense against the virus and will not develop chickenpox again. **Sensitized** is the term for having had previous contact with an antigen. If you are sensitized to an antigen, when you contact it again, you will have an immune response. All people who are immune to a disease have first experienced sensitization.

4–8

The **immune response** has two parts. First is the initial antigen contact that causes lymphocytes and other components to act and destroy the antigen. This is called the **primary response,** or the **first response.** This is when sensitization takes place. Antibodies are produced in certain amounts over a certain time period. The B cells involved in this first stage of antibody production are now called **memory cells.** If that same antigen is ever encountered again, the second part of the response is called the **anamnestic** or **secondary response.** "Anamnestic" is from the Greek language and means "memory." The clonal line of B cells that were involved in the first defense recognizes and "remembers" the antigen

TABLE 4–1. TYPES OF IMMUNITY

Natural Immunity	Acquired Immunity
Host is not susceptible	Host is susceptible
Response not required	Active immunity 　Natural (disease) 　Artificial (vaccination)
	Passive immunity 　Natural (fetomaternal) 　Artificial (immune serum or gammaglobulin)

(hence, the name memory cell). The difference between the primary and anamnestic responses is in the amount of antibody produced and how long it takes. These memory cells were previously programmed or already patterned to make this antibody. Therefore there is little to no "down time" while the antibody is produced again. So the secondary response is much faster than the primary one. Also, much more antibody is made during the secondary response. The result of this difference is that the antigen is destroyed before disease can occur.

4–9

Immunity may or may not be the result of an immune response by the host. This is apparent when you consider the types of immunity that are explained in this frame and shown in Tables 4–1 and 4–2.

1. **Active Immunity.** The host has contacted an antigen and formed antibodies against it. This can develop in two ways. In natural active immunity, there is an actual encounter with the antigen and the experience of some degree of disease. Artificial active immunity, or **vaccination,** on the other hand, involves receiving the antigen into the body parenterally or orally. Antigens in a vaccine are either "killed" or "attenuated," which means weakened beyond the ability to cause disease. The antibodies made by the host in this instance are the same as if the disease had developed naturally. Another term used to describe this process is **immunization.**

2. **Passive immunity.** The host has not contacted an antigen or formed any antibodies, but antibodies are present. The important difference from active immunity is that passive immunity is only *temporary* and an anamnestic response will *not* occur. Since the host did not produce the antibodies, there are no memory cells to call upon. These antibodies are present from two sources. In natural passive immunity, maternal antibodies cross the placenta into the fetus' circulation before birth. In artificial passive immunity, antibodies can be injected into someone exposed to a known antigen for temporary protection until their own response is adequate.

TABLE 4–2. CLASSES OF BODY DEFENSE

Specific	Nonspecific (Innate)
Natural	Physical properties
Acquired	Barriers (skin, mucous membrane)
Humoral	Secretions
Cell mediated	Temperature
	pH
	Cilia
	Inflammation and phagocytosis
	Complement system (alternative pathway)

4—10

The primary cells of the immune response are the lymphocytes, one of the five types of white blood cells in the circulation. Lymphocytes originate from lymphoid tissue such as lymph nodes, and are found in lymphoid organs such as the spleen and tonsils. The bone marrow is an important site of both origin and housing of lymphocytes. There are two kinds of lymphocytes, the **B cell** and the **T cell.** There are thousands of different types of receptors on lymphocyte surfaces. Antigens attach to these receptors and stimulate a response. This attachment is what is meant by a cell "recognizing" or "knowing" that a material is an antigen. It has been estimated that the varying arrangements of receptors can produce up to ten million different antibodies. If an antigen enters the body, chances are that there is a cell somewhere that has a matching receptor. B cells and T cells are each the parent of their own line and each line can produce clones. Clones are identical daughter cells made through mitosis and cell division. Each line is specific for only one antigen and is, therefore, antigen specific. Each clone will also be specific.

4—11

The response of B cells is called humoral immunity. Humoral refers to the fluids or circulation. B cell products, antibodies, are released into the circulation and that is why it is called humoral immunity. B cells undergo the following activities.

1. Antigen stimulates the B cell by interacting with the receptor.
2. This B cell is the mother of the line of clones to be produced.
3. The mother B cell goes through several changes (blast transformation).
4. The changed or transformed B cell divides and subsequent generations divide.
5. These daughter cells mature into **plasma cells.** There are many plasma cells or clones compared to the original stimulated B cell.
6. Each clone or plasma cell produces antibody. In this way, much more antibody is made against the antigen than could have been made by the original B cell.

These activities make up the primary response. Figure 4–1 shows the effectiveness of this response in making more antibody than originally possible.

4—12

Not all B cells become plasma cells. Some that are also stimulated by the antigen become dormant and contain information about the antigen. If the antigen is encountered again, this dormant cell "remembers" it. This is the memory cell mentioned earlier. Now the secondary response begins. Because of previous programming, the memory cells go through the same activities to produce plasma cells and antibody except the response is much faster and the amount of antibody is greater.

4—13

Antibodies are a plasma protein like albumin but in lesser amounts than albumin. They are actually called **immunoglobulins.** Globulin is the kind of protein and "immuno" refers to their function. Their structure is polypeptides that are chains of many amino acids. Two "light" chains and two "heavy" chains make up the antibody. The end of this molecule is called the **hypervariable region.** This means the end has many different possibilities of configuration. These differences in arrangement of amino acids at the end are responsible for the unique specificity of the antibody for the antigen. This part is sometimes called the **Fab,** which means the antigen-binding fragment. Figure 4–2A presents the basic structure of an antibody. Antibodies are produced starting at about 6 weeks after birth.

4—14

There are 5 classes of antibodies. **Ig** is the abbreviation standing for immunoglobulin. The first class is G or **IgG.** (It is pronounced by each individual letter, I-G-G.) IgG is the most abundant, consisting of about 80 percent of plasma antibodies. This is the class that is produced during the secondary or anamnestic response. This Ig can neutralize bacterial toxins directly or can opsonize particulate antigens. This means the antibody attaches to the particle and makes phagocytosis easier. Macrophages then ingest the antigen–antibody pair. This attachment also stimulates or activates the complement system.

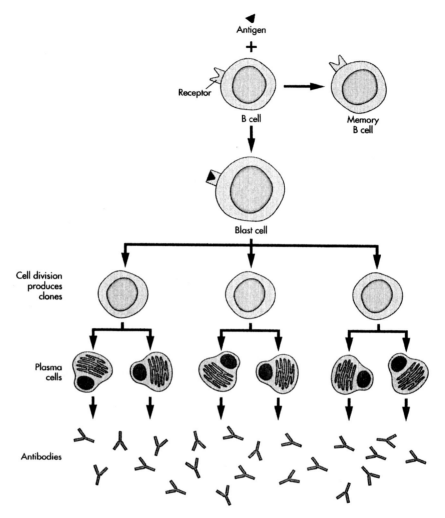

Figure 4–1. B lymphocyte transformation after stimulation by an antigen.

The next class is **M** or **IgM.** M could stand for macro because this molecule is very large. It is five times the size of an IgG. IgM is made during the primary response so it is this antibody found in the circulation first. The size of IgM makes it especially useful against larger antigens. It is like five IgG molecules bound together so there are many more sites to bind to antigen. Because of its size, IgM is confined to the intravascular space. The structural differences between IgG and IgM are shown in Figure 4–2B.

IgA is the antibody secreted into some body fluids such as tears, saliva, and respiratory secretions. It is found along mucosal barriers and adds to that protective function. It works to inactivate antigens before they can enter the body systems. **IgE** is an important antibody that is part of the hypersensitivity or allergy reaction. IgE is attached to tissue cells called **mast cells.** When the IgE and mast cell complex contacts an antigen, IgE causes the mast cell to release several chemical mediators, including histamine. Histamine is a commonly known mediator associated with allergies. Table 4–3 compares the different immunoglobulins.

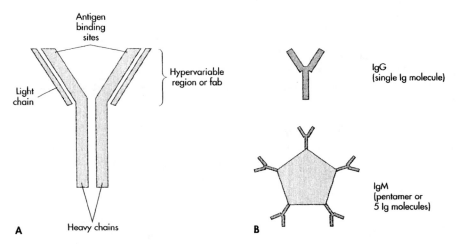

Figure 4–2. A. Basic immunoglobulin (antibody) structure. **B.** Structural comparison between IgG and IgM molecules.

4–17

The second type of lymphocyte is called a T cell. The various types of T cells can be classified as **effector** cells and **regulator** cells. Effectors cells are involved in actions against antigens and regulator cells control the process. Effector cells are activated by antigens and interactions with macrophages. These activated cells are then sensitized, as are activated B cells. Sensitized effector T cells are **cytotoxic T cells** or **killer T cells.** Their effect is direct because the cells destroy the antigens, rather than a product such as an antibody from a B cell. Receptors on the killer T cell surface bind to the antigen. One mechanism of destruction is the release of a kind of poison from the killer T cell. One killer T cell can destroy many antigens. It is important to note that the specificity of killer Ts is just as targeted as an antibody.

4–18

Because T cells directly destroy antigens, this immunity is called cell-mediated. The antigens targeted by cytotoxic T cells include some bacteria, body cells that have been invaded by viruses, neoplastic or cancer cells, and transplantation cells. Another type of cytotoxic cell is the **natural killer T cell.** It is called natural because it appears no stimulation by antigen is required for it to act. The natural killer T cell is especially useful in looking for and destroying cells that have the potential to become cancerous. It is constantly on the lookout for cancer cells to destroy. This function is called **immune surveillance.**

TABLE 4–3. PROPERTIES OF IMMUNOGLOBULINS

	Location	Size	Function	Complement Fixation	Crosses Placenta
IgG	Body fluids (most abundant)	Single Ig molecule	Secondary response to antigen	Yes	Yes
IgM	Intravascular	Pentamer (5 Ig molecules)	Primary response to antigen	Yes	No
IgA	Seromucous secretions	Dimer (2 Ig molecules)	Antigen neutralization on mucous membrane surfaces	Classical—no Alternative—yes	No
IgE	Body fluids or on mast cells	Single Ig molecule	Cause allergies, response to parasites	No	No
IgD	Lymphocyte surface	Single Ig molecule	Antigen receptor?	No	No

4–19

There are two major regulator cells. The first is the **helper T cell.** As the name implies, it assists in several functions. It delivers information about an antigen to B cells. It does this by the release of several chemical mediators called **lymphokines.** The action of lymphokines helps B cells to transform into plasma cells and make antibody. Helper cell lymphokines act on macrophages, which phagocytize antigens, and play an important role with killer T cells (see Frame 4–24). These lymphokines also assist the activities of killer or cytotoxic T cells. There are proteins on the surface of helper T cells that have been named **CD4** proteins. **CD8** is the marker on both cytotoxic T cells and suppressor T cells. There are twice as many CD4 cells as CD8 cells and these numbers are the **CD4 to CD8 ratio.** In the disease AIDS, CD4 cells are greatly decreased. This creates less helping function, which affects B cells, killer T cells, and macrophages. It also leaves more suppressor cells, which decreases the immune response.

4–20

Suppressor T cells, as the name indicates, suppress or decrease the normal immune response. They are CD8 cells. CD8 cells tell the B cells to stop making antibody. This is a necessary function because the immune response must be controlled and stopped when it is appropriate. Recall from Chapter 2 that normal defense mechanisms can be a source of injury if they become uncontrolled. Suppressor T cells also are important in preventing antibodies directed against self, or autoantibodies. It is thought that a breakdown in this mechanism is partly responsible for autoimmune diseases. The relatively greater number of CD8 or suppressor cells that are present in AIDS contribute to the immune vulnerability of the patient.

4–21

The **macrophage,** which is so important in the inflammatory response as a scavenger, is also important in the immune response. The macrophage will phagocytize or ingest a recognized antigen very effectively. Once inside, the antigen is put through several chemical changes that break it down. This is called **antigen processing.** The processed antigen then resurfaces onto the macrophage outer membrane. The macrophage takes the altered antigen to a T cell for recognition. This stimulates the activities of the various kinds of T cells. This operation is called **antigen presentation** because the antigen is presented to T cells for destruction. Figures 4–3 and 4–4 illustrate the development, relationships, and function of immune cells.

4–22

The next several frames refer to events of humoral immunity. Once an antibody joins with an antigen, this forms an **immune complex.** It is a relatively large molecule that usually includes other parts, such as complement, as well as the antigen–antibody pair. The importance of the presence of an immune complex is that it triggers the remaining steps of the immune response. The goal, as you know, is destruction or elimination of harmful foreign material. Immune complexes can also trigger responses that we classify as diseases because the body is harmed. Here, once again, mechanisms designed to be protective can backfire.

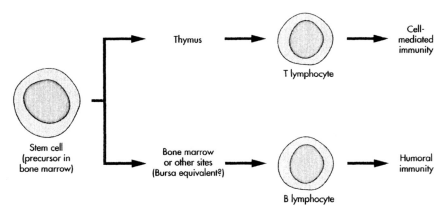

Figure 4–3. Development of immune cells.

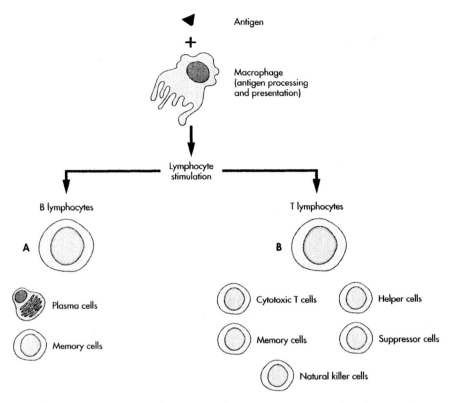

Figure 4–4. Relationship and function of immune cells. **A.** B lymphocytes. Plasma cells: antibodies (IgG, M, A, E, and D). Memory cells: anamnestic or secondary response. Antigens: bacteria, proteins, polysaccharides, haptens, viruses, toxins, parasites. **B.** T lymphocytes. Cytotoxic or killer cells: direct antigen destruction. Memory cells: anamnestic or secondary response. Natural killer cells. Helper cells. Suppressor cells. Antigens: intracellular bacteria, viruses, neoplastic (cancer) cells, transplanted cells, fungi, protozoa, parasites.

4–23

Agglutination is the clumping together of several antibodies and attached antigens. The antigens are solid particles, or are particulate. Examples are bacteria, which are single cell organisms, and red blood cells. This clumping is assisted by the fact that each IgG antibody has two binding sites and IgM has ten sites. This makes it easy to grab onto more than one antigen at a time. The value of agglutination is that it acts as an opsonin. Bacteria coated with or bound with antibody are more attractive to phagocytic cells. If the antigen is not solid matter, but is dissolved substance, the interaction with antibody is called **precipitation.** Another way to refer to this kind of antigen is to say it is soluble. Once antibody binds, the immune complex is now insoluble. It is no longer dissolved but now is a particle on which cells can act. **Neutralization** is the process by which antibodies combine and inactivate toxins from bacteria. This is the origin of the term **antitoxin.** Antibodies against circulating viruses, or antiviral antibodies, also work by neutralization. Figure 4–5 compares these interactions.

4–24

Our next subject is the effects of immune complex formation, which is complement activation and cell-mediated cytotoxicity. Frame 4–2 mentioned complement as part of the non-specific response. It is not directed against any particular antigen. It is stimulated classically by immune complexes. It is a system or series of nine plasma proteins. **Complement activation** is sometimes called the **complement cascade** because it is a series of reactions in sequence. Each reaction creates a product that goes on to create another product, and so forth. It is similar to setting up a formation of dominos and knocking them all down by knocking over the first one. By-products, or fragments, are also created that bring the total

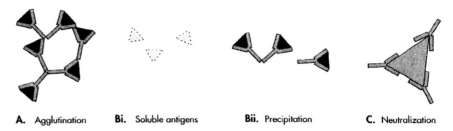

Figure 4–5. Antigen–antibody interactions. **A.** Agglutination–particles adhere or stick together. **Bi.** Soluble antigens. **Bii.** Precipitation–particles fall from solution. **C.** Neutralization–harmful effects are inactivated.

number of parts to 14. Three results of complement activation are cell lysis, binding of organisms to cells, and contributions to the inflammatory response.

Complement activation can take place through one of two pathways. Each pathway produces three separate parts or units. The **recognition unit** and the **activation unit** are different for each pathway. The **membrane attack unit** is the same for both. The units are various combinations of the nine proteins and their fragments. The classic pathway is stimulated by the presence of immune complexes (joined antibody and antigen). The units are made by the cleaving of the whole proteins into their active fragments. Cleaving means separate into two. The alternative pathway does not depend on immune complexes. It is started by chemicals such as toxins from some organisms. The final membrane attack unit is what binds to cell membranes and forms open channels or puncture sites. These holes cause the cell to lyse or burst open and be destroyed. An excellent example of cell lysis due to complement action is antibody-coated red blood cells destroyed during a mismatched blood transfusion. Please refer to Figure 4–6 for an overview of complement activation and its effects.

Additional consequences of complement involvement include the following.

1. Creation of **anaphylatoxin,** which are fragments that increase histamine release and vascular permeability.
2. **Immune adherence,** which is binding of complement to soluble immune complexes and then to cells. This helps in removal by phagocytosis. This is described as **opsonization.**
3. **Chemotaxis,** as mentioned earlier.
4. Activation of **kinins,** which are more chemical mediators that assist inflammation by chemotaxis and histamine release.

The last two topics of normal immunology deal with how cellular antigens come about and how they are recognized by immune cells. Realize that we are talking about *human body tissue* having proteins on their surfaces that are called antigens. We are not talking about foreign material and pathogens. Body tissue antigens are produced by the **major histocompatibility complex** or **MHC,** a set of genes located on chromosome 6. These genes control the expression of antigens on our cells that are considered "self" by immune cells. The term "major" refers to the reactions these antigens cause, which are very strong. This complex was first discovered in mice. It was also uncovered in humans by the demonstration of antibodies in serum that reacted against antigens on the surface of white blood cells. For this reason the MHC in people is often called the **HLA** system, which means **human leukocyte antigen.** The genes of the MHC produce the HLA. These products are specific proteins on cell surfaces that act as markers. When immune cells, especially T cells, come in contact with a cell, these markers are checked by interaction with T cell receptors. This process verifies if the suspect cell is self or non-self.

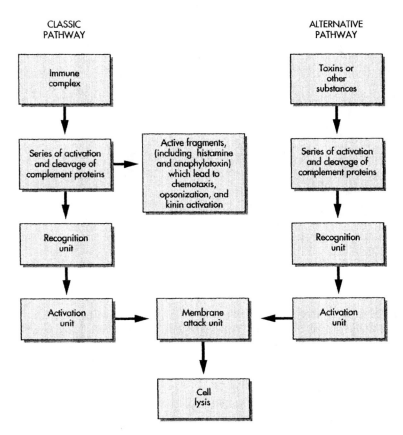

Figure 4–6. Complement activation.

4-28

The specific combination of genes for each person is called a **haplotype.** The set of genes making up a haplotype is inherited as a single unit. The genetics involved in this inheritance is why family members tend to match each other more closely than people from the general population. This similarity is why transplant success is greater among relatives than among unrelated individuals. There are three classes of MHC antigens. Only class I and II are important in transplant rejection so we will limit our discussion to those. Class I is widely distributed and is found on all nucleated cells of the body. These antigens are recognized or checked by cytotoxic or CD8 T cells. Class II is restricted mainly to B cells and macrophages. They are recognized by CD4 cells or helper T cells. They are important in the interactions that take place between these three cells during the immune response. The major histocompatibility complex is shown in Figure 4–7.

4-29

The reason for learning about the MHC is because of its use in transplantation. The word "histocompatibility" in MHC means "tissue match." The HLA antigens between donor and recipient must be matched as closely as possible. This matching process is often called **typing** and the kind of antigens present is the **type.** Immune cells will check the transplanted tissue for "self" or "non-self" classification. Strongly non-self tissue will be rejected very efficiently. If the recipient has many of the antigens that are present in the donor tissue, the graft may not be recognized as foreign. Because of the thousands of antigens and different combinations, there are degrees of matches. This means that the results could range anywhere from a perfect fit to barely close enough. Success of transplantation depends directly on the degree of the fit. This fit is often called **histocompatibility.** The ABO blood antigen system is like the MHC. ABO genes are responsible for the antigens on the surface of red blood cells (RBCs). When a blood transfusion is needed, these antigens must be matched between donor and recipient. For a transplant, ABO matching is also required because of the amount of blood present in the donor tissue.

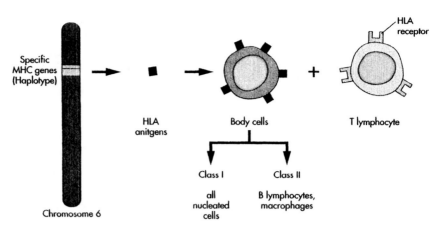

Figure 4–7. Major histocompatibility complex.

4-30

Another use for information on the MHC is the association of some diseases with a specific haplotype. In cases of **ankylosing spondylitis** the haplotype HLA B27 is often found. Ankylosing spondylitis is a disorder of the spinal column. It is a chronic joint disease of the vertebrae that results in stiffening and fusion of the spine. Certain haplotypes are often linked with type I diabetes mellitus, as well as other diseases. All this suggests that there is a genetic influence toward developing some disorders.

SECTION ▶ 11. HYPERSENSITIVITY

4-31

1. hypersensitivity
2. four

Normal immune function is a defensive action and neutralizes potentially harmful antigens. By definition, **hypersensitivity** is the same mechanism that causes harm to tissues during the course of the immune reaction. Hypersensitivity is a very good example of a protective mechanism that leads to damage. It is an over reaction of standard procedures. Hypersensitivity includes allergies but it is a more specific term since other hypersensitivities are different from allergies. This over response is classified into four types. Types I, II, and III are controlled by antibodies, or are a humoral response. Type IV is mediated by T cells. Immune responses that damage tissues are called _____(1). There are _____(2) different types of hypersensitivity.

▶ TYPE I HYPERSENSITIVITY

4-32

This is also called **anaphylactic-atopic allergy, IgE-mediated response,** and **immediate hypersensitivity.** Immediate refers to a quick reaction and IgE is the antibody involved. Atopy, allergy, and anaphylaxis are more common terms. Some sources say "allergy" should only be used in cases of IgE directed responses. The signs of type I are the signs of inflammation. Keep in mind that the events of inflammation and the elimination of antigen by antibody are closely related. Recall that exudation brings antibodies to the scene (see Chap. 2). Type I is like inflammation because vasoactive chemicals (inflammatory mediators) are released from cells. These substances include histamine and **slow-reacting substance of anaphylaxis (SRS-A).** Only some people react to the antigens that cause allergy. These antigens are called **allergens.** The immune response to allergens is not universal, as it is for other antigens such as foreign protein. This predisposition to react to allergens is probably genetic. These individuals produce IgE instead of IgG. The timing of type I hypersensitivity is _____(1). The antibody responsible for type I is _____(2). The signs of type I look like _____(3). The two processes, _____(4) and _____(5), are closely linked because of the release of _____(6) chemicals. Antigens in type I hypersensitivity are called _____(7) and the tendency to react to them is probably due to _____(8).

1. immediate
2. IgE
3. inflammation
4. type I hypersensitivity
5. inflammation
6. vasoactive
7. allergens
8. genetics

4–33

People who are genetically programmed to have *local* reactions to allergens are **atopic** and the condition is **atopy.** The most commonly known atopy is **allergic rhinitis** or hay fever. Rhinitis is inflammation of the nasal passages or the nose, even though hay fever also affects the eyes. The tissues of the nasal passages are the site of the reactions. The allergens are environmental and include plant pollens, animal dander, and dust. **Asthma** (see Chap. 11) is atopy to environmental allergens that affect the bronchi, or air passages, in the lungs. The reactions of allergy are a primary and secondary response. When the allergen is first contacted, IgE is formed and it attaches primarily to mast cells (and other cells). This is the sensitization stage. The secondary response begins when the IgE–mast cell complex meets the allergen again. The interaction between the cell bound IgE and allergen sends the signal to the mast cell to **degranulate.** This means the tiny sacs or **granules** in the cytoplasm break open. The granules contain the chemicals. Histamine is released and has the same inflammatory effects that you studied in Chapter 2. The inflammation and edema are responsible for the signs of hay fever. Figure 4–8 illustrates the primary and secondary responses of type I hypersensitivity. Genetically influenced local reactions to allergens are called _____(1). A very common form of atopy is hay fever or _____(2). Hay fever allergens are not pathogens but come from the _____(3). During the primary response to an allergen, _____(4) is produced. It binds to _____(5) cells. In the secondary phase, further contact causes mast cells to release chemicals when they _____(6). The signs of hay fever are due to the effects of the chemical _____(7).

1. atopy
2. allergic rhinitis
3. environment
4. IgE
5. mast
6. degranulate
7. histamine

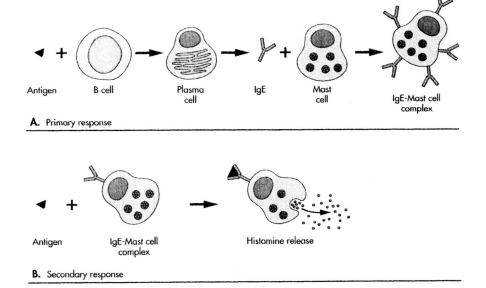

Figure 4–8. Type I hypersensitivity (anaphylactic–atopic allergy). **A.** Primary response–first exposure to antigen. **B.** Secondary response–next exposure to antigen.

4-34

1. urticaria
2. pruritus
3. site

Other kinds of local type I reactions are caused by some drugs and some foods. These do not involve the nasal passages. Food and drug allergies can cause reactions in the skin. **Urticaria** is a commonly known sign and is hives. Often along with hives is itching or **pruritus.** Food allergies can also affect the gastrointestinal system through cramps and diarrhea. The mechanisms are all the same as allergic rhinitis. The difference is the site or place of reaction (skin or gut). The medical term for hives is _____(1). The term for itching is _____(2). The difference between hay fever and other local allergies is the _____(3) of reaction.

4-35

1. Atopy
2. anaphylaxis
3. fatal
4. body

Atopy is local allergy and **anaphylaxis** is systemic allergy. Anaphylaxis is from the Greek meaning "against" ("ana") and "protection" ("phylaxis"). This is the most severe example of a protective function turning against the body. True anaphylaxis is easily fatal if not treated aggressively. The vasoactive substances exert their effects on several systems. Imagine the events of inflammation throughout the body. Persons who are anaphylactic have extreme effects to small doses of allergens. The common allergens to cause this are some drugs like penicillin and insect stings from bees or wasps. Some foods such as strawberries affect susceptible individuals this way. *Any* substance injected into the bloodstream has the potential to cause anaphylaxis. _____(1) is local allergy and _____(2) is systemic allergy. Anaphylaxis which is not treated can be _____(3). Vasoactive chemicals affect the whole _____(4).

4-36

1. edema
2. hypo
3. permeability
4. edema
5. hypotension
6. heart
7. circulatory
8. respiratory
9. laryngeal
10. bronco
11. dyspnea

In anaphylaxis, the chemical mediators of inflammation and allergy, especially histamine, cause great increases in capillary permeability. The fluid loss into the tissues can be tremendous. From previous chapters you know that excess fluid in the tissues is called _____(1). The decreased intravascular fluid creates decreased blood pressure which is _____(2) tension (see Chap. 3). This low blood pressure, or hypotension, leads to decreased output from the heart and shock. Circulatory failure can be one cause of death. The events of anaphylaxis are often called **anaphylactic shock.** Two other fatal possibilities are laryngeal edema and bronchospasm. In humans the anaphylactic shock organ, or the system most quickly affected, is the respiratory system. The smooth muscle around the bronchi of the lungs contract in response to chemical mediators. This closes down the air passages and causes **dyspnea,** or very difficult breathing. Edema builds to dangerous amounts in the larynx and can shut down this part of the air passages completely. It is this internal suffocation that is most recognized as anaphylaxis, and affected individuals need emergency intervention to survive. Figure 4–9 outlines these events. Anaphylactic shock begins with massive increase in capillary _____(3) which causes fluid loss in the tissues or _____(4). This loss creates low blood pressure or _____(5), which in turn causes decreased output from the _____(6). Failure of the _____(7) system results in death. Other fatal effects involve the _____(8) system and is seen as _____(9) edema and _____(10) spasm. Both of these events cause difficulty in breathing or _____(11).

▶ TYPE II HYPERSENSITIVITY

4-37

This is also called **cytotoxic hypersensitivity** or **antibody-dependent cell-mediated cytotoxicity** (ADCC). The destruction of antigens results in lysis of cells carrying the antigens. It is called antibody dependent because first antibody must bind to the antigens on the cell membranes and this is the signal for destruction. There are two mechanisms that lead to cell lysis. In the first mechanism the events are the following.

1. An antigen (such as a drug) binds to blood cells or the antigen is already present on cell membranes. The most common example of this is a transfusion of incompatible blood cells into a patient.

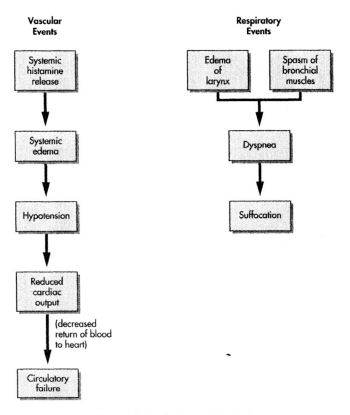

Figure 4-9. Events of anaphylactic shock.

2. The corresponding antibody will attach to the antigen.
3. This antigen–antibody complex activates complement through the classic pathway.
4. The cell is lysed or destroyed by the complement membrane attack unit.

Type II hypersensitivity can occur with the first exposure to the antigen. In other words, there may not be a need for the primary response to be followed by the secondary response. This would be in cases where the host already has the antibody, such as a mismatched blood transfusion. Type II hypersensitivity is called _____(1) cell-mediated cytotoxicity because the message for destruction is started when _____(2) binds to the _____(3) on the cell _____(4). The first type II mechanism involves activation of _____(5) once the _____(6) complex is formed. The targeted cell is lysed by the complement _____(7).

1. antibody-dependent
2. antibody
3. antigen
4. membrane
5. complement
6. antigen–antibody
7. membrane attack unit

4-38

The second type II mechanism events are as follows.

1. Antibody complexes with the cell membrane antigen.
2. Complement is *not* activated. Instead, the complex acts as a chemotaxin and phagocytic WBCs are drawn to the area.
3. The WBCs recognize the foreignness of the antigen–antibody complex.
4. The WBCs directly cause cell lysis or the coated cell is destroyed by phagocytosis.

1. complement
2. WBCs
3. chemotoxin
4. WBCs
5. lysis
6. phagocytosis

Figure 4-10 illustrates the types of responses in type II hypersensitivity. The difference between this type II mechanism and the first mechanism is _____(1) is not activated. Instead _____(2) are drawn to the area by the complex, which acts as a _____(3). The targeted cells are destroyed by the _____(4) through cell _____(5) or by _____(6).

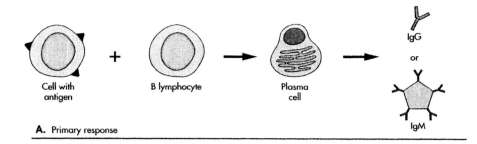

A. Primary response

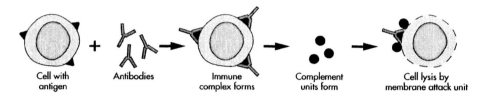

B. Secondary response - Complement activation

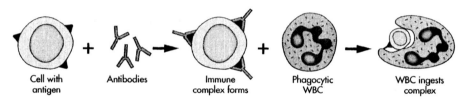

C. Secondary response - Phagocytosis

Figure 4–10. Type II hypersensitivity (antibody-dependent cell-mediated cytotoxicity). **A.** Primary response—first exposure to antigen (sensitization). **B.** Secondary response and complement activation—next exposure to antigen. **C.** Secondary response and phagocytosis.

4-39

One kind of type II hypersensitivity is related to incompatible blood transfusions. It is **hemolytic disease of the newborn** or **HDN.** The **RH** or **D** antigen on the RBC membranes is the culprit. If a mother is D negative (does not have the D antigen) and her fetus is D positive (has the antigen), HDN will occur. It is like a mismatched transfusion except here the "transfused" blood is blood that comes from the fetus and enters into the mother's circulation. It enters through the circulatory system of the placenta. The mother becomes sensitized when the D cells first enter her blood. This relatively large sensitizing dose takes place when the placenta separates and bleeds during delivery. She responds by making anti-D antibody. There are no ill effects on this first incompatible child because it has already been born. However, if she has another Rh positive baby, the secondary or anamnestic response "remembers" the D antigen and makes a great deal of anti-D. The secondary response takes place before birth because a few times during pregnancy there are small amounts of mingling of blood between the mother and fetus. This is called a **fetomaternal bleed** and is normal. But if the mother was previously sensitized, this small amount is more than enough to produce anti-D quickly. This now creates danger for the unborn child. Maternal anti-D enters the baby's circulation and begins to destroy the RBCs. In severe cases, the baby can become very anemic to the point of **hydrops fetalis.** Some sources call this **erythroblastosis fetalis.** In hydrops fetalis the severe anemia can cause congestive heart failure and death. If the baby survives until birth the immediate danger is brain damage due to **kernicterus.** This is the buildup of bilirubin in brain neurons. Bilirubin is a breakdown product of destroyed RBCs and the unprocessed form is toxic to tissue cells. The liver must process the bilirubin and make it harmless but the newborn liver is not very good at this. Severe cases require an **exchange transfusion** that instills an entirely new supply of blood into the baby without the antibody or the bilirubin.

4–40

In hemolytic disease of the newborn, the antigen causing the reaction is _____(1). The mother _____(2) has / does not have (choose one) the antigen. The baby _____(3) has / does not have (choose one) the antigen. At delivery there is a large mingling of incompatible baby blood with the mother. This mixing together is called a _____(4). This large fetomaternal bleed causes the mother to become _____(5) as part of the primary response. By this we mean she makes _____(6), that is directed at the baby's RBCs. The next incompatible child (_____(7) positive) creates a _____(8) response in the mother when there are small bleeds during pregnancy. The secondary response creates large amounts of anti-D that quickly enter the baby's circulation and destroy the baby's _____(9). This destruction can cause severe anemia before birth. The events of anemia that cause heart failure and death are called _____(10) or _____(11). After birth, the concern is the large amounts of _____(12) which can build up in the tissues. When this happens in the brain cells it is called _____(13) and can result in permanent _____(14) damage.

1. Rh or D
2. does not have
3. has
4. fetomaternal bleed
5. sensitized
6. anti-D
7. Rh or D
8. secondary
9. RBCs
10. hydrops fetalis
11. erythroblastosis fetalis
12. bilirubin
13. kernicterus
14. brain

▶ TYPE III HYPERSENSITIVITY

4–41

Type III hypersensitivity is also known as **immune complex-mediated hypersensitivity** or **Arthus-type hypersensitivity.** In this condition antigens are circulating free in the bloodstream and antibodies bind to them. For some reason these complexes then lodge in vessel walls. Complement binds to the complex as it sticks to the inside of the vessel. Activation of complement and resulting destruction causes damage to the tissue there, specifically to the endothelial cells. Endothelial cells make up the lining of vessels. This complex attachment and immune-mediated destruction creates a fairly severe local inflammation. This is known as **acute vasculitis,** which describes inflammation of a blood vessel. This vasculitis often causes local necrosis of the walls of arterioles and capillaries, as shown in Figure 4–11. Because blood supply is interrupted, the tissue supplied by the vessel can suffer ischemia. Another contributing factor is that these complexes are chemotactic to WBCs, especially the complement portion. When WBCs arrive and begin to do their job, the release of lytic enzymes from their lysosomes further injures the area. These complexes can also activate blood factors that cause coagulation. Small **thrombi** formation (clots) can lead to **thrombosis,** which is the blockage of small vessels by clots. Thrombosis is another means for ischemia to develop. Refer to Figure 4–12 for an illustration of these events. Immune complex-mediated hypersensitivity occurs when _____(1) that are in the circulation are bound by _____(2). This forms a complex that _____(3) to _____(4) walls. The lining cells of the vessels, which are _____(5) cells, are injured when complement is activated to destroy the antigen. The inflammation in the vessels is called _____(6). This inflammation or vasculitis can interfere with local blood supply and cause _____(7) of the tissue that is fed by the vessel. Two more factors that add to the damage are the release of lytic _____(8) from _____(9) that were drawn to the area, and possible activation of _____(10) factors. This activation can lead to clot formation or _____(11). If the clots block the vessel this is called _____(12). The blockage, or thrombosis, can make the ischemia worse.

1. antigens
2. antibodies
3. attaches
4. vessel
5. endothelial
6. acute vasculitis
7. ischemia
8. enzymes
9. WBCs
10. coagulation
11. thrombi
12. thrombosis

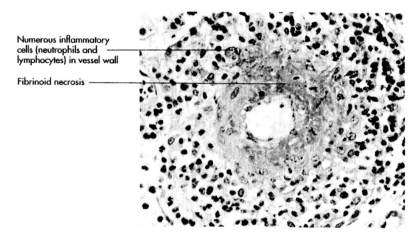

Numerous inflammatory
cells (neutrophils and
lymphocytes) in vessel wall

Fibrinoid necrosis

Figure 4–11. Necrotizing vasculitis involving small vessels—typical of immune complex injury. *(From Chandrasoma and Taylor, Concise Pathology, 2nd ed., Appleton & Lange.)*

4–42

1. glomerulonephritis
2. Group A streptococci
3. local
4. immune complex

Type III immune injury can be localized or systemic. It is not known why only certain sites in the body attract these complexes to attach. Joints are one local site of attachment and injury. Another fairly common place is in the kidneys, in the capillary bed of the glomeruli. The inflammation there is called **glomerulonephritis** (inflammation of the glomeruli in the nephron). Figure 4–13 is a tissue picture taken with an electron microscope that shows immune complexes deposited along the basement of a glomerular capillary. A common reason for immune complex deposits in the glomeruli is infection with Group A streptococcus. Generally it is associated with "strep throat." Group A streptococcus will be discussed in Chapter 5 on infectious disease. Ischemic damage from kidney vasculitis is the main injury. Inflammation of the capillary bed in the nephron of the kidney is called _____(1). It is often associated with infections by _____(2). Streptococcal glomerulonephritis is an example of _____(3) local / systemic (choose one) type III _____(4) mediated hypersensitivity.

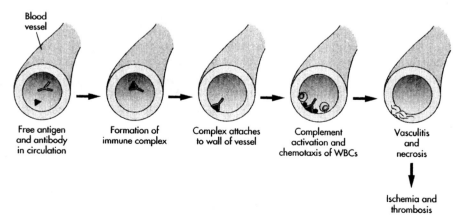

Blood vessel

Free antigen and antibody in circulation → Formation of immune complex → Complex attaches to wall of vessel → Complement activation and chemotaxis of WBCs → Vasculitis and necrosis → Ischemia and thrombosis

Figure 4–12. Type III hypersensitivity (immune complex-mediated hypersensitivity).

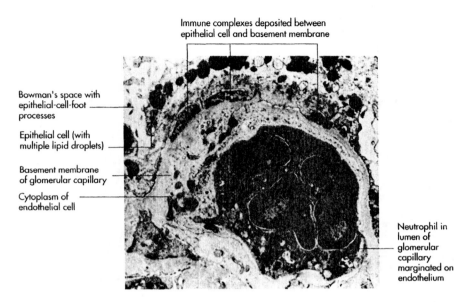

Immune complexes deposited between
epithelial cell and basement membrane

Bowman's space with
epithelial-cell-foot
processes

Epithelial cell (with
multiple lipid droplets)

Basement membrane
of glomerular capillary

Cytoplasm of
endothelial cell

Neutrophil in
lumen of
glomerular
capillary
marginated on
endothelium

Figure 4–13. Electron micrograph of a small area of glomerular capillary, showing electron-dense immune complexes deposited in the area between the basement membrane and the epithelial cell. These immune complexes contain antigen, IgG, and fixed complement factors. *(From Chandrasoma and Taylor,* Concise Pathology, *2nd ed., Appleton & Lange.)*

▷ TYPE IV HYPERSENSITIVITY

4–43

The final class of hypersensitivity, type IV, is also known as **delayed cell-mediated hypersensitivity.** Some sources call this **tuberculin hypersensitivity.** The first three types were mediated by soluble (dissolved in the blood) antibody and recruited the help of polymorphonuclear WBCs. Type IV is directed only by cells, mainly the T lymphocytes and also the macrophages. The mechanism is just like the normal response of these cells to foreign antigens (see Fig. 4–14). Type IV is called delayed because it takes at least 12 hours to develop and usually up to 48 hours. The site of immune destructive activity is the skin where the antigen enters the body in small amounts. Therefore this is where the injury is seen. Inflammation, sometimes severe, is caused by the activity of T cells, macrophages, and the chemical mediators released by both cells. Histological examination of the tissue demonstrates some necrosis of the inflamed tissue and infiltration by lymphocytes and macrophages. Type IV hypersensitivity is called delayed because reactions can take as long as _____(1) hours to be seen. The difference between type IV and the first three types is the activity is directed only by _____(2) and not by _____(3) and PMNs. The cells of type IV reactions are _____(4) and _____(5). The site of immune injury is the _____(6). The injury itself is _____(7). Some tissue death or _____(8) can be seen microscopically.

1. 48
2. cells
3. antibodies
4. T lymphocytes
5. macrophages
6. skin
7. inflammation
8. necrosis

4–44

The mechanism of type IV hypersensitivity is just like the antigen destruction that occurs in tuberculosis infection, viral infection, fungal infections, and parasite infestations. The inflammation in these cases is often chronic. Because of this the kind of inflammation is classified as granulomatous. The necrosis that goes along with the inflammation is caseous. If you will stretch your memory back to Chapter 2, you may recall features of granulomatous inflammation and caseous necrosis. In granulomatous inflammation the localized swelling is called a _____(1). That area is loaded with _____(2) and _____(3) lymphocytes. The kind of necrosis produced is _____(4). Caseous necrosis is firm and has a _____(5) consistency.

1. granuloma
2. macrophages
3. T
4. caseous
5. cheesy

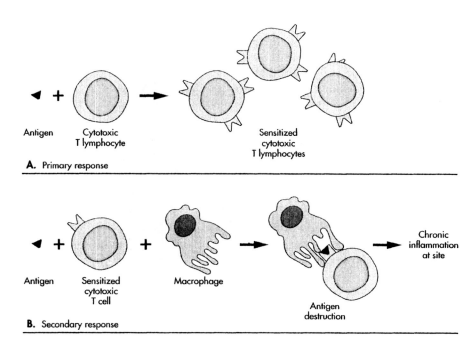

Figure 4–14. Type IV hypersensitivity (delayed cell-mediated hypersensitivity). **A.** Primary response—first exposure or sensitization to antigen. **B.** Secondary response—next exposure or anamnestic response.

4-45

1. inflammation
2. type IV
3. contact dermatitis
4. type IV

The characteristic reaction of type IV hypersensitivity forms the basis for the **TB test.** If a person has been exposed to the tuberculosis bacteria, a local nodule is formed at the site of injection of TB bacilli. The nodule formation is called a **tuberculin reaction,** which is why type IV is sometimes called tuberculin hypersensitivity. Since tuberculosis causes a characteristic type IV skin reaction, the TB test is fairly reliable. In addition to the TB test, other reactions that are type IV hypersensitivities include the rejection of transplants. A broad category of type IV reactions is **contact dermatitis.** You will often see this called allergic contact dermatitis. However if you go with the guideline of restricting allergy to IgE reactions, it should be called contact dermatitis. There are many examples of this category. Poison ivy and poison oak are two plant antigens that commonly cause contact dermatitis. (You should be able to define "dermatitis" as meaning _____(1) of the skin. Contact means the antigen has touched the skin.) Other antigens that cause contact dermatitis are as variable as the susceptibility of each person. Culprits identified include soaps and laundry detergents, perfumes, jewelry, dyes, plastics, chemically treated clothing, and more. The lesions on the skin range from slightly red to itchy, blistering areas with edema. Transplant rejections are _____(2) hypersensitivities. Inflammation of the skin caused by antigens on the skin is best called _____(3). This is also _____(4) hypersensitivity.

4-46

Table 4–4 compares the features of hypersensitivity reactions. This should help you to recall what you have learned about the four types. There are several immune injury conditions that don't fall neatly into one of the four categories you have just learned. Some conditions may be a combination of the different mechanisms. Autoimmune diseases are most likely not to be a specific classification. In closing this section let's compare some features of hypersensitivity with normal immune reaction. *Hypersensitivity:*

1. Affects only some people, so genetics probably plays a part.
2. The immune response causes tissue damage while eliminating the antigen.
3. The dose of antigen is not related to the severity of reaction. This means a small dose causes just as much reaction as a larger dose.
4. Antigens may not be pathogens, but a normal part of the environment.

TABLE 4–4. A COMPARISON OF THE FEATURES OF HYPERSENSITIVITY

	Mechanism	Mediator	Injury	Antigen Site
Type I	IgE–mast cell complex degranulation, histamine release	IgE	Local inflammation (atopy), systemic inflammation (anaphylaxis)	Atopy–respiratory passages, anaphylaxis–systemic
Type II	Antibody complexes with antigen on cell surface, complement activation	IgG or IgM	Cell lysis or phagocytosis	Circulation
Type III	Immune complex deposits in vessel walls	IgG or IgM	Necrotizing vasculitis, ischemia	Circulation, blood vessel walls
Type IV	Direct antigen destruction by immune cells	Cytotoxic T cells, macrophages	Chronic inflammation (granulomatous)	Skin

In contrast, *normal immune reaction:*

1. Affects all people the same way (everyone reacts the same way to the antigens).
2. The immune response is protective (destroys antigen) and doesn't cause tissue injury.
3. The degree of reaction depends on the amount of antigen present (it is directly proportional).
4. Antigens are usually pathogens or foreign substances in the bloodstream.

A protective immune response made by all people against a pathogen is _____(1) immune reaction. A damaging response made by only some people against an environmental substance is _____(2).

1. normal
2. hypersensitivity

II. REVIEW QUESTIONS

1. Hypersensitivity can be BEST described as:
   a. immune function that eliminates potentially harmful antigens
   b. immune function that causes injury to host tissues
   c. immune function that is uncontrolled
   d. immune function that is absent in most people

2. Hypersensitivity directed by lymphocytes, not antibodies is:
   a. type I
   b. type II
   c. type III
   d. type IV

3. Hypersensitivity directed by IgE antibody is:
   a. type I
   b. type II
   c. type III
   d. type IV

4. Type I hypersensitivity is also known as:
   a. antibody-dependent cell-mediated cytotoxicity
   b. delayed cell-mediated hypersensitivity
   c. immune complex-mediated hypersensitivity
   d. anaphylactic-atopic allergy

1. b–immune function that causes injury to host tissues

2. d–type IV

3. a–type I

4. d–anaphylactic–atopic allergy

5. a–allergic rhinitis

6. c–systemic allergy

7. c–cell lysis after complement activation

8. b–ADCC type II hypersensitivity

9. a–endothelial cell damage

10. false

11. d–antigens make surface contact with the skin

12. b–T lymphocytes and macrophages

13. a–granulomatous

5. A common example of local atopy is:
   a. allergic rhinitis
   b. autoimmune hemolytic anemia
   c. glomerulonephritis
   d. contact dermatitis

6. Anaphylaxis is:
   a. localized acute vasculitis
   b. local allergy
   c. systemic allergy
   d. granulomatous inflammation

7. One mechanism of destruction of antigens in type II hypersensitivity or ADCC is:
   a. mast cell degranulation
   b. phagocytosis by lymphocytes
   c. cell lysis after complement activation
   d. granuloma formation

8. Hemolytic disease of the newborn is an example of:
   a. systemic allergy type I hypersensitivity
   b. ADCC type II hypersensitivity
   c. delayed cell-mediated type IV hypersensitivity
   d. immune complex type III hypersensitivity

9. Tissue injury caused by type III hypersensitivity results from:
   a. endothelial cell damage
   b. mast cell degranulation
   c. inflammation of the skin
   d. cell lysis

10. True or false: In type III immune complex hypersensitivity, the PRIMARY injury to tissues is thrombosis and ischemia. _____

11. Type IV delayed cell-mediated hypersensitivity is usually a skin reaction because:
   a. free antigens in the circulation are bound by antibody and these complexes attach to the skin
   b. the skin is the "shock organ" in humans for this kind of hypersensitivity
   c. antigens enter through the nasal passages and migrate to the skin through the circulation
   d. antigens make surface contact with the skin

12. Cells involved in type IV hypersensitivity are:
   a. B lymphocytes and macrophages
   b. T lymphocytes and macrophages
   c. B lymphocytes and PMNs
   d. T lymphocytes and PMNs

13. The chronic inflammation in type IV reactions is:
   a. granulomatous
   b. caseous
   c. coagulative
   d. none of the above

14. A *common* example of type IV hypersensitivity is:
    a. tuberculosis
    b. allergic rhinitis
    c. serum sickness
    d. contact dermatitis

14. d–contact dermatitis

III. IMMUNODEFICIENCY ◀ SECTION

4-47

Immunodeficiency is that part of immune activity described as "under responsive." Hypersensitivity is described as _____(1) responsive. **Anergy** is a word sometimes used to mean immunodeficiency. Anergy is a poor response or no response to antigens. It means the opposite of anamnestic, which is a vigorous response. **Immunosuppression** is another term that can be used, since it means the immune system is prevented from normal response.

1. over

▶ NONSPECIFIC IMMUNOSUPPRESSION

4-48

There are several causes for the immune system to be depressed. The first is **iatrogenic immunosuppression.** This is depression of the immune response by steroids or other drugs. A common reason for intentionally suppressing this system with drugs is transplantation. Immune destruction needs to be kept under control so a transplant is not rejected. Steroids work well since they decrease immune response in several ways. Medical terms for steroids are **glucocorticoid** and **corticosteroid.** They are named after the body's natural steroid, **cortisol.** Cortisol is made by the adrenal cortex. Commonly used steroids are prednisone, prednisolone, and dexamethasone. The immune suppressing function of steroids is dose related. At lower doses, steroids decrease inflammation. At higher doses the same drug goes beyond decreasing inflammation to immune suppression. Other drugs that do the same thing are **cytotoxic** drugs like cyclophosphamide and cyclosporine. Cyclophosphamide is a cancer chemotherary and cyclosporine is used in transplants. These drugs interfere with T cell activity. In transplant rejection therapy, cytotoxic drugs must be given for the life of the patient. If not, T cells bounce back and may reject the transplant. Cancer chemotherapy is a very common immunosuppressant but that is not the intent. It is an unfortunate side effect. The drugs, and procedures like **irradiation,** can kill healthy lymphoid tissue along with cancer cells. Whether for transplant success or cancer treatment, the effect on the patient is increased susceptibility to infections. Patients must be closely monitored for any indication of infection and treated immediately and aggressively. ("Aggressive" treatment refers to the potency of a drug, the route of administration, and length of treatment.) Two common uses for iatrogenic immunosuppression are to increase the success of a _____(1) and to try to eliminate _____(2). A class of drug similar to natural body steroid is called _____(3) or _____(4). Steroids will decrease either _____(5) or function of the _____(6) system depending on the _____(7). Drugs that prevent T cell activity are called _____(8) drugs. The most important consideration in iatrogenic immunosuppression is that the patient is _____(9) to _____(10).

1. transplant
2. cancer
3. glucocorticoids
4. corticosteroids
5. inflammation
6. immune
7. dose
8. cytotoxic
9. susceptible
10. infection

4-49

Other immunosuppression is naturally occurring. In elderly people the ability to mount an immune response diminishes with time. Levels of antibodies can be decreased because of poor production. In malnutrition the protein necessary for antibody production can be lacking, also causing low antibody levels. Lower than normal antibody levels are called **hypogammaglobulinemia.** These conditions are not severe in themselves but can add to existing problems. Premature babies, while having some passive protection from the

1. hypogammaglobulinemia
2. fighting
3. secondary

mother, are at risk for infection because of poorly functioning immune systems. People who have an infectious illness are **immunologically challenged,** which means that their immune system is very active in fighting the disease. Since any resource is limited there comes a point where, if a second infection should occur, it could overwhelm the system and make the patient much sicker. Besides a primary illness, cancer can also cause this scenario. Especially cancers involving the blood cells (leukemia) or lymphoid tissue (lymphomas). Immunosuppression associated with age or malnutrition is due to low antibody levels called _____(1). The idea of being immunologically challenged means that the immune system is _____(2) against an existing disease. If another disease agent should challenge the immune system a _____(3) disease could develop.

▶ INHERITED IMMUNODEFICIENCY

------- 4-50 --

1. antibody
2. hypoplasia
3. agammaglobulinemia
4. newborns or babies
5. fatal
6. infection

An **immunodeficiency** implies there is something inadequate about the immune system itself. This is different from being suppressed by outside factors. Inherited deficiencies are genetic defects which are **congenital,** or present at birth. Inherited immunodeficiencies are not common but are often fatal early in life. These babies are extremely vulnerable to infection by pathogens and even nonpathogens. There are two kinds of deficiencies. The first involves the B lymphocytes. There seems to be **hypoplasia** (underdevelopment) of the lymphoid tissue that produces B cells. Since B cells make antibodies, the resulting problem is lack of antibodies or immunoglobulins. The levels are much lower than the hypogammaglobulinemia state we discussed in the last frame. With very few B cells the antibody level is extremely low to almost nonexistent. This is called **agammaglobulinemia.** (The prefix "a" means without.) B lymphocyte immunodeficiency is a defect in humoral immunity. It is considered a **sex-linked** genetic condition because it occurs in male babies. Since humoral immunity is responsible for controlling most bacteria, it is bacterial infections that plague these individuals. Pneumonia is commonly seen. The signs of this condition (one severe infection after another) develop when passive immunity from the mother wears off, usually around 3 to 6 months of age. Inherited immunodeficiency can involve B lymphocytes, which make _____(1). Lack of B cells appears to be related to _____(2) of lymphoid tissue. Extremely low antibody levels are called _____(3). The population this condition appears in are _____(4). The condition is often _____(5) early in life. Death occurs from recurring _____(6). Mechanisms of inherited immunodeficiency are summarized in Figure 4–15.

------- 4-51 --

1. T lymphocytes
2. B
3. plasma
4. antibodies
5. thymus
6. severe combined immunodeficiency

The other kind of deficiency is a defect in cellular immunity. You should know that this must mean there is a lack of _____(1). Babies with this condition have **thymic hypoplasia** so T cells are not processed as they should be. The kinds of infections in these cases are related to the protection cellular immunity is supposed to give. These infections are by viruses, fungi, protozoans, and some intracellular bacteria. The odd thing about T lymphocyte deficiency is it often causes B cell problems as well. If helper T cells are lacking, as they often are, there will be a deficiency of immunoglobulin as well. Remember helper T cells stimulate _____(2) cells and assist them to change into _____(3) cells. Plasma cells then make _____(4). So you can see the relationship here. Lack of T cell function also causes lack of B cell function. When there is definite involvement of both sides of the immune response (B or humoral and T or cellular) this is called **severe combined immunodeficiency** or **SCID.** Cases of SCID experience more severe infections more often and this condition is fatal sooner than just humoral deficiency or cell-mediated deficiency. T lymphocyte deficiency is seen in cases of underdevelopment of the _____(5). When both humoral and cellular immunity are insufficient, the combination is called _____(6).

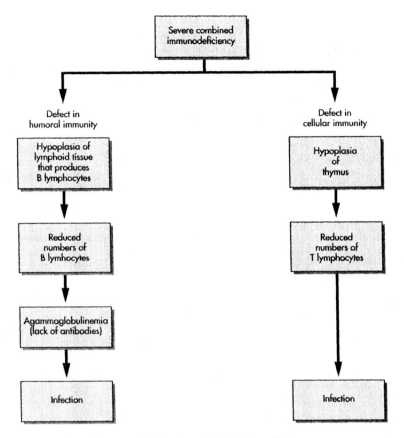

Figure 4–15. Mechanisms of inherited immunodeficiency.

▶ ACQUIRED IMMUNODEFICIENCY

4–52

Acquired immunodeficiency means that the condition is not inborn but developed later due to outside factors. By far the most common and significant condition is **acquired immunodeficiency syndrome** or **AIDS.** This is a viral disease that destroys the immune system. The presence of AIDS shows us the tremendous importance of the daily work and protection of the immune system. The virus does not attack organs like the liver or heart. Instead it wipes out immune protection, and death is secondary to unusual infections. These infections are often caused by organisms we come into contact with every day. But without the immune system, these same opportunistic organisms are able to easily cause death. From this you should be able to appreciate the role of constant vigilance played by humoral and cellular immunity. The virus is **human immunodeficiency virus** or **HIV-I.** There is a related strain, **HIV-II.** HIV-II is still primarily confined to some parts of Africa. Understand the difference between having HIV and having AIDS. Having HIV is testing positive for antibodies to the HIV antigen (the virus). A positive HIV test means the virus has entered the body. The individual is not sick. Having AIDS means the infection with the virus has progressed to the point of clinical signs. The person is unable to remain healthy. In most cases other infections and wasting progress to death. The medical definition of AIDS is the presence of specific kinds of infections or unusual cancers in a person who is HIV positive. AIDS stands for _____(1). HIV stands for _____(2). The target of destruction for the HIV virus is the _____(3). Death results from unusual _____(4) caused by opportunistic _____(5). AIDS is medically defined as the presence of _____(6) or _____(7) in a _____(8) person.

1. acquired immunodeficiency syndrome
2. human immunodeficiency virus
3. immune system
4. infection
5. organisms
6. specific infections
7. unusual cancers
8. HIV positive

4–53

1. pneumocystis
2. pneumonia
3. Kaposi's sarcoma
4. protozoa
5. normal people
6. disease
7. endothelial
8. blood vessels

AIDS was first identified in the early 1980s in young, otherwise healthy, homosexual men. These men were dying of strange infections or rare cancers. Pneumonia caused by **pneumocystis** or cancer called **Kaposi's sarcoma** was most commonly the cause of death. Pneumocystis is a protozoa that can be found in the respiratory tract of most normal people and does not cause disease because of normal immune response. Kaposi's sarcoma is a rare cancer of the endothelial cells of blood vessels. The presence of these two disorders formed the basis of the early definition of AIDS. Tracing back clues to the origin, it is believed that the virus originated in Africa and spread among specific populations until it reached the United States. Other populations identified with the disease included drug addicts who used needles, hemophiliacs who received blood-based treatments, and the sex partners of these groups. These populations emerged because of the way HIV is transmitted. Today, any population is at risk and includes heterosexual men, women, and babies. AIDS was first identified in homosexual men who had infections with _____(1), which caused _____(2). A rare cancer called _____(3) was also identified. Pneumocystis is a _____(4) found in most _____(5) and does not cause _____(6). Kaposi's sarcoma is cancer of the _____(7) cells of _____(8).

4–54

1. blood
2. semen
3. openings
4. mucous
5. wounds
6. body fluids

HIV is transmitted in body fluids. The virus has been recovered from many kinds of fluids but it is generally agreed infectivity is confined to the blood and semen. The virus does not penetrate intact skin. It enters natural body openings such as the genital tract or can enter through other mucosal surfaces. The presence of even a microscopic tear or wound in the skin or any mucosa can be a port of entry. Since such wounds may not be known, body surfaces contacting the fluid of another person should be protected. Specific examples of transmission are sexual contact, shared needles, perinatal (mother to baby), blood products (transfusions, Factor VIII for hemophiliacs), and unprotected contact with infected fluids by a health care worker. It has never been shown that HIV is transmitted by casual contact (kissing, hugging), airborne routes, or fomites (objects in a household like dishes, toilets, food). Therefore living with an HIV positive person is in itself not considered a risk. However, note that objects like a razor or toothbrush, which might contain blood should *never* be shared. HIV is primarily transmitted through two body fluids, _____(1) and _____(2). HIV enters the body through natural _____(3) that are lined with _____(4) membranes. It may also gain entry through _____(5). Transmission of the virus is only by direct contact with _____(6) that are known to be infective, such as blood and semen.

4–55

The way AIDS develops, or the pathogenesis, is by destruction of helper T lymphocytes as shown in Figure 4–16. The virus binds to the CD4 proteins on the T cell surfaces. It enters and replicates inside the cell. HIV kills the cell when virus numbers reach a certain concentration and it buds out of the T4 lymphocyte. The virus proceeds to other T4 lymphocytes. This happens on a scale that becomes greater as time goes by. Monocytes and macrophages are thought to act as a reservoir or holding tank for the virus. It lives inside these cells and can be transported to various body parts to attack lymphocytes there. This transport probably explains the presence of HIV in the central nervous system of clinically ill patients. With depletion of helper T4 lymphocytes, the effects are suppression of the immune system by:

1. Decreased antigen recognition and mounting of an immune response.
2. Decreased B cell activation.
3. Decreased antibody production.
4. Decreased cytotoxic T cell killing activity.
5. Decreased macrophage response.
6. Relatively more suppressor T cells.

Recall all of the roles the helper T cell plays and it is easy to understand these effects. It is no wonder the cause of death is opportunistic infection or cancer cells. With fewer helper T4

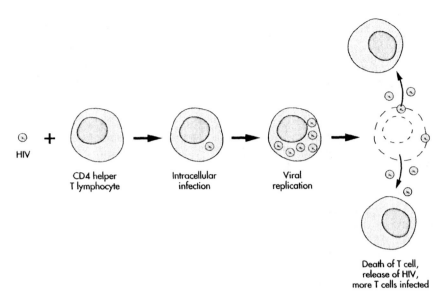

Figure 4–16. Pathogenesis of HIV infection.

cells, and therefore more suppressor T8 cells left, the CD4 to CD8 ratio is decreased or reversed. There is much less *stimulation* of the immune system and much more *suppression*. The CD4 to CD8 ratio can be used to assess the status of an HIV positive person. HIV destroys the immune system by killing _____(1). It can also live in and be transported by _____(2) and _____(3). The effects of T cell destruction lead to severe _____(4) of the immune system. The ratio of _____(5) to _____(6) cells is decreased or _____(7).

1. T4 lymphocytes
2. macrophages
3. monocytes
4. suppression
5. CD4 cells
6. CD8
7. reversed

4-56

The clinical course of HIV infection has been divided into 7 stages. The **incubation period** (time from infection to illness) is very long. These stages were developed by performing CD4 T lymphocyte counts, examining CD4 T lymphocyte function at various times and by the presence of opportunistic infection. **Stage 0** is initial infection with the virus. **Stage 1** is seroconversion, which is when the HIV test is first positive. Some people have temporary flu-like illnesses at this time. In **stage 2,** there may be chronic **lymphadenopathy** which is enlarged lymph nodes for a long time. Enlargement is from all the activity between the virus and lymphocytes. Stage 2 can last for 3 to 5 years. Affected individuals appear otherwise healthy. In **stage 3,** there is a drop in the CD4 lymphocyte count that continues. This may last about a year and a half. During all of this time virus numbers escalate to a critical threshold that causes enough immune destruction to begin to see signs. The risk of spreading HIV is tremendous through these stages if the person is unaware they have the virus. The infectivity of body fluids from a person in later stages is greater because of the greater number of virus particles. Stages of HIV infection are based upon studies of _____(1) lymphocytes. Initial infection is stage _____(2). A positive HIV test is stage _____(3). Stage 2 shows enlarged _____(4). A drop in CD4 count is part of stage _____(5).

1. CD4 T
2. 0
3. 1
4. lymph nodes
5. 3

4-57

People in **stage 4** of infection have severely impaired cell-mediated immunity that manifests as a lack of response to antigen skin tests. General signs of illness begin here. There is unexplained weight loss, continued diarrhea, fatigue, mood changes, and fever. In **stage 5** opportunistic infections appear. **Thrush** is almost universal. Thrush is a fungus infection of the mouth caused by **candida.** (Remember, T cells are responsible for immunity against fungi, protozoa, and neoplastic cells.) Other fungus and viral infections like herpes are common.

1. 4
2. weight
3. diarrhea
4. fatigue
5. mood
6. fever
7. 5
8. thrush
9. body surfaces
10. mucous
11. internal organs
12. Weight
13. pneumocystis
14. dementia

These infections involve body surfaces and mucous membranes. Stage 5 can last 1 to 2 years. **Stage 6** is marked by infections that involve internal organs as the disease moves inward. Protozoan and viral infections predominate as the CD4 count bottoms out. The weight loss seen now is extreme compared to earlier and there is wasting away as some organs begin to atrophy. Some of the unusual disease manifestations are:

1. Pneumocystis pneumonia (fully half of AIDS patients develop this).
2. Toxoplasmosis of the brain.
3. Lymphomas or other rare cancers of the brain or spinal cord.
4. Cryptosporidiosis of the intestinal tract.
5. Cryptococcus meningitis.
6. Systemic histoplasmosis.
7. Cytomegalovirus infection.
8. Rare cancers.
9. AIDS encephalopathy. Also very common, this is degeneration of the brain caused by HIV. It is commonly called **AIDS dementia complex.** Dementia is mental confusion with loss of memory and personality change.

Stage 6 lasts no longer than 2 years before the patient expires. From stage 0 to 6 can be as long as 10 years or more, with the average being about 8 years. These stages are summarized for you in Table 4–5. Stage _____(1) is where the first insidious signs of AIDS begins to appear. Signs include _____(2) loss, _____(3), _____(4), _____(5) changes, and _____(6). In stage _____(7), a fungal infection of the mouth called _____(8) is usually seen. Infections in stage 5 are usually confined to _____(9) and _____(10) membranes. In stage 6, infections move to _____(11). _____(12) loss is extreme. Two of the most common conditions seen are _____(13) pneumonia and AIDS _____(14) complex.

4–58

There are several means of prevention of HIV transmission. Blood products are all tested for HIV-I and this is very effective against transfusion-associated HIV infection. The FDA and CDC (Centers for Disease Control) say that HIV-II is not a threat to the United States at this time. Testing for HIV-II is not required. However most blood banks take precautions in their donor selectivity, and tests for HIV-I appear to be cross reactive for HIV-II as well. Factor VIII, a treatment for hemophilia, is heat treated to destroy the virus and this is also very effective. It remains the responsibility of the general public to control risk associated behavior. Of course sexual activity is the major risk. The only *safe* sex is abstinence. Beyond that there is only "safer" sex. Safer refers to the relative state of taking some precautions instead of none. Precautions should include the use of condoms at all times, being selective in choice of partners, and testing. The association of alcohol or drug use with throwing pre-

TABLE 4–5. STAGES OF AIDS PATHOGENESIS

Stage	Events	Manifestation
0	Infection by HIV	None
1	Seroconversion to positive HIV antibody test	None
2	Lymphadenopathy	Enlarged lymph nodes
3	CD4 lymphocyte count declines	None?
4	Impaired cell-mediated immunity	No response to antigen skin tests, weight loss, diarrhea, fatigue, mental effects, fever
5	Superficial opportunistic infections	Thrush (Candida fungal infection of the mouth)
6	Systemic opportunistic infections and cancer	Extreme weight loss and wasting, pneumocystis pneumonia, AIDS dementia complex, fungal infections, protozoal infections, viral infections, neoplasia, death

caution to the wind is obvious. Most people think they don't have to worry about the contaminated needles of an intravenous drug user. But don't forget about the other uses of needles for the general public—acupuncture, electrolysis, and tattooing. Any certified practitioner of these services should be using disposable needles on only one client. A vaccine against HIV is not soon in coming. Two reasons for this are the several strains of HIV that exist and the mutations the virus undergoes. Making a vaccine against an antigen is a little like the lock-and-key theory of antibody and antigen complexes. Imagine making a key for a lock and every time you try to use it the lock has been changed.

4-59

One risk of HIV transmission in the health care workplace is a needle stick. However studies have shown the chances of contracting HIV from a needle with HIV positive blood is *very* small. Being splashed in the face with body fluids is also a potential risk, as is a hand wound contacting the fluid. For these reasons, the Centers for Disease Control has **universal precautions** that go along with safety guidelines from OSHA (Occupational Safety and Health Administration). Since OSHA is a federal agency following these guidelines is the law. It is the employers' responsibility to provide safety training that must include, but is not limited to:

1. Hand-washing guidelines.
2. Protective equipment (gloves, face shields, gowns, laboratory equipment).
3. Proper "sharps" disposal (for needles and other sharp objects that could cause a laceration).
4. Education about the pathogenesis of HIV and AIDS.
5. Biohazard warning labels for risk areas and on HIV positive specimens.

Every health care professional should follow these precautions. The statistics about workers contracting the virus from patients are *not* cause for alarm. Professionals should remember their primary purpose, to care for every patient. Ideally this issue should be addressed by each person before entering this profession.

III. REVIEW QUESTIONS

1. A term meaning the opposite of an anamnestic or normal immune response is:
   a. immunodeficiency
   b. immunosuppression
   c. anergy
   d. any of the above

2. Corticosteroids, cytotoxic drugs, and irradiation are examples of:
   a. acquired immunodeficiency
   b. iatrogenic immunosuppression
   c. inherited immunodeficiency
   d. none of the above

3. The most common side effect of iatrogenic immunosuppression is:
   a. anemia
   b. thrombocytopenia
   c. infection
   d. kidney toxicity

4. Hypogammaglobulinemia may be seen in (choose all that apply):
   a. the elderly
   b. cancer patients
   c. premature babies
   d. patients with a serious primary infection

1. d–any of the above

2. b–iatrogenic immunosuppression

3. c–infection

4. a–the elderly; c–premature babies

5. d–agammaglobulinemia

6. c–deficient cell-mediated immunity

7. d–acquired immunodeficiency syndrome

8. human immunodeficiency virus

9. a–blood; b–semen

10. b–skin

11. d–any of the above

12. a–helper T lymphocytes

13. c–immune suppression

5. Inherited immunodeficiencies affecting B lymphocytes demonstrate:
   a. hypoplasia of the thymus
   b. hypogammaglobulinemia
   c. deficient cell-mediated immunity
   d. agammaglobulinemia

6. Inherited immunodeficiencies affecting T lymphocytes demonstrate:
   a. hypoplasia of lymphoid tissue
   b. hypogammaglobulinemia
   c. deficient cell-mediated immunity
   d. agammaglobulinemia

7. The most common immunodeficiency seen today is:
   a. severe combined immunodeficiency
   b. inherited immunodeficiency
   c. iatrogenic immunodeficiency
   d. acquired immunodeficiency syndrome

8. The full name of the virus that causes AIDS is:

   _____

9. Body fluids shown to transmit the HIV virus are (choose all that apply):
   a. blood
   b. semen
   c. tears
   d. saliva

10. The HIV virus does NOT enter the body through:
    a. wounds
    b. skin
    c. the genital tract
    d. mucous membranes

11. The HIV virus is NOT transmitted by:
    a. kissing
    b. food or utensils
    c. the air
    d. any of the above

12. The HIV virus primarily destroys:
    a. helper T lymphocytes
    b. B lymphocytes
    c. macrophages
    d. suppressor T lymphocytes

13. The overall effect of HIV pathogenesis is:
    a. immune overstimulation
    b. immune misdirected stimulation
    c. immune suppression
    d. any of the above

14. Seroconversion to positive HIV status marks:
    a. stage 0
    b. stage 1
    c. stage 2
    d. stage 3
    e. stage 4
    f. stage 5
    g. stage 6

15. The greatest risk of unknowingly spreading HIV occurs before:
    a. stage 0
    b. stage 1
    c. stage 2
    d. stage 3
    e. any of the above

16. Thrush is seen in stage _____ of HIV infection.

17. Of all the possible types of infection, cancers, or other signs of AIDS the two most common are:
    a. pneumocystis pneumonia
    b. cryptococcus meningitis
    c. toxoplasmosis of the brain
    d. AIDS dementia complex

14. b–stage 1

15. e–any of the above

16. 5

17. a–pneumocystis pneumonia; d–AIDS dementia complex

IV. AUTOIMMUNITY

▶ AUTOIMMUNITY

4–60

Autoimmunity is reacting to "self"-antigens. It is an immune response that is directed against various body tissues. Antibodies made against self-antigens are **autoantibodies.** In Frame 4–6 we discussed the concept of tolerance. Tolerance is recognizing tissue or cells as belonging to the individual. They are not foreign and an immune attack does not occur. In autoimmunity there is a breakdown in this tolerance. Both antibodies and T cells will attack self-antigens (see Fig. 4–17). It's like being allergic to yourself. The mechanism of autoimmunity includes several of the hypersensitivity mechanisms. There are circulating immune complexes that lodge in tissue and cause damage (type _____(1)), antibody-dependent cytotoxicity that lyse cells (type _____(2)), and direct T-cell-mediated destruction (type _____(3)). To really define autoimmunity, we must say the reaction between host antigens and antibodies or T cells causes injury to the host. This injury is seen as various diseases that will be mentioned soon. The basis for the injury or disease is the inflammation that results from an immune response. Therefore, autoimmune diseases can be inflammatory conditions. Recall from Chapter 2 how inflammation itself can interfere with normal body function. When host antibodies or immune cells attack the host's own tissues, this is called _____(4). The antibodies in this case are specifically called _____(5). Autoimmune diseases often demonstrate their presence by causing _____(6) at the site, which can interfere with normal _____(7).

1. III
2. II
3. IV
4. autoimmunity
5. autoantibodies
6. inflammation
7. function

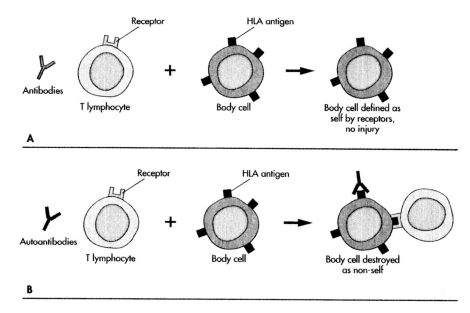

Figure 4–17. Autoimmunity. **A.** Normal immune response. **B.** Misdirected immune response (autoimmune disease).

4-61

1. unknown

You should be aware that classifying a disease as autoimmune is sometimes questionable. Diseases that are considered idiopathic, which means the cause is _____(1), are sometimes called autoimmune just because autoantibodies have been found in the blood of the patient. These autoantibodies may in fact be responsible for the condition or it may be a coincidental finding. Classifying a condition as autoimmune can be convenient if no other cause can be found. Autoimmunity is still just a theory when trying to explain some disease states. There are a few criteria that help define true autoimmune disease. They are listed as follows.

1. The injured area demonstrates the presence of antibodies that react with tissue antigens there.
2. There are chronic inflammatory cells (macrophages) and immune cells (T cells and plasma cells) also present.
3. Clinically, the condition shows signs consistent with autoimmune disease. Since autoimmune disease is inflammatory, signs of inflammation such as pain and fever are common.
4. The condition improves with the use of steroids or immunosuppressants as treatment.

4-62

No one knows for certain how autoimmunity develops, but current theories are summarized in the following list.

1. There is a defect in the fetal process of eliminating lymphocytes that react against self.
2. Helper T cells sometimes stimulate B cells to make autoantibodies if the determinants on foreign antigens are very similar to body tissue antigens.
3. There are structural changes to cell surfaces as a result of injury or stimulation from a virus. These changes produce an antigen that is altered and therefore no longer recognized as self. Another reason could be HLA antigens that used to be hidden from the surface are now exposed by the changes and considered new to the body, or foreign.

▶ AUTOIMMUNE DISEASES BY SYSTEM

4-63

This and the following frames will cover some diseases that are either accepted to be autoimmune or strongly suspicious of being autoimmune. These diseases will be discussed in greater detail in the following chapters.

Cardiovascular disorders include:

1. **Rheumatic fever** (type III hypersensitivity mechanism). This is a hypersensitivity reaction to the bacteria group A streptococci, commonly known as strep throat. In some people the antibodies made against the bacteria also cross-react with some body tissue. The areas affected are the joints and heart valves, so it is seen as arthritis and heart disease.
2. **Pernicious anemia.** Antibodies against **intrinsic factor,** which comes from the stomach lining, prevent binding with vitamin B_{12}, which is required for red blood cell production. The result is B_{12} deficiency and anemia.
3. **Autoimmune hemolytic anemia.** Antigens on the surface of red blood cells are the target of autoantibodies. The RBCs are lysed and destroyed through the type II ADCC mechanism. As numbers of RBCs fall, anemia results.
4. **Immune-mediated thrombocytopenia** (type II hypersensitivity mechanism). HLA antigens on the surface of platelets are the target of autoantibodies. Platelets are important in blood coagulation, so as numbers of platelets fall, bleeding is a result.

Gastrointestinal disorders. Autoantibodies have been found in cases of **ulcerative colitis,** which produces erosions or ulcers in the large intestine or colon. **Primary biliary cirrhosis** and **chronic active hepatitis** are suspected to have some autoimmune component.

In rheumatic fever the tissues that are injured are the _____(1) and _____(2) because antibodies against _____(3) also react with these tissues. Pernicious anemia is a result of _____(4) deficiency. This is because antibodies against _____(5) interfere with the role of vitamin B_{12} in _____(6) production. Type II ADCC destruction of red blood cells is the basis of _____(7) anemia. Bleeding can occur in _____(8) because numbers of _____(9) are decreased.

1. joints
2. heart
3. group A streptococci
4. vitamin B_{12}
5. intrinsic factor
6. red blood cell
7. autoimmune hemolytic
8. immune-mediated thrombocytopenia
9. platelets

4-64

Endocrine disorders include:

1. **Type I juvenile diabetes mellitus.** There is a link between some HLA antigens of the beta islet cells of the pancreas and autoantibodies. It is believed these cells are destroyed and since they make insulin, diabetes is a result. Insulin is required for glucose to enter body cells. Insulin deficiency leads to high blood glucose and the complications of diabetes.
2. **Hashimoto's thyroiditis.** The antigen is thyroglobulin, a protein in cells of the thyroid gland. Follicles, which are packets of hormone producing cells, are infiltrated with immune cells and destroyed. The result is a deficiency of thyroid hormone, or hypothyroidism.

Musculoskeletal disorders include:

1. **Myasthenia gravis.** Acetylcholine receptors at neuromuscular junctions serve as the antigen for autoantibodies. The complex blocks neuromuscular transmission. Acetylcholine is the chemical messenger that stimulates muscle contraction. The inability of this chemical to be received causes signs of extreme muscular weakness and interference with functions such as swallowing.
2. **Rheumatoid arthritis.** In this relatively common disorder, it is believed that long-term exposure to some antigens such as viruses causes normal IgG to be altered. This changed IgG becomes an autoantibody and attacks synovial membrane in the joints. The inflammation can be quite severe and is chronic. Chronic inflammation gradually erodes the

1. beta
2. pancreas
3. insulin
4. elevated or increased
5. follicles
6. thyroglobulin
7. Hashimoto's thyroiditis
8. acetylcholine receptors
9. Neurotransmission
10. weakness
11. functions
12. rheumatoid factor
13. synovial membrane
14. inflammation
15. joint surface

joint surface, causing permanent deformity and loss of use. In rheumatoid arthritis the autoantibodies are easily identified in serological tests and have been named **rheumatoid factor.**

In juvenile type I diabetes, tissue destroyed by autoantibodies are the _____(1) cells of the _____(2). These cells make _____(3) so the patient is lacking in this hormone and the blood glucose is _____(4). Hypothyroidism can develop when immune cells invade thyroid _____(5) and attack the protein _____(6). The name of this condition is _____(7). The antigen in myasthenia gravis is _____(8). _____(9) is blocked and the signs are muscle _____(10) and interference with other _____(11). Autoantibodies in rheumatoid arthritis are called _____(12). The destruction is of the _____(13) in the joints. The presence of chronic _____(14) eventually erodes the _____(15).

4-65

1. glomerulonephritis
2. Goodpasture's
3. basement membrane
4. pemphigus
5. bullous
6. layers
7. systems
8. connective tissue
9. nuclear

Kidney disorders include **acute glomerulonephritis** (type II hypersensitivity mechanism). Post-infection with streptococcal bacteria was an example of type III immune complex hypersensitivity damage. It should not be confused with autoimmune glomerulonephritis. In **Goodpasture's syndrome** there is an antibody formed that targets the basement membrane of the glomerulus or capillary bed. At the same time, capillaries in the lungs also serve as antigens, and the result is signs of lung disease. It is uncertain if it is the same antibody or two different ones.

Skin disorders. Antibodies target various layers of the skin in **pemphigus vulgaris** and **bullous pemphigoid.** In pemphigus vulgaris the intracellular substance of the upper layers (stratified squamous epithelium) is the antigen. In bullous pemphigoid the lesion is in deeper layers. The antigen is the basement membrane under the epidermis. Both disorders cause **bulla** or blisters.

Connective tissue disorders. These autoimmune diseases are sometimes called **mixed connective tissue disease** or **multisystem diseases** and are hard to classify as one particular disorder. They affect a variety of systems. Two examples are **dermatomyositis** and **scleroderma** (also known as systemic sclerosis). Dermatomyositis affects skin and muscle and is often found with some internal malignancy. Scleroderma can affect only the skin or also internal organs, especially the GI tract and kidneys. In both conditions the antigen is thought to be nuclear material such as RNA so it is logical that there will be many manifestations. **Systemic lupus erythematosus (SLE)** is a mixed connective tissue disease you will study in the following frames. The examples of autoimmune disease given here are by no means inclusive. Table 4–6 summarizes the diseases to which you were introduced. An example of autoimmune kidney disease is acute _____(1) in the condition _____(2) syndrome. The antigen is the _____(3) of the glomerulus. Skin diseases in which the lesions are blisters are _____(4) vulgaris or _____(5) pemphigoid. Different _____(6) of the skin are affected by antigen–antibody interaction. Dermatomyositis and scleroderma are difficult to categorize exactly since they affect several _____(7). The most likely antigen in mixed _____(8) disease or multisystem disease is _____(9) material.

4-66

Systemic lupus erythematosus is a multisystem disease. The antigens in SLE appear to be the DNA, RNA, and organelles of cells. There are several autoantibodies implicated in this disease. The mechanism of damage to tissues includes types II, III, and IV hypersensitivity. A good descriptive phrase is "diffuse collagen vascular disease." In deciphering this phrase you will see SLE is a widespread disorder affecting the collagen in connective tissue and blood vessels. Lupus erythematosus can be a local disorder affecting only the skin. This is called the **discoid form.** Here we will only consider the systemic form that is by far more serious. It is widespread inflammation caused by breakdown of collagen and vessel lining. SLE is most often seen in relatively young women (20 to 40). The severity of the signs and

TABLE 4–6. EXAMPLES OF AUTOIMMUNE DISEASES

	Site of Injury	Antigen
Rheumatic fever	Heart, joints	Cardiac and joint tissue by streptococcal antibody
Pernicious anemia	RBC development due to vitamin B_{12} deficiency	Intrinsic factor
Autoimmune hemolytic anemia	Red blood cells	Surface blood group antigens
Immune-mediated thrombocytopenia	Platelets	Surface HLA antigens
Rheumatoid arthritis	Joint surface	Altered IgG
Myasthenia gravis	Skeletal muscle	Acetylcholine receptors
Type I juvenile diabetes	Pancreas	Beta islet cells
Hashimoto's thyroiditis	Thyroid	Thyroglobulin
Goodpasture's syndrome	Kidney and lung	Basement membrane
Pemphigus vulgaris, bullous pemphigoid	Skin	Intracellular substance and basement membrane
Dermatomyositis, scleroderma	Connective tissue, muscle, organs	Many
Systemic lupus erythematosus	Collagen, skin, blood vessels, kidney, heart, joints	Many

speed of onset can vary greatly from case to case. A very characteristic sign is the presence of a "butterfly rash" on the face that is shown to you in Figure 4–18. This is a red rash across the nose and cheeks. Joint and muscle involvement produces pain and fever. The patient experiences cytopenia or decreased numbers of white blood cells. They are left vulnerable to infection such as pneumonia. Degeneration appears in the endocardium or lining of the heart and heart valves. As organs become infiltrated with cells of chronic inflammation, failure can occur. This especially is seen in the kidneys and sometimes the heart. As the brain is affected, psychosis or behavior disorder is not uncommon. Diffuse collagen vascular disease describes the condition _____(1). Widespread degeneration of collagen and blood vessels causes chronic _____(2). Organs become overwhelmed with _____(3) of chronic inflammation. Two organs prone to failure in SLE are the _____(4) and the _____(5). A characteristic sign is a _____(6) on the face.

1. systemic lupus erythematosus
2. inflammation
3. cells
4. kidneys
5. heart
6. butterfly rash

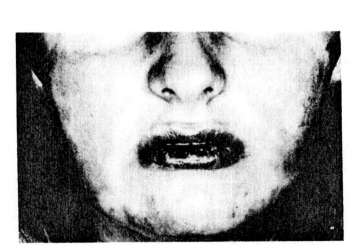

Figure 4–18. Butterfly rash of systemic lupus erythematosus. (From Kent and Hart, *Introduction to Human Disease*, 3rd ed., Appleton & Lange.)

IV. REVIEW QUESTIONS

1. Autoimmunity is:
   a. over response to foreign antigens
   b. misdirected response to self-antigens
   c. over response to self-antigens
   d. misdirected response to foreign antigens

2. Tissue injury in autoimmune disease is primary due to:
   a. chronic inflammation
   b. ischemia
   c. necrosis
   d. granulomatous inflammation

3. Please match the autoimmune diseases in the left column with the information in the right column:
   a. rheumatoid arthritis
   b. Hashimoto's thyroiditis
   c. rheumatic fever
   d. bullous pemphigoid
   e. acute glomerulonephritis
   f. pernicious anemia
   g. juvenile diabetes
   h. myasthenia gravis

   1. ____ blisters on the skin
   2. ____ antigen is glomerular basement membrane
   3. ____ antibody is called rheumatoid factor
   4. ____ antigen is intrinsic factor
   5. ____ antigen is pancreatic beta cells
   6. ____ leads to hypothyroidism
   7. ____ may occur after strep throat
   8. ____ causes muscle weakness

4. Dermatomyositis, scleroderma, and systemic lupus erythematosus are examples of
   _____ autoimmune disease:
   a. endocrine
   b. musculoskeletal
   c. mixed connective tissue
   d. dermal or skin

5. Two primary tissue targets in SLE are:
   a. blood vessels
   b. collagen
   c. skin layers
   d. glomerular basement membrane

6. A characteristic superficial sign of SLE is a _____ on the face.

7. In SLE, organ infiltration with immune cells and degeneration can lead to failure of which two organs most commonly?
   a. heart
   b. liver
   c. brain
   d. kidney

8. Antigens in SLE are most likely:
   a. cellular DNA
   b. cellular RNA
   c. cellular organelles
   d. all of the above

Answers (margin):

1. b–misdirected response to self-antigens
2. a–chronic inflammation
3. 1. d–bullous pemphigoid; 2. e–acute glomerulonephritis; 3. a–rheumatoid arthritis; 4. f–Pernicious anemia; 5. g–juvenile diabetes; 6. b–Hashimoto's thyroiditis; 7. c–rheumatic fever; 8. h–myasthenia gravis
4. c–mixed connective tissue
5. a–blood vessels; b–collagen
6. butterfly rash
7. a–heart; d–kidney
8. d–all of the above

▶ **SECTION II**

Hypersensitivity is excessive immune response by either antibodies or T cells that occurs in some people. In the process of eliminating an antigen, body tissues are injured. Inflammation is part of hypersensitivity, and is a major contributor to the signs of disorder. Type I or anaphylactic-atopic allergy is directed by IgE. Atopy is local allergy that can affect the upper respiratory tract, skin, or intestinal tract. When IgE that is bound to mast cells contacts an allergen, the mast cell degranulates and releases histamine and other vasoactive chemical mediators. The most common atopy is allergic rhinitis or hay fever. Atopy affecting the skin may produce urticaria (hives) or pruritus (itching). Type I hypersensitivity that affects several systems, or is systemic, is called anaphylaxis. This is a life-threatening condition because of the inflammatory vascular changes that compromise intravascular blood volume, blood pressure, and cardiac output. Circulatory failure or hypovolemic shock may cause death in what is known as anaphylactic shock. Also, changes in the respiratory tract such as bronchial constriction and laryngeal edema cause dyspnea or difficult breathing. Suffocation is a possibility without treatment.

Type II hypersensitivity is antibody-dependent cell-mediated cytotoxicity (ADCC). Antigens are found on cell surfaces. Antibody binds to the antigen and creates an immune complex that is adhered to the cell surface. When complement is activated by the complex, this results in lysis of the cell. Primary and secondary exposure is not necessary to activate this mechanism. Sometimes complement is not activated by the immune complex but instead draws phagocytes through chemotaxis. The phagocytes destroy the targeted cells by ingesting them. Conditions such as anemia or thrombocytopenia can result, depending on the cell line involved and the amount of destruction. Drug reactions are often type II hypersensitivities, as are blood transfusion reactions and hemolytic disease of the newborn. When receiving incompatible blood, the natural ABO antigens incite a reaction from the opposite naturally occurring antibodies. The type II destruction causes signs in the patient associated with vascular compromise and organ ischemia. HDN is similar to an incompatible transfusion except the antigen is Rh or D. The source of the D antigen is the fetus. During fetomaternal bleeding, the antigen enters the mother's circulation and she makes anti-D antibody. In future pregnancies, this anti-D can be a severe threat to the baby's red blood cells. Hydrops fetalis is severe anemia that can cause heart failure. Excess toxic bilirubin from RBC destruction can cause kernicterus or brain damage.

Type III hypersensitivity is immune complex-mediated hypersensitivity. Once formed in the circulation, the antigen–antibody pair attaches to vessel endothelial cells. Subsequent destruction of the immune complex causes inflammation of the vessels. This is called acute vasculitis. Side effects that accompany the inflammatory damage include ischemia to organs supplied by the affected vessels and thrombus formation. Thrombi can block small vessels and worsen damage from ischemia. Type III immune complex damage can occur systemwide but most often it affects joints and the kidneys. Glomerulonephritis can be associated with group A streptococcal infections when immune complexes deposit there. Serum sickness is a systemic type III reaction that was seen when patients were given immune serum from animals. Generalized vasculitis was a side effect as patients reacted against foreign animal proteins in their bloodstream. Rheumatoid arthritis and systemic lupus erythematosus are type III autoimmune mechanisms.

Type IV is delayed cell-mediated hypersensitivity. It differs from the first three because it does not involve antibodies but instead relies on T lymphocytes. The mechanism of antigen elimination is like the normal immune response. The skin is the site of reaction, producing granulomatous inflammation and damage. Transplant rejections are type IV hypersensitivities. A common type IV reaction is contact dermatitis, where many environmental substances can be the antigens. Hypersensitivity in general can be compared to normal immune response by examining the population affected, the damage to the body, the kinds of antigens causing it, and the severity of reaction.

◀ CHAPTER SUMMARY

► SECTION III

Anergy and immunosuppression are terms indicating lack of normal response or immuno-deficiency. Nonspecific causes are suppression of the immune system in general by factors outside of the immune system. Examples are iatrogenic immunosuppression, old age, mal-nutrition, immaturity, and primary disease states. Specific immunodeficiency includes both inherited and acquired states. Inherited problems are due to hypoplasia of immune cell pro-ducing tissues. It may be B lymphocytes and therefore antibodies that are affected, or it may be T lymphocytes that are deficient. Agammaglobulinemia describes the severe lack of anti-bodies when humoral immunity is involved. Cellular immunity deficiencies often affect B-cell function and the combination is called severe combined immunodeficiency. Acquired immunodeficiency syndrome or AIDS is the most common acquired state of deficient immune response. It is caused by human immunodeficiency virus-I. The disease AIDS is defined as unusual infections or cancers in a person who has a positive HIV test. In AIDS, the patient has progressed to the point of almost total immune suppression and is defense-less against opportunistic organisms. Two uncommon conditions first seen in AIDS patients, and on which the definition is based, were pneumocystis pneumonia and Kaposi's sarcoma. HIV is primarily spread through blood and semen. It enters the body through mucosal lined openings or through broken skin. Contracting HIV only occurs by touching those body sur-faces with blood or semen of an infected person. HIV specifically targets the helper T lym-phocyte for destruction. Monocytes and macrophage may act as reservoirs or carriers of the virus. Because of all the functions of the helper T cells, many aspects of immune function are wiped out. As numbers of helper T cells decline, the CD4 to CD8 ratio also decreases to the point of reversal. The incubation period for AIDS is several years. In the seven stages of AIDS pathogenesis, signs don't begin until stage 4. Superficial infections like thrush appear in stage 5. Internal infections mark stage 6. Almost any type of infection by protozoans, bac-teria, or viruses can be seen. Common manifestations are pneumocystis pneumonia and AIDS dementia complex.

► SECTION IV

The concept of autoimmunity is that antibodies are formed that do not recognize body anti-gens as self. Since this recognition is lacking, the autoantibodies target the tissue as though it were foreign. Autoimmune disease is associated with chronic inflammation because anti-gen destruction causes inflammation. Several of the hypersensitivity mechanisms can be found in the development of autoimmune disease. To avoid classifying a disease as autoim-mune because no other cause can be found, criteria act as guidelines to help define autoim-mune disease. We can only theorize why autoantibodies develop.

Cardiovascular autoimmune disorders include rheumatic fever, where antibodies to group A streptococci also attack heart and joint tissue; pernicious anemia, in which antibod-ies destroy red blood cell precursors; and autoimmune hemolytic anemia and immune-mediated thrombocytopenia, where RBCs and platelets are destroyed because of their sur-face antigens. Some gastrointestinal disorders such as ulcerative colitis, biliary cirrhosis, and chronic active hepatitis may be immune mediated. Hormone imbalances such as hypothy-roidism in Hashimoto's thyroiditis and juvenile diabetes develop when antibodies destroy thyroid follicle protein and pancreatic beta cells, respectively.

In musculoskeletal disorders, myasthenia gravis is extreme muscle weakness and loss of function, and results when acetylcholine receptors are blocked by antibodies. Rheumatoid factor antibody is found in cases of rheumatoid arthritis where chronic inflammation destroys joint surfaces. Goodpasture's syndrome causes acute glomerulonephritis when glomerular basement membrane serves as the antigen. The lungs are also affected. Destruc-tion of different skin layers causes bulla-type lesions in pemphigus vulgaris and bullous pemphigoid. The mixed connective tissue diseases, or multisystemic autoimmune diseases, include dermatomyositis, scleroderma, and systemic lupus erythematosus. In SLE, there is widespread damage to collagen in connective tissue and to blood vessel lining, earning this condition the label diffuse collagen vascular disease. A butterfly rash is usually seen on the faces of the affected young female population. Some results of the systemic destruction include infections secondary to cytopenia, internal organ infiltration, psychosis, and heart or kidney failure. SLE antigens are found in most body cells and include nuclear proteins and organelles.

Common Pathogens and Infectious Disease

▶ OBJECTIVES

SECTION I

Define all highlighted terms.

Give the proper terminology to describe bacterial morphology based on gram stain and microscopic examination.

Describe laboratory procedures used to diagnose bacterial infection, including the purpose of each.

Explain the concepts of secondary infection and opportunistic infection.

Contrast the difference between bacterial colonization and bacterial infection.

Cite the most common source of infection.

Relate the various concepts of sepsis, septicemia, and septic shock to each other.

Outline the events of septic shock and its pathogenesis.

Distinguish between disinfection and sterilization.

Compare the differences in diagnostic procedures for viruses versus bacteria.

Relate viral cytopathic effect in vitro to viral disease in vivo.

SECTION II

Define all highlighted terms.

Describe the effects of pyogenic bacteria.

List possible complications of *Streptococcus pyogenes* infection and explain the mechanisms behind them.

Identify *Salmonella* as a cause of food poisoning, cite the most common source of this bacteria, and explain preventive measures.

State the most common bacterial venereal disease.

Explain the significance of infection by *Neisseria gonorrhoeae* and list all possible results of gonorrhea.

Relate clinical signs of syphilis to each stage of the disease.

Describe the consequences of end-stage syphilis.

Indicate the general mechanism by which the *Clostridium* genus causes disease.

Relate each *Clostridium* bacteria to its particular disease, and explain the mechanism for each disease.

List primary and secondary sites of infection by *Mycobacterium tuberculosis*.

Describe how plague and Lyme disease are spread and their clinical features.

SECTION III

Define all highlighted terms.
Discuss the characteristics of viruses, including physical properties and life cycle.
Relate viral disease to viral life cycle in host cells.
Understand the defense mechanisms against viruses.
For each viral disease most commonly affecting children, describe the clinical appearance, cite organs or structures involved, and list unique features.
State the most common adult viral disease.
Differentiate viral URI and influenza, including clinical signs.
Recall the significance of delivery and birth by a woman with active herpes simplex type II.
Understand the significance of cytomegalovirus infection.
State the causative agent of infectious mononucleosis.

SECTION IV

Define all highlighted terms.
Associate *Chlamydia* species with their particular diseases and describe the diseases.
List two clinical features of rickettsial disease, state the name given to these diseases, and describe their transmission.
Equate the rash seen in rickettsial disease to the mechanism of production.
Equate each fungal organism with the disease caused by the organisms, including clinical and common names.

SECTION V

Define all highlighted terms.
Contrast diarrhea and dysentery and name a protozoan responsible for dysentery.
Describe the source and spread of amebiasis and giardiasis.
Explain the transmission of *Plasmodium* species and the pathogenesis of malaria.
List results of chronic malaria.
Explain the danger of toxoplasmosis infection in a pregnant woman or the immunosuppressed.
Explain trichomoniasis.
Indicate the significance of pneumocystosis in immunosuppressed populations.
Describe how intestinal parasites cause disease.
List helminthic infection acquired by eating undercooked meats.
Identify hydatid disease, name the source, and explain the cause of death.

SECTION ▶ 1. GENERAL PRINCIPLES OF INFECTIOUS DISEASE

▶ THE NATURE OF INFECTIOUS DISEASE

5-1

A **microorganism** is a living organism that cannot be seen with the naked eye, with the exception of some intestinal parasites. They can only be seen with a microscope. Microorganisms include **bacteria, viruses, fungi, chlamydia, rickettsia,** and **protozoa.** A **pathogen** is any microorganism that can and does cause disease. This is in contrast to the concept of **normal flora.** Another word for normal flora is **commensal.** Normal flora refers to microorganisms that naturally inhabit different parts of the body and *usually* don't cause disease. (We'll get back to this when we talk about opportunistic infections.) These body parts include the skin, mouth, respiratory tract, and the intestines. One very important function of having "normal" bacteria in your body is to prevent pathogens from easily taking over. This is accomplished in two ways. First, the presence of normal bacteria can prevent pathogens from attaching to the same surface. Second, the normal bacteria compete with pathogens for nutrients. The **virulence** of a pathogen is the degree to which the organism can cause injury.

Put another way, it's the strength in causing disease. A virulent pathogen makes you very ill while a less virulent pathogen does not. The term **"infection"** is commonly understood to mean the disease that is caused by the pathogen. However, technically, it can mean just that the organism has gained entry into the body and is multiplying there. This multiplying and carrying on of life processes is called **colonization.** So an organism that has colonized, and therefore infected the body, may or may not cause signs of disease. The infection may be **subclinical,** or not have visible signs or effects. Whether or not an infection is subclinical or **clinical** (obvious illness) depends on the virulence of the organism, the dose of the organism, the strength of the host's immune defense, and an effective inflammatory response.

.... 5-2 ....

Bacteria that inhabit some body parts on a regular basis are called _____(1). Their presence can prevent harmful bacteria that cause _____(2) from colonizing. A microorganism that doesn't belong in the body and causes disease is called a _____(3). A strong pathogen that causes serious illness is described as _____(4). The entry of microorganisms into the body and multiplying in the tissue is the strict definition of _____(5). Whether or not an infection is _____(6) (shows signs of illness) or is not even noticeable [_____(7)] depends in part on effective functions of host _____(8) defense and _____(9) response.

1. normal flora
2. disease
3. pathogen
4. virulent
5. infection
6. clinical
7. subclinical
8. immune
9. inflammatory

▷ PRIMARY AND SECONDARY INFECTION

.... 5-3 ....

A primary infection is the type we have been talking about so far. Think of primary here as meaning first. Primary disease refers to any *predisposing* disorder. In this example, when another infection develops on top of the first one, that is a **secondary** infection. It is certainly possible that if a host is compromised by fighting one infection and a second pathogen is introduced, a secondary infection can develop. It would be in addition to, or on top of, the first, or primary, infection. Another concept in secondary infections is **opportunistic** infections. This specifically means the additional infection is caused by a miroorganism that usually doesn't cause disease by itself. This could be a microorganism foreign to the body that is not very virulent. But, if given the opportunity (hence the name), it can cause clinical infection. This opportunity can arise in two ways. First, as already mentioned, the host can be very involved fighting a virulent or strong pathogen. The immune system has limited resources like any other entity. If stretched far enough, gaps develop that allow an opportunistic organism to slip through and gain a hold. Normally, the immune response would render such an organism harmless, but in this case it may go unchecked. This relationship is shown Figure 5–1.

.... 5-4 ....

In addition to being overburdened, it is possible that the immune system is suppressed. Overuse of immunosuppressive steroids can lead to an opportunistic infection. If the cause is immunosuppression, an opportunistic infection can exist without a primary infection. In this case, the opportunistic infection *is* the primary infection. The most common cause of immunosuppression is AIDS. As you learned in Chapter 4, opportunistic infection is largely the cause of death in AIDS. Often, normal flora can cause opportunistic infection. Even though these organisms are normal inhabitants, one of the reasons they don't cause disease is because the immune system keeps their numbers to a harmless level. Immunosuppression can allow these numbers to increase to disease-producing levels. The factor relating to numbers that determines if disease occurs is called the **dose.** Another reason for the dose of normal flora to reach pathogenic levels is an obstruction. Often in obstruction, the washing away of bacteria cannot occur. An example is urethral obstruction leading to cystitis, or bladder infection. An initial infection is classified as a _____(1) infection. An additional infection is then classified as a _____(2) infection. A secondary infection can be caused by an organism that doesn't usually produce disease. This is classified as a (an) _____(3) infection because the organism takes advantage of the opportunity.

1. primary
2. secondary
3. opportunistic

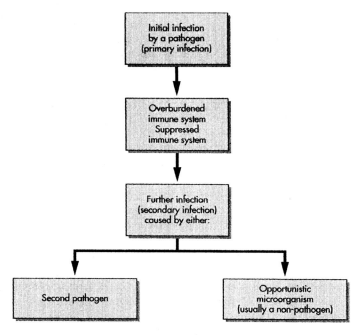

Figure 5–1. Relationship between primary and secondary infection.

4. immune
5. infection
6. suppressed
7. normal flora
8. numbers

Two ways this can develop is if the _____(4) system is overburdened with fighting another _____(5), or if it is _____(6). Commensals, or _____(7), can cause secondary infection if their dose or _____(8) are allowed to reach pathogenic proportions.

► PATHOGENESIS OF INFECTIOUS DISEASE

5–5

1. congenital
2. endogenous
3. exogenous
4. exogenous
5. environment

There are three sources of pathogens. First is **congenital** (present at birth), which is the least common. Organisms may gain entry to the fetus through maternal circulation or during passage through the birth canal. Second is an **endogenous** source, which means the organisms are already within the body. (Endogenous means within.) This happens when normal flora from one part of the body are introduced to an irregular site. Examples are when upper respiratory bacteria enter the lungs, and when intestinal bacteria contact the urinary or genital tracts. The most common source is **exogenous,** which means from outside of the body. These environmental sources are many. One is other infected persons. Disease transmitted from one person to another is called **infectious** or **contagious.** Another is **carriers** (those having a disease but not sick). **Fomites** are another source. A fomite is an inanimate object that harbors pathogens. Some pathogens are hardy enough to withstand the environment for a period of time. Examples of fomites are dishes and utensils, doorknobs, clothing, or any surface. Three classifications of pathogen sources are _____(1), _____(2), and _____(3). The most common is _____(4), and the organisms are coming from the _____(5).

5–6

Another kind of exogenous source is called **nosocomial.** Nosocomial infections are commonly associated with the hospital environment. Technically, any group housing situation can be a source of nosocomial infection. In hospitals, staphylococcal (staph) infections can be a big problem. Hospital patients are usually compromised with some primary disease that leaves their defenses vulnerable. Cleanliness is very important to minimize transmission of organisms from fomites. Carriers can pass organisms to those who are debilitated. Surgical and burn patients are susceptible to wound infection, primarily from staph organisms. Infections acquired by hospital patients or others in group housing are called _____(1) infections.

There are a variety of ways a pathogen can be transmitted and enter the body. These avenues can be grouped together as either through the skin when it is damaged, or through the natural passages, such as the respiratory or alimentary tracts. Some of the specific means of entry are in the following list.

1. Direct injection into an open wound.
2. Contamination where the organism is deposited on the skin surface and the skin later becomes damaged.
3. Sexual contact, as in the case of venereal disease.
4. Contamination of the hands from a fomite and then transfer to a body passage.
5. Inhalation of infected droplets from an infected person produced by coughing or sneezing. Dust in the air acts as a fomite if it carries dried infected particles.
6. Ingestion of contaminated food or water, or hand-to-mouth practices.
7. Bites from **vectors,** which are insects that carry an infectious organism. Examples are malaria from the mosquito, plague from rodent fleas, and Lyme disease from deer ticks.

Two main means that organisms use to enter the body are through damaged _____(1) or through natural body _____(2).

Once a pathogen enters the body it may become localized or spread. The inflammatory response may be able to contain the pathogen. If not, it may spread to cause systemic disease. What determines if a pathogen can be contained or if it causes systemic disease? There are several factors that come into play. One is the natural ability of the pathogen to cause injury. This strength is called _____(1). A virulent organism is more likely to become problematic than a weaker organism. Also important is the dose of the pathogen. Small numbers may be easily destroyed by the immune and inflammatory responses, while a very large dose may overcome these defenses. Site of entry is a factor. Direct entry into the bloodstream, perhaps in an invasive dental procedure, is an example of possible systemic involvement. The host's ability to destroy the organism requires an efficient immune and inflammatory response. Anything interfering with these responses allows the organism to cause more destruction. Necrotic, or dead, tissue supports the colonization and growth of pathogens because the tissue is an excellent source of nutrients. This allows multiplication, and once numbers of the pathogen reach a certain point, dose comes into play. Also, since necrotic tissue lacks blood supply, antibodies and phagocytes are unable to reach the site of colonization to destroy the bacteria. Finally, ischemic tissue is susceptible to successful invasion because the decreased blood supply means decreased inflammatory and immune response to the area. Factors of spread *relating directly to the pathogen* include strength or _____(2) of the organism and the numbers present or the _____(3). *Host factors* are efficient functioning of the _____(4) and _____(5) responses; the presence of dead or _____(6) tissue; and decreased blood supply to the area, which is called _____(7).

▶ DEFENSE AGAINST INFECTION

The body is constantly subjected to contamination by potentially harmful microorganisms. Healthy people are able to resist infection in a variety of ways. Once a microorganism gains entry, three things can happen. The organism may die or be killed. Second, it may live but be prevented from causing disease by the immune system. Often in this case, immunity can develop and antibodies will be effective in fighting future infections with the same pathogen. The last result is that the pathogen is successful in producing injury.

5-10

1. presence
2. nutrients
3. opsonization

The defenses that the body has to protect itself include the following.

1. Physical integrity of the **skin.** This is considered the *first line of defense.* The outer, tough layer of keratin on the epithelium of the skin is an effective barrier to penetration. Infection occurs only if this barrier is injured.

2. **Decontamination,** where the organism is removed from the body surface. This is accomplished through **mechanical** means, where organisms are shed with flakes of keratin or washed away by body fluids such as tears, saliva, urine, and respiratory mucus. **Biologic** decontamination takes the form of resident normal flora. Remember, commensal organisms interfere with pathogen colonization by their mere _____(1), which blocks adhesion by pathogens. They also interfere by competing for _____(2) that the pathogens need to survive. The third form of decontamination is **chemical,** where certain body secretions are lethal to microorganisms. Examples are the very acid pH of the stomach secretions and an enzyme called **lysozyme.** Lysozyme in secretions like tears lyse, or burst, some microorganisms.

3. Inflammation with its fibrin wall, phagocytosis, and hydrogen peroxide can be effective in destroying organisms should they breach the epithelial barrier.

4. The immune response works along with inflammation to destroy the disease agent. Remember, coating of foreign organisms with antibody, which eases phagocytosis, is a process called _____(3). Also, complement can be effective in lysing the pathogen.

5-11

1. skin
2. does not
3. decontamination
4. mechanical
5. biological
6. chemical
7. mechanical
8. normal flora
9. commensals
10. chemical
11. inflammatory
12. immune

The first line of body defense against invasion by microorganisms is the _____(1). When this layer is intact, infection _____(2) does / does not (circle one) occur. Removal of microorganisms from body surfaces is called _____(3). This takes place through three general methods, _____(4), _____(5), and _____(6). Shedding of organisms with keratin flakes or washing away are examples of _____(7) decontamination. Biologic decontamination is accomplished by resident bacteria called _____(8) or _____(9). Body secretions lethal to some organisms make up _____(10) decontamination. Two important defense responses that destroy invading microorganisms are the _____(11) response and the _____(12) system.

▶ SEPSIS

5-12

1. generalized
2. systemic
3. sepsis

Sepsis is severe generalized or systemic infection that can cause shock and death. Sepsis occurs when body defenses are overcome by the virulence and numbers of the invading pathogen. It is the most serious consequence in the breakdown of defenses. It is most likely to develop in individuals with previously compromised responses. Severe trauma, preceding or primary disease, and immunosuppression are some things that weaken defense responses. **Bacteremia,** or **viremia,** literally means bacteria or viruses in the bloodstream (**"emia"** means blood). In most cases, pathogens gaining access to the circulation are quickly destroyed and bacteremia or viremia is a temporary, harmless condition. Sepsis occurs when the bacteremia is not resolved. **Septicemia** specifically means toxins from pathogens in the circulation, which serve to poison the systems. Another correct term is **toxemia.** A common reason for septicemia is toxins from gram-negative bacteremia. In an overwhelming infection, or due to weakened defenses, bacteremia involving gram-negative organisms can turn into life-threatening septicemia. Sepsis or septicemia can lead to **septic shock,** which contributes greatly to fatality. Shock is failure of the circulatory system leading to low blood pressure, ischemia, and possibly organ failure and death. In septic shock the cause of the blood vessel changes is the reaction to the poisonous toxins. When body defenses break down or are overcome by pathogens, a severe _____(1) or _____(2) infection can develop, called _____(3). Often, some organisms make their way into the bloodstream and are quickly dispatched by defense responses. This temporary presence of bacteria or viruses in the blood is called _____(4) or _____(5). Prolonged bacteremia with toxemia defines _____(6). The usual cause of death in septicemia is septic _____(7). Blood _____(8) react badly to the _____(9) in the circulation, leading to shock.

4. bacteremia
5. viremia
6. septicemia
7. shock
8. vessels
9. poisonous toxins

5-13

In shock there is insufficient perfusion of the tissues with blood. In Chapter 2 you learned that inadequate blood supply is called _____(1). This causes decreased oxygen to the area or _____(2). Ischemia and hypoxemia cause cell injury and a certain amount of cell death. Worsening of the situation will damage or kill greater areas until an entire organ is involved. Signs of septicemia start with pyrexia. The common term for pyrexia is _____(3). Following fever, if septic shock develops, *a cardinal sign is hypotension.* Hypotension means low _____(4). Because of the low blood pressure, tissues are not supplied or perfused with blood as they should be. Small vessels all over the body are damaged by widespread inflammation. This microvascular injury due to systemic inflammation is responsible for organ failure. Multiple organ failure leads to death. The organs commonly responsible are the kidneys, liver, lungs, and brain.

1. ischemia
2. hypoxia
3. fever
4. blood pressure

5-14

The pathogenesis of septic shock lies in the systemic inflammatory response to severe bacteremia or toxemia. Recall that the inflammatory response starts with changes in blood _____(1). Vasodilation, increase in permeability, and loss of fluid into the tissues usually happen in isolated areas. These reactions lower local blood pressure, so it is easy to understand why widespread vascular changes lead to systemic hypotension. **Tachycardia,** or rapid heartbeat, is an important sign of systemic hypotension. The heart is trying to compensate for inadequate pressure by beating faster and moving more blood through the tissues. Unfortunately, this is not a compensatory mechanism that is effective for long. The basis for hypotension in septic shock lies in the widespread _____(2) response. Inflammation starts with changes in _____(3) that result in lower local blood pressure. When this happens on a system-wide basis, the generalized low blood pressure is called _____(4). An attempt at compensation is made by the heart as it beats _____(5) to bolster circulation. The term for this rapid heartbeat is _____(6). An overview of sepsis and septic shock is shown in Figure 5-2.

1. vessels
2. inflammatory
3. blood vessels
4. hypotension
5. faster
6. tachycardia

5-15

The etiology, or _____(1), of sepsis and septic shock can be any of many microorganisms, including bacteria and some fungi. The most common organisms isolated in these cases are *Pseudomonas aeruginosa, Escherichia coli,* and *Staphylococcus aureus.* In the next section you will be introduced to these organisms. An important note is in regards to *nosocomial sepsis.* This would mean the infection was acquired while the patient was in the _____(2). There are several invasive procedures that are performed on a regular basis that are important to the treatment of the patient. However, since they are invasive, a *breach in aseptic technique* or *immunosuppression* provides an opportunity for organisms to enter the bloodstream. Examples of invasive treatment techniques are indwelling venous or arterial catheters and intravenous injections.

1. cause
2. hospital

▶ ENVIRONMENTAL CONTROL OF MICROORGANISMS

5-16

Controlling microorganisms in the environment is a great help to body defenses. There is less work to be done and a greater chance of success. Control is primarily through chemical and mechanical means. There are two classifications of control. First is **disinfection,** which reduces the numbers of organisms to relatively harmless levels. (Remember, dose or numbers is one factor in determining if infection occurs.) Disinfection kills most pathogens and other organisms. However, it does not kill all of them. Something that does survive are bacterial **spores.** Spores are extremely resistant, dormant forms of some bacteria with a tough

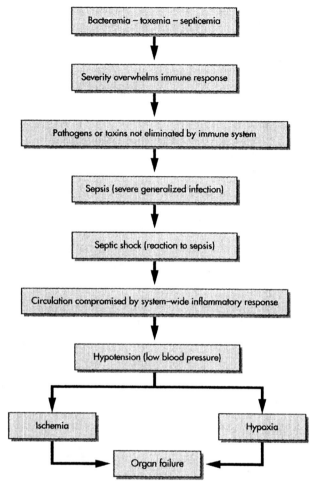

Figure 5–2. Pathogenesis of sepsis and septic shock.

1. body defenses
2. disinfection
3. damaging
4. environment
5. antiseptics

outer coat. There are two kinds of disinfectants. One is a chemical, which is corrosive, or would damage living tissue. Examples are formalin and bleach. These caustic disinfectants are used on inanimate objects and in the environment. Less toxic chemicals that can be used on tissues are called **antiseptics.** Examples are iodine and alcohol. To disinfect living tissues, such as a wound, is called **antisepsis.** Control of environmental microorganisms is helpful to the process of _____(1). Killing most organisms and therefore reducing numbers is _____(2). A corrosive disinfectant is one that is _____(3) to living tissues and should be used only in the _____(4). Disinfection of living tissues is accomplished with the use of _____(5).

5-17

The other class of control is **sterilization.** In contrast to disinfection, sterilization kills *all* microorganisms present. An object totally free of microorganisms is **sterile.** Spores are also killed. The most common method of sterilization is **autoclaving.** In this process, steam is produced to penetrate every microscopic nook and cranny. The specific requirements that cause sterilization are that the steam produces a temperature of 121 degrees Celsius and pressure of 15 pounds per square inch. These conditions must exist for a minimum of 15 minutes. If any of these parameters vary, sterilization cannot be depended upon. The device that creates these conditions is called an **autoclave.** A method of organism control that kills all living things, including spores, is _____(1). This is usually done through the process of _____(2). In this process, _____(3) is produced at a temperature of _____(4) and pressure of _____(5). To cause sterilization, this must last at least _____(6) minutes.

1. sterilization
2. autoclaving
3. steam
4. 121 degrees Celsius
5. 15 pounds per square inch
6. 15

Cleaning is removal of the gross, or visible, matter present such as soil or organic matter. Organic matter includes fecal material, vomitus, and blood. Cleaning is a vital prerequisite to disinfection or sterilization. The presence of soil and organic matter serves to protect or shield the organisms from the agents of control. **Sanitization** generally means disinfection during housekeeping procedures. The hospital environment should be both clean and sanitary. **Aseptic technique,** or **asepsis,** is a procedure designed to prevent or minimize contact between living tissue and pathogens that could cause infection. In surgery, aseptic technique means handling of all sterile material in a manner that maintains sterility. In general practice, asepsis is also important in preventing spread of infectious disease and in treating wounds. This extremely important concept uses many forms of control, not the least of which is frequent hand washing. Before disinfection or sterilization, it is important to _____(1) to remove visible matter. This is because visible matter interferes with _____(2) or _____(3). Disinfection during housekeeping procedures is _____(4). Ways of preventing infection by protecting vulnerable tissue is part of _____(5) technique. In these procedures, exposure to or transmission of _____(6) is kept to a minimum.

1. clean
2. disinfection
3. sterilization
4. sanitization
5. aseptic
6. pathogens

I. REVIEW QUESTIONS

1. A microorganism that causes disease is a:
   a. commensal organism
   b. pathogen
   c. normal flora
   d. fomite

2. Normal flora describes (choose all that apply):
   a. microorganisms usually present on many body surfaces
   b. microorganisms also called commensals
   c. microorganisms generally causing disease
   d. secondary disease producers
   e. pathogens transmitted by carriers

3. The strength or ability of a microorganism to cause disease is described as:
   a. colonization
   b. infection
   c. opportunistic infection
   d. virulence

4. Which of the following statements BEST describes an opportunistic infection?
   a. primary infection by a pathogen
   b. secondary infection by an additional pathogen
   c. infection by a weak pathogen or normal flora when the immune system is overburdened or suppressed
   d. infection by a virulent pathogen when the immune system is overburdened or suppressed

1. b–pathogen

2. a–microorganisms usually present on many body surfaces; b–microorganisms also called commensals

3. d–virulence

4. c–infection by weak pathogens or normal flora when the immune system is overburdened or suppressed

5. b–exogenous

6. a–fomite

7. c–nosocomial

8. b–broken skin; d–natural body openings

9. a–virulence; b–dose; c–entry; d–inflammatory and immune; e–necrotic; f–ischemia

10. 1. c–chemical decontamination; 2. e–inflammation; 3. f–immune response; 4. a–skin; 5. d–biologic decontamination; 6. b–mechanical decontamination

11. d–sepsis

12. bacteremia

5. The most common source of infection is:
   a. endogenous
   b. exogenous
   c. congenital
   d. carriers

6. An inanimate object that can harbor pathogens and transmit infection is a:
   a. fomite
   b. carrier
   c. vector
   d. commensal

7. Infection acquired in a group housing situation such as a hospital is called:
   a. endogenous
   b. contagious
   c. nosocomial
   d. virulent

8. Pathogens generally enter the body through (choose all that apply):
   a. intact skin
   b. broken skin
   c. the bloodstream
   d. natural body openings
   e. all of the above

9. Several factors determine if an infection can be contained or becomes systemic. Please supply the missing words to explain these factors:
   a. the strength of the pathogen or its _____
   b. the numbers of microorganisms or the _____
   c. how the microorganisms gains access or the site of _____
   d. effective functioning of host defense by the _____ and _____ response
   e. the presence of dead or _____ tissue
   f. decreased blood supply to an area or _____

10. Please match the body defenses against infection in the left column with their descriptions in the right column:
    a. skin
    b. mechanical decontamination
    c. chemical decontamination
    d. biologic decontamination
    e. inflammation
    f. immune response

    1. ____ lethal body secretions
    2. ____ fibrin wall and phagocytosis
    3. ____ opsonization and complement
    4. ____ first line of defense
    5. ____ normal flora
    6. ____ shedding or washing away

11. When pathogens are able to overcome all body defenses and cause severe systemic infection with possible shock and death, this is called:
    a. septicemia
    b. bacteremia
    c. toxemia
    d. sepsis

12. Write the term that means bacteria in the bloodstream or circulation:

    _____.

13. Bacteremia that is not eliminated by defense mechanisms and leads to toxins in the blood is called:
    a. septicemia
    b. sepsis
    c. septic shock
    d. none of the above

14. Generalized reaction by the blood vessels to toxins, which causes severe hypotension, describes:
    a. septicemia
    b. sepsis
    c. septic shock
    d. toxemia

15. Please match the terms describing control of microorganisms in the left column with their definition in the right column:
    a. sterilization
    b. antisepsis
    c. sanitization
    d. disinfection
    e. cleaning
    f. aseptic technique

    1. ____ removes visible soil or organic matter
    2. ____ kills most microorganisms
    3. ____ disinfects living tissue
    4. ____ disinfects objects
    5. ____ kills all microorganisms
    6. ____ decreases infection through procedures that minimize contact with pathogens

13. a–septicemia

14. c–septic shock

15. 1. e–cleaning; 2. d–disinfection; 3. b–antisepsis; 4. c–sanitization; 5. a–sterilization; 6. f–aseptic technique

II. BACTERIAL INFECTIONS ◀ SECTION

5-19

Since bacteria are only one of several kinds of microorganisms, there must be more to their definition than a living entity too small to be seen without a microscope. A **bacterium** is a single-celled microorganism that is more primitive than fungi or protozoa. This is because they are **prokaryotic** cells, which means they do not have a true nucleus. The structural membrane is missing. Reproduction is asexual, which means there is no need for joining of male and female genetic material. They grow by **binary fission,** or splitting in two. **Bacteria** (the plural of bacterium) lack important organelles, such as mitochondria, found in higher forms of life. There are also differences in cell walls. Bacterial cell walls are usually rigid because of peptidoglycans and do not contain sterol. In summation, bacteria are the simpler of the microorganisms. (A virus has even fewer structures, but is not a cell.)

5-20

Several bacterial pathogens are described as **pyogenic.** That means they cause an inflammatory response that leads to the production of pus. In Chapter 2 you learned that pus is made of dead neutrophils, bacteria, and debris. Exudate that contains pus is called _____(1) exudate. Another word that describes the presence of purulent exudate is suppuration. In a suppurative infection, much of the tissue damage is from neutrophilic enzymes. Bacteria that cause the formation of purulent exudate or pus are called _____(2).

1. purulent
2. pyogenic

▶ MAJOR PYOGENIC GRAM-POSITIVE COCCI

5-21

The first organisms we will consider are the **staphylococci.** In lay terms these organisms are called staph. The staphylococci are gram-positive cocci in clusters. ***Staphylococcus epidermidis*** is normal skin flora. Rarely, it is implicated in nosocomial infections associated with invasive procedures in debilitated patients. The most virulent is ***Staphylococcus aureus.*** It is

1. *Staphylococcus aureus*
2. nosocomial

common practice to refer to bacteria by the first letter of the genus, followed by the species name. So *Staphylococcus aureus* is called *S. aureus*. *S. aureus* is found as an inhabitant on the skin of some healthy people, or can be harbored as a pathogen in the nasal passages of others who are carriers of this bacteria. *S. aureus* infections are a major problem in hospitals where many of the health care workers can pass the organisms to vulnerable patients. The most virulent of the *Staphylococcus* organisms is _____(1). Because it can be transmitted by hospital personnel, it is a major cause of hospital-acquired, or _____(2), infections.

5–22

1. skin
2. mucous membranes
3. pustule
4. incision
5. bacteremia or septicemia
6. abscesses

S. aureus lesions can involve superficial sites (skin or mucous membranes) or can be internal in some organs. Skin lesions are familiar to most people and include acne pustules, boils, and abscesses. A stye is a staph infection of an eyelash. Impetigo is a skin infection of children composed of blisters and pustules. Folliculitis, or infection of hair follicles, is caused by *S. aureus*. Surgical incisions are prime candidates for *S. aureus* infection. There are some strains of this bacteria that produce a spreading factor called **hyaluronidase,** which enables them to move through tissues once they have gained access through broken skin. Hyaluronidase is an enzyme that dissolves the glue of connective tissue, leaving space for movement. *S. aureus* that gains access to the circulation, or to some organs directly, can produce disease of the body systems. Examples are bronchopneumonia (lungs), enterocolitis (intestines), osteomyelitis (bones), and phlebitis (veins). *S. aureus* is an important cause of septicemia. As these pyogenic bacteria cruise the general circulation, they can cause abscesses of organs they pass through. Important examples are liver abscess and kidney abscess. Superficial *S. aureus* infection involves the _____(1) or _____(2). An example is the small sac of pus seen in acne, which is called a (an) _____(3). A wound that must be protected from *S. aureus* infection is a surgical _____(4). If *S. aureus* enters the bloodstream, the general term for this is _____(5). A consequence of *S. aureus* septicemia is the formation of _____(6) in organs like the kidney or liver.

5–23

1. toxin

Another aspect of *S. aureus* infection has to do with toxin production. It is the effect of the poisonous toxin that makes the person ill. Food poisoning is discussed in later frames. **Toxic shock syndrome** is a condition that was first described in children. Recently, it became associated with the use of some tampons by menstruating women. It is thought that the bacteria somehow grow in the tampon and produce a toxin that is absorbed into the bloodstream. The tissue that sloughs and causes bleeding in menstruation is susceptible to bacterial invasion. Signs of this systemic toxemia include high fever and diarrhea with possible hypotension and kidney impairment. In addition to tissue infection, *S. aureus* can cause illness by producing a (an) _____(1).

5–24

1. *Streptococcus pyogenes*
2. group A hemolytic
3. beta hemolytic
4. acute pharyngitis
5. circulation

The **streptococci** are the next group to be considered. Streptococci appear as gram-positive cocci in chains. The first virulent species we will study are the **group A hemolytic streptococci.** They are also called **beta hemolytic streptococci.** This is because of the particular type of hemolysis they exhibit when cultured on blood agar. Beta hemolysis is a clear zone around the colonies resulting from hemolysis of blood cells and breakdown of the products. The particular species we will examine here is *Streptococcus pyogenes* or *S. pyogenes*. This bacteria is responsible for the well-known condition of strep throat. Infection of the throat by *S. pyogenes* causes **acute pharyngitis.** In children, this infection can travel to involve the middle ear, producing **otitis media.** The importance of strep throat lies in possible complications. In **scarlet fever,** the organisms produce systemic illness if a toxin they produce is absorbed into the circulation. One of the effects of the toxin is to create a rash in the skin because of the action on blood vessels. This red rash is responsible for the name of the disease. The bacterium responsible for strep throat is _____(1). Descriptive names for this same bacterium, based on its reaction on blood agar, include _____(2) streptococci and _____(3) streptococci. The medical term for strep throat is _____(4). Toxins that are absorbed into the _____(5) and cause a

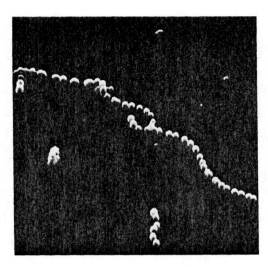

Figure 5–3. Scanning electron micrograph of *S. pyogenes* showing typical chain formation. *(From Greenwood et al, Medical Microbiology, 14th ed., Churchill Livingstone.)*

---

red _____(6) on the skin cause general illness in the disease _____(7). Figure 5–3 is an electron micrograph showing the arrangement of *S. pyogenes* in a chain.

6. rash
7. scarlet fever

Two more serious complications are **rheumatic fever** and **poststreptococcal glomerulonephritis.** These diseases are due to the reaction to the infection by the immune system. For reasons not well understood, host tissue is damaged by antibodies made against the bacteria. "Cross-reaction" could describe this phenomenon. This is an example of hypersensitivity that you studied in Chapter 4. Technically, they can be considered autoimmune diseases as well (host antibody injuring host tissue). Poststreptococcal glomerulonephritis is an inflammatory condition of the kidneys, specifically affecting the glomeruli. Rheumatic fever affects the joints and the heart. The joints become swollen and painful as a result of antibody injury to the synovial membranes lining the joints. The injury naturally results in inflammation. The valves of the heart are also damaged by immune system activity. However, this damage does not become apparent until perhaps years later when the defective valves can no longer do their job. This causes impairment of heart function. Upper respiratory infection with *Streptococcus* _____(1) has been associated with a kidney disease called _____(2). It can also be also a forerunner of _____(3) fever, which injures the _____(4) and the heart _____(5). These two consequences of *S. pyogenes* infection are thought to be due to reaction to the bacteria by the _____(6). This reaction could be classified as overreactive or _____(7), or possibly as autoimmune.

S–25

1. *pyogenes*
2. poststreptococcal glomerulonephritis
3. rheumatic
4. joints
5. valves
6. immune system
7. hypersensitivity

Streptococcus pneumoniae is a little different morphologically from *S. pyogenes*. It is a gram-positive coccus, but it appears in pairs. This kind of arrangement is called **diplococcus.** Another name for this organism is **pneumococcus.** It is part of the oral normal flora, particularly the throat. Children are susceptible to ear infections by this bacteria (otitis media), and it has been isolated in cases of pneumonia. Figure 5–4 shows the appearance of *S. pneumoniae* in the sputum of a patient with pneumonia. These lower respiratory infections can lead to meningitis if the patient experiences septicemia. One microorganism that is normal flora of the urogenital tract is ***Enterococcus.*** *Enterococcus* was thought to be streptococcus group D, so you may still see it referred to in the literature that way. However, we know now it is not one of the streptococci. Enterococci have been associated with opportunistic infections of the urogenital tract. A gram-positive diplococcus isolated in cases of ear infection or pneumonia is likely to be _____(1). This organism is also called

S–26

1. *Streptococcus pneumoniae*

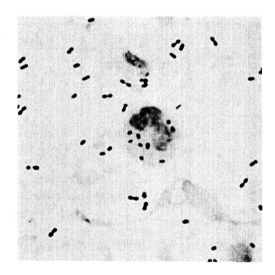

Figure 5–4. *S. pneumoniae* in the sputum of a patient with pneumonia. *(From Ryan,* Sherris Medical Microbiology, *3rd ed., Appleton & Lange.)*

2. pneumococcus
3. enterococci
4. has

_____(2). Normal flora of the urogenital tract that look like the streptococci are _____(3). This microorganism _____(4) has / has not (choose one) been found in urogenital infections. Table 5–1 summarizes the diseases associated with the major pyogenic gram-positive cocci.

▶ MAJOR PYOGENIC GRAM-NEGATIVE DIPLOCOCCI

5–27

There is only one microorganism we will consider in this category, *Neisseria meningitidis.* As the name implies, it causes meningitis. Meningitis is inflammation of the meninges, the membrane covering the brain and spinal cord. This organism is different from previous ones in that it is **intracellular.** With proper staining, it can be seen inside polymorphonuclear white blood cells, or PMNs. It appears as a pair of red or pink cocci in the cytoplasm of these cells ("diplo" means two). It arrives there by phagocytosis but is not destroyed. Another term assigned to describe this organism is **meningococcus.** The gram-negative diplococcus caus-

TABLE 5–1. PYOGENIC GRAM-POSITIVE COCCI OF MAJOR MEDICAL IMPORTANCE

Bacteria	Associated Diseases
Staphylococcus aureus	Nosocomial infection in debilitated patients
	Skin infections (acne, boils, abscesses, styes, impetigo, folliculitis)
	Systemic infection (bronchopneumonia, enterocolitis, osteomyelitis, phlebitis)
	Septicemia and organ abscess
	Toxemia (food poisoning, toxic shock syndrome)
Streptococcus pyogenes	Acute pharyngitis
	Otitis media
	Scarlet fever
	Rheumatic fever
	Poststreptococcal glomerulonephritis
Streptococcus pneumoniae	Otitis media
	Pneumonia
	Septicemia
	Meningitis
Enterococci	Urogenital tract infection

ing meningitis is _____(1). The term describing the usual location of this microorganism is _____(2). The cells in which *N. meningitidis* are found are _____(3). *N. meningitidis* is also called _____(4).

1. *Neisseria meningitidis*
2. intracellular
3. polymorphonuclear cells (PMNs)
4. meningococcus

5-28

N. meningitidis can be an oral commensal. More virulent strains are responsible for **epidemic meningitis,** which means it is contagious. It is spread through the airborne route. It is an opportunistic organism, gaining hold in suppressed or strained immune systems, or in children. A sore throat and fever are followed by a stiff, sore neck as the organism gains access to the meninges through the circulation. Bacteria in the bloodstream is called _____(1). The mortality rate can be quite high. Since meningococcal meningitis is contagious, it is sometimes referred to as _____(2). Since *N. meningitidis* affects vulnerable populations, it is classified as a (an) _____(3) organism.

1. bacteremia
2. epidemic meningitis
3. opportunistic

▷ MAJOR PYOGENIC GRAM-NEGATIVE BACILLI

5-29

These bacilli or rods are made up of a group of organisms with several common names. They are normal flora of the intestines and colon. For this reason, in addition to being called intestinal bacteria, they are called **enteric bacilli** and **coliforms.** These gut organisms play useful roles as participants in production of certain vitamins, such as B and K. The two categories of causes of infection by enteric rods are as opportunists and as invaders of other body sites. Other body parts can be contaminated by coliforms in a variety of ways. They can be introduced to the urogenital tract through unsanitary practices or sexually. Wounds can become contaminated by lack of proper aseptic technique or by the patient. Opportunistic infections arise when coliforms invade the bloodstream of susceptible individuals, which includes hospital patients. Gram-negative rods can cause a threatening septicemia in these patients. An endotoxin from these organisms produces **endotoxic shock** or septic shock. Of the coliforms, *E. coli* is often the cause of septic shock. Another mechanism of septic shock is **perforation,** or a hole or tear, of the intestines or colon. These organisms immediately cause severe **peritonitis,** infectious inflammation of the peritoneum that lines the entire abdominal cavity. The size of this membrane allows it to absorb endotoxins at a rapid pace. Aggressive treatment is vital to prevent fatal endotoxic shock.

5-30

Intestinal bacteria are often called _____(1) or _____(2). They are commensals with useful roles. Infection occurs when they are introduced to other body _____(3), or if they act as _____(4) in debilitated people. Two common sites that can become infected with coliforms are the _____(5) tract and _____(6) that are exposed by poor management. If gram-negative rods of the intestines enter the circulation, they can cause serious _____(7), leading to _____(8) or _____(9). Perforation of the gut leads to infectious _____(10). The danger here is _____(11) following absorption of toxins.

1. enteric bacilli
2. coliforms
3. sites
4. opportunists
5. urogenital
6. wounds
7. septicemia
8. endotoxic shock
9. septic shock
10. peritonitis
11. fatal endotoxic shock

5-31

The specific coliforms include *Escherichia coli* and the genuses of *Klebsiella, Proteus,* and *Pseudomonas. E. coli* is associated with urinary tract infections (UTIs), genital tract infections, diarrhea, and abscesses. In female UTI or genital infection, the organisms ascend, or move up, from the perineum. Therefore, this is called an **ascending infection.** Ascending infections are not limited to *E. coli. Proteus* and *Pseudomonas* are other enteric bacteria isolated from cases of urogenital tract infections. *Pseudomonas* especially likes growing in wounds, where it produces a characteristic greenish pus. Patients with burns must be carefully guarded from this infection. Necrotizing pneumonia can be produced by bacteremia from *Pseudomonas* or *Klebsiella.* The infection of the lung tissue produces large areas of

1. *Escherichia coli*
2. *Proteus*
3. *Pseudomonas*
4. *E. coli*
5. *Pseudomonas*
6. *Pseudomonas*
7. *Klebsiella*

5-32

necrosis or tissue death. In the following sentences, associate these infections with the enteric rods often responsible. Urinary or genital tract infections are caused by _____(1), _____(2), and _____(3). Diarrhea is caused by _____(4). Wound infection is caused by _____(5) and necrotizing pneumonia by _____(6) and _____(7).

Salmonella are gram-negative rods found in the intestines of poultry and other animals. A type of food poisoning is caused by *Salmonella enteritidis. S. enteritidis* causes gastroenteritis, or stomach and intestinal disease. One source of salmonella gastroenteritis or **salmonellosis,** is direct contamination of water or food by these animal coliforms. Most common is the contamination of meat, especially poultry, during processing. Also, any person ill with salmonellosis or a carrier can shed the organism in their stool and be a source of contamination. Food handlers that might be ill or be carriers should not prepare food or should take special precautions not to contaminate the food. Home preparation of poultry dishes requires sanitary practices that minimize the possibility of salmonellosis.

5-33

1. salmonellosis
2. *enteritidis*
3. water
4. food
5. poultry
6. processing
7. salmonellosis
8. carrier

Gastroenteritis caused by *Salmonella* is called _____(1). The species associated with this condition is S. _____(2). Sources of this bacteria include direct contamination of _____(3) or _____(4) by the intestinal contents of animals, specifically _____(5). A common way this can occur is during meat _____(6). Other sources are people with active _____(7), or a _____(8). Table 5–2 summarizes the pyogenic gram-negative rods of medical importance.

5-34

These last few pyogenic gram-negative rods are presented for your information and are less likely to be routinely encountered. *Shigella* is a species that causes serious intestinal disease in other parts of the world due to unsanitary conditions and poor hygiene. In the United States, it is present but not as great a problem. A virulent species is *Shigella dysenteriae,* and it results in dysentery. **Dysentery** looks like severe diarrhea at first, but the damage is on a deeper level. Diarrhea may involve secretion of excess fluid into the bowels, making the stool runny, or superficial invasion of the intestinal lining by microorganisms. In dysentery there is deep invasion of the bowel walls by microorganisms. This damaging infection, combined with toxins from some organisms, causes sections of the intestinal lining to slough off and be passed in the stool. Present in the stool, which differentiates it from diarrhea, is pus, blood, and mucus. The patient experiences severe cramping and **tenesmus** (frequent straining of the bowels). The excessive loss of fluid and other materials cause dehydration and debilitation.

5-35

Haemophilus influenzae is a small, gram-negative rod, also called a **coccobacillus.** A coccobacillus is a very short rod. This bacterium was misnamed when it was thought to be the cause of influenza in children some years ago. (We now know influenza is caused by a virus.) *H. influenzae* is a child's disease involving upper respiratory infection (**nasopharyngitis**), otitis media, and possible meningitis. It is most dangerous when **acute epiglottitis** develops. There is swelling of the epiglottis that can obstruct air passages. *H. influenzae* can cause opportunistic infection in debilitated adults.

TABLE 5–2. PYOGENIC GRAM-NEGATIVE BACILLI OF MAJOR MEDICAL IMPORTANCE

Bacteria	Associated Diseases
Coliforms	
Escherichia coli	Endotoxic septic shock, urogenital tract infection, diarrhea, abscesses
Klebsiella	Necrotizing pneumonia
Proteus	Urogenital tract infection
Pseudomonas	Urogenital tract infection, wound infection, necrotizing pneumonia
Salmonella	Salmonellosis (gastroenteritis)

5-36

One respiratory infection of adults is **legionellosis** or **Legionnaires' disease.** The causative agent is **Legionella pneumophila.** This bacteria was identified relatively recently (1976) during an outbreak at an American Legion convention. The pneumonia produced by this pathogen is not to be taken lightly, since there is about a 15 percent mortality rate. The organism is breathed directly into the lungs, and the source is usually air conditioning equipment. The cooling unit is damp and warm, which is the perfect breeding ground for *L. pneumophila.*

► VENEREAL INFECTION CAUSED BY BACTERIA

5-37

A **venereal infection** is infection of the genitals that is transmitted only through genital contact. This is in contrast to **sexually transmitted disease,** or **STD,** which is *primarily* spread through sexual activity but other routes are possible. The two venereal diseases we will consider are gonorrhea and syphilis. Gonorrhea is caused by *Neisseria gonorrhoeae.* Like *Meningococcus,* this *Neisseria* is also an intracellular gram-negative diplococcus. Gonorrhea is much more common than syphilis. In fact, it is still the most commonly reported communicable disease in the United States. **Asymptomatic** cases, or those with no visible signs or symptoms, are chiefly responsible for the continuance of gonorrhea. Twenty percent of males and more than 50 percent of females are asymptomatic sufferers of gonorrhea. Genital infection transmitted only by genital contact defines _____(1). The most common bacterial venereal disease is _____(2), and it is caused by _____(3). An important reason gonorrhea persists in society is because of _____(4) cases.

1. venereal disease
2. gonorrhea
3. *Neisseria gonorrhoeae*
4. asymptomatic

5-38

Detecting gonorrhea in males is a relatively simple matter. Signs are hard to miss. Men experience burning urination and have a purulent exudate or discharge from the penis. The infection is an **acute urethritis,** or the sudden onset of infectious inflammation of the urethra. The penile discharge is stained and examined microscopically for the presence of gram-negative diplococci in the cytoplasm of PMNs. Figure 5–5 demonstrates the presence of *N. gonorrhoeae* in the neutrophils of a urethral discharge. Early diagnosis and treatment makes gonorrhea in men a curable and relatively benign condition. In females it can be much different, with serious consequences. Women do not develop the obvious acute urethritis as readily. Early cases are often unnoticeable. But as *N. gonorrhoeae* travels up the female reproduc-

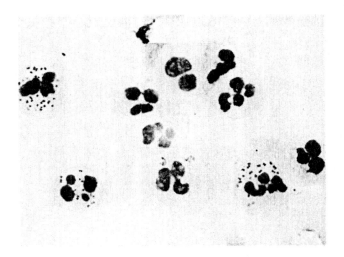

Figure 5–5. Gram stain of a urethral exudate of an acute case of gonorrhea in a male. *(From Ryan,* Sherris Medical Microbiology, *3rd ed., Appleton & Lange.)*

tive tract, it infects the fallopian tubes causing **salpingitis.** This infectious inflammation of the fallopian tubes can lead to fibrosis or scarring. The scar tissue interferes with the fertilization process so that the female may be sterile. If fertilization does occur, it may be outside of the fallopian tubes. This is an **ectopic pregnancy** in the abdomen instead of the uterus. If purulent infection continues with production of abscesses, this chronic condition is called **pelvic inflammatory disease,** or **PID.** PID further contributes to infertility.

5–39

1. signs
2. urethritis
3. burning
4. discharge
5. penis
6. unnoticeable
7. fallopian
8. salpingitis
9. scarring
10. ectopic
11. pelvic inflammatory disease

Men with gonorrhea are usually diagnosed and treated before there is any permanent damage because _____(1) are obvious. The injury by *N. gonorrheae* is acute _____(2). The signs of this infection are _____(3) urination and a purulent _____(4) from the _____(5). In women, early cases may be _____(6), or show no signs. As the condition progresses, infection of the _____(7) tubes, or _____(8), is common. The inflammation and resulting _____(9) is a cause of sterility. Pregnancy that does occur may be outside of the reproductive tract, and this is called _____(10) pregnancy. Chronic gonorrhea in women produces _____(11).

5–40

1. pharyngeal gonorrhea
2. septicemia
3. septic
4. gonococcal conjunctivitis
5. treated

Oral–genital contact is responsible for gonorrhea of the throat, or **pharyngeal gonorrhea.** Another possible manifestation of this disease is septicemia, occurring in menstruating females. The sloughing of the endometrium (uterine lining) and subsequent bleeding provides an avenue for entry into the bloodstream. This systemic involvement can produce **septic arthritis,** or infectious inflammation of the joints. An actively infective woman can give birth to a newborn with infection of the eyes, or **gonococcal conjunctivitis.** Gonococcal conjunctivitis, if untreated, can lead to ulcers of the cornea and blindness. For this reason, all newborns are routinely treated at birth with antibiotics or silver nitrate placed into the conjunctival sacs. In addition to infection of the adult reproductive tract, gonorrhea has other manifestations. In the throat it is called _____(1). Systemic involvement is in the form of _____(2), with possible _____(3) arthritis. Newborns of infected mothers are susceptible to the dangerous infection, _____(4). All babies should be _____(5) at birth to prevent this.

5–41

1. *Treponema pallidum*
2. a spiral or coil
3. less
4. more
5. fatal

Syphilis is caused by the microorganism *Treponema pallidum. T. pallidum* is not a coccus or bacillus, but a **spirochete.** The morphology of a spirochete, or what it looks like, is a spiral or coil. Several hundred years ago, when syphilis was introduced into Europe from Columbus' New World, the organism was much more virulent than it is today. The various stages were more severe, and it was often fatal. For this reason, this common disease was called the Great Pox. It is not such a devastating disease today, and it is much less common than gonorrhea. However, it is still a more dangerous disease than gonorrhea. Syphilis is a chronic infection that still has the ability to kill in later stages. Fortunately, in both men and women, it is relatively easy to diagnose and treat. The organism _____(1) causes syphilis. Morphologically, it looks like _____(2). Syphilis is _____(3) common than gonorrhea, but it is _____(4) dangerous. The end stages of syphilis can be _____(5).

5–42

The clinical course of syphilis is divided into three stages. **Stage 1** is the **primary stage.** About 3 weeks after exposure, a lesion develops at the site of entry. This is usually the genital region but may be around the mouth. The lesion is a **chancre** which becomes an ulcer. This is pictured in Figure 5–6A. The chancre is highly infectious and is teeming with the spirochetes. Because the ulcer is painless, it may be missed or mistaken for something else. Internal chancres are not noticeable. The primary stage lasts about 2 to 3 weeks. Blood tests may be positive by the end of this stage, but could also be negative. The best way to diagnose it at this stage is by **dark-field microscopy.** This requires the identification of the chancre for what it is, so the organisms can be obtained from the lesion. Dark-field microscopy is direct examination of a specimen from the lesion, using a special attachment so the organ-

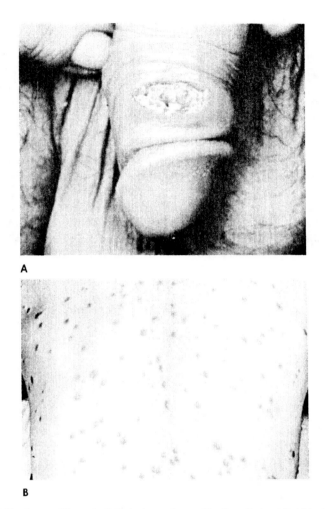

A

B

Figure 5–6. A. Syphilitic chancre of the penis. **B.** Rash of secondary syphilis. *(From Kent and Hart,* Introduction to Human Disease, *3rd ed., Appleton & Lange.)*

ism can be seen. Treatment cures the infection. Untreated cases advance to the next stage. *T. pallidum* is a very invasive organism. Stage 1 of syphilis is the _____(1) stage. The lesion is a _____ (2), which looks like (a) an _____(3). Blood tests in the primary stage may be _____(4) or _____(5). If the chancre is correctly identified, the diagnostic test of choice is _____(6).

1. primary
2. chancre
3. ulcer
4. positive
5. negative
6. darkfield-microscopy

5–43

Untreated cases advance to **stage 2,** or the **secondary stage.** The chancre has healed, the patient feels well, and the infection is unapparent. The secondary stage can last from several weeks to a year. *T. pallidum* spreads through out the body via the circulation and grows in various sites. Stage 2 is marked by a **syphilitic rash** that develops on many parts of the body, including the palms and feet. This is shown in Figure 5–6B. The rash is painless, doesn't itch, and is not characteristic. This means that it could be mistaken for another condition. The rash is not as infective as the chancre, but organisms can be transmitted by contact with the rash. The patient usually has complaints of nonspecific illness as well. Blood tests during the secondary stage are positive, and specimens from the rash can be examined with dark-field. Again, treatment cures the infection. In untreated cases, the infection becomes latent or dormant. About one third of these advance to the next stage, which has life-threatening effects. Meanwhile, the patient again feels fine after stage 2. Because the primary and secondary stages can be missed, routine blood tests are important to control the disease. Stage 2 of syphilis is called the _____(1) stage. The organisms

1. secondary

2. spread
3. rash
4. positive
5. one third

5–44

1. scarring
2. tertiary
3. cardiovascular
4. central nervous
5. vasculitis
6. syphilitic aortitis
7. fibrosis
8. aneurysm
9. neurosyphilis
10. paralysis
11. blindness
12. insane dementia

5–45

5–46

1. gastroenteritis
2. vomiting
3. diarrhea
4. food preparation

have _____(2) throughout the body. Stage 2 is marked by the onset of a (an) _____(3) that can appear everywhere. Blood tests are _____(4). About _____(5) of untreated secondary cases will advance to the most serious stage.

The last and most serious stage is **stage 3,** or the **tertiary stage.** Remember, the organism is system-wide now. *T. pallidum* can injure several body systems, but the most significant are the cardiovascular and nervous systems. In cardiovascular damage, the primary lesion is **vasculitis,** or inflammation of the blood vessels. This vasculitis especially affects the aorta. It is sometimes called **syphilitic aortitis.** You have learned that continued inflammation leads to a lot of fibrosis or _____(1). This scar tissue of chronic inflammation replaces the elastin in the aortic walls. The aorta absorbs a tremendous amount of pressure from blood ejecting from the heart and elastin (elastic fibers) is vital in being able to bounce back. The fibrotic wall becomes weak under the pressure. This defect can lead to rupture, or an **aneurysm,** and fatal hemorrhage. In the nervous system, **neurosyphilis** develops. Vasculitis of vessels supplying the central nervous system (CNS) leads to death of certain regions from lack of blood supply. Necrosis of the brain and spinal cord cause the signs of paralysis, blindness, and insane dementia. Interference with motor function and voluntary muscles produce a characteristic staggering gait that has been often referred to in historical literature. Stage 3 develops anywhere from 3 to 25 years after the primary stage. Treatment must occur before this permanent damage is done to the body. Stage 3 of syphilis is the _____(2) stage. The two most seriously affected body systems are the _____(3) and _____(4) systems. The injury to both of these is an underlying _____(5) involving the blood vessels. Aortic involvement is sometimes called _____(6). The end result of the scarring or _____(7) of the wall is rupture or a (an) _____(8). Vasculitis of CNS vessels has been called _____(9). Three signs of this are _____(10), _____(11), and _____(12).

Diagnosis of syphilis depends on dark-field examination of chancre or rash specimens, or on blood tests. These tests are routine in many circumstances. The tests are based on serology, using the patient serum that has antibody to *T. pallidum* and reacting it with various antigens. The **screening tests** are done initially, and if they are positive, then **definitive tests** are performed. A screening test is generally nonspecific. This means that other antibodies or serum components could react and cause a **false positive.** Therefore, a positive screening test calls for a definitive test, which *is* specific for the disease in question. Screening tests are performed first because of ease, availability, and expense. A negative screening test for syphilis usually ends there. Treatment of syphilis is not difficult since resistance is not a problem and the infection responds well. However, reinfection *is* a problem if someone is exposed again because immunity is almost nonexistent. For unknown reasons, the organisms must be present a long time to cause an effective immune response.

▶ TOXINS IN BACTERIAL INFECTIONS

Some illnesses caused by bacteria are not directly related to colonization, inflammation, and damage to tissues. They are a reaction to toxins produced and secreted by the bacteria (**exotoxin**) or to toxins released from inside the organisms when they die (**endotoxin**). The first example of this is **food poisoning.** This condition is associated with unsanitary or unsafe food preparation practices. Food poisoning causes **acute gastroenteritis,** a sudden upset of the stomach and intestines, with vomiting and diarrhea. Food poisoning should be suspected when several people who have eaten the same food develop vomiting and/or diarrhea soon after. Food poisoning causes the condition acute _____(1), and the signs are _____(2) and _____(3). Food poisoning develops because of unsafe _____(4) practices.

5–47

Two organisms that cause food poisoning due to toxins are *S. aureus* and the agent of botulism. *S. aureus* is a very common contaminant and is associated with both an unclean environment and carriers. Food with this organism, left at room temperature, guarantees illness. The organism itself may cause gastroenteritis from uncooked foods, or a toxin from it can cause sickness after the food is cooked. Many people mistakenly think that cooking food destroys all potential disease-causing agents. While the microorganisms are indeed often destroyed, many toxins are **heat stable** and not destroyed by cooking. *S. aureus* and its toxin target the stomach and upper intestines so signs of illness begin very soon after ingestion (1 to 4 hours). Another agent of food poisoning that does *not* produce a toxin is *Salmonella,* as you learned earlier. The mechanism of illness in this case is dose of the pathogen. *Salmonella* multiplies and grows well in contaminated foods at room temperature. This leads to numbers that, once ingested, overcome local defenses and cause illness. Because *Salmonella* affects the *lower* intestinal tract, it can take up to 48 hours before diarrhea develops. This may develop sooner, but usually not as quickly as *S. aureus* poisoning. This timing helps to differentiate the two organisms when food poisoning cases are investigated. Because we are not concerned with toxins in *Salmonella* contamination, cooking foods well and a sanitary preparation environment are good means of prevention.

5–48

A common contaminant of foods that produces a toxin is _____(1). Food poisoning due to *S. aureus* is caused by the organism itself or by a _____(2) from it. Cooking does _____(3) destroy the toxin because it is heat _____(4). Signs of *S. aureus* gastroenteritis develop in _____(5) hours after ingestion of contaminated food. In *Salmonella* food poisoning, the mechanism of injury is not toxicity, but _____(6) related. As *Salmonella* sits in food, it _____(7) to numbers that overcome defenses. Signs of *Salmonella* food poisoning develop up to _____(8) hours later because it affects the _____(9) intestines. This timing helps to separate it from cases of _____(10) gastroenteritis.

1. *S. aureus*
2. toxin
3. not
4. stable
5. 1 to 4
6. dose
7. multiplies
8. 48
9. lower
10. *S. aureus*

5–49

Other disorders due to toxin production are tetanus, gas gangrene, botulism, and diphtheria. Tetanus and gas gangrene are more likely to be encountered than botulism and diphtheria. This is because of commercial food preparation and immunization, respectively. Tetanus, gas gangrene, and botulism are caused by a group of gram-positive rods known as **clostridia.** These are commensals of animal intestines and often found in soil. For this reason, dirty wounds and food grown in contaminated soil are sources of infection. The clostridia are **anaerobes,** which mean they grow in the absence of oxygen. This helps to explain the development of infection in deep necrotic wounds or growth in improperly canned foods. The clostridia also form **spores** that are dormant stages of the bacteria that are extremely resistant to environmental conditions, such as heat, drying, and disinfection. Therefore, clostridia-contaminated soil remains infective for very long periods, and cooked foods are still infective. Gram-positive rods causing tetanus, gas gangrene, and botulism are classified as _____(1). The development of infections by these organisms is partly due to growth in the absence of _____(2). This characteristic is described by the term _____(3). Highly resistant dormant forms of clostridia are called _____(4), and this characteristic also contributes to the pathogenesis of infection.

1. clostridia
2. oxygen
3. anaerobe
4. spores

5–50

The clostridia that produces tetanus is ***Clostridium tetani.*** **Tetanus** is a rigid paralysis that affects the muscles because of the action of tetanus toxin on neuromuscular junctions. The toxin binds to nerve cells and produces painful, continual contraction of skeletal muscle, so that voluntary relaxation of the muscles cannot occur. Tetanus due to *C. tetani* is associated with wounds received outside, or anytime a wound becomes contaminated with dirt. The significance of this disorder is that the wound in question can be trivial, that is, so small as to be disregarded. Puncture wounds are commonly cause for concern, as they should be. The

1. *Clostridium tetani*
2. rigid
3. paralysis
4. neuromuscular
5. wounds
6. puncture
7. dead or necrotic
8. lockjaw
9. trismus

deeper the wound, the better the growing conditions for *C. tetani*. Wounds with deep layers of dead tissue are also excellent growth sites, since there is no blood supply or oxygen associated with necrosis. After the organisms grow and produce an exotoxin, this exotoxin is absorbed from the wound and travels to the spinal cord. Tetanus affects the entire body, but life-threatening rigidity develops in the muscles of mastication, or chewing, and in the respiratory muscles. For this reason, tetanus is commonly referred to as **lockjaw.** The medical term for rigid paralysis of the jaw muscles is **trismus.** The organism that causes tetanus is _____(1). Clinically, tetanus is seen as a _____(2) _____(3) due to the action of the toxin on _____(4) junctions. Tetanus develops when _____(5) are contaminated with soil. Wounds classically associated with tetanus are deep _____(6) wounds, or those with _____(7) tissue. Tetanus of the jaw muscles is commonly called _____(8), and is medically referred to as _____(9).

5-51

1. debridement
2. respiratory
3. prevention
4. debridement
5. vaccination
6. tetanus antitoxin or toxoid
7. incubation period

Development of trismus and fatal respiratory paralysis is inevitable, so the only real treatment is prevention. Wounds should be meticulously cleaned out and all necrotic tissue removed. In Chapter 2 you learned that this process of removing dead tissue was part of the procedure called _____(1). This debridement physically removes *C. tetani* from the site before it produces exotoxin. Another vital prevention technique is vaccination with **tetanus antitoxin,** sometimes called **tetanus toxoid.** This antitoxin is an antibody against the exotoxin that prevents attachment to nerve cells. Because of the long **incubation period** (time from exposure to clinical signs), administering this inoculation after potential exposure is effective prevention. Tetanus toxoid is given routinely to all who present for treatment of wounds because of the fatal outcome should tetanus develop. One cause of fatality in tetanus is _____(2) paralysis, so that the patient can no longer breathe. Treatment of tetanus is mainly through _____(3). Cleaning and _____(4) of wounds is the first step in prevention, and should be followed by _____(5) with _____(6). There is time after exposure to give the immunization because the _____(7) is long.

5-52

1. *Clostridium perfringens*
2. spores
3. oxygen
4. necrotic
5. gas
6. pressure
7. spread

Before we discuss *gas* gangrene, know that gangrene in general can be caused by non-clostridial organisms that do not make exotoxin. These are **saprophytic** anaerobic organisms whose function it is to decompose dead tissue. This is most commonly found in contaminated necrotic tissue that has died because of vessel occlusion or blockage. **Gas gangrene** is specifically caused by *Clostridium perfringens,* as well as a few other clostridia. In the necrotic tissue of deep wounds, anaerobic *C. perfringens* grows extremely well. Injured muscle tissue of the limbs that has little or no blood supply makes a perfect incubator. The decreased oxygen tension allows the spores to germinate, or come out of the dormant state, into a full life cycle. As it grows and multiplies, *C. perfringens* produces gas from the breakdown or fermentation of muscle carbohydrates. The gas causes further tissue death in the area because of the tremendous pressure. It has a characteristic foul smell. This sets up a cycle of spread, as more tissue dies from the gas pressure and becomes further breeding ground. Tissue death specifically from pressure is called **pressure necrosis.** The agent causing gas gangrene is _____(1). The _____(2) can germinate because the _____(3) tension is very low or absent in _____(4) tissue. *C. perfringens* produces a (an) _____(5) that causes _____(6) necrosis and a bad stench. The reaction to the gas allows the organisms to advance or _____(7) further.

5-53

The exotoxin of *C. perfringens* is actually an enzyme that is secreted and kills the surrounding tissue. The enzyme can be described as a toxic necrotizing enzyme. This also is a factor in the spread of this destructive bacteria through neighboring tissue. A zone of necrosis is continually produced around the infection that allows the bacteria to move to new sites in tissue that previously was healthy. Enzymatic decomposition of muscle proteins, with its own foul smell, is called **putrefaction.** Combined with gas production, clinically this is seen as bloating or distention of the affected limb. **Crepitation,** or crackling sounds, can be heard upon palpation of the area, due to the gas bubbles in the muscle. To stop the vicious cycle of gas gangrene, vigorous debridement, antibiotics, and antitoxin are necessary. Amputation is required in advanced cases, because there is too much tissue destruction for treatment to be effective. The exotoxin can also be absorbed, producing fatal toxemia and septic shock. That is another reason for amputation. The exotoxin of *C. perfringens* is a (an) _____(1) that _____(2) surrounding tissue. This contributes to the _____(3) of gas gangrene because new _____(4) tissue is always being produced. This allows the bacteria to move to different areas. This enzymatic, bad-smelling destruction of the muscle is called _____(5). Clinical signs of gas gangrene include bloating or _____(6) of the area and noise when it is felt, called _____(7). To prevent death from _____(8) shock, _____(9) may be required.

1. enzyme
2. kills
3. spread
4. necrotic
5. putrefaction
6. distention
7. crepitation
8. septic
9. amputation

The last two microorganisms that generate disease through toxicity are not as prevalent as they once were, but you should be aware of them. These are the agents of botulism and diphtheria. **Botulism** is caused by ***Clostridium botulinum.*** Food grown in soil containing spores of *C. botulinum* must be carefully processed, since the spores are not destroyed by cooking. Historically, botulism has been associated with improper home canning. Today's commercial processing makes this disease much less likely. In foods where the spores have germinated, a toxin is produced that is deadly. The toxin is extremely potent, and even a tiny amount can cause death. It also targets the neuromuscular junction, causing paralysis. The paralysis includes the muscles of respiration, and death is by **asphyxiation,** or suffocation.

Diphtheria is due to the gram-positive rod or bacilli ***Corynebacterium diptheriae.*** It used to be fairly prevalent, especially in children. The word diphtheria is from the Greek, meaning hide, skin, or leather. It describes a **pseudomembrane** that is formed in the throat. Diphtheria begins with pharyngitis or throat infection. This infection is not invasive and remains on the surface of the mucous membranes. A strong exotoxin that accompanies this disease may be absorbed, causing toxemia. Locally, the toxin kills the underlying membrane in the pharynx. Along with the necrosis is a typical inflammatory reaction, leading to neutrophil accumulation and debris. Much fibrin is created, and this binds together all of the cells and dead tissue so that they do not slough off. It remains on the surface of the throat and makes up the tough, leathery pseudomembrane. This membrane is adhered to the throat, and attempt at removal causes bleeding. This is different from the film of exudate that can occur in strep throat, which is easily removed. The pseudomembrane of diphtheria can even cause suffocation. The systemic effects of the toxemia include necrosis of the myocardium (heart muscle) and congestive heart failure, and nerve degeneration leading to paralysis. Because of the degree of fatality associated with this condition, all children should be immunized against diphtheria. The relative success of the vaccination program has greatly decreased the incidence of this infection. Table 5–3 lists bacterial infections with toxin production.

TABLE 5–3. TOXINS IN BACTERIAL INFECTION

Bacteria	Disease Produced by Toxins
Staphylococcus aureus	Food poisoning
Clostridium botulinum	Botulism
Clostridium tetani	Tetanus
Clostridium perfringens	Gas gangrene
Corynebacterium diphtheriae	Diphtheria

► MISCELLANEOUS BACTERIAL INFECTIONS

5-56

Of the final diseases you will learn about, the ones most likely to be encountered are tuberculosis, plague, Lyme disease, and *Campylobacter* enteritis. The other conditions appear with less incidence because of control factors such as childhood vaccination, living conditions, and our knowledge of the pathogenesis of the diseases.

5-57

1. lungs
2. *Mycobacterium tuberculosis*
3. air
4. unsanitary
5. resistance

Mycobacterium tuberculosis is the causative agent of **tuberculosis.** Until recently, this disease has been well controlled in the United States. Tuberculosis, or TB, is on the rise because of AIDS patients, the living conditions of the homeless, and illegal immigrants from countries where TB is more prevalent. The lungs are the primary organ affected, and the bacilli are spread by coughing only in an active case. Droplets in the air may be inhaled directly by another, or after sputum dries and turns to dust, it is infective in that manner. Another mycobacterium, *M. bovis,* produces TB in cows, and in the past, unpasteurized milk was a source of infection. Historically, TB has been a major killer. It thrives and is easily passed in crowded, unsanitary living conditions. Patients with the disease were labeled as having "consumption" because of the wasting away they experienced. Children were more susceptible, and today the elderly seem to be targeted more. Natural, or innate, resistance to *M. tuberculosis* is high in healthy adults. Many people harbor latent (noninfective) bacilli. Some may develop TB when the immune system is hampered. Tuberculosis is generally a disease of the _____(1). It is caused by _____(2). It is spread by the _____(3) borne route. TB is a disease seen in _____(4) living conditions. Most healthy adults have high levels of _____(5) to *M. tuberculosis.*

5-58

1. granulomatous
2. macrophages
3. epithelioid
4. giant
5. tubercle
6. calcified

The lesions in the lungs represent a cycle of spread and healing. The response to the active bacilli is granulomatous inflammation. The following description should sound familiar to you from Chapter 2. Macrophages infiltrate the area and ingest the mycobacteria. They are then modified to become epithelioid cells. Some merge to become giant cells. This cellular collection forms a nodule in the tissues that is called a **tubercle.** The tubercle undergoes caseation necrosis. Caseous necrosis is described as cheesy. Healed nodules calcify when calcium salts are deposited there. These calcified areas look very characteristic on a chest x-ray. This process is illustrated in Figure 5–7. Surviving organisms may spread to other areas. Entire lung lobes may be destroyed. The body responds to *M. tuberculosis* invasion with _____(1) inflammation. The principal cells are _____(2) that turn into _____(3) cells. Some join together to form _____(4) cells. The final nodule is called a _____(5). These are easy to recognize on an x-ray because the nodules become _____(6).

5-59

1. hemoptysis
2. cachectic
3. circulation or blood-stream (bacteremia)

TB sufferers have a chronic cough that may produce blood depending on the amount of lung destruction. Coughing up blood is called **hemoptysis.** There is a low-grade fever, constant fatigue, and considerable weight loss. This **cachectic** look is responsible for the old term "consumption." The final degree of lung destruction and resulting death depends on the patient's resistance and state of immune system. The factors that determine if an individual exposed to *M. tuberculosis* develops TB are the same as in other diseases. The factors are dose of the pathogen, its virulence, age and general health of the patient, and his or her immune state. Persons with active cases of tuberculosis may experience spread of the disease to other organs through bacteremia. The most common secondary sites of TB are bone, kidney, and brain. A patient with tuberculosis may cough up blood. This is called _____(1). The amount of weight loss is responsible for the term describing their physical appearance, which is _____(2). Secondary tuberculosis may develop in other organs by spread of the organisms in the _____(3). The initial screening test for tuberculosis is the **tuberculin test.** This in an injection into the skin of **purified protein derivative,** or **PPD,** from the tubercle bacilli cell wall. People previously exposed to *M. tuberculosis* will have sensitized T cells that produce a hypersensitivity response that is visible in the skin as a red nodule.

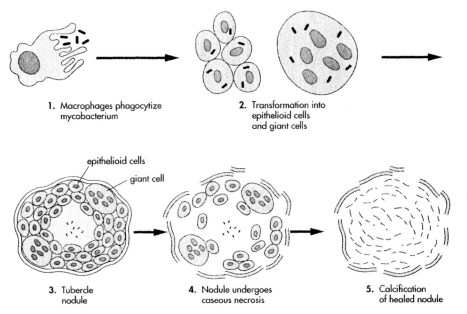

1. Macrophages phagocytize mycobacterium

2. Transformation into epithelioid cells and giant cells

epithelioid cells

giant cell

3. Tubercle nodule

4. Nodule undergoes caseous necrosis

5. Calcification of healed nodule

Figure 5-7. The formation of lung lesions (tubercles) during tuberculosis.

A disease of great historical significance is **plague.** It is caused by a gram-negative rod known as **Yersinia pestis.** *Y. pestis* can be an extremely virulent organism. In the Middle Ages it was called the Black Death and almost wiped out the European population. It is still found in parts of the United States in the southwest and a few other western states. Properly diagnosed plague is easily resolved with antibiotics. The microorganism _____(1) causes the disease plague.

Plague is a disease of rats. Fleas on the rodents carry *Y. pestis* and are responsible for the spread of this infection. Humans contract the disease when an infected flea bites them and injects the organisms through the skin. The lymph nodes that drain the bitten area swell to great proportions. In this swollen condition, the nodes are referred to as **buboes.** This is why plague is also called **bubonic plague.** The buboes are infected with *Y. pestis* and become great bags of pus or suppuration. Eventually, they break the skin surface and drain. The patient becomes bacteremic and massive organ infection results. There is extensive necrosis and hemorrhage. Death from septicemia is rapid. Another form of the disease is **pneumonic plague.** In this form the infection is spread directly from one person to another through the airborne route. The sputum is very infectious. Pneumonic plague is just as rapidly fatal, if not more so. The natural host for plague is the _____(1). It is transmitted to humans by _____(2) from the rodents who carry _____(3). The organism is injected into the skin by a _____(4) from an infected flea. Swollen lymph nodes that drain the area are called _____(5). The lymph nodes become bags of _____(6) from the infection. *Y. pestis* enters the _____(7) and then causes massive infection in internal organs. Death is from _____(8). Direct spread of *Y. pestis* from person to person through the air is the form of the disease called _____(9).

Lyme disease was first diagnosed as a rare form of arthritis that appeared in several children in New Lyme, Connecticut. It is now known to be an infectious disease caused by the spirochete **Borrelia burgdorferi.** This spirochete is present in the deer tick. Insects that harbor and transmit infectious organisms from one host to another are called **vectors.** The rat flea that spreads plague is a vector. The usual means of transfer by vectors is by biting the new host and injecting the microorganism. In this case, ticks that usually feed off deer, if attached

5-60

1. *Yersinia pestis*

5-61

1. rat or rodent
2. fleas
3. *Y. pestis*
4. bite
5. buboes
6. pus
7. circulation
8. septicemia
9. pneumonic plague

5-62

1. *Borrelia burgdorferi*
2. deer ticks
3. vector

to humans, transmit *B. burgdorferi*. The causative agent of Lyme disease is _____(1). This spirochete is found in _____(2). This insect is called a (an) _____(3) because it is responsible for the spread of an infectious agent to humans.

5-63

1. flu
2. rash
3. bull's eye
4. heart
5. nerves
6. arthritis

Lyme disease, if untreated and advanced, can manifest through three stages. Most cases are mild and confined to the first stage, either by treatment or an effective immune response. Signs and symptoms include fever, headache (flu-like symptoms), and a characteristic rash that looks like a bull's-eye target. Populations most susceptible are those out in wooded areas in the summer, like children, outdoor sports enthusiasts, and hobbyists. The few cases that do advance can affect the heart and nerves in stage two and cause crippling arthritis in stage three. Treating Lyme disease with a course of antibiotics is simple and effective and will avoid potentially serious consequences. The most common illness caused by Lyme disease are symptoms that resemble the _____(1) and a classic _____(2) that looks like a _____(3). Treatment will prevent advances that adversely affect the _____(4) and _____(5), or cause _____(6).

5-64

1. enterocolitis
2. upper
3. lower
4. animals
5. water
6. animals
7. mouth
8. meat
9. pain
10. diarrhea

An infection of the bowels caused by a gram-negative rod of the genus *Campylobacter* is *Campylobacter enterocolitis*. Enteritis is inflammation of the small or upper intestines. Colitis is inflammation of the colon or lower intestines. The acute diarrhea caused by *Campylobacter* is not uncommon. *Campylobacter* is an animal intestinal commensal, so sources of infection include water from streams contaminated by the feces of animals. Also, handling of domestic animals like dogs or cats can contaminate the hands. Ingestion of the bacteria could then result from hand-to-mouth practices. As in cases of *Salmonella* contamination, processed meat can be a source of *Campylobacter* and another reason for food poisoning. *Campylobacter* enterocolitis involves a toxin that causes abdominal pain and moderate to severe diarrhea for about a week. *Campylobacter* causes _____(1), which is infection of the _____(2) and _____(3) bowels or intestines. This organism comes from the intestines of _____(4). Sources of infection are _____(5) from streams, handling domestic _____(6) followed by hand-to-_____(7) practices, and _____(8) contaminated during processing. Signs of *Campylobacter* enteritis are nonspecific and include abdominal _____ (9) and moderate to severe _____(10).

5-65

An organism related to the *Campylobacter* genus is **Helicobacter.** For a while it has been known that *Helicobacter* can live and cause injury in the stomach through several mechanisms. It is not destroyed by the very acid pH. Its ability to attach to the stomach wall is remarkable, and it secretes several products that can eat through the gastric mucosa and lining. Recently, it has been taken very seriously as a major contributing factor to gastric ulcers. Not every case of gastric ulcer can be attributed to *Helicobacter,* but its role is being closely examined. The part this organism plays can help explain some factors, like why some people are more susceptible than others and why treatments don't always work. Antibiotics to eliminate *Helicobacter* are becoming part of treatment for gastric ulcer.

5-66

The remaining bacterial infections are less likely to be encountered in this country because of the control factors mentioned earlier. They are presented for your information. **Bordetella pertussis** causes **pertussis** or **whooping cough.** *B. pertussis* is a gram-negative bacilli found in the bronchial mucosa. When acting as a pathogen, it produces bronchitis or pneumonia that is characterized by a type of breathing described as "whooping." Whooping cough used to be a serious disease of small children. Today, cases that do exist are so mild that most are not diagnosed as such. This is due to the prevalence of the childhood vaccine **DPT,** or **diphtheria-pertussis-tetanus.**

Brucellosis or **undulant fever** is due to one of several *Brucella* bacteria, with *Brucella abortus* being the most common. This organism is responsible for animal disease found in cattle, sheep, and goats. There is a fairly high rate of infection in cattle in this country by *B. abortus*. In the past, brucellosis was more common because of drinking unpasteurized milk. *B. abortus* is passed through cow's milk and also contaminated meat. Pasteurization of milk has greatly decreased brucellosis. This condition is not fatal but is very inconveniencing because of the length of time that the patient has bouts of being unwell. Also, the persistent fever causes confusion with other serious diseases and interferes with proper diagnosis. This is a chronic condition involving months to years of waves of fevers (hence, the name undulating). There is persistent weakness, muscle pain, and general feelings of misery.

5–67

Vibrio cholerae is a comma-shaped, gram-negative bacillus that causes **cholera.** This disease is spread through drinking water that has been contaminated with infective feces. Toxins that accompany this disease produce tremendous amounts of watery diarrhea. So much body water is lost through the small intestines that the cause of death is usually dehydration in untreated cases. Up to 20 percent of body weight in fluids can be lost in a 24-hour period. The stool in cholera has been described as "rice water" because of its extreme fluid consistency. The stool is teeming with *V. cholerae* and highly infectious. Unsanitary conditions are the reason for epidemics. While treatment should include antibiotics, life-saving measures are those that replace lost water and electrolytes.

5–68

Typhoid fever is another infectious intestinal disease. The agent is *Salmonella*, specifically *Salmonella typhi.* The source of this organism is actively infected people or apparently healthy carriers. Carriers harbor *S. typhi* in the gallbladder and periodically shed the organisms, causing outbreaks. Other people are infected by ingesting tainted water or food or by hand-to-mouth practices. Carriers that are food handlers are especially a problem. Flies can also transmit the bacteria from feces to food that is unprotected. Signs of typhoid fever include fever, headache, lethargy, abdominal pain, and a "pea soup" diarrhea. Lymphoid tissue along the intestines is attacked. If ulceration and perforation of the tissue occurs, hemorrhage will cause blood to be seen in the stool. In some cases bacteremia and toxemia develop.

5–69

The last bacteria to be discussed is *Mycoplasma.* (Don't confuse this with *Mycobacterium.*) *Mycoplasma* are different from the previous bacteria because they are the simplest and smallest of these microorganisms. They do not have a rigid cell wall, only a cell membrane. They also lack some of the organelles. In children and young adults, *Mycoplasma pneumoniae* is a cause of pneumonia. Before *M. pneumoniae* was recognized as the cause, the disease was called primary atypical pneumonia and a virus was considered the agent. Another term for this particular respiratory disease is walking pneumonia. As that name implies, *Mycoplasma* pneumonia is not particularly debilitating in otherwise healthy individuals. Those affected have a low-grade cough, some shortness of breath, and fatigue.

5–70

II. REVIEW QUESTIONS

1. Bacteria that cause infections with purulent exudate are described as:
    a. pathogenic
    b. pyogenic
    c. prokaryotic
    d. producers of toxins

2. The source of *Staphylococcus aureus* is (choose all that apply):
    a. animal intestines
    b. human intestines
    c. skin
    d. nasal passages

1. b–pyogenic

2. c–skin; d–nasal passages

3. a–hospital patients

4. f–all of the above

5. c–*S. pyogenes*

6. d–*S. pyogenes*

7. b–immune system hyper-
sensitivity

8. a–arthritis; c–damage to
heart valves

9. a–*N. meningitidis*

10. c–airborne route

3. Populations particularly at risk for serious *S. aureus* infection are:
   a. hospital patients
   b. hospital workers
   c. children
   d. elderly

4. *S. aureus* infections are associated with:
   a. skin pustules
   b. organ abscesses
   c. bone infection
   d. bronchopneumonia
   e. toxin production
   f. all of the above

5. The streptococcus associated with acute pharyngitis or "strep throat" is:
   a. *S. pneumoniae*
   b. *S. viridans*
   c. *S. pyogenes*
   d. enterococci

6. Scarlet fever, rheumatic fever, and glomerulonephritis are possible complications of streptococcal infection by:
   a. *S. viridans*
   b. *S. pneumoniae*
   c. enterococci
   d. *S. pyogenes*

7. The mechanism that causes injury in poststreptococcal glomerulonephritis and rheumatic fever is:
   a. toxins from the bacteria
   b. immune system hypersensitivity
   c. bacterial colonization of the organs
   d. septicemia

8. Rheumatic fever results in (choose all that apply):
   a. arthritis
   b. bone infection
   c. damage to heart valves
   d. kidney failure

9. The pyogenic gram-negative diplococci that causes meningitis is:
   a. *N. meningitidis*
   b. *N. gonorrhoeae*
   c. *H. influenzae*
   d. *E. coli*

10. Epidemic meningitis is spread by:
    a. contaminated food
    b. hand-to-mouth practices
    c. airborne route
    d. contaminated drinking water

11. Epidemic meningitis affects:
    a. any healthy individual
    b. weakened individuals
    c. animals and humans
    d. none of the above

12. The habitat of coliform bacteria is:
    a. skin
    b. nasal passages
    c. intestines
    d. mouth

13. Coliforms cause infection by:
    a. being introduced to another body site
    b. airborne passage
    c. hand-to-mouth practices
    d. all of the above

14. Infection by enteric bacteria can result in (choose all that apply):
    a. peritonitis after perforation of the intestines
    b. septicemia
    c. endotoxic shock
    d. damage to heart valves
    e. meningitis
    f. arthritis

15. *Salmonella* gastroenteritis is the result of:
    a. bacteremia
    b. contaminated drinking water
    c. unsanitary conditions
    d. food poisoning

16. Salmonellosis is most commonly associated with:
    a. food that has been left at room temperature
    b. contaminated poultry
    c. uncooked food
    d. contaminated drinking water

17. The most common bacterial venereal disease is caused by:
    a. *Treponema pallidum*
    b. *Neisseria meningitidis*
    c. *Neisseria gonorrhoeae*
    d. *Haemophilus influenzae*

18. The primary reason gonorrhea is still prevalent is because of:
    a. asymptomatic females
    b. symptomatic females
    c. asymptomatic males
    d. symptomatic males

19. Consequences of undiagnosed gonorrhea in females include:
    a. sterility
    b. salpingitis
    c. ectopic pregnancy
    d. pelvic inflammatory disease
    e. all of the above

11. b–weakened individuals

12. c–intestines

13. a–being introduced to another body site

14. a–peritonitis after perforation of the intestines; b–septicemia; c–endotoxic shock

15. d–food poisoning

16. b–contaminated poultry

17. c–*Neisseria gonorrhoeae*

18. a–asymptomatic females

19. e–all of the above

20. a–*Treponema pallidum*

21. 1. a–more; 2. d–easier

22. b–an ulcer called a chancre

23. c–a common-looking rash

24. c–vasculitis

25. a–aneurysm

26. b–central nervous system

27. b–toxin production

28. a–*Staphylococcus aureus*

20. Syphilis is caused by:
   a. *Treponema pallidum*
   b. *Neisseria gonorrhoeae*
   c. Legionella pneumophila
   d. none of the above

21. Syphilis is 1. _____ serious than gonorrhea, but can be
    2. _____ to diagnose than gonorrhea
   a. more
   b. less
   c. harder
   d. easier

22. Stage 1 of syphilis is characterized by:
   a. a unique-looking rash
   b. an ulcer called a chancre
   c. fever and headache
   d. burning urination

23. Stage 2 of syphilis is characterized by:
   a. a unique-looking rash
   b. an ulcer called a chancre
   c. a common-looking rash
   d. vasculitis

24. Stage 3 of syphilis is characterized by:
   a. high fever and disorientation
   b. syphilitic rash
   c. vasculitis
   d. arthritis

25. A fatal consequence of syphilitic aortitis is:
   a. aneurysm
   b. heart failure
   c. extreme anemia
   d. blockage of the aorta

26. Another body system involved in end-stage syphilis is the:
   a. respiratory system
   b. central nervous system
   c. immune system
   d. digestive system

27. The mechanism of injury in some food poisonings, tetanus, gas gangrene, and botulism is:
   a. bacteremia
   b. toxin production
   c. colonization and inflammatory damage to tissues
   d. hypersensitivity reactions

28. Toxin production and the onset of gastroenteritis shortly after eating best describes food poisoning by:
   a. *Staphylococcus aureus*
   b. *Staphylococcus epidermidis*
   c. *Salmonella enteritidis*
   d. *Salmonella typhi*

29. Food poisoning that is delayed in onset and is associated with dose of the pathogen instead of toxin is due to:
    a. *Staphylococcus aureus*
    b. *Staphylococcus epidermidis*
    c. *Salmonella enteritidis*
    d. *Salmonella typhi*

30. Clostridial infections have as their source:
    a. meat contaminated in processing
    b. carriers who periodically shed the organisms
    c. soil contaminated with human feces
    d. soil contaminated with animal feces

31. Two important characteristics of clostridia that contribute to the pathogenesis of infections by them are (choose two):
    a. they are anaerobes
    b. they are aerobes
    c. they form spores
    d. they do not form spores

32. Clostridial infections that result in fatal muscle paralysis are (choose two):
    a. tetanus
    b. botulism
    c. gas gangrene
    d. diphtheria

33. Tetanus by *C. tetani* results from:
    a. eating contaminated foods
    b. direct contact with another infected person
    c. wounds contaminated with spore-laden soil
    d. hand-to-mouth practices

34. Deep wounds or necrotic tissue grow clostridia very well because:
    a. they are anaerobes
    b. they form spores
    c. they are aerobes
    d. they are resistant to body defenses

35. Exotoxin from *C. tetani:*
    a. travels to the spinal cord and affects neuromuscular junctions
    b. travels to the lungs and directly paralyzes respiratory muscles
    c. causes mass necrosis of tissue in the surrounding area
    d. causes toxic shock

36. The pathogenesis of gas gangrene by *C. perfringens* is production of foul-smelling 1. _____, which puts extreme pressure on surrounding tissues and causes it to 2. _____. (A) an 3._____ is secreted, which is an enzyme. This breaks down more tissue and allows the bacteria to 4._____. This decomposition of muscles is called 5._____. The bloated limb will make crackling sounds when felt and this is called 6._____. Systemic effects causing death are due to 7._____.

    enzymes   localize
    gas   spread
    crepitation   trismus
    die   putrefaction
    toxic   bacteremia
    exotoxin   septic shock

---

29. c–*Salmonella enteritidis*

30. d–soil contaminated with animal feces

31. a–they are anaerobes; c–they form spores

32. a–tetanus; b–botulism

33. c–wounds contaminated with spore-laden soil

34. a–they are anaerobes

35. a–travels to the spinal cord and affects neuromuscular junctions

36. 1. gas; 2. die; 3. exotoxin; 4. spread; 5. putrefaction; 6. crepitation; 7. septic shock

37. a–airborne contact with an active case

38. d–granulomatous inflammation with epithelioid and giant cells

39. c–tubercle

40. d–all of the above

41. 1. d–*Yersinia pestis;*
    2. e–rats

42. b–rat flea

43. a–lymph node

44. 1. c–rat to person;
    2. b–person to person

37. Tuberculosis is spread through:
    a. airborne contact with an active case
    b. airborne contact with someone who has a positive test for TB
    c. latent carriers
    d. pasteurized milk

38. Tuberculosis lesions in the lungs are a result of:
    a. suppurative inflammation, with neutrophils and macrophages
    b. granulomatous inflammation, with neutrophils and lymphocytes
    c. suppurative inflammation, with epithelioid and giant cells
    d. granulomatous inflammation, with epithelioid and giant cells

39. In tuberculosis, the nodule that is formed is called a:
    a. chancre
    b. calcified nodule
    c. tubercle
    d. none of the above

40. Common secondary sites of tuberculosis are:
    a. bone
    b brain
    c. kidney
    d. all of the above

41. Plague is caused by 1. _____ and is primarily a disease of 2. _____.
    a. *Borrelia burgdorferi*
    b. cattle
    c. humans
    d. *Yersinia pestis*
    e. rats
    f. fleas

42. Plague is transmitted to humans by the vector:
    a. deer tick
    b. rat flea
    c. dog flea
    d. cattle tick

43. In plague, buboes describe swollen, infected:
    a. lymph nodes
    b. bite wounds
    c. limbs
    d. any of the above

44. In bubonic plague, the spread is 1. _____. In pneumonic plague, the spread is 2. _____.
    a. flea to rat
    b. person to person
    c. rat to person
    d. flea to person

45. Fatality in plague is due to:
    a. bacteremia
    b. respiratory paralysis
    c. toxin production
    d septicemia

46. Lyme disease is transmitted by the:
    a. deer tick
    b. rat flea
    c. dog flea
    d. cattle tick

47. Signs of Lyme disease are flu-like symptoms and a:
    a. chancre
    b. tubercle
    c. pustule with a black surface
    d. bull's-eye rash

48. Untreated, advanced Lyme disease can result in:
    a. damage to heart valves
    b. paralysis
    c. arthritis
    d. blindness

49. *Campylobacter* enterocolitis causes:
    a. dehydrating "rice water" diarrhea
    b. abdominal pain and diarrhea
    c. gastric ulcers
    d. death due to toxic shock

45. d–septicemia

46. a–deer tick

47. d–bull's-eye rash

48. c–arthritis

49. b–abdominal pain and diarrhea

III. VIRAL INFECTIONS ◄ SECTION

5–71

Before we cover specific viral diseases, you need to learn general concepts regarding viruses. The spectrum of injury caused by a virus can range from almost none to explosive. Host cells that have been invaded by a virus defines a viral infection, while noticeable injury is what we call viral disease. The presence of a virus in host cells without apparent injury is a latent infection. Usually, a virus is species specific and adapted to one host, such as a particular animal or humans. In addition to host specificity, viruses can also show tissue specificity and parasitize only those cells.

▶ DEFINITION AND PROPERTIES OF A VIRUS

5–72

A **virus** is an obligate intracellular parasite. This means it is required to be inside cells to survive. A virus is too small to be seen with a regular light microscope. A virus is not a cell. It doesn't have a cell membrane, or a wall like bacteria. It doesn't have organelles for replication, ATP energy production, nor enzyme production. It has *either* DNA or RNA nucleic acids, but not both. All of these functions are provided by the host cell. The virus uses the host cell, often to death, and gives nothing in return, so it is a true parasite. A virus is rightly called a particle. A virus particle is called a **virion.** A virion is illustrated in Figure 5–8. It is made up of just two, sometimes three, parts. The inner **core** is the DNA or RNA nucleic acids. The outer coat is a protein called a **capsid.** Some viruses, like herpes simplex, have an **envelope** that surrounds the capsid. A virus can only live _____(1) a host cell.

1. inside

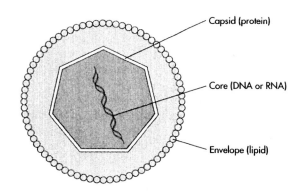

Figure 5–8. Components of a virion.

2. host
3. intracellular parasite
4. cell
5. capsid
6. envelope
7. DNA
8. RNA

It uses the host cell to survive, usually at the expense of the _____(2) cell. These two properties are described in the phrase obligate _____(3), which describes a virus. A virus is a particle, not a _____(4). That is because it lacks many vital structures. The outer protein coat of a virus is a _____(5). Some viruses have an additional covering called a (an) _____(6). The inner core contains _____(7) or _____(8).

5–73

Replication or multiplication takes place in five basic steps. (Keep in mind that this explanation is greatly simplified, and that the details are quite different between RNA and DNA viruses.) The life cycle begins with the **attachment** of a virus to the target host cell surface. Then, there is **penetration** of the cell surface and the virus enters into the cytoplasm. The virus **uncoats** or sheds its coat to free the nucleic acids inside. The **eclipse phase** begins, which is true replication. The virus uses host ribosomes to transcribe (read and decode) the virus' nucleic acid. New viral DNA or RNA and protein for a new coat are manufactured. Next, these parts are **assembled** into a new virion (core and coat). Thousands or even millions of new virions can be made by the hostage host cell. Finally comes **release** of the new virions from the host cell with the purpose of finding and attacking more host cells for more multiplication. This release can be in the form of budding and pinching off. This type of release may not kill the host cell and is responsible for the outer envelope that is made of host cell membrane. More often, the damaged host cell will rupture or lyse and be destroyed. Host cells that are blown to pieces by viral release form the basis of the mechanism of injury in viral diseases.

5–74

1. attachment
2. host cell
3. penetration
4. uncoats
5. ribosomes
6. assemble
7. virion
8. release
9. lysed

The life cycle and replication of a virus begins with its _____(1) to the surface of a _____(2). It enters the cell through _____(3). Nucleic acids in the viral core are set free when the virus _____(4). The nucleic acid then interacts with host cell _____(5), which decipher the message for new nucleic acid production. After the nucleic acids and new proteins are made, the parts _____(6) into a new _____(7). The virus leaves the cell in a process called _____(8). The mechanism of injury in viral disease is related to release when the host cell is ruptured or _____(9).

▶ **RESULTS OF VIRAL INFECTION**

5–75

There are several reactions by the body of the host to invasion by virions. The reproduction and release of virions damage cells. This can be in the form of degeneration or outright death or necrosis. Tissues and organs that are invaded by viruses will show the effect of massive destruction first at the cellular level. The cumulative effect will be seen as impairment of overall function of that tissue or organ. As usual, tissue damage or necrosis will result in inflammation. The cells of viral-induced inflammation are macrophages and lymphocytes, with no pus formation. Damage may continue due to the process of inflammation. One result of viral infection of host cells is damage, which is _____(1) or _____(2) of the host cell. As great numbers of cells are injured, visible effects are seen at the _____(3) or _____(4) level. This injury causes _____(5) that is mediated by macrophages and lymphocytes. Inflammation itself may cause _____(6).

1. degeneration
2. death
3. tissue
4. organ
5. inflammation
6. injury

5-76

Some viral nucleic acids will mix in with host genetic material. The host cells are not especially injured, but are certainly altered as they reproduce. The continued presence and reproduction of the virus along with the host cell is a **latent** infection. It is subclinical, or lacking visible signs of injury. Unknown factors can later cause the infection to erupt or become apparent. In chickenpox, after the clinical course, some virions can become latent in host cells. Later stimulation can result in a disease called shingles. Still other viruses can persist in the same host cells and reemerge from time to time in a chronic infection. A good example of this is herpes simplex, which normally resides in nerve cells in between episodes of clinical signs.

5-77

Results of viral infections include rapid death of the patient, complete recovery in a short time, latent infection activated later, chronic recurring clinical episodes, susceptibility to serious secondary bacterial infection, and tumor production. Some viruses are known to cause cancer in lab animals.

▶ SPECIFIC DEFENSES AGAINST VIRUSES

5-78

Our defense against viruses is similar to defense against other foreign invaders. Both arms of the immune response are activated. In humoral defense, you know that _____(1), or immunoglobulins, are produced. These are specific for the invader. The immune response is very effective against some viruses, and immunity does result. Examples are the chickenpox and measles, where a second disease due to these viruses does not develop. Other viruses give a poor response; that is, immunity does not develop. The most likely explanation for this is the dozens or more of different strains of the same virus. Each strain is just different enough that the immune system doesn't recognize it, and the virus continues unstopped. The common cold is a good example of this. In response to viral invasion, the humoral aspect of the immune system manufactures _____(2), or antibodies, to fight the virus. Lack of immunity to future infection by the same virus is probably due to the many different _____(3) of the same virus. In this case, the immune system does not _____(4) the virus as being the same.

1. antibodies
2. immunoglobulins
3. strains
4. recognize

5-79

In cell-mediated immunity, T lymphocytes are vital in stopping or destroying viruses. This key role is really highlighted in cases of deficient T-cell function, where a common, simple viral infection can cause death. These specific cytotoxic T cells directly kill or destroy host cells that have been infected, thus providing containment of the virus. A very important product from lymphocytes is the lymphokine interferon. Interferon prevents the virus from spreading to other cells because it directs host cells to make proteins that prevent replication of the virus. There is no hope for the host cell already infected. However, containment is often effective because a virus must multiply to cause injury on a noticeable scale. Cell-mediated immunity is directed by _____(1). These cells directly kill _____(2) cells infected with a _____(3). A virus-fighting lymphokine from these T cells is _____(4). This chemical mediator works by preventing further _____(5) of the virus in other cells. It does this by causing the _____(6) to make a _____(7) that does not allow replication of viral material.

1. cytotoxic T cells
2. host
3. virus
4. interferon
5. replication
6. host cells
7. protein

5-80

1. inhalation
2. ingestion
3. lesions
4. insect
5. viremia

Transmission of viral agents is primarily through inhalation, or the respiratory system, or through ingestion. Direct contact with a lesion on the skin or mucous membranes is another means, as in herpes simplex transmission. Viruses may also be injected through the skin by the bite of an infected vector. Once entry is gained, the virus may cause local injury only. It can also enter the bloodstream, and this **viremia** is responsible for organs becoming infected. Injury to an organ is seen as disorder or even failure of whatever system is affected. Systemic viral infections are the presence of virions replicating in multiple tissues or organs, having gained access through viremia. A virus enters the body primarily through _____(1) or _____(2). Direct contact with _____(3) and _____(4) bites are also ways of entry. Organs can be invaded if the virus enters the bloodstream, and this is called _____(5).

▶ VIRAL DISEASES AFFECTING CHILDREN

5-81

Some viral diseases are considered a child's affliction because these are the infectious agents that lead to an effective immune response. Because immunity usually develops for the life of the individual, first-time exposure and disease are often seen in children. This does not mean an adult cannot, for example, catch the measles or chickenpox. But the majority of adults have already harbored the infectious virus as children and do not develop the same disease again. Adults who have not experienced these childhood diseases are susceptible to infection.

5-82

Measles is caused by the virus **rubeola.** Transmission is airborne, through infected droplets from the nose or mouth. Measles is very contagious. Signs and symptoms of measles affect the eyes, skin, and respiratory system. A high fever is accompanied by pain of the eyes and **photophobia,** or extreme sensitivity to light. Cough is common and pneumonia is a possibility. In persons with compromised cell-mediated immunity, system-wide complications may arise. The most characteristic sign of measles is a **maculopapular rash.** This is shown in Figure 5–9A. A macule is a red blotch, and a papule is a tiny bump. The rash is a combination of these. Persons with this rash are contagious until the rash is gone. Vaccination against rubeola is important and effective. Another virus called **rubella** causes **German measles.** German measles is commonly called rubella to separate it from rubeola. Rubella is also a respiratory and skin affliction, including a similar rash. However, the signs and symptoms are milder and there are no known complications. Vaccination is just as important as in measles, because rubella is a potent **teratogen.** A teratogen is an agent capable of causing birth defects or deformities. Rubella, if contracted by a woman in her first trimester of pregnancy, produces congenital heart defects, as well as other defects in the child. The virus directs the infected fetal cells to reproduce and grow abnormally.

5-83

1. rubeola
2. photophobia
3. macules
4. papules
5. are
6. rubella
7. birth defects
8. teratogen
9. vaccination

The virus _____(1) causes measles. The eyes become sensitive to light, and this is called _____(2). Respiratory signs go along with a skin eruption characterized by red blotches or _____(3), and tiny bumps, or _____(4). Persons with the rash _____(5) are / are not (circle one) contagious. German measles is often called _____(6). Rubella is a mild disease, but it is important because it can cause _____(7) in children. This ability to cause deformity is described by the term _____(8). To prevent this, _____(9) is important.

5-84

Varicella is the agent of **chickenpox.** It is a herpesvirus. This is also a respiratory disease with airborne transmission. Fever and malaise, or lethargy, accompany a skin eruption. It is different from the measles rash, as you can see in Figure 5–9B. For one thing, it is itchy or **pruritic.** For another, the eruptions include papules and vesicles (blisters) and a crust when these have opened. All three stages of the rash can be found at any one time. Scratching of the lesions must be kept to a minimum to prevent secondary bacterial infection of the open

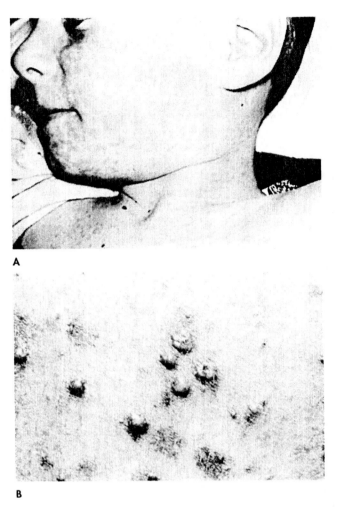

Figure 5–9. A. The macular (flat) rash of measles. **B.** The papular (raised) rash of chickenpox. (*From Kent and Hart,* Introduction to Human Disease, *3rd ed., Appleton & Lange.*)

sores and scarring. Cases of chickenpox should be isolated until the skin lesions are gone. Birth defects in the child are also possible if a pregnant woman contracts varicella in the first 6 months of pregnancy. There is no vaccine for chickenpox. **Shingles** is a condition that can develop in persons who have had the varicella virus. Latent varicella virus is called **zoster** virus. Sometimes the agent is called varicella-zoster to indicate it is the same agent. If the chickenpox virus becomes dormant in nerve cells, it can later be stimulated and cause painful skin eruptions along the skin supplied by the infected nerve. Often, the face is involved. **Herpes zoster** is also a name for this agent of shingles. We will discuss more about the latencies of herpesviruses later. Shingles probably develops after cases of chickenpox in those persons whose immune response was less effective than normal.

Chickenpox is caused by the _____(1) virus. It is also a respiratory disease with skin effects. The rash in chickenpox is pruritic or _____(2), which is different from measles. The lesions include vesicles, which are _____(3), and crusts. Treatment of chickenpox should include relief of _____(4), as scratching could lead to secondary _____(5) infection and scars. In some people, varicella becomes dormant and is called by the name _____(6). It hides out in _____(7) cells and may cause painful eruptions of the _____(8) along the tracts of the infected _____(9). The development of this condition, known as _____(10), is probably linked to inadequate _____(11) response.

5–85

1. varicella
2. itchy
3. blisters
4. itching
5. bacterial
6. zoster
7. nerve
8. skin
9. nerve
10. shingles
11. immune

5-86

1. signs
2. salivary glands
3. parotitis
4. orchitis
5. sterility

The **mumps** virus affects more people than it seems because many cases are subclinical. Subclinical means _____(1) are not readily apparent. This respiratory infection usually targets the parotid salivary glands. However, cases involving the pancreas (a similar glandular tissue), ovaries, and testicles are known. Fever accompanies painful swelling of the parotid gland **(parotitis).** Headache is common and earache may develop. As in all the previous viral diseases, it is self-limiting (the disease is resolved and the patient recovers without specific treatment). Adult males who have not had mumps as a child have an unrealistic fear of the disease as causing sterility. **Orchitis,** or testicular swelling, may certainly develop. But the condition must cause severe atrophy of both testicles, or be bilateral, to cause sterility. Most often, the condition is unilateral (one sided) or involves one testicle. The mumps virus usually affects the parotid _____(2). This infection of the glands is described as _____(3). Testicular involvement, which is called _____(4) is given too much credit for causing _____(5).

▶ VIRAL DISEASES AFFECTING THE GENERAL POPULATION

5-87

1. upper respiratory infection
2. rhinovirus
3. adenovirus
4. coronavirus
5. hand-to-face practices
6. fomites
7. strains or serotypes

The most common by far of the viral diseases are the ones causing **upper respiratory infection,** or **URI.** The "common cold" can be due to several viruses. **Rhinovirus, adenovirus,** and **coronavirus** seem the most responsible. Familiar symptoms and signs include nasal discharge, congestion, sneezing, cough, fever, and sore throat. The sneeze is responsible for transmission, as well as fomites with hand-to-face practices. We are always susceptible to URI viruses because of the *many* different strains or serotypes. Immunity doesn't have a chance to develop in the face of constantly changing antigens. A common cold is properly called a (an) _____(1). Three agents associated with URI are _____(2), _____(3), and _____(4). The contagious nature of URI is perpetuated by _____(5) and inanimate objects or _____(6). Immunity to URI does not develop because of many differnt _____(7).

5-88

1. influenza
2. myalgia
3. bronchi
4. pneumonia
5. secondary bacterial

A more serious viral URI is **influenza.** This disorder is often seen in epidemics. A variant called the Asian flu can cause death among the old or debilitated. Signs include those of a head cold but with **myalgia,** or muscle pain and aches. The chest often hurts. Tracheobronchitis can lead to pneumonia. Secondary bacterial pneumonia is the most common reason for fatality. These cases are excellent examples of when antibiotics should be included in treatment of a viral disease. There are three recognized types of influenza virus, types A, B, and C. Type A is most responsible and is very good at mutating into virulent strains, which prevents immunity from occurring. More serious than the common cold is the viral URI, _____(1). Muscle pain, or _____(2), occurs with general signs of illness. Tracheobronchitis, infection of the trachea and _____(3), can lead to _____(4). Usually, death in cases of pneumonia is because of _____(5) infection.

5-89

1. hantavirus pulmonary syndrome

A relatively new and fairly uncommon virus is **hantavirus.** It causes **hantavirus pulmonary syndrome,** or **HPS.** Even though it is uncommon, it has been newsworthy because about 50 percent of cases are fatal. One particular hantavirus has been named **sin nombre virus.** The rural areas of the western United States seem to be endemic areas, but it has been found elsewhere. HPS is a respiratory disease spread by the vector deer mice that carry the virus. Hantavirus is spread to people when they breathe air contaminated with dried rodent urine, saliva, or feces. Hand-to-mouth practices and rodent bites are also means of transmission. The virus survives in dust or dirt but is easily killed with disinfectants. Signs are general and flu-like, with high fever and pain in several parts of the body. The primary symptom is difficulty breathing caused by fluid buildup in the lungs. No cure or vaccine is available. Hantavirus causes HPS, or _____(1). The vector that spreads the virus is _____(2) or other rodents. Transmission is by inhaling or _____(3) aerosolized dried urine or _____(4) of the rodents. The most important symptom of HPS is difficulty _____(5) because of _____(6) in the lungs.

2. deer mice
3. breathing
4. feces
5. breathing
6. fluid

5–90

Viral gastroenteritis is sometime called intestinal flu. Two of several agents are **calicivirus** and **rotavirus.** Rotavirus is a major cause of gastroenteritis in young children, producing high fever, vomiting, and diarrhea. **Norwalk agent** is a calicivirus causing epidemics in group situations such as schools, nursing homes, restaurants, and camps. Transmission is person to person through fecal contamination and it is also waterborne. Vomiting and diarrhea are followed by recovery, with no long-term immunity. Intestinal flu is properly known as _____(1). Two causative agents are _____(2) and _____(3). Transmission is through _____(4) contamination and in _____(5). Predominant signs are _____(6) and _____(7).

1. gastroenteritis
2. calicivirus
3. rotavirus
4. fecal
5. water
6. vomiting
7. diarrhea

5–91

The next three agents, HSV, CMV, and EBV are all **herpesviruses.** Herpesviruses are known for their tendency to become latent and may produce recurring infections. An example already presented was varicella-zoster of chickenpox and shingles. As a group, the herpesviruses are the most widely spread viruses in the population. Figure 5–10 is an electron micrograph of the herpes simplex virus.

5–92

Herpes simplex virus (HSV) types I and II are very widespread. They are transmitted by direct or indirect contact with sores. HSV type I affects the mouth region, and HSV type II is a venereal disease of the genitals. Both of these exhibit two stages of infection. The primary, or first, infection may or may not be noticed. Noticeable cases are those with painful open sores or ulcer-type lesions, characteristic of HSV. In women, HSV II may ascend to produce painful **cervicitis,** or infection of the cervix. Worse case scenario is in those with T-cell deficiency where the virus can become internally systemic, causing **visceral herpes simplex.** Babies born to mothers with an active case of HSV II are susceptible to this visceral type, with fatal organ necrosis the result. Cesarean section is called for in known active cases of maternal HSV II. After primary infection, HSV becomes dormant in nerves that supply the original area of lesions. Secondary, or recurrent, infections are seen as further outbreaks of the ulcers, known as "cold sores" or "fever blisters" in HSV I. The lesions start out as vesicles that break open, ulcerate, and may form a crust. Secondary outbreaks are set off

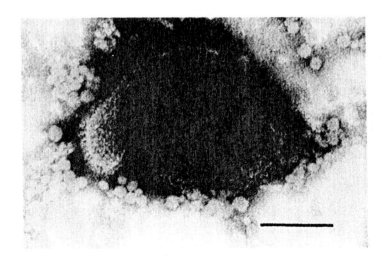

Figure 5–10. Electron micrograph of herpes simplex virus. *(From Greenwood et al, Medical Microbiology, 14th ed., Churchill Livingstone.)*

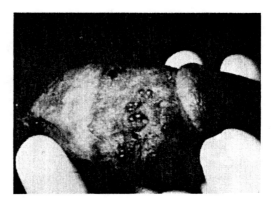

Figure 5–11. Vesicles of genital herpes. *(From Ryan,* Sherris Medical Microbiology, *3rd ed., Appleton & Lange.)*

1. herpes simplex virus
2. mouth
3. genitals
4. primary
5. T-cell
6. babies
7. visceral herpes simplex
8. nerves
9. ulcer

by things like stress, fever, sunlight, and other obscure causes. The appearance of genital herpes is shown in Figure 5–11. Acyclovir is currently used topically on the lesions to decrease the severity of symptoms and frequency of attacks. There is no cure. HSV stands for _____(1). Type I is associated with the _____(2). Type II is associated with the _____(3). The _____(4) infection may or may not be noticeable. A serious sequela can occur in persons with defective _____(5) function, or in newborn _____(6). HSV can cause _____(7), which is necrosis of internal organs. Dormant HSV is found in the _____(8) associated with the original site of entry. The primary sign of a secondary outbreak is the presence of a characteristic _____(9) that can be relived with acyclovir.

5–93

1. cytomegalovirus
2. fetuses
3. premature babies
4. chemotherapy
5. AIDS
6. CMV negative

Most people have had contact with **cytomegalovirus**, or **CMV**. It is named after its effect on living cells, and it causes host cells ("cyto") to enlarge or get big ("megalo"). CMV infection does not cause noticeable problems in healthy people. The significance of this infection is in regards to susceptible populations. These are unborn fetuses, premature babies, and the immunosuppressed. This group includes those suppressed by therapy for cancer or organ transplants (chemotherapy), and those with AIDS. Fetuses are susceptible to brain damage or death, and others are plagued by pneumonia and severe secondary bacterial infections. CMV can be transmitted through the blood, and transfusions are often necessary for these populations at risk. Finding *CMV-negative* blood for transfusion, or organs for transplantation, presents a problem since many people are CMV positive. CMV stands for _____(1). It can cause a formidable infection in certain populations such as _____(2), _____(3), and the immunosuppressed. Examples of immunosuppression are those undergoing _____(4) for cancer or transplants, or those with the disease _____(5). Blood transfusions for these groups need to be _____(6).

5–94

1. Epstein–Barr
2. airborne
3. oral
4. weakness
5. weeks to months
6. liver
7. cancer

The **Epstein–Barr virus** is the causative agent of **infectious mononucleosis.** Teenagers and young adults are most often affected. Transmission is airborne or through direct oral contact. Signs include sore throat, enlarged regional lymph nodes, and extreme fatigue. This weakness can last through several weeks or months. Disease of the liver has been traced to cases of mononucleosis and is thought to be due to the latency of this herpesvirus in liver cells. EBV has also been associated with two cancers, Burkitt's lymphoma (tumor of the neck and jaw) and nasopharyngeal carcinoma. Infectious mononucleosis is caused by _____(1). Viral transmission is _____(2) or by direct _____(3) contact. Sore throat and enlarged lymph nodes accompany extreme _____(4) that can last _____(5). EBV has been linked to disease of the _____(6) and to _____(7). The common viral agents and their diseases are summarized in Table 5–4.

TABLE 5–4. VIRAL PATHOGENS AND ASSOCIATED DISEASES

Virus	Associated Diseases
Rubeola	Measles
Rubella	German measles
	Birth defects
Varicella	Chickenpox
Varicella-zoster	Shingles
Mumps	Mumps
Rhinovirus	Upper respiratory infection (URI)
Adenovirus	
Coronavirus	
Influenza, types A, B, C	Influenza
Hantavirus	Hantavirus pulmonary syndrome
Calicivirus/Rotavirus	Viral gastroenteritis (intestinal flu)
Herpes simplex virus type I	Oral herpes (cold sores)
Herpes simplex virus type II	Genital herpes
Cytomegalovirus	Pneumonia
	Secondary bacterial infection in vulnerable populations
Epstein–Barr	Infectious mononucleosis

▶ MISCELLANEOUS VIRAL DISEASES

The causative agent of acquired immunodeficiency syndrome is HIV, or _____(1), which was presented in Chapter 4. **Chronic fatigue syndrome** (CFS) is a debilitating disorder whose actual cause is largely unknown. Several viruses are suspected. Individual predisposing factors also play a part. It has been called "yuppie flu" but is properly named **myalgic encephalomyelitis.** It is generally seen in young adults. There are a variety of symptoms, but as the name implies, weakness and fatigue for extended periods is the hallmark. For quite a while, CFS was considered a disease not of organic origin, but psychosomatic. This was particularly frustrating for sufferers of the disorder. Diagnosis today of CFS is based on the presence of persistent fatigue of at least 6 months' duration, and the presence of at least 6 of the general signs that can be seen. These signs include fever, sore throat, bronchitis, myalgia (muscle pain), arthralgia (joint pain), irritability, depression, or other personality effects.

5–95

1. human immunodeficiency virus

Respiratory syncytial virus is named for its effect on living cells where host cells fuse together into giant cells, or a syncytium. This virus causes signs of a common cold in an adult. However, in infants it poses a threat of severe bronchitis or pneumonia. RSV is the most common cause of pneumonia in infants less than 6 months old. Another respiratory virus is **parainfluenza,** which, as the name implies, is like influenza. It primarily strikes infants, causing the condition known as **croup.** It is actually laryngotracheobronchitis, infectious inflammation of the larynx, trachea, and bronchi. Parainfluenza causes a hoarse cough and some respiratory distress that can lead to pneumonia.

5–96

The **Ebola** and **Marburg** viruses have made sensational headlines in recent years as particularly devastating diseases. They are primarily confined to Africa, and person-to-person transmission has not been reported. The source of these viruses are monkeys and other primates, as well as their tissues used in vitro. The fatality in this disease is due to severe shock from widespread, explosive hemorrhage. The exportation of monkeys for use in laboratories has been associated with cases in other parts of the world. Another fatal virus of animal origin is **rabies.** While rabies in humans is not common, the unpleasant demise makes it well known. Normal host animals in the wild include the fox, skunk, raccoon, and bat. Domestic animals are also susceptible. The excitement phase of this disease is characterized by spasms

5–97

and convulsions. Hydrophobia is the name given to the condition where the patient experiences painful laryngeal spasms when trying to drink water. This is followed by paralysis and death. Bites from infected animals are the means of exposure.

5–98

Polio, or **poliomyelitis,** is also known as **infantile paralysis.** This is an enteric infection (fecal transmission) that leads to viremia and invasion of the central nervous system. The neurons controlling motor activity, including breathing, are especially affected. Many cases are actually subclinical, with only about 2 percent progressing to the well-known paralysis and death. Effective vaccination against all three strains of poliovirus have made this disease largely a thing of the past. Cases still persist outside the United States. Another serious viral infection outside the United States is **yellow fever.** The virus of yellow fever is spread by the bite of a mosquito vector. The virus has an affinity for the liver and multiplies in liver cells. Hepatic, or liver, necrosis and kidney failure are causes of death. The intense jaundice, or yellow coloring of the skin, is responsible for the name of the disease.

III.   REVIEW QUESTIONS

1. b–an intracellular parasite

2. false

3. f–release

4. d–all of the above

5. d–the numbers of strains or
   varieties of the same virus
   that are not recognized later

6. b–these diseases result in
   permanent immunity as
   adults

1. A virus is:
    a. an extracellular parasite
    b. an intracellular parasite
    c. free living in the environment
    d. either free living or found in host cells

2. True or false: A virus either replicates on its own or uses host cell organelles to reproduce. _____

3. Disease or injury caused by viruses is most likely related to the _____ phase of the life cycle:
    a. attachment
    b. penetration
    c. uncoating
    d. eclipse
    e. assembly
    f. release

4. Defense against viral disease is mediated by:
    a. antibodies
    b. cytotoxic T cells
    c. interferon
    d. all of the above

5. Lack of permanent immunity against a virus is due to:
    a. small doses of the virus that are not enough to elicit an immune response
    b. deficient response by the person's immune system
    c. the nature of the immune response, which never can provide immunity for any virus
    d. the numbers of strains or varieties of the same virus that are not recognized later

6. Some viral diseases are considered a child's disease because:
    a. weak immune function makes only children susceptible to them
    b. these diseases result in permanent immunity as adults
    c. adults are not susceptible to them
    d. children are the natural host for these viruses

7. Photophobia, or sensitivity to light, is associated with:
   a. measles
   b. German measles
   c. chickenpox
   d. mumps

8. The significance of rubella, or German measles, is that it causes:
   a. birth defects
   b. retardation in children with the disease
   c. meningitis in adults with the disease
   d. none of the above

9. Two characteristics of a chickenpox rash are (choose two):
   a. macules
   b. ulcers
   c. vesicles
   d. pruritus

10. A latent infection following chickenpox which causes skin eruptions is:
    a. zoster
    b. parotitis
    c. shingles
    d. smallpox

11. Mumps *most commonly* result in:
    a. parotitis
    b. orchitis
    c. pancreatitis
    d. male sterility

12. The most common viral disease of adults is:
    a. influenza
    b. infectious mononucleosis
    c. gastroenteritis
    d. upper respiratory infection

13. A viral disease of adults associated with respiratory signs, muscle pain or myalgia, and secondary bacterial pneumonia, and that may cause death in epidemics is:
    a. influenza
    b. infectious mononucleosis
    c. gastroenteritis
    d. upper respiratory infection

14. A respiratory viral disease spread by deer mice that causes fluid in the lungs and death in half the cases is:
    a. rhinovirus infection
    b. hantavirus pulmonary syndrome
    c. Norwalk agent infection
    d. visceral herpes simplex

15. Vomiting and diarrhea are seen in:
    a. URI
    b. hantavirus pulmonary syndrome
    c. influenza
    d. viral gastroenteritis

7. a–measles

8. a–birth defects

9. c–vesicles; d–pruritus

10. c.–shingles

11 a–parotitis

12. d–upper respiratory infections

13. a–influenza

14. b–hantavirus pulmonary syndrome

15. d–viral gastroenteritis

16. a–mouth; b.–genitals; c–two;
    d–ulcers; e–systemic;
    f–nerves; g–is not

17. a–it is often in blood or
    transplant organs intended
    for populations susceptible to
    CMV

18. c–Epstein–Barr

16. Use the terms listed below to complete these sentences. Herpes simplex type I affects the a. _____, while HSV type II affects the b. _____. Both of these viruses have c. _____ stages of infection. Lesions associated with HSV are d. _____. Visceral herpes simplex is e. _____ and may be fatal. HSV lies dormant in f. _____ that supply the area of original entry. HSV g. _____ curable.

cervicitis	local	systemic
is	genitals	muscles
mouth	nerves	is not
two	three	ulcers

17. The significance of cytomegalovirus infection is:
    a. it is often in blood or transplant organs intended for populations susceptible to CMV
    b. it is a virulent pathogen for any population
    c. it is uncommon and therefore immunity does not exist
    d. it is often in the environment of populations susceptible to CMV

18. Infectious mononucleosis is caused by:
    a. varicella
    b. herpes zoster
    c. Epstein–Barr
    d. rhinovirus

SECTION ▶ IV. CHLAMYDIAL, RICKETTSIAL, AND FUNGAL INFECTIONS

5–99

1. inside
2. intracellular
3. DNA
4. RNA
5. metabolism

Chlamydia and **rickettsia** are both bacteria, but with some differences from the common pathogens we have studied. They are smaller than the conventional bacteria but larger than viruses. They can be seen with a light microscope. They contain *both* DNA and RNA but are strict intracellular pathogens. They are metabolically deficient compared with free-living bacteria and use host cells for much of their metabolism. Chlamydia and rickettsia live _____(1) host cells and so are called _____(2) pathogens. Their nuclear material consists of both _____(3) and _____(4). They use host cell organelles for much of their _____(5).

▶ CHLAMYDIAL INFECTIONS

5–100

Chlamydia trachomatis, or *C. trachomatis,* causes a variety of infections. The first is **trachoma,** which is a chronic infection of the lining around the eye, or the conjunctiva. This **conjunctivitis** usually spreads to involve the surface of the cornea. Growth of blood vessels over the corneal surface and scars from the infection can lead to blindness. Trachoma is not an important concern in the United States, but worldwide, it is a common cause of blindness. In another manifestation caused by the same organism, it is a venereal disease. It causes **chlamydial urethritis** and **cervicitis.** *C. trachomatis* is a common cause of male nongonococcal urethritis. In females, subclinical infection of the cervix is responsible for maintaining the infection in the population. Like gonorrhea, infected persons who are asymptomatic can easily spread a disease. *Chlamydia* infection has been identified as a leading cause of sterility in women. If a woman who has an active case of chlamydial cervicitis gives birth, the eyes of the newborn are usually infected. This condition is often called **neonatal ophthalmia.** The eyes of adults may become infected with the venereal strain due to hand-to-face practices or through community activities. For this reason, it is sometimes referred to as "swimming pool conjunctivitis." Another species is *C. psittaci.* It causes disease in psittacine birds, which is the parrot family. This disease is called **psittacosis.** (It can affect other birds, in which case it is called **ornithosis**.) People can catch the disease from these animals. Therefore, psittacosis is classified as a **zoonotic** disease. (**Zoonosis** is another term to describe a disease transmitted from animals.) Psittacosis causes pneumonia in people who have inhaled dust from an area contaminated with infected droppings. It is generally seen in those who work with or contact infected parrots.

5-101

A chlamydial conjunctivitis that often leads to blindness is caused by the agent _____(1). The disease is named _____(2). The venereal strain of *C. trachomatis* causes _____ (3). Eye infection of a newborn from a mother with chlamydial _____(4) produces the condition named _____(5). The eyes of _____(6) can also become infected from certain practices. Chlamydial urethritis is _____(7) common / uncommon (choose one) in men. The species that primarily affects birds is _____(8). The disease is most commonly called _____(9). It is classified as a _____(10) disease because it is contagious from _____(11). Psittacosis causes _____(12) in people.

1. *C. trachomatis*
2. trachoma
3. chlamydial urethritis and cervicitis
4. cervicitis
5. neonatal ophthalmia
6. adults
7. common
8. *C. psittaci*
9. psittacosis
10. zoonotic
11. animals
12. pneumonia

▶ RICKETTSIAL INFECTIONS

5-102

Rickettsia are organisms that have a preference for the endothelium of blood vessels. This vasculitis causes hemorrhage in the small vessels of the skin. The hemorrhage is universally seen as a rash. Therefore, the majority of rickettsial diseases have a rash as one of their signs. Rickettsial diseases are generally **febrile**, or causing fever. Therefore, fever is another hallmark of rickettsial infection. They used to be more of a problem in poor living conditions in which people and vermin would cohabitate. Epidemics were caused by this virulent pathogen and, given the right conditions, could occur again. *Rickettsia* cause a group of similar illnesses, and they are given the name **typhus**. (Do not confuse this with typhoid fever.) Rickettsia are transmitted by vectors. The vectors for typhus are both lice and rat fleas. In typhus there is high fever, intense headache, other associated aches and pains, and prostration (great weakness). The vasculitis becomes systemic and, as it affects the central nervous system, causes stupor and death. Typhus has always been a historical scourge associated with war, poverty, and famine. One form of typhus is **Rocky Mountain spotted fever**, which describes both a geographical association and a physical sign. RMSF is transmitted by ticks. A zoonotic rickettsial disease is **Q fever**, an infection of cows and sheep. It may be seen in people as a result of drinking tainted milk or working with these animals. Q fever can cause pneumonia or hepatitis in people.

5-103

Rickettsia prefer to attack the _____(1) or blood _____(2). When small vessels in the skin _____(3), it causes the characteristic sign of a _____(4). A second common sign of rickettsial disease is the presence of a _____(5). Several similar illnesses due to *Rickettsia* are grouped together as _____(6). This disease is transmitted by _____(7) and _____(8). The tick transmits a form of typhus called _____(9).

1. endothelium
2. vessels
3. hemorrhage
4. rash
5. fever
6. typhus
7. lice
8. rat fleas
9. Rocky Mountain spotted fever

FUNGAL INFECTIONS

5-104

Fungi are microorganisms that are more biologically complex than bacteria. They metabolize organic matter in their environment. Fungi may reproduce by either asexual or sexual processes. Fungi grow in two different manners; one form is a yeast and the other is a mold. A **yeast** reproduces or grows by a simple **bud** that extends out from the parent cell. **Mold** growth involves the formation of **hyphae**, which are filamentous branch-like structures that form an intertwining network. Reproductive structures from the hyphae include **conidia** (asexual) and **spores** (sexual).

5-105

1. hospital

A disease caused by a fungus is called a **mycosis** or **mycotic disease** ("myco" refers to fungus). Fungi do not cause the acute illnesses seen in bacterial and viral infections. The infection is chronic and can be disseminated internally or be superficial on the skin. Fungi are everywhere in the air, so contraction of fungal disease is not difficult in the right situation. One of these situations is the indiscriminate use of antibiotics that kill commensal organisms and allow fungi to overgrow. This is an opportunistic infection, as many fungal infections are. An increasing problem is a nosocomial opportunistic infection. Nosocomial means the infection was acquired while a patient was in the _____(1). Many patients today are treated aggressively for cancer or in preparation for transplants. Therefore, the use of immunosuppressive drugs is a major contributing factor. The decreased immune response of these and naturally suppressed patients gives rise to disease by organisms that normally don't cause disease. The existence of AIDS results in an increased incidence of mycosis. Also, today's extended life spans of debilitated patients allow mycosis to be seen more frequently than in the past. In short, mycotic disease is gaining importance because of immunosuppression, due to either treatments or AIDS, and because of otherwise weakened individuals.

5-106

The majority of mycoses are medically unimportant skin infections. We will consider the few that create significant disease. Many of these organisms have a specific geographic distribution, and so the mycotic disease is usually confined to certain parts of the country. These mycoses can be divided into two groups, the systemic or internal disease caused by genuine pathogens, and the superficial conditions caused by opportunists.

5-107

1. uncommon
2. resistance
3. respiratory
4. inhaled
5. chickens
6. pigeons

Histoplasmosis is caused by the agent *Histoplasma capsulatum.* Histoplasmosis is endemic in the northeast and central United States, especially around the Mississippi Valley. Skin tests show that the majority of the population has been infected at one time or another. The fungus is inhaled in dust. Local mild infections are common. Much less common is the systemic form that is often fatal. It is a progressively destructive disease resulting in areas of necrosis in several major organs. Factors leading to the systemic form include a very heavy dose of the organism or the poor resistance of the very young, the elderly, or compromised individuals. Histoplasmosis can occur in epidemics, and this is associated with soil contaminated by infected animals. The most common reservoirs of *H. capsulatum* are pigeons and chickens. This mycosis should be suspected if a group of people with a common history show respiratory signs. The suspicious history is usually having worked in a contaminated environment, such as around chicken coops or pigeon nesting areas. The signs of histoplasmosis are cough, fever, weakness, and aches and pains. It can also be asymptomatic in a healthy person. Life-threatening histoplasmosis is _____(1) common / uncommon (choose one). Poor _____(2) is a major factor in systemic histoplasmosis. The milder form involves the _____(3) system, since the agent is _____(4) in dust. This disease can appear in a group of people who have all been working around _____(5) or _____(6).

5-108

Coccidioidomycosis is caused by *Coccidioides immitis.* It is fond in the southwest, with spores found in sandy soil. Several species of animals can be infected and contaminate an area. After inhalation, typical respiratory signs are cough, fever, chest pains, and headache. **Cryptococcosis** is a mycosis caused by *Cryptococcus neoformans.* This is also a respiratory disease but it is more dangerous because it prefers the meninges and brain, so chronic meningitis can be a result if it is not treated. *C. neoformans* is an opportunist, so weak populations are targeted. *Blastomyces dermatitidis* is the agent of **blastomycosis.** It is found in several parts of the world. The superficial form is more common, with papules and ulcers forming over large areas. The systemic form results from the organisms entering the circulation **(fungemia)** and traveling to the lungs or other organs. Systemic blastomycosis can be very destructive to organ tissue.

5-109

Candida albicans results in **candidiasis.** *Candida* prefers moist areas and is normal flora of the mucus membranes of the mouth and genitals. It is only an opportunist but is in the spotlight because of its prevalence in AIDS patients. Recall from Chapter 4 that oral candidiasis is called thrush and is a hallmark infection in these patients. It forms characteristic white patches in the mouth. Fungemia is possible, with endocarditis resulting. Endocarditis is infection of the lining of the heart. *C. albicans* causes _____(1). *Candida* is normal flora of the _____(2). Candidiasis is found in patients with _____(3). It produces infection of the _____(4), and is specifically called _____(5). It may enter the circulation, a condition called _____(6).

1. candidiasis
2. mouth and genitals
3. AIDS
4. mouth
5. thrush
6. fungemia

5-110

We will finish our study of mycotic disease by talking about the **dermatomycoses,** or cutaneous fungal infections. These skin conditions are commonly called **ringworm,** even though they are not due to a parasitic "worm." The term "ring" comes from the characteristic red lesions on the skin that are round red patches. Ringworm is very contagious, so it is not uncommon for entire households to be affected. These fungi are transmitted very well by fomites, so environmental decontamination is an important part of their eradication. Direct contact with the lesions is also a means of transmission. Ringworm can be difficult to clear up, since it resists treatment. It is an opportunist in the weakened or stressed, and in children. It is a zoonosis since pets such as dogs or cats can harbor the fungus. Ringworm of the scalp in children is called **tinea.** The causative fungi is *Trichophyton,* and its name means it grows in hair follicles. Tinea results in bald patches on the head. Another dermatomycosis is caused by **epidermophyton,** leading to interdigital infection of the toes. (Interdigital means between the toes or fingers.) It is commonly called **athlete's foot** because of the means of transmission. This organism is found in environments such as around swimming pools, gyms, and locker rooms. Epidermophyton is very prevalent. Dermatomycosis means fungal infection of the _____(1). Two common cutaneous mycoses are known in lay terms as _____(2) and _____(3). The lesion in ringworm is _____(4) and red. Ringworm is easily transmitted through the _____(5). Since it can be transmitted from animals, it is a _____(6). Ringworm of the scalp in children is called _____(7) and it causes _____(8) patches on the head. Athlete's foot is mycosis of the _____(9). It is common in environments such as pools, _____(10), or _____(11). Table 5–5 summarizes diseases caused by *Chlamydia, Rickettsia,* and fungi.

1. skin
2. ringworm
3. athlete's foot
4. round
5. environment
6. zoonosis
7. tinea
8. bald
9. toes
10. gyms
11. locker rooms

TABLE 5–5. MAJOR DISEASES CAUSED BY *CHLAMYDIA, RICKETTSIA,* AND FUNGI

Pathogen	Associated Diseases
Chlamydia trachomatis	Trachoma (conjunctivitis)
	Urethritis
	Cervicitis
	Neonatal ophthalmia
Chlamydia psittaci	Psittacosis
Rickettsia	Typhus
	Rocky Mountain spotted fever
	Q fever
Fungi	
Histoplasma capsulatum	Histoplasmosis
Coccidioides immitis	Coccidioidymycosis
Cryptococcus neoformans	Cryptococcosis
Blastomyces dermatitidis	Blastomycosis
Candida albicans	Candidiasis
	Thrush
Trichophyton	Ringworm
Epidermophyton	Interdigital dermatitis (athlete's foot)

1. c–both DNA and RNA

2. d–any of the above

3. b–zoonotic

4. d–endothelium of vessels

5. a–fever; c–rash

6. c–vectors

7. a–typhus

8. d–opportunistic infection in increasingly vulnerable populations

IV. REVIEW QUESTIONS

1. Viruses, *Chlamydia,* and *Rickettsia* have all been described as intracellular parasites. *Chlamydia* and *Rickettsia* are different from viruses because they have:
   a. neither DNA nor RNA
   b. only DNA
   c. both DNA and RNA
   d. only RNA

2. *C. trachomatis* causes infection of the:
   a. eyes
   b. urethra
   c. cervix
   d. any of the above

3. Psittacosis is a respiratory disease that is classified as a _____ disease.
   a. venereal
   b. zoonotic
   c. mycotic
   d. viral

4. The site of attack by *Rickettsia* is the:
   a. epithelium of the skin
   b. endothelium of the skin
   c. epithelium of the vessels
   d. endothelium of the vessels

5. Two characteristic signs of *Rickettsia* disease are (choose two):
   a. fever
   b. chest pain
   c. rash
   d. conjunctivitis

6. *Rickettsia* are transmitted by:
   a. inhalation (airborne route)
   b. fomites
   c. vectors
   d. animals

7. The general name for febrile rickettsial diseases is:
   a. typhus
   b. Rocky Mountain spotted fever
   d. ornithosis
   d. Q fever

8. The growing significance of fungal infection today is because of:
   a. emergence of virulent strains due to mutation
   b. increased exposure to fungi
   c. lack of drugs that are effective in halting the infections
   d. opportunistic infection in increasingly vulnerable populations

9. Histoplasmosis is a disease affecting the 1. _____ system, and it is contracted by working around 2. _____.
   a. parrots
   b. digestive
   c. respiratory
   d. pigeons or chickens
   e. nervous
   f. sheep or cows

10. *Candida albicans* is:
    a. normal flora of the skin
    b. a virulent pathogen
    c. an environmental contaminant
    d. normal flora of mucous membranes

11. Thrush is actually:
    a. oral candidiasis
    b. respiratory candidiasis
    c. intestinal candidiasis
    d. infection of the nervous system by *C. albicans* seen only in AIDS patients

12. Ringworm is a:
    a. skin infection by a worm-like parasite
    b. dermatomycosis
    c. fungal infection of the intestines
    d. none of the above

13. Sources of ringworm include (choose all that apply):
    a. locker rooms
    b. fomites in an infected household
    c. infected animals
    d. children who are carriers
    e. all of the above

14. Tinea is:
    a. ringworm of the scalp
    b. ringworm affecting only animals
    d. dermatomycosis caused by epidermophyton
    d. athlete's foot

9. 1. c–respiratory; 2. d–pigeons or chickens
10. d–normal flora of mucous membranes
11. a–oral candidiasis
12. b–dermatomycosis
13. b–fomites in an infected household; c–infected animals
14. a–ringworm of the scalp

V. PROTOZOAL AND HELMINTHIC INFECTIONS ◀ SECTION

We conclude our study of microscopic pathogens with the protozoa and helminths. Protozoa are single-celled organisms that parasitize animals and humans. They are higher life forms than the previous organisms because they have a well-defined, distinct nucleus. They are all motile (as are some bacteria) by way of cilia, flagella, or ameboid movement. They cause several exotic diseases that will not be covered in this text. The more commonly known disorders are presented in the following frames.

▶ PROTOZOAL INFECTIONS

Entamoeba histolytica produces a condition known as **amebiasis** or **amebic dysentery.** Recall from the discussion about cholera that dysentery is intense diarrhea with deeper injury to the intestinal lining that causes loss of blood, mucus, and bits of tissue with the watery stool. Amebic dysentery has a much higher incidence outside the United States. The pathogenesis is as follows. The **cyst** stage of this parasite is infectious because it can withstand the acid of the stomach. It is ingested with food or water that has been somehow contaminated with infectious feces. The **trophozoite** stage of development invades the mucosa of the large intestine or colon. This results in catarrhal, or bloody, inflammation and ulcers in the colon. Dysentery (bloody diarrhea with mucus) is the obvious sign of this infection. In addition to profuse diarrhea, fever and abdominal pain are present. It is also possible, with entry into the circulation, that the liver is invaded and abscesses result. For unknown reasons, only a minority of people are susceptible to this clinical form. Most cases are asymptomatic carriers. Carriers are mainly responsible for the spread of cysts, through their stool. Water may be contaminated, or food touched by handlers or even flies may be contaminated. Obviously, this is a disease associated with unsanitary conditions or carelessness.

1. amebiasis
2. amebic dysentery
3. blood
4. mucus
5. tissue
6. minority
7. cyst
8. large intestine or colon
9. food
10. water
11. carriers

Entamoeba histolytica causes _____(1) or _____(2). Dysentery is intense diarrhea with the presence of _____(3), _____(4), and even bits of _____(5). Amebic dysentery affects the _____(6) majority / minority (choose one) of the people who swallow the infective stage. The infective stage is the _____(7). The site of damage by the trophozoite stage is the _____(8). The cyst form of *E. histolytica* is ingested with contaminated _____(9) or _____(10). Those most responsible for this contamination are _____(11) who are not sick themselves.

1. *Giardia lamblia*
2. water
3. wild animals
4. small intestine or jejunum
5. diarrhea
6. asymptomatic

Giardiasis is caused by *Giardia lamblia.* This is more commonly found in this country than amebiasis because wild animals are the reservoir. All municipal or city water supplies are tested and treated for *Giardia. Giardia* lives in the intestines of several animals, such as beavers, and easily finds its way into rivers, streams, and lakes. The cyst stage of this parasite is also the infective one, withstanding stomach pH. However, the trophozoite attaches to the jejunum of the small intestine. It can produce an acute diarrhea or, less commonly, intermittent chronic diarrhea. This chronic condition may lead to malabsorption and malnutrition, since it interferes with intestinal function. Many cases are asymptomatic. The causative agent of giardiasis is _____(1). This protozoa can be found in the _____(2) supply. It arrives there through the feces of _____(3). The site colonized by the trophozoite is the _____(4). It can cause _____(5), or often show no signs or be _____(6).

Malaria is still a significant problem and major cause of death in tropical regions of the world. It is caused by four different species of the genus *Plasmodium.* Malaria is transmitted by a mosquito vector, specifically the female *Anopheles.* The mosquito bite injects this parasite into the victim's bloodstream. It travels to the liver to multiply during the incubation period of the disease. An infective form, the **sporozoite,** leaves the liver and enters the red blood cells (RBCs) in circulation. In great numbers, the sporozoites multiply inside the RBCs. They become **merozoites** that burst out of the RBCs and invade other RBCs. This cycle of invasion, multiplication, and rupture of the blood cells continues. Of course, the rupture of the RBCs is called lysis. Lysis of red blood cells is further defined as **hemolysis.** The release and hemolysis of the cells is directly related to the **paroxysm** of signs in malaria. A paroxysm is a "sudden fit." These fits are rigor, or rigidity of the body, and fever. The fever demonstrates the three classic stages, and includes chills, shaking, and sweating. These are reactions to RBC hemolysis and parasites in the blood. Malaria is a disease the affects the _____(1) cells. It is caused by the genus of protozoal parasites known as _____(2). Malaria is transmitted by the female anopheles _____(3). An insect that transmits disease is a _____(4). Sudden fits of signs are due to _____(5) of RBCs and parasites in the _____(6). Hemolysis is _____(7) of the red blood cells. These fits are called _____(8) and include _____(9) and _____(10).

1. red blood
2. *Plasmodium*
3. mosquito
4. vector
5. hemolysis
6. blood
7. rupture, bursting, or lysis
8. paroxysms
9. rigor
10. fever

5-116

One species of *Plasmodium* causes what is known as malignant malaria, or blackwater fever. In this condition there is massive intravascular hemolysis and death. The other forms are more common and follow a chronic course of infection. The first attacks are worse, and lessen in severity as time goes by. The parasites live in the liver and continue to produce episodes throughout the life of the victim. The effects of this continual destruction of RBCs are anemia, debilitation, cachexia (weight loss), and a variety of secondary diseases because of weakened resistance. Treatment to prevent malaria is with quinine and several related compounds that kill the immature forms in the circulation. Diagnosis of malaria can be made with a routine blood smear. The organisms can be seen inside the RBCs, often in the form of a ring. This is illustrated in Figure 5–12. The usual course of infection in malaria is _____(1) acute / chronic (choose one). Ongoing hemolysis of RBCs leads to _____(2), _____(3), and _____(4). Patients are susceptible to many _____(5) diseases. On a blood smear, *Plasmodium* can be seen _____(6) red blood cells.

1. chronic
2. anemia
3. debilitation
4. cachexia
5. secondary
6. inside

5-117

Toxoplasma gondii is an animal parasite, especially of the cat. It causes **toxoplasmosis.** *T. gondii* is passed in the feces and remains infective in the environment for many days. Humans may be infected if it is ingested through hand-to-mouth practices. While this is primarily an intestinal infection, the parasite may invade other body tissues, including the central nervous system. Many people have been infected, as shown by the presence of antibodies in as high as 50 to 70 percent of the population in some areas of the country. Very few people become ill because of it. In the minority that do become symptomatic, effects range from mild fever to brain involvement or encephalitis (inflammation of the brain). It is a concern in immune-compromised populations (AIDS patients, chemotherapy recipients), where it can cause rapid fatal encephalitis. This is another example of opportunistic infection in the debilitated. Another major concern is **transplacental transmission.** An infected pregnant woman who is asymptomatic herself can pass the organisms to the fetus through the circulation supplying the placenta and fetus. Serious effects on the fetus include abortion, congenital brain infection, and injury to the eyes (chorioretinitis). The destruction of the brain can leave the infant mentally retarded, if it survives.

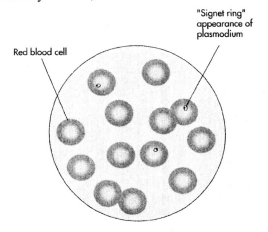

Figure 5–12. *Plasmodium* organisms in red blood cells in malaria.

5-118

1. toxoplasmosis
2. cat
3. digestive
4. infected
5. ill or symptomatic
6. encephalitis
7. deficient or compromised
8. pregnant
9. children
10. transplacental
11. brain
12. retardation

T. gondii is responsible for _____(1), and the natural host for this parasite is the _____(2). *T. gondii* enters humans through the _____(3) system. Many people have actually been _____(4), but few have become _____(5). The most serious consequence of toxoplasmosis is brain infection or _____(6). Three vulnerable populations include the immune _____(7), _____(8) women, and young _____(9). A fetus may acquire the infection through _____(10) transmission. Infection of the _____(11) can result in mental _____(12) or death.

5-119

1. itching
2. intestines
3. diarrhea
4. fluids
5. vagina
6. sexual intercourse
7. males
8. *Pneumocystis carinii*
9. AIDS
10. chemotherapy

Cryptosporidium is the agent of **cryptosporidiosis,** an intestinal disease resulting in diarrhea in humans. *Cryptosporidium* is an intestinal parasite of some animals and so can be seen among animal handlers. Children are another relatively common population to have cryptosporidiosis. In AIDS patients, a severe cholera-like diarrhea results in substantial, life-threatening fluid loss. A common sexually transmitted disease is **trichomoniasis,** caused by *Trichomonas vaginalis.* As the name implies, the condition is vaginitis, or infection of the vagina. Signs include pruritus, which means _____(1), and profuse watery vaginal discharge. In men, a mild urethritis may be present. The condition is propagated through male asymptomatic carriers. **Pneumocystosis** is a protozoal pneumonia that was occasionally seen in sickly infants. Today, it is a significant cause of death in AIDS patients. It is caused by *Pneumocystis carinii. P. carinii* is an inhabitant of the respiratory tract of many healthy people. It is an opportunist for any immune-deficient population, including chemotherapy recipients. Pneumocystosis in these patients manifests as fatal pneumonia. Cryptosporidiosis is a disease of the _____(2), causing _____(3). In AIDS patients, it may result in extreme loss of _____(4). Trichomoniasis in women is an infection of the _____(5), and is transmitted through _____(6). Urethritis may be seen in infected _____(7), though most are carriers. Fatal opportunistic pneumonia is caused by the organism _____(8). Those susceptible to pneumocystosis include _____(9) patients and recipients of _____(10).

▶ HELMINTH INFECTIONS

5-120

A **helminth** is what is commonly known as a parasitic "worm," usually of the intestines. Helminths are more complex than protozoa. They are two cells thick instead of one. Adults are visible without a microscope, and indeed can be several meters long. Even though the adults live primarily in intestines, different stages of development produce organisms that can be very migratory. Immature forms can travel widely through the body. These parasite infections are uncommon in the United States today because of improved sanitary measures. They are associated with unsanitary conditions, overcrowding, and warm climates. Eggs passed in feces cannot survive cool or cold climates.

5-121

1. hookworm
2. feet

Ancylostomiasis, or **hookworm disease,** is caused by the parasite *Ancylostoma duodenale.* It used to be a problem in the South and today is still prevalent in warm climates of the world. This worm occupies the duodenum and jejunum. It attaches to the intestinal mucosa using four hooklets or little teeth. It sucks blood from the host through this mucosa, and a heavy infection can result in anemia. Hookworm embryos are in the soil, and they penetrate the skin of bare feet. They travel through the blood to the lungs and migrate up the trachea, at which time they are swallowed. They then mature in the GI tract and attach to the small intestines. *Ancylostoma duodenale* causes _____(1) disease. The site of entry into the body is usually bare _____(2). The final destination of the parasite is

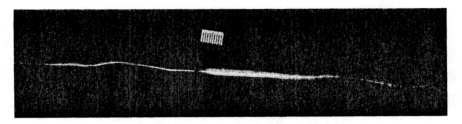

Figure 5–13. *Ascaris lumbricoides*—an adult roundworm. *(From Walter, An Introduction to the Principles of Disease, 3rd ed., Saunders.)*

the _____(3), where they attach and suck _____(4). This activity can result in _____(5).

3. small intestine or duodenum and jejunum
4. blood
5. anemia

Ascariasis, or **roundworm disease,** is due to *Ascaris lumbricoides.* An adult roundworm is shown in Figure 5–13. The eggs in soil can contaminate vegetables. The infection is acquired by eating raw contaminated vegetables. Adult roundworms inhabit the intestines, and this condition is seen more frequently in children. As in any intestinal parasite, diarrhea may be present. Heavy infection can result in intestinal obstruction. Another similar infection is **trichuriasis,** or **whipworm disease,** caused by *Trichuris trichuria.* (Common names indicate physical characteristics of the worms. *Trichuris* resembles a small whip.) These eggs are also ingested with fecal-contaminated material. In addition to diarrhea, abdominal pain and bleeding may be present. The most common sign of intestinal parasite infection is _____(1). Infections are acquired by _____(2) material that is contaminated with feces containing helminth _____(3).

1. diarrhea
2. eating or ingesting
3. eggs

Enterobiasis is commonly known as **pinworm disease.** The agent, *Enterobius vermicularis,* can be a common intestinal parasite of children and can be passed in households by objects like bedclothes. The source is also eating contaminated raw fruits or vegetables. Instead of eggs passing in the stool, the adult is passed and resembles white thread. This relatively harmless but annoying parasite causes irritation and intense itching around the anus. Adult pinworms in the stool look like _____(1). Enterobiasis most commonly affects _____(2) but can be passed to other family members. The common phrase for enterobiasis is _____(3).

1. white thread
2. children
3. pinworm disease

Trichinella spiralis is a parasite of both animals and humans. The usual route of infection is that an infected rat is eaten by a pig, the pork of that animal is consumed by a human, and **trichinosis** results. The disease occurs in humans when pork is undercooked, or heated to less than 131°F. After developing in the intestines, *Trichinella* invades several organs. However, it can only survive in muscle tissue, which may include the heart. The parasite exists as embryos in the muscle and they cause **myositis,** which is painful inflammation with hardening and swelling. Fever often accompanies the muscle pain or myalgia. Fatal cardiac involvement has been reported. *Trichinella* is acquired by eating _____(1) that has not been _____(2) thoroughly. The site of injury in this infection are the _____(3) tissues, with possible infection of the _____(4). Signs include muscle inflammation, or _____(5), and fever.

1. pork
2. cooked or heated
3. muscle
4. heart
5. myositis

The **tapeworms** are a group of worm parasites that are physically different from the previous parasites, which were all rounded and whole. Adult tapeworms are pictured in Figure 5–14. Tapeworms are flat and segmented. Their bodies are divided into distinct compartments that are shed individually in the stool. An entire segment is passed, filled with eggs. This differs from the free eggs passed by adult roundworms. The various tapeworms together are called **taenia,** with individual species having different hosts. They cause diarrhea and occasional abdominal pain, and heavy loads can obstruct the intestines.

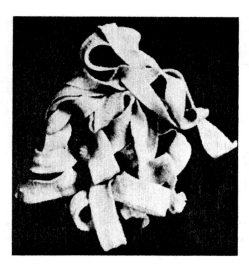

Figure 5–14. Adult tapeworms. *(From Walter,* An Introduction to the Principles of Disease, *3rd ed., Saunders.)*

5-126

The tapeworm diseases are commonly called by the animals in which they are found. The first is the **beef tapeworm,** or *Taenia saginata,* found in cattle. Cattle infection is common in this country. The eggs of this intestinal parasite are swallowed by the cattle, and maturing forms migrate and become cysts in the muscle. Human infection occurs by eating undercooked beef. The **pork tapeworm,** or *T. solium,* is acquired through undercooked pork. This parasite has a tendency to migrate and spread to visceral organs, including the brain. Infection by the **fish tapeworm,** or *Diphyllobothrium latum,* is also acquired through raw or undercooked fish. The **dog tapeworm,** or *Echinococcus granulosus,* has a different, more serious consequence. Dogs or wolves become infected by eating infected sheep. Humans get the disease by eating raw foods from soil contaminated with canid feces. In humans it is called **hydatid disease.** It is named after the presence of **hydatid cysts** that the parasites form in various tissues. Hydatid cysts can be commonly found in the liver and other vital organs. They can reach a great size and cause death by obstructing the function of the organ and causing pressure necrosis in the organ.

5-127

1. taenia
2. segments
3. animals
4. eating or ingesting
5. beef
6. pork
7. fish
8. dog
9. hydatid
10. cysts
11. size

As a group, tapeworms are called _____(1). They pass their eggs in flat parts of their body known as _____(2). Common names are associated with the _____(3) they parasitize. Infection in humans occurs by _____(4) undercooked _____(5), _____(6), or _____(7). The most dangerous infection is by the _____(8) tapeworm. It causes _____(9) disease in humans, which is the presence of hydatid _____(10) in body organs. Death can occur due to the massive _____(11) of these cysts. Table 5–6 summarizes diseases caused by protozoa and helminths.

TABLE 5–6. DISEASES CAUSED BY PROTOZOAL AND HELMINTHIC INFECTION

Pathogen	Associated Diseases
Protozoa	
Entamoeba histolytica	Amebiasis (amebic dysentery)
Giardia lamblia	Giardiasis
Plasmodium	Malaria
Toxoplasma gondii	Toxoplasmosis
Trichomonas vaginalis	Trichomoniasis
Cryptosporidium	Cryptosporidiosis
Pneumocystis carinii	Pneumocystosis
Helminths	
Ancylostoma duodenale	Hookworm disease
Ascaris lumbricoides	Roundworm disease
Trichuris trichuria	Whipworm disease
Enterobiasis vermicularis	Pinworm disease
Trichinella spiralis	Trichinosis
Taenia	Tapeworm disease
Echinococcus granulosus	Hydatid disease

V REVIEW QUESTIONS

1. Amebic dysentery is caused by:
   a. a helminth, *Ascaris lumbricoides*
   b. a protozoan, *Plasmodium*
   c. a protozoan, *Entamoeba histolytica*
   d. a helminth, *Trichuris trichuria*

2. Amebic dysentery causes inflammation and ulcers of the:
   a. duodenum
   b. colon
   c. jejunum
   d. anus

3. The continued presence of amebic dysentery is due to:
   a. shedding of cysts by asymptomatic carriers
   b. flies
   c. soil contaminated by animal feces
   d. shedding of cysts by the clinically ill

4. Giardiasis is associated with:
   a. food contaminated by asymptomatic carriers
   b. raw vegetables contaminated by egg-infested soil
   c. water contaminated by asymptomatic carriers
   d. water contaminated by wild animal feces

5. Giardiasis causes:
   a. diarrhea in the minority that are infected
   b. anemia due to blood loss
   c. diarrhea in the majority that are infected
   d. anemia due to red blood cell rupture

1. c–a protozoan, *Entamoeba histolytica*
2. b–colon
3. a–shedding of cysts by asymptomatic carriers
4. d–water contaminated by wild animal feces
5. a–diarrhea in the minority that are infected

6. b–a protozoan, *Plasmodium*

7. b–mosquito vector

8. a–rigidity; b–fever

9. c–parasites in the circulation; d–destruction of RBCs or hemolysis

10. d–all of the above

11. b–AIDS patients; c–the fetus of a pregnant woman; e–patients undergoing immunosuppressive therapy

12. b–brain

13. b–vagina of women; c–urethra of men

6. Malaria is caused by:
   a. a protozoan, *Toxoplasma gondii*
   b. a protozoan, *Plasmodium*
   c. a helminth, *Echinococcus granulosus*
   d. a helminth, *Ancylostoma duodenale*

7. Malaria is transmitted through:
   a. transplacental transmission
   b. mosquito vector
   c. egg-infested feces
   d. hand-to-mouth practices

8. Episodes of active malaria are clinically seen as (choose all that apply):
   a. rigidity
   b. fever
   c. diarrhea
   d. weight loss
   e. anemia

9. Malarial paroxysms are related to (choose all that apply):
   a. destruction of liver cells or hepatocellular lysis
   b. rigor
   c. parasites in the circulation
   d. destruction of red blood cells or hemolysis

10. Results of continued episodes of active malaria are:
    a. weight loss
    b. anemia
    c. decreased resistance to secondary disease
    d. all of the above

11. Toxoplasmosis is a danger to (choose all that apply):
    a. pregnant women
    b. AIDS patients
    c. the fetus of a pregnant woman
    d. anyone who becomes infected
    e. patients undergoing immunosuppressive therapy

12. The injury in toxoplasmosis primarily affects the:
    a. liver
    b. brain
    c. intestines
    d. red blood cells

13. Trichomoniasis is protozoal infection of the (choose all that apply):
    a. cervix of women
    b. vagina of women
    c. urethra of men
    d. testis of men

14. Fatal pneumonia in immune-deficient populations, caused by an opportunist, best describes:
    a. cryptosporidiosis
    b. amebiasis
    c. ancylostomiasis
    d. pneumocystosis

15. The main injury associated with hookworm disease is:
    a. diarrhea
    b. abdominal pain
    c. blood loss
    d. intestinal obstruction

16. Roundworm and whipworm disease are acquired by ingesting:
    a. contaminated water
    b. contaminated raw foods
    c. undercooked meats
    d. any of the above

17. Pinworm disease is associated with:
    a. anal irritation
    b. diarrhea
    c. abdominal pain
    d. intestinal obstruction

18. Trichinosis is acquired by ingesting:
    a. contaminated water
    b. contaminated raw foods
    c. undercooked meats
    d. any of the above

19. The main injury associated with trichinosis is:
    a. myositis
    b. encephalitis
    c. anemia
    d. pneumonia

20. Infection by the *Taenia* species is acquired by ingesting (choose all that apply):
    a. contaminated water
    b. contaminated raw foods
    c. undercooked meats
    d. all of the above

21. Hydatid disease is produced by the *Taenia* commonly known as the:
    a. fish tapeworm
    b. pork tapeworm
    c. dog tapeworm
    d. beef tapeworm

22. Death in hydatid disease is caused by the presence of enlarged _____ in vital organs.

14. d–pneumocystosis

15. c–blood loss

16. b–contaminated raw foods

17. a–anal irritation

18. c–undercooked meats

19. a–myositis

20. b–contaminated raw foods; c–undercooked meats

21. c–dog tapeworm

22. hydatid cysts

CHAPTER SUMMARY ►

► **SECTION I**

A pathogen is a microorganism that causes disease. Normal flora, or commensals, are normal inhabitants of the body and only cause disease as opportunists. The virulence of a pathogen is its ability to cause disease. Virulence, dose of an organism, and the immune and inflammatory responses all determine if infection leads to disease. A primary infection may allow a secondary infection to develop, either by another pathogen or by an opportunistic organism. An opportunistic organism may be a commensal. Exogenous, or environmental, is the most common source of pathogens. Sick individuals, carriers, and fomites are part of exogenous sources. Nosocomial infections are associated with group housing, especially hospitals. Pathogens enter the body through broken skin or natural body passages. Spread beyond the site of entry depends on pathogen factors (virulence, dose, site of entry) and host factors (necrotic or ischemic tissue, immune and inflammatory responses). Defense against infectious disease includes intact skin, decontamination (mechanical, biological, chemical), inflammation, immune response, and chemical mediators. Sepsis is overwhelming systemic infection produced by bacteremia or viremia. Toxemia or septicemia can lead to death because of septic shock. Septic shock is failure of the circulatory system, and therefore major organs, in reaction to toxins. Environmental control of microorganisms is accomplished by disinfection or sterilization. Disinfection decreases the numbers of harmful organisms except for spores. Sterilization destroys all microorganisms and spores. Cleaning removes gross material and should precede all disinfection and sterilization. Aseptic techniques are procedures designed to prevent or minimize contact between living tissue and microorganisms.

In diagnosing bacterial disease, the first diagnostic procedure is the Gram stain and microscopic exam. From this, bacteria are classified as gram positive or negative and their morphology is identified. This physical classification determines the manner in which the bacteria are tested for identification. Viruses require an electron microscope to be seen and are not stained. Bacteria and viruses are cultured, or grown, in artificial conditions (in vitro). For bacteria, synthetic media provides nutrients and support for growth. Bacteria grow on agar in separate colonies, specific for each bacteria, which allow for isolation for testing. Bacteria are identified through the biochemical reactions they produce in test media that contain indicators. They may also be identified through immunology. Viruses must be grown in living cells or tissues, which are cell or tissue cultures. They may be identified according to their cytopathic effect. Live animal inoculation and immunology are also methods to diagnose specific viruses. Bacterial infections are treated with antibiotics. An antibiotic may be bactericidal (kill the organisms) or bacteriostatic (inhibit their growth). It may be specific for gram-positive or -negative organisms, or be broad spectrum (effective against both). The best antibiotic for a particular infection is determined through sensitivity testing. An antibiotic becomes ineffective if a bacteria has developed resistance to it. Antiviral drugs are relatively few because of lack of selective toxicity. Host cells may be destroyed along with the virus.

► **SECTION II**

Pyogenic bacteria cause the formation of pus during the inflammatory response. Pyogenic gram-positive cocci include *Staphylococcus* (in clusters) and *Streptococcus* (in chains). *Staphylococcus aureus* is a common pathogen, often implicated in nosocomial infection. *S. aureus* may cause infection of the skin, associated structures, and wounds. Some *S. aureus* secrete hyaluronidase, which allows movement through the tissues. *S. aureus* can infect several body systems or cause septicemia. *S. aureus* can produce toxin-associated food poisoning or toxic shock syndrome. *Streptococcus pyogenes* (group A hemolytic or beta hemolytic) causes acute pharyngitis, or strep throat. Complications of *S. pyogenes* infection include scarlet fever, rheumatic fever, and poststreptococcal glomerulonephritis. *Streptococcus viridans, S. pneumoniae,* and enterococci are normal flora and have been identified as opportunists in some infections. *Neisseria meningitidis* is a pathogen that causes meningitis. Epidemic meningitis is spread by the airborne route. It especially affects immune-vulnerable populations, with a high mortality rate. Pyogenic gram-negative bacilli include the coliforms or enteric rods of the intestines. These commensals cause disease as opportunists in a vulnerable individual, or by being introduced to another body site. Septicemia due to gram-negative rods can lead to fatal endotoxic shock, especially by *E. coli. Salmonella* is a poultry intestinal commensal that can cause food poisoning (gastroenteritis or salmonellosis). Water and food are the sources of contamination. Human carriers are also a source.

Venereal disease is infection of the genitals through sexual contact. *Neisseria gonorrhoeae* is the causative agent of gonorrhea. Asymptomatic cases, especially in females, perpetuate this disease. Men usually have obvious signs of urethritis with a discharge, while women may experience silent infection that can lead to salpingitis. Salpingitis is a cause of sterility and ectopic pregnancy. Pelvic inflammatory disease accompanies chronic gonorrhea. Syphilis is caused by the spirochete *Treponema pallidum*. It is less common than gonorrhea but has life-threatening complications. Stage 1, or the primary stage, is marked by a contagious chancre, or ulcer, at the site of entry. The secondary stage manifests as a syphilitic rash. The rash is nonpruritic and common looking. The rash is somewhat contagious. The tertiary stage, or stage 3, advances to serious vasculitis, significantly affecting the cardiovascular and central nervous systems. Death can occur due to aneurysm in syphilitic aortitis. Necrosis of the brain or spinal cord in areas causes neurosyphilis and the signs paralysis, blindness, and insanity. Some bacterial infections are characterized by the effects of toxins from the pathogens.

Food poisoning may be due to the toxins of *S. aureus,* which are heat stable and not destroyed by cooking. Clostridia are anaerobic animal intestinal organisms found in soil. They grow best in necrotic or deep wounds, or in poorly canned foods. They are known for forming spores that remain infective for long periods under adverse conditions. Tetanus, or lockjaw, is produced by *C. tetani* and results in fatal paralysis. *C. perfringens* is the agent of gas gangrene. Enzymatic exotoxin and advancing gas are part of this mechanism as it causes putrefaction of muscle tissue. *Mycobacterium tuberculosis* is spread through the air and primarily affects the lungs, although bone, kidneys, and brain are secondary sites. TB is associated with poor living conditions and vulnerable populations. Of the people who manifest AIDS, TB is likely to develop as part of the spectrum of secondary diseases. TB lesions, especially in the lungs, are called tubercles and are a result of chronic granulomatous inflammation. Cachexia and hemoptysis are common signs of TB prior to death. Plague is caused by *Yersinia pestis*. It is spread through rats and their fleas. Affected, swollen lymph nodes are called buboes and break the skin surface with suppurative exudation. Bacteremia, systemic organ infection with necrosis and hemorrhage, and septicemia proceed death. Pneumonic plague is the form that is spread via the air from person to person. Lyme disease, caused by *Borrelia burgdorferi*, is spread through deer ticks. Stage 1 is mild and flu-like, with a characteristic bull's-eye rash. Untreated, advanced Lyme disease can affect the heart and nerves (stage 2) or lead to arthritis (stage 3). *Campylobacter enterocolitis* is a bacteria that can cause infectious inflammation of the small and large intestines.

▶ SECTION III

A virus is an intracellular parasite. The virus must use the host cell to reproduce. Viral activities often lead to death of the host cell and form the basis for disease of the body. Results of viral infection include degeneration or necrosis of cells, tissues, or organs, or latency with either subclinical or recurring signs. Numbers of and changes in strains of viruses often prevent immunity from developing. Viruses are primarily contracted through the respiratory and digestive systems, with vectors and direct lesion contact also being means of exposure. Children's viral diseases are so called because immunity does develop and these individuals do not become ill again as adults. Measles (rubeola) is most characterized by a widespread maculopapular rash. German measles, or rubella, is a teratogen (causes birth defects) if it is contracted by a pregnant woman. Chickenpox (varicella-zoster) is a herpesvirus. Chickenpox has an itchy or pruritic rash with vesicles (blisters). In some people the virus becomes dormant in nerves and later causes painful skin eruptions in the condition named shingles.

Mumps infection is relatively common and usually causes painful inflammation of the parotid salivary glands (parotitis). Other organs that may be involved are the pancreas, ovaries, and testes, with male sterility a remote, unlikely possibility. URI, or upper respiratory infection, is the most common adult viral affliction. Immunity to the common cold doesn't develop because of the numbers of viral strains. Influenza is a more severe respiratory infection, with death possible in the elderly or otherwise weakened.

Another potentially fatal viral disease is hantavirus pulmonary syndrome. Hantavirus is transmitted by body fluids and feces of rodents. HPS is characterized by fluid in the lungs. Intestinal flu is actually viral gastroenteritis. Group situations and fecal contamination set the stage for transmission. Herpesviruses have latent, chronic tendencies. Herpes simplex virus type I produces "cold sores" or "fever blisters" around the mouth. HSV type II affects the genitals and is a venereal disease. HSV lesions are ulcers which may be painful. HSV I and II lesions recur in the same areas indefinitely and hide in nerve cells meanwhile. Cytomegalovirus is a very common, harmless virus in the general population. It may cause death in weak newborns and for those immunosuppressed by therapy or disease. Infectious mononucleosis is caused by the Epstein–Barr virus. Airborne transmission and direct oral contact are the means of propagation among young adults, who become fatigued for a long while.

► SECTION IV

Chlamydia and *Rickettsia* are both bacterial intracellular pathogens. *C. trachomatis* causes trachoma, eye infection involving the cornea with potential blindness. In its venereal form it causes urethritis, cervicitis, and neonatal ophthalmia if newborn eyes become infected. *C. psittaci* leads to psittacosis (or ornithosis), a bird disease infectious also for the human respiratory tract. Rickettsial disease is marked by fever and a red skin rash. These typhus diseases are associated with poor living conditions and may cause death in epidemics. Rocky Mountain spotted fever is tick-borne, and Q fever is a zoonotic disease from ruminants. Fungal infections are a concern among immunosuppressed or debilitated people as opportunistic infections. *Histoplasma capsulatum* is responsible for the respiratory infection histoplasmosis. People working around animal reservoirs, especially chickens and pigeons, are susceptible. Coccidioidomycosis, cryptococcosis, and blastomycosis are other environmental fungi capable of producing disease, usually of the respiratory tract. *Cryptococcus neoformans* may advance to meningitis. *Blastomyces dermatitidis* can lead to systemic organ lesions. *Candida albicans* is an oral normal flora of the mucous membranes. It is of most concern in cases of AIDS where it causes opportunistic infection of the mouth, or thrush. The dermatomycoses (fungal skin infections) are commonly known as ringworm and athlete's foot. Ringworm is a contagious, resistant zoonosis often affecting children. Athlete's foot is contagious in locker room environments.

► SECTION V

Entamoeba histolytica causes amebiasis or amebic dysentery (bloody diarrhea with mucus). Carriers play an important part in water and food contamination. Giardiasis, due to *G. lamblia,* is a water-borne cause of diarrhea associated with contamination by animal feces. Several species of *Plasmodium* cause malaria. It is spread by the female *Anopheles* mosquito. Patients experience paroxysmal episodes of shaking and fever with each cycle of release of *Plasmodium* from the RBCs, which causes hemolysis. Anemia and general debilitation are the result of this chronic infection. The cat parasite *Toxoplasma gondii* is the agent of toxoplasmosis. This common infection is asymptomatic in most people but of major concern in the immunosuppressed and in pregnant women (transplacental transmission to the fetus). Trichomoniasis is a common STD affecting the vagina in women or urethra in men. Pneumocystosis is an opportunistic pneumonia due to *Pneumocystis carinii*. Its prevalence today is seen among AIDS patients as a common cause of death.

A helminth is a parasite commonly known as a "worm." The intestines are most commonly parasitized, but other body parts may be involved. Hookworm disease is due to *Ancylostoma duodenale,* a parasite of warm climates. Hookworms attach to small intestine mucosa with hooklets and draw blood, occasionally causing anemia. *Ascaris lumbricoides* produces roundworm disease, with diarrhea a likely result and obstruction a possibility. Whipworm disease is due to *Trichuris trichuria,* leading to diarrhea and possibly pain and bleeding. Pinworm disease is caused by *Enterobiasis vermicularis,* which resembles white thread. Adults lay eggs at night around the anus, causing irritation and itching. Trichinosis is infestation by *Trichinella spiralis* that leads to cysts in the muscles. Undercooked pork is the source. Tapeworms also are acquired by eating undercooked meats, with each tapeworm being specific for the source or animal host. *T. saginata* is the beef tapeworm. *T. solium* is the pork tapeworm. *D. latum* is the fish tapeworm. *Echinococcus granulosus,* or the dog tapeworm, causes hydatid disease, and fatality is associated with the size of the hydatid cysts.

CHAPTER 6

Central Concepts of Neoplasia

▶ OBJECTIVES

SECTION I

Define all highlighted terms.

Describe the difference between a differentiated and a nondifferentiated cell.

Compare and contrast the terms "hypertrophy" and "hyperplasia."

Give an example of a tissue exhibiting atrophy and a possible reason for the atrophy.

Distinguish between the concepts of hypoplasia aplasia, and agenesis.

Describe how neoplastic tissue would appear when viewed with a microscope.

Describe a tumor and why it is characterized as a space-occupying lesion.

Distinguish between a solid tumor and a diffuse tumor, and give an example of each.

Explain the differences between a benign tumor and a malignant tumor.

Explain the phenomena of metastasis and invasion.

Distinguish between the terms "primary tumor" and "secondary tumor."

Distinguish between a carcinoma and a sarcoma, and give an example of each.

Describe the method by which tumors are named.

Describe the process of chemical carcinogenesis.

Describe the process by which therapeutic radiation kills tumor cells.

Define the term "oncogenic viruses," outline a way by which these viruses might cause cancer, and give several examples of cancers that are caused by viruses.

As they relate to malignancy, distinguish between the terms "initiator" and "promoter."

Cite the contributions the following have to an individual's likelihood of developing a malignancy: family background, environmental pollutants, hormones, and the immune system.

Compare and contrast the epigenetic and the genetic theories of carcinogenesis.

List the three defined stages in carcinogenesis, and describe what is happening in each.

Distinguish between the terms "grading" and "staging" as they pertain to malignancy, and define the four grades of malignancy.

SECTION II

Define all highlighted terms.

Describe the concept of pressure necrosis, and list several of its consequences.

Explain why the following conditions may indicate a malignancy: pathologic bone fracture, hemorrhage, infection, anemia, anorexia, cachexia, and paraneoplastic syndrome.

Describe two natural defense mechanisms against cancer.

SECTION ▶ 1. GENERAL ASPECTS OF NEOPLASIA

▶ TERMINOLOGY OF CELLULAR GROWTH PATTERNS

6–1

Before we begin our study of neoplasia, a brief review of various cell growth activities is in order. Most of these terms should be familiar to you from your study of normal physiology. Many cells of the body are constantly undergoing reproduction, maturation, and other changes as part of the normal replacement process. All cell lines go through the process of **differentiation,** which is a primitive nonspecialized cell that matures into a specific cell type. These specific cell types develop according to function. So some primitive cells, or **stem cells,** become muscle cells, others become nerve cells, and so forth. A cell that is **nondifferentiated** is one that has remained in that earliest stage, or perhaps has regressed back. This process is illustrated in Figure 6–1. Neoplastic, or cancer, cells are less differentiated (more primitive) or completely nondifferentiated.

6–2

The word root **"plasia"** is important to understand and will be used frequently in the following frames. It means growth or form depending on its use. It refers to the growth or formation of cells and therefore tissue. **Hyperplasia** is an increased ("hyper") *number* of cells that leads to increased mass in that particular tissue. Hyperplastic cells are normal size. Hyperplasia results from many different stimuli. **Hypertrophy,** on the other hand, is increased *size* of individual cells, which leads to increased size of the affected tissue. Hypertrophied tissue has a normal number of cells. Various stimuli are also responsible for hypertrophy, and the most recognizable is enlarged skeletal muscle in response to work or strenuous exercise. Organs affected by hypertrophy are visibly or palpably enlarged, and are described with the suffix **"megaly."** An enlarged spleen is splenomegaly, enlarged heart muscle is cardiomegaly, and so forth. (You will be introduced to these terms again when we study specific body systems in Part Two of this text.) Both hyperplasia and hypertrophy can exist within the same tissue. The important point about these growth patterns is that microscopically these cells have a *normal appearance.* They are easily recognizable as to what type they are. You will soon see the significance of this when discussing concepts of neoplasia.

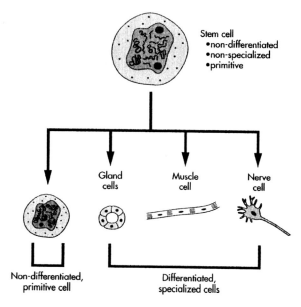

Figure 6–1. The process of differentiation.

6-3

The opposite changes also occur with cells, where there is a decrease in size or in number. Both of these situations can be described as **atrophy.** Atrophied tissue is visibly smaller. Think of it as withering away. The most commonly understood example of this is a limb whose musculature is meager after a cast has been removed. Disuse of a body part causes atrophy, as does poor blood supply or poor innervation. Hyperplasia, hypertrophy, and atrophy are illustrated in Figure 6–2. The next three terms are associated with interference in the development of an embryo or fetus. These conditions are congenital in that they are present at birth. **Hypoplasia** is a decreased number of cells leading to less tissue mass than normal. **Aplasia** means a complete lack of a cell line. (The prefix "a" means without.) **Agenesis** is lack of a particular organ, with "genesis" referring to development or creation.

6-4

Now we arrive at terms that are more associated with abnormal growth patterns or possible disease processes. When examined microscopically, cells that look abnormal are called **atypical** or **dysplastic.** The most important structure that is used to determine what is normal is the *nucleus,* although cytoplasmic changes are also noted. Since the nucleus holds the genetic material and is responsible for future generations, abnormality here means deviant instructions for growth and other activities. Word forms also referring to these conditions are **atypia** and **dysplasia.** A related term is **anaplasia,** which is translated as "without form." It is similar to dysplasia in that the cell has an abnormal appearance. However, it specifically means that the cell has reverted back to its nondifferentiated or primitive form. These three terms are used often in describing abnormal preneoplastic or neoplastic tissue. Be certain at this point that you understand their meanings. Figure 6–3 should increase your understanding. A cell that looks abnormal may be described as either _____(1) or _____(2). The most important structure in determining what is normal is the _____(3). Atypia or dysplasia that specifically is of primitive, regressed cells is called _____(4). These anaplastic cells are non_____(5).

1. atypical
2. dysplastic
3. nucleus
4. anaplasia
5. differentiated

6-5

"Neo" means new, so **neoplasia** would mean _____(1). An important notation is that this is not only new growth or formation, it is abnormal and serves no useful purpose. Certainly, in the processes of repair and regeneration, normal new growth is necessary and functional. The growth associated with neoplasia is uncontrolled or unrestrained and progressive. There is often no stop mechanism. The pattern of resulting tissue is haphazard because it lacks the normal coordination of reproducing tissue. A neoplastic growth can be described as having gone "haywire," with no end in sight. This growth is often responsible for the signs of neoplastic disease. A **tumor** is a solid, localized mass or lump that the new growth produces. Historically, a suffix assigned to describe swelling in general was **"oma,"** which can lead to some confusion. A "lumpoma" referred to any kind of swelling or lump. This could be a pocket of blood (hematoma), the presence of a granuloma, or even a cyst or abscess. A solid neoplastic growth, or tumor, is a space-occupying lesion. A lesion is a physical abnormality or injury, and a tumor has mass and takes up space. Other types of masses or lumps are also space-occupying lesions. The most basic definition of neoplasm is that it

1. new growth

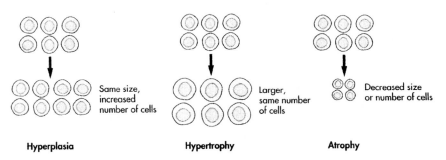

Figure 6–2. Normal cellular growth patterns.

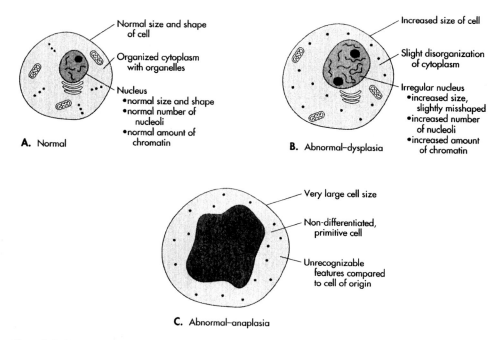

Figure 6–3. Abnormal cellular growth patterns. **A.** Normal. **B.** Abnormal. Described by the terms "atypical/atypia" or "dysplastic/dysplasia." **C.** Abnormal. Described by the terms "anaplastic" or "aplasia."

2. abnormal
3. function
4. controlled
5. coordination
6. tumor

is new growth that is _____(2) normal / abnormal (choose one) and has no useful _____(3). The growth of a neoplasm is un_____(4). The pattern is random because it lacks _____(5). A solid mass that is neoplasm is called a _____(6). Figure 6–4 shows some changes that occur in a neoplastic cell, as opposed to a normal cell.

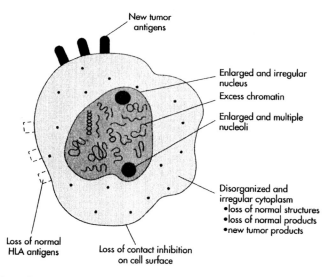

Figure 6–4. Some abnormalities in a neoplastic cell. *(Adapted from Chandrasoma and Taylor, Concise Pathology, 2nd ed., Appleton & Lange.)*

In contrast to tumors, there is another presentation of neoplasia and that is **diffuse.** This means the new abnormal growth is not confined to a local mass. Examples include neoplasia of the white blood cells (leukemia) in which the bone marrow is affected, and infiltration of the stomach wall or intestines. This infiltration produces very thickened walls in these organs, not a mass. Neoplasia whose growth is spread out, instead of tumor producing, is called _____(1).

1. diffuse

The relationship of neoplasia to **cancer** is that benign forms are not cancer, while malignant forms are cancer. Benign and malignant forms have different characteristics. A benign neoplasia is slow growing, usually encapsulated with cells that stick together, doesn't invade local tissue, doesn't spread to other body parts, and, once removed, does not recur. The capsule and adherent cells make removal fairly easy. Benign neoplasia is not associated with disease and death unless its location interferes with some vital function. Such a space-occupying lesion in the brain could cause death or obstruction if it is in the intestines. Malignant neoplasia has the opposite characteristics. It grows faster and does not have a capsule so removal is more difficult. It doesn't "peel out" as well. Also, malignant cells do not adhere to each other well so shedding of cancerous cells to local areas and into the blood are common. Recurrence after removal is also a possibility. Cancer *is* locally invasive. It spreads into surrounding tissue with long projections. This type of extension is responsible for the term "cancer," which comes from the Latin cancri, which means crab. The projections or extensions were thought to resemble the claws of a crab. Figure 6–5 contrasts the features of a benign and malignant tumor. Figure 6–6 is an excellent example of these differences as found in biopsy specimens. The cells of cancer look very abnormal and primitive and are called anaplastic. In some cases of hyperplasia, if the cells look atypical or dysplastic, the condition may be classified as premalignant. The slight abnormality may develop into anaplasia and malignancy. A very important characteristic of cancer, or malignancy, is **metastasis.** Metastasis is spread to other body parts through the blood or lymph circulation and the establishment and growth of new tumors. These distant new growths are called secondary tumors as opposed to the primary site of origin. An example is breast cancer as a primary malignancy and spread to the lungs as the secondary malignancy.

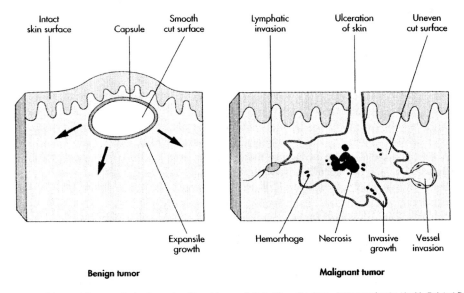

Figure 6–5. Contrasted features of a benign and malignant tumor. *(Adapted from Damjanov,* Pathology for the Health-Related Professions, *Saunders.)*

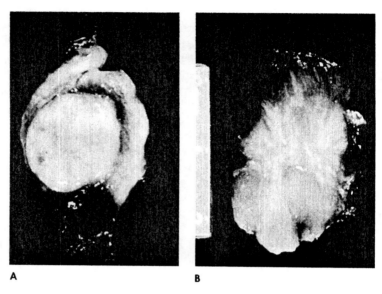

Figure 6–6. Excisional biopsy specimens of breast neoplasms. **A.** Spherical, encapsulated, benign neoplasm. **B.** Invasive, crab-like streaks of a breast cancer. *(From Kent and Hart,* Introduction to Human Disease, *3rd ed., Appleton & Lange.)*

6–8

1. cancer
2. benign
3. malignant
4. invade
5. spread
6. invade
7. anaplastic
8. metastasis
9. blood
10. grow
11. secondary tumors

Only malignant neoplasia is called _____(1). Several characteristics separate _____(2) and _____(3) neoplasia. Probably the two most important attributes of benign neoplasia is that it doesn't _____(4) local tissue, nor does it _____(5) to the rest of the body. Malignancy *does* _____(6) the local area with long, finger-like projections. The cells of cancer are described as _____(7). Spread of malignant cells to other body parts is called _____(8). This is accomplished through the _____(9) supply or the lymph system. An important part of the definition of metastasis is that, once elsewhere, the cancer will establish itself and _____(10) there. These distant new growths are called _____(11).

► CLASSIFICATION OF NEOPLASIA

6–9

Classifying neoplasia is useful in treatment of patients, for statistical study, and for research purposes. The best way to categorize neoplasia seems to be by the cell line or tissue of origin. The two largest categories of tissue in the body are epithelial and connective, or mesenchymal. Most neoplasia arises from these two tissues. You already know the aspects that classify a neoplasia as either benign or malignant. In general, *malignant* neoplasia or tumors of epithelial origin are called **carcinoma.** Epithelial tissue includes internal organs and glands as well as linings of body cavities. *Malignant* neoplasia of connective tissue origin is called **sarcoma.** Connective tissue includes bone, muscle, and blood. Following this rule, either carcinoma or sarcoma together with the name of the affected tissue identifies cancer. A few miscellaneous categories exist. Tumors of very specialized tissue may be given their own name. Glial cells are connective tissue of the brain. Cancer of these cells is not called a sarcoma, but a glioma. Some cancers are so undifferentiated (extreme anaplasia) that one can't tell what the tissue or cell origin is because of the bizarre appearance of the cells. In these cases, electron microscopy or testing for specific cell membrane markers can help to classify the cancer. A side note is that cancer of melanocytes (malignant melanoma) is classified as uncertain origin because melanocytes don't fit neatly into any one tissue type. Clas-

TABLE 6–1. CLASSIFICATION AND NOMENCLATURE OF NEOPLASIA

Epithelial Tissue Origin	Connective Tissue Origin
Benign: Tissue of origin followed by "oma"	*Benign:* Tissue of origin followed by "oma"
Example: adenoma (gland)	Examples: chondroma (cartilage), lipoma (adipose or fat)
Malignant: Tissue of origin and "carcinoma"	*Malignant:* Tissue of origin and "sarcoma"
Examples: adenocarcinoma (gland), squamous cell carcinoma (skin), hepatocellular carcinoma (liver)	Examples: chondrosarcoma (cartilage), osteosarcoma (bone)

sifying neoplasia is done on the basis of cell or tissue _____(1). Cancer that develops from epithelial tissue is called _____(2). Malignancy of connective tissue origin is called _____(3). Cases in which the cells are very undifferentiated, or very _____(4), require additional techniques to classify them because the cells don't resemble any particular tissue.

1. origin
2. carcinoma
3. sarcoma
4. anaplastic

6–10

Benign tumors are named according to the involved tissue, with the addition of the suffix "oma." Malignant tumors are named according to the involved tissue, and either carcinoma or sarcoma is added. Take a moment to study Table 6–1, which will help you to visualize these rules for naming the different types of neoplasia. Based on these rules, a benign neoplasia of the bone would be called an _____(1). Breast cancer (glandular tissue) is rightly called mammary_____(2). Malignancy of skeletal muscle is called rhabdomyo_____(3).

1. osteoma
2. carcinoma
3. sarcoma

► ETIOLOGY OF MALIGNANT NEOPLASIA

6–11

In the mysterious and frightening world of cancer, there are two categories of causes of malignant neoplasia. In one category are known or proven causes, and in the other are factors that are suspected to play a role in the development. The distinction between these two categories is often blurred, with some agents falling into both categories. It is important to remember that cancer is a *process,* and is one that leads to disease in the latest stages. There are many factors in cancer, known or theorized, and many steps in the complex production of a malignancy. By the end of this topic, it should be apparent that the cause of malignancy is probably a combination of a variety of elements. There are more things that are suspected to cause cancer than there are proven.

6–12

Compared to all of the agents and elements that are believed to be linked to cancer, the known causes are few. These causes are **carcinogens** and **radiation.** A carcinogen is a chemical that is capable of causing cancer. This cancer may be of the skin, if the carcinogen is topical (on the skin surface), or it may be internal, if the agent is inhaled or ingested. There are even compounds that are *not* carcinogens until a step in normal metabolism converts them into one. Both carcinomas and sarcomas have been created by carcinogens. In identifying carcinogens, a procedure called the Ames test shows if a compound can cause mutations in the DNA structure of normal cells. (We will consider more about mutation in Frame 6–23 on initiation.) A positive test is vital information for use in public health administration. As with many suspected causes, the latency period associated with carcinogens is long (usually many years). The latency period of a malignancy is like the incubation period of an infectious disease. It is the period starting from the initial exposure and injury to the time when a condition can be clinically demonstrated (usually by signs of disease). The tar in cigarette smoke is a well-known carcinogen, producing bronchiogenic carcinoma, or lung cancer. Other examples of specific carcinogens will be considered under environmental factors (Frame 6–19). A chemical that causes cancer is called a _____(1). This cancer

1. carcinogen

2. skin
3. internal
4. test
5. DNA mutation

may be on the surface of the _____(2), or be _____(3). Carcinogens are identified by the Ames _____(4). It identifies the ability of the agent to cause _____(5) in normal cells.

6-13

1. atomic particles
2. electromagnetic waves
3. DNA
4. abnormal

Radiation is a physical agent capable of producing tumors of the skin and viscera (internal organs) and leukemia. Sources of radiation are x-rays, nuclear weapons, nuclear power plants, radioactive compounds, and even radiation that in the past was part of therapy for another condition. The danger from diagnostic x-rays is very small, because radiation damage is dose related. The more exposure that exists, the greater the damage. Therefore, technicians and radiologists working with x-rays are really the susceptible populations and take precautions against exposure. Another susceptible population is pregnant women, especially in the first trimester when the embryo can be harmed. Radiation is a stream of atomic particles (electrons, neutrons, protons, alpha particles) that are transmitted through the air in electromagnetic waves. These waves of energy enter cells and interact with nuclear material, damaging the DNA by creating breaks in the helical structure. This damaged genetic material will produce abnormal cells if it is not repaired. Ultraviolet light from the sun is a form of radiation known for its ability to cause cancer of the skin (malignant melanoma and squamous cell carcinoma). Radiation-induced cancer occurs when or if the damage to DNA is greater than the body's abilities to repair it. Radiation is a stream of _____(1) that transmit through the air in _____(2). Radiation causes cancer by damaging the _____(3) of cells. Damaged nuclear material will produce _____(4) daughter cells.

6-14

1. associated
2. higher

The remainder of the possible causes that we will discuss have to be classified as highly suspect rather than known. The first of these are viruses. Viruses are *known* to cause neoplasia in lab animals and even in some human cell cultures. But beyond that there are only associations of some viruses with specific cancers. That means that the incidence of that cancer is much higher in people with a particular virus than in the general population. Examples are Epstein–Barr virus and Burkitt's lymphoma, herpes simplex II virus and cervical cancer, hepatitis B virus and primary hepatocellular carcinoma, and HTLV-1 with adult T-cell leukemia or lymphoma. So does that mean that a woman with herpes is going to get cancer? Or that a case of mononucleosis by Epstein–Barr will lead to cancer? Of course not. It isn't nearly as clear-cut as smoking and lung cancer. However, many cases of these particular malignancies have been found to be infected with these viruses. Viruses have been accepted as one of the many factors that are highly probable in the development of malignancy. This further underscores the fact that there are few cases of cancer that are proven to be of a single cause. Some viruses are _____(1) with particular cancers, because the incidence of these cancers is _____(2) in infected individuals than in noninfected individuals.

6-15

1. oncogenic
2. oncogene

Studies in laboratory animals have identified more than 20 viruses that cause malignancy in the animals. These tumor-producing viruses are called **oncogenic** viruses. (The prefix "onco" refers to cancer, such as oncology [study of cancer] and oncologist [physician who specializes in cancer].) So oncogenic means cancer creating. This is done through **oncogenes,** which are viral nucleic acid material (DNA or RNA) that cause malignant transformation of host cells when they incorporate with host cell DNA. Oncogenes induce tumor production. In other words, these are genes from a virus that transform a normal cell into a cancer cell, or malignant neoplastic cell. Going back to the definition of a neoplastic cell, it is a very abnormal mutation that grows wildly without a stop mechanism. A virus that has been shown to cause cancer in lab animals is called an _____(1) virus. The genetic material of the virus that transforms host cells into mutants is called an _____(2).

6-16

Oncogenes are believed to work in the following manner. The nucleic acid or genetic material in the core of a virus integrates with, or becomes a part of, the nucleic acid of the infected host cell. This creates an abnormal chromosome, being part host DNA and part virus DNA or RNA. This combination of genetic material produces abnormal daughter cells when the infected cells replicate. The daughter cells have mutated and often there is uncontrolled growth. This is because the virus can inactivate a protein in cells (p53) that normally controls growth. This process of mutation and unrestrained replication is called **cell transformation.** Proof of integration into host genes is demonstrated by **vertical transmission** in which offspring of infected parents inherit the same altered genetics. A prevalent theory of viral infection leading to cancer production rests on the concept of mixing viral _____(1) with host _____(2). Once this occurs, replication produces daughter cells that have _____(3). In addition to this abnormality, there is uncontrolled _____(4). This process has been named _____(5).

1. nucleic acid
2. DNA
3. mutated
4. growth
5. cell transformation

6-17

In many cases, it is thought that a virus acts as an **initiator.** This is an agent that begins or sets the stage for later malignancy. The abnormality of the infected cells may be classified as preneoplastic. During a long latency period, other factors may enter into the equation until, finally, malignancy exists. These other factors that add to the development of cancer are called **promoters.** Some viruses themselves may be promoters. In the absence of promoters, it is unknown if malignancy will still develop.

6-18

Genetics as a cause of cancer is almost proven in lab animals, but in humans all we have to go by is **familial** tendencies. A familial condition is one that runs in certain families. Rare cancers have been traced through some family lines, showing a startlingly high incidence among close relations. However, statistical studies of various races and populations do _not_ implicate genetics as a primary cause of cancer. Most likely, heredity predisposes an individual to susceptibility to the suspected factors. For example, this may explain malignancy following viral infection in some people. This predisposition may account for why these factors cause cancer only in some people and not in others. One example of genetic predisposition or susceptibility is seen in women with breast cancer. The incidence of breast cancer among the female relatives of the victim has been shown to be higher than the general population. A woman whose mother or grandmother has breast cancer has a higher risk for developing this malignancy. Genetic makeup _____(1) is / is not (choose one) a direct cause of cancer. The significance of heredity is that it seems to make some people more _____(2) to developing cancer. This susceptibility is in relation to the other theorized causes of _____(3). Therefore, genetics is considered a contributing factor in malignant neoplasia.

1. is not
2. susceptible
3. cancer

6-19

The environment can be listed in both categories of causes because in it there are proven carcinogens, suspected carcinogens, and other factors. Some known carcinogens may be contacted during occupational exposure. There are many examples of this, and they include work with tar and petroleum distillates, aniline dyes, radioactive compounds, vinyl chloride of plastics, and heavy metals. Suspicious agents found in the general environment include agricultural chemicals and food preservatives like nitrite, asbestos in buildings, industrial waste, air pollution, car exhaust, and perhaps household chemicals. The environment contains both _____(1) and _____(2) carcinogens. Exposure to known carcinogens may occur though industrial work or one's _____(3). Other exposures are possible through day-to-day living.

1. known
2. unknown
3. occupation

6-20

Hormones are thought to play a role in specific malignancies, especially of the male and female reproductive organs. Subtle relations have been demonstrated between women with high or prolonged estrogen levels and breast or endometrial cancer. These tumors of the reproductive system appear to be dependent on the sex hormones for growth. For instance, removing the ovaries can cause regression of mammary carcinoma, even if only temporarily. Administration of estrogen in men with prostate carcinoma causes inhibition of this

TABLE 6–2. PROVEN AND SUSPECTED CAUSES OF MALIGNANT NEOPLASIA

Proven Causes	Suspected Causes

Chemical carcinogens
  Tobacco tar
  Industrial chemicals
	Viruses
	  Oncogenic viruses (oncogenes)

	Genetics Possible predisposing factor

Radiation
  Nuclear activity
  Radioactive compounds
	Environment
	  Suspected carcinogens

	Hormones Sex hormones in reproductive malignancy
	Chronic tissue injury Possible promotors of a primary initiator
	Severe immune deficiency Deficiency of T cells

1. hormones
2. growth

6–21

testosterone-dependent tumor. In cancer of the reproductive organs, _____(1) are considered suspicious factors in its development. The relationship seems to be dependency on the hormones for _____(2).

For a long while, chronic infection or chronic irritation was considered a factor in cancer production. The rationale was that the insult, being present through many cell generations, finally resulted in mutations. Certainly, there are links between cirrhosis and liver cancer and chronic skin ulcers and squamous cell carcinoma. But most likely, these chronic conditions act as promoters of some primary initiator and should be considered a contributing factor, rather than a primary cause. Immune deficiency is another suspected factor in neoplasia, especially when T lymphocytes are deficient. Recall from Chapter 4 that T cells constantly survey the body for abnormal cells. Slight mutations do occur and this is normal. However, these abnormal cells are identified and destroyed by the T cells. Hence, an inadequacy of T cells can lead to the survival of abnormal cells. This accounts for the frequency of rare cancers in AIDS patients. These proven and suspected causes of malignancy are summarized for you in Table 6–2.

▶ PATHOGENESIS OF MALIGNANT NEOPLASIA

6–22

1. carcinogenesis
2. normal
3. expression
4. DNA material

Carcinogenesis is the development or creation of neoplasia, and is commonly understood to mean malignant neoplasia. The latent period for carcinogenesis is very long. There are currently two theories to explain how cancer develops. The first is the **epigenetic theory,** in which *normal* genetic material, or DNA blueprints, are *expressed* abnormally. By expression we mean the transcription and translation processes carried out during the cell reproduction process. This abnormal reading and deciphering of the DNA causes the cell to differentiate abnormally. When viral nucleic acids incorporate into host cell DNA, this might occur. Also, carcinogenic agents could cause this by gene interference. In the **genetic theory,** it is believed that there is an actual change or mutation in the DNA itself, so naturally the expression would deviate from the normal. Again, a viral oncogene or chemical alteration might explain this. The development of malignant neoplasia is called _____(1). In the epigenetic theory of carcinogenesis, it is thought the DNA material is _____(2), but the _____(3) is abnormal. The genetic theory holds that the _____(4) is abnormal because of an alteration.

There appear to be three stages in carcinogenesis. The first is **initiation.** This is the first, or initial, event that begins the journey to malignancy. Some factor, such as a carcinogen or a virus, begins the process by causing the changes discussed in Frame 6–22. Remember, the basis of neoplasia is abnormality in cells and growth due to abnormal genetic material or expression. These genetic changes lead to mutant clones that can later transform into malignancy. Initiation can be thought of as relating to initial exposure. It does not mean malignancy is certain to develop. Remaining stages must be successfully completed by the abnormal cells, and they must grow and survive. Initiation is the first step in converting to neoplasia. A carcinogen binding to DNA can cause errors in replication, and daughter cells are dysplastic. Dysplasia, if diagnosed, is to be watched since it is a precursor to anaplasia. The dysplastic cells proliferate or multiply as if some autonomous growth potential had been conferred upon them. By this we mean that the growing mass of abnormal cells does not follow the rules but takes on a life of its own. The first step in carcinogenesis is _____(1). This is the beginning of _____(2) cell production. This abnormality is because of _____(3) changes. The clones or daughter cells are described as being _____(4). These dysplastic cells _____(5) in an uncontrolled manner.

1. initiation
2. abnormal
3. genetic
4. dysplastic
5. grow

The next phase is **promotion.** It is important in that it acts as a necessary factor in whether or not malignancy develops. The alterations stemming from initiation may not amount to anything were it not for promotion. Promotion can be compared to a catalyst in chemical reactions. It speeds things up and heavily supports the reaction. If initiation is the beginning event, promotion is the support through the long latency period. A promoter can be any of the factors we discussed under the causes of cancer. Carcinogens can be both initiators and promoters. It can be difficult to say which factors started the road to cancer and which kept it going. During the process of promotion, the cells move from dysplasia toward anaplasia. The growth rate is increased because the cells divide more quickly under the influence of a promoter. A promoter then is a factor that supports the formation of a malignant tumor. Looking at the combined effects of initiation and promotion, we have an increased production of mutant cells. In the long promotion stage, the condition is considered precancerous. Removal of causative factors at this point may provide a chance of reversion to normal. The phase of carcinogenesis that continues the effects of initiation is _____(1). This provides fuel to the fire throughout the _____(2) period. A carcinogen can act as both a (an) _____(3) and a _____(4). Cell characteristics during promotion change from dysplasia and lean more towards _____(5) in this gradual process. The growth rate is _____(6).

1. promotion
2. latency
3. initiator
4. promoter
5. anaplasia
6. increased

The last stage is **progression,** where malignancy exists. The cell morphology is definitely anaplastic. There is a spurt of growth, with invasion and metastasis. The more anaplastic the cells, or the more poorly differentiated and primitive the cells, the faster the growth and spread. This is because the mutant cells are further away from control and normalcy than are more differentiated cells. Cancer often is not diagnosed until this time, which is really very late in the whole process. (However, clinically it may be early.) The stage in which malignancy can be identified is called _____(1). The cells are _____(2), with the degree of primitive de-differentiation related to the rate of _____(3) and _____(4). Examine Figure 6–7 to be sure you understand the stages of carcinogenesis.

1. progression
2. anaplastic
3. growth
4. spread

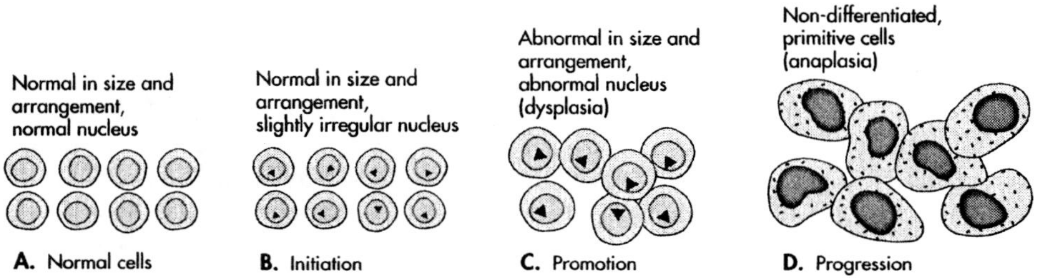

Figure 6–7. Stages of carcinogenesis. **A.** Normal cells. **B.** Initiation. Cancerous agent affects DNA, causing changes in nucleic acids. **C.** Promotion. Repeated exposure or additional agents. **D.** Progression. Malignant cells with potential for invasion and metastasis.

6–26

Once cancer exists, there are further stages in its activities. In cancer involving squamous epithelium, there is a time when the malignancy has not moved past the basement membrane. It is temporarily contained within the epithelium and has not broken through to the underlying tissue. This very localized form is called **cancer in situ.** This can be seen in early lesions of the cervix, mouth, and larynx.

6–27

Direct spread of cancer is in the form of **invasion** along tissue planes and through natural spaces, in the claw-like manner described earlier. The tumor becomes attached to adjacent structures like overlying skin and underlying muscle. Therefore, cancerous tumors are usually not moveable, in contrast to benign tumors like a lipoma. At this point death is possible *if* tumor causes obstruction of a passage like the ureters or the esophagus, if it ulcerates an area containing a large vessel resulting in fatal hemorrhage. Extensions of cancerous tumors also invade lymphatic vessels, arteries, and veins. This is vital because it gives the malignancy a chance to metastasize. This vessel invasion consists of long cords of cells extending from the mother mass. In actual **metastasis,** clumps of tumor cells from the invading cord break off and travel to other parts of the body through the vessels. They implant elsewhere at some distant site and grow into new secondary tumors. These secondary tumors are referred to as **metasta*ses*.** The process of metastasis and the existence of metastases are responsible for death in malignancy. This body-wide spread limits the effectiveness of any treatment and hope for survival. Carcinoma in situ, invasion, and metastasis are diagrammed in Figure 6–8. Figure 6–9 depicts metastases, or secondary tumors, in the liver that have traveled there from a primary malignancy.

6–28

1. invasion
2. attached
3. is
4. vessels
5. metastasis
6. break off
7. vessels
8. grow
9. metastases

Direct spread of cancer through solid tissue or spaces is called _____(1). Malignant tumors that have invaded the local site are usually not moveable because they have _____(2) to nearby tissues. Death _____(3) is / is not (choose one) possible from local invasion only. Cords of tumors cells also enter lymphatic and blood _____(4). This sets the stage for _____(5). In metastasis, groups of tumor cells _____(6) and travel to distant sites through the _____(7). They settle and _____(8) in the new location. These secondary tumors are called _____(9). The most common site for secondary cancer, or metastases, is the liver. The lungs are the second most common. Cancer of the breast, prostate, and lung are drawn to bone. The brain is also a secondary site for lung cancer.

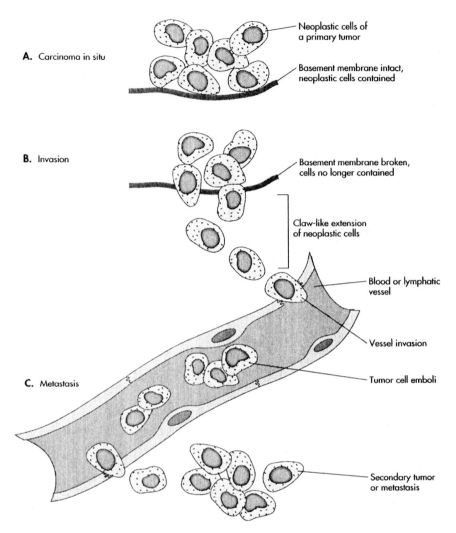

A. Carcinoma in situ

Neoplastic cells of a primary tumor

Basement membrane intact, neoplastic cells contained

B. Invasion

Basement membrane broken, cells no longer contained

Claw-like extension of neoplastic cells

Blood or lymphatic vessel

Vessel invasion

C. Metastasis

Tumor cell emboli

Secondary tumor or metastasis

Figure 6–8. **(A)** Carcinoma in situ, **(B)** invasion, and **(C)** metastasis of malignant neoplasia.

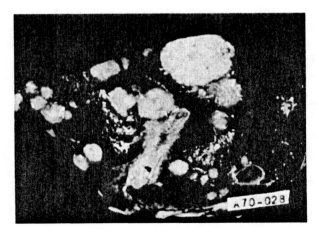

Figure 6–9. A liver studded with metastatic cancer (secondary tumors or metastases). *(From Kumar et al, Basic Pathology, 5th ed., Saunders.)*

▶ GRADING AND STAGING OF MALIGNANT NEOPLASIA

Grading and staging of cancer is a classification process that is helpful in determining prognosis and treatment. **Grading** is a histologic, or tissue-based, method used by pathologists when they examine biopsy (tissue) or cytology (cell) specimens. What is being looked for is differentiation. Through microscopic exam, the severity of a malignancy can be assessed by the degree of dysplasia or anaplasia present. Remember that anaplastic cells have de-differentiated or regressed from a normal mature form. The growth rate can be loosely determined by the number of mitotic cells present. Recall that mitosis is the process of cell division, so increased numbers mean the cells are reproducing faster. Grading of malignancy is done based on _____(1) examination of _____(2) or _____(3). It is performed by _____(4). The severity of malignancy is correlated with the amount of _____(5) or _____(6) present, and with the growth rate that is based on numbers of _____(7) cells.

The following are the recognized grades of malignancy.

1. Grade I. Cells are well differentiated (closely resemble tissue of origin), with few mitoses. Prognosis is good.
2. Grade II. Cells are moderately differentiated (some structural similarity to parent tissue), with moderate mitoses. Prognosis is fair.
3. Grade III. Cells are poorly differentiated (little resemblance to their origin), with many mitoses. Prognosis is fair to poor.
4. Grade IV. Cells are de-differentiated (bizarre and primitive with unrecognizable origins), with many mitoses. Prognosis is poor.

Grading is somewhat subjective and the correlation between grade and prognosis is affected by other considerations like the location and type of malignancy. The least abnormal cells and the best prognosis is seen in grade _____(1). The most abnormal cells and worst prognosis are seen in grade _____(2).

Staging is a classification based on clinical findings by the physician, often an oncologist. Whereas grade relates to malignancy, stage relates to degree of spread. It is based on the size of the primary tumor and the amount of metastasis or secondary tumors. The rules of staging vary with the specific type of tumor but generally follow the "TNM" protocol. T refers to tumor size (1 to 4), N refers to numbers of lymph nodes affected (local invasion), and M means the extent of metastasis. Staging usually has a better correlation with prognosis. Staging is based on _____(1) findings and is related to the degree of _____(2). It is based on the size of the _____(3) and the extent of _____(4). The protocol uses the designation _____(5).

I. REVIEW QUESTIONS

1. Cells that appear abnormal are described as (choose all that apply):
   a. atypical
   b. anaplastic
   c. dysplastic
   d. neoplastic

2. Primitive-looking cells that are nondifferentiated are described as:
   a. atypical
   b. anaplastic
   c. dysplastic
   d. neoplastic

3. Neoplasia means _____.

4. A tumor is a:
   a. swelling such as a hematoma
   b. neoplastic mass
   c. lump such as a granuloma

5. Please match the type of neoplasia in the left column with the characteristic in the right column:
   a. benign neoplasia
   b. malignant neoplasia

   1. ___ encapsulated
   2. ___ cells shed easily
   3. ___ local invasion
   4. ___ slow growing
   5. ___ distant spread
   6. ___ more likely to cause death
   7. ___ easily removed

6. Neoplasia is classified according to:
   a. degree of anaplasia
   b. benign or malignant characteristics
   c. tissue of origin
   d. rate of growth

7. Benign neoplasia is named by the suffix a. _____. Malignant neoplasia is named by the affected tissue and either b. _____ or c. _____. Malignant neoplasia of connective tissue is called d. _____. An origin in epithelial tissue is called e. _____.

8. Proven causes of cancer include (choose all that apply):
   a. viruses
   b. radiation
   c. genetics
   d. environment
   e. carcinogens
   f. hormones

9. Suspected causes of cancer include (choose all that apply):
   a. viruses
   b. radiation
   c. genetics
   d. environment
   e. carcinogens
   f. hormones

10. A chemical known to produce malignant neoplasia is called a _____.

11. A virus that causes cancer or tumors in lab animals is:
    a. oncogenic
    b. carcinogenic
    c. a promoter
    d. an initiator

3. new growth

4. b–neoplastic mass

5. 1. a–benign; 2. b–malignant; 3. b–malignant; 4. a–benign; 5. b–malignant; 6. b–malignant; 7. b–benign

6. c–tissue of origin

7. a–"oma"; b–carcinoma; c–sarcoma; d–sarcoma; e–carcinoma

8. b–radiation; e–carcinogens

9. a–viruses; c–genetics; d–environment; f–hormones

10. carcinogen

11. a–oncogenic

12. b–cell transformation

13. c–initiation

14. c–DNA

15. b–promotion

16. d–initiation and promotion

17. b–local spread versus distant spread with secondary growths

18. a–metastases; b–secondary growths or tumors

19. b–Grading follows the TNM rule of classification.

12. Oncogenes create abnormal DNA material and mutant daughter cells in the process of:
   a. oncogenesis
   b. cell transformation
   c. promotion
   d. carcinogenesis

13. The first stage of carcinogenesis is:
   a. promotion
   b. progression
   c. initiation
   d. oncogenesis

14. In the first stage of carcinogenesis the targeted structure is the:
   a. nucleus
   b. RNA
   c. DNA
   d. growth regulation protein

15. The change from dysplasia toward anaplasia occurs in:
   a. initiation
   b. promotion
   c. progression
   d. cell transformation

16. The result of an increased production of abnormal or dysplastic cells is the combined effort of:
   a. carcinogenesis and cell transformation
   b. promotion and progression
   c. initiation and progression
   d. initiation and promotion

17. The differences between invasion and metastasis is:
   a. remaining in tissue versus entering vessels
   b. local spread versus distant spread with secondary growths
   c. attachment to nearby structures versus mobility
   d. all of the above

18. The result of metastasis is (choose all that apply):
   a. metastases
   b. secondary growths or tumors
   c. movement along tissue planes
   d. obstruction of body passages

19. Choose the INCORRECT statement:
   a. Grading and staging of malignancy are used to determine prognosis.
   b. Grading follows the TNM rule of classification.
   c. Staging is related to degree of spread and is determined clinically.
   d. Grading is related to differentiation and growth rate and is determined histologically.

II. CLINICAL ASPECTS OF NEOPLASIA

▶ THE EFFECTS OF MALIGNANT NEOPLASIA

In this first part of Section II, we will talk about the signs and symptoms of cancer and the mechanisms that lead to death. Keep in mind the very long time frame in the development of cancer. The effects of cancer, as seen clinically, do not appear until late in the course of this disease.

Since a tumor is a mass, a tumor is a space-occupying _____(1). The presence of such a lesion causes **pressure** or **obstruction.** The amount of pressure or obstruction will depend on the size of the tumor and its location in the body. Speaking only of pressure, this effect produces **pressure necrosis** of surrounding normal tissue. This means that the normal tissue dies because of the pressure. Both mechanical means and interference in blood supply cause this death. Tiny vessels become closed off and oxygen cannot reach the area. Necrosis associated with the presence of a large tumor is also found inside the tumor itself. This is because the center of the mass eventually "starves" as the mass outgrows its blood supply. Obstruction is the blockage of one of the body's natural passageways or hollow organs. In this case, a benign tumor can be the culprit. Examples of passages that can be obstructed are the respiratory system and the urinary system. If the bronchi become obstructed, a common sign of this is a persistent cough, since the irritation stimulates nerve endings and the cough reflex. If the urethra or bladder is obstructed, the patient has difficulty passing a normal urine stream. This is called **dysuria.** The intestines and stomach are good examples of hollow organs that may become occluded. Intestinal obstruction is a life-threatening condition since it may lead to rupture and often fatal peritonitis. Malnutrition and even starvation can develop if blockages in the esophagus or stomach interfere with the passage of food. Both pressure and obstruction cause pain, a common denominator in cancer cases.

1. lesion

The physical manifestation of a tumor as a mass can cause either _____(1) or _____(2). In significant amounts of pressure, the surrounding tissue will _____(3). This is called _____(4). Necrosis can be found both _____(5) and outside of a large, malignant mass. A benign mass can also be the cause of _____(6) of a natural passageway or a _____(7) organ. The following signs can be seen with obstruction of bronchi in the respiratory system = _____(8), the urethra in the urinary system = _____(9), intestines in the GI system = rupture and _____(10), and the esophagus or stomach in the GI system = _____(11) or _____(12).

1. pressure
2. obstruction
3. die
4. pressure necrosis
5. inside
6. obstruction
7. hollow
8. coughing
9. dysuria
10. peritonitis
11. malnutrition
12. starvation

    Not all obstruction is due to a mass *inside* the passageway or organ. If the mass exists outside the area in question, it can still cause blockage by compressing the area from the outside. A good example of this is adenocarcinoma of the head of the pancreas (see Chap. 13), where this mass compresses the common bile duct exiting from the liver.

The **destruction** of surrounding normal tissue by a malignancy is well demonstrated by **pathologic fractures** of bone. Both primary cancer and secondary metastases (from the lungs, breast, or prostate), weakens bone so much that it breaks at the slightest injury. The fracture itself is usually slight, just a hairline, and the presenting complaint by the patient is pain in the bone. Upon x-ray, the finding of such a fracture should alert the physician to look for an occult (hidden) malignancy. A pathologic fracture can be an important first finding in some cases of cancer. In general, the destructive effects of malignancy cause pain, especially when nerve endings are invaded or pressure is put on the nerves. As you would expect, the body responds to the presence of damaged tissue with the process of inflammation, which further contributes to pain. In bone, the destruction of tissue is demonstrated by the

1. pathologic fractures
2. secondary metastases
3. malignancy or cancer
4. pain

occurrence of _____(1). This damage can be due to both primary malignancy or _____(2). (Recall that primary means the original site, so here we mean bone cancer.) The importance of finding a pathologic fracture is that the physician should look for possible hidden _____(3). A very common symptom of cancer is _____(4) due to a variety of reasons.

······ 6–36 ······

1. bleeding
2. malignant
3. erode
4. ulcerate
5. blood vessel

Another important signal that should alert physicians to the possibility of cancer is unexplained bleeding or **hemorrhage.** A few examples are blood in the urine, sputum, or vomitus. One mechanism that causes bleeding is the erosion of any free surface by the malignancy. (By a free surface we mean the skin, lining of a natural passageway, or hollow organ.) This erosion or ulceration is a distinguishing characteristic of malignant neoplasia. Ulcers that don't heal are another red flag of cancer. A second mechanism that causes bleeding is the erosion into nearby blood vessels. Hemorrhage, or _____(1), that has no apparent cause is an important finding that may be due to _____(2) neoplasia. A malignancy will _____(3) or _____(4) a free surface and cause bleeding in this manner. Another way hemorrhage may be caused is if the cancer erodes into a _____(5).

······ 6–37 ······

1. skin
2. mucous membranes
3. infection
4. occult malignancy or hidden cancer
5. dose or numbers
6. decontamination
7. immune
8. debilitated

Infection is a dangerous consequence of malignant neoplasia and is a common cause of death in cancer patients. (A patient experiencing repeated bouts of infection should be examined for malignancy, as well as immunosuppresive disease.) There are several ways infection can be acquired. Ulcerated surfaces are vulnerable, having lost the first line of defense, which is intact _____(1) or _____(2) (see Chap. 5). Obstruction of passageways usually leads to infection, such as pneumonia in bronchial obstruction or cystitis of the bladder in urethral obstruction. You learned in Chapter 5 that dose is one factor in the development of infection. In an obstruction, the numbers of microorganisms increase to significant levels because mechanical decontamination is impaired. Once these numbers are beyond the control of the immune system and phagocytes, infection results. Other reasons for infection are an impaired immune response because of the demands of fighting the malignancy, poor nutritional status or debilitation, and even chemotherapy, which wipes out white blood cells. A common cause of death in cancer patients is _____(3). It can also be an important signal of _____(4). In obstruction, the mechanism that leads to infection is the _____(5) of microorganisms, because mechanical _____(6) is impaired. Other factors in the development of infection are a weakened _____(7) response, being run down or _____(8), and cancer treatments.

······ 6–38 ······

1. anemia
2. cachexia
3. anorexia
4. tumor or malignant mass
5. steal
6. normal

Anemia often develops in cases of advanced malignancies. There are many reasons for this, including chronic bleeding, poor nutrition, metastases in the bone marrow that crowd out normal cells, and chemotherapy, which depresses red blood cell production and blood clotting. A common visible effect of cancer is **cachexia,** a very thin, wasted appearance. Again, this is due to several factors. Most patients with advanced cancer have **anorexia,** or loss of appetite, because of pain, side effects of therapy, or because of generally feeling very sick. Naturally, this would cause weight loss. Other factors to explain this generalized atrophy include **tumor necrosis factor** or **TNF.** TNF is secreted from macrophages and is intended to kill tumor cells. However, it also interferes with normal fat metabolism. A very important reason for cachexia is the malignant mass itself. Remember that the tumor is made of very rapidly growing cells. Growth and cell division take energy derived from nutrients. As the tumor grows it becomes extremely "hungry" for nutrition and literally steals it from the rest of the body. The tumor grows at the expense of the body. The continual synthesis of new tumor cells leads to the starvation of normal cells. In cancer, chronic bleeding and other causes can lead to _____(1). A wasted, emaciated appearance is properly termed _____(2). Loss of appetite or _____(3) will contribute to cachexia. A direct cause of cachexia is the behavior of the _____(4). The tumor cells _____(5) nutrients from _____(6) cells and cause the normal cells to _____(7). The reason for the monopoly of nutrients by the tumor is because of its rapid _____(8).

7. starve
8. growth

6-39

In some cases, there may be excessive hormone production if the neoplasia affects an endocrine gland. An example is hyperadrenocorticalism, or excessive steroid production because of an adenoma of the adrenal glands. Generally, this is seen with *benign* neoplasia because the cells are more differentiated and therefore closer to normal in appearance and function. (The undifferentiated cells of a malignancy are unlikely to be able to function at all, so hormone production is not likely.)

6-40

An interesting phenomenon in cancer is the occasional presence of a **paraneoplastic syndrome.** In this instance, some tumors seem to be able to make and secrete chemicals that act *like* hormones. Even though they are not hormones, they are similar enough so that they interact with receptors on normal tissue and produce the same results. These substances are counterfeit chemical messengers. Cortisol (steroid) and insulin are two hormones that can be mimicked by some tumors. Cases in which these hormones seem to be increased should also be investigated for occult malignancy.

6-41

There are some findings that have historically been common in cancer cases but have no basis for explanation. Great weakness of the muscles is an example. It is theorized that autoimmune injury may be the reason. From the description of the common effects of cancer on the body, it should be apparent that there are many mechanisms at work that are often closely related. Together, they are responsible for the demise of the patient. Examine Table 6–3 for a review of the clinical effects of cancer.

▶ DEFENSE AGAINST NEOPLASIA

6-42

The first line of defense against neoplasia is the immune system. Based on what you learned in Chapter 4, you know the type of cell that destroys neoplastic cells is the _____(1). The importance of this function is seen in cases of defective immune response where cancer often appears. The most common immunodeficiency disease that can result in unusual cancers is _____(2). Normally, **immune surveillance** is performed by killer T lymphocytes, which seek out and destroy non-self foreign cells. Neoplastic cells are certainly modified enough to be recognized as foreign. Interleukin-2, a chemical mediator, or lymphokine, from T lymphocytes, also plays a role in tumor cell destruction. This property has been investigated as a means of immunotherapy. Injections of interleukin-2 (IL-2) has maintained the killing ability of T lymphocytes in lab animals. Lymphokine-activated killer cells, or LAK, are T cells that have been stimulated by IL-2. Recent

1. T lymphocyte
2. AIDS

TABLE 6–3. CLINICAL EFFECTS OF MALIGNANT NEOPLASIA

Effect	Result
Pressure	Necrosis of surrounding tissue and pain
Obstruction	Blockage of passageways or hollow organs, pain, and infection
Tissue destruction	Weakening, pain, and inflammation
Erosion and ulceration	Hemorrhage and infection
Stressed immune system and debilitation	Infection
Anemia	Further debilitation
Anorexia	Further debilitation and cachexia
Tumor growth	Competition for nutrients starves normal cells
Paraneoplastic syndrome	Activity of hormone-like substances

3. immune
4. deficiency
5. cancer
6. Killer
7. immune surveillance
8. interleukin-2

------ 6-43 ------

1. anti-oncogenes
2. tumor suppressor genes
3. replication
4. lost
5. mutation

experiments in immunotherapy have tried in vitro production of LAK cells by incubating T cells with IL-2, and then infusing them into the subject. The most important defense against neoplasia is the _____(3) system. Persons with immune _____(4) often have a higher incidence of _____(5). _____(6) T lymphocytes perform a function called _____(7) to seek out and destroy neoplastic cells. Lymphokine-activated killer cells are those that have been stimulated by _____(8) to maintain their killing function.

Another line of defense is genetics, where certain genes are called **anti-oncogenes** or **tumor suppressor genes.** You learned that oncogenes are genes that cause cancer, so an anti-oncogene is one that would help prevent cancer. Genetic defense works differently from immune defense. In immunity, the action is offensive or working against abnormal cells that are already present. In genetic defense, the action is defensive or working to prevent the development of abnormal cells in the first place. A tumor suppressor gene helps ensure that cell replication follows normal patterns and produces a normal cell through differentiation. Production of an abnormal or neoplastic cell can occur in the *absence* of a tumor suppressor gene. This absence can come about through random or point mutations that lose or inactivate some genes. Frame 6–16 mentioned p53 as an antitumor gene, where it was thought that a viral mechanism could inactivate it. The p53 gene regulates normal proliferation, so its loss results in abnormal growth, which partly defines neoplasia. The loss of p53 has been demonstrated in some cases of colorectal cancer. Genetic defense against neoplasia is in the form of genes called _____(1) or _____(2). The function of these genes is to ensure normal cell _____(3). If an anti-oncogene is _____(4), an abnormal cell can be produced. A genetic means for this loss is by random _____(5).

------ 6-44 ------

Research is always being conducted to find compounds that inhibit tumor production by known carcinogens in lab animals. The anti-oxidant vitamins may hold some promise. They are beta carotene (vitamin A precursor), vitamin C, and vitamin E. Anti-inflammatory steroids are being examined for the same effect. Some holistic sources claim melatonin as somewhat effective. The best defense is prevention by avoiding known carcinogens, as presented in the next section.

II. REVIEW QUESTIONS

1. a–pressure necrosis;
   d–pressure; e–obstruction

2. 1. e–destruction;
   2. c–pathologic fracture

1. The physical property of a tumor or mass, that of a space-occupying lesion, can produce which of the following effects (choose all that apply)?
   a. pressure necrosis
   b. cachexia
   c. anemia
   d. pressure
   e. obstruction
   f. hemorrhage

2. Weakened bone that breaks at the slightest injury is the result of 1. _____ of tissue by malignant neoplasia. The break itself is called a 2. _____.
   a. fracture
   b. pressure
   c. pathologic fracture
   d. infection
   e. destruction

3. Signs and symptoms in a patient that might be the result of *occult* malignancy include (choose all that apply):
   a. bleeding
   b. pressure necrosis
   c. pathologic fracture
   d. obstruction
   e. recurring infection
   f. cachexia

4. Erosion into blood vessels or ulceration of surfaces by cancer is responsible for:
   a. hemorrhage
   b. pain
   c. weight loss
   d. coughing

5. A common cause of death in cancer patients is:
   a. obstruction
   b. anemia
   c. cachexia
   d. infection
   e. paraneoplastic syndrome

6. The mechanism for infection to develop in cases of *obstruction* is:
   a. impaired chemical decontamination that leads to increased numbers of microorganisms
   b. impaired mechanical decontamination that leads to increased numbers of microorganisms
   c. a greater dose of microorganisms because the presence of tumor cells stimulates the multiplication of the organisms
   d. impaired ability of the immune system in cancer cases

7. Cachexia means:
   a. loss of appetite
   b. severe weight loss
   c. bleeding
   d. difficulty passing urine

8. The mechanism for cachexia caused directly by a malignant tumor is:
   a. accelerated consumption of nutrients by the mass, which deprives the remainder of the body of nutrition
   b. accelerated metabolism in general, stimulated by the presence of malignancy
   c. anorexia
   d. tumor necrosis factor

9. Effects of a benign tumor may include (choose all that apply):
   a. paraneoplastic syndrome
   b. obstruction
   c. anemia
   d. excessive hormone production
   e. pressure
   f. infection

3. a–bleeding; c–pathologic fracture; e–recurring infection

4. a–hemorrhage

5. d–infection

6. b–impaired mechanical decontamination that leads to increased numbers of microorganisms

7. b–severe weight loss

8. a–accelerated consumption of nutrients by the mass, which deprives the remainder of the body of nutrients

9. b–obstruction; d–excessive hormone production; e–pressure

10. Defense against neoplasia that involves killer T lymphocytes takes place during a process called:
    a. interferon activation of killer T cells
    b. lymphokine activation of killer T cells
    c. immunostimulation
    d. immune surveillance

11. Cancer has been linked to:
    a. immunodeficiency
    b. immunostimulation
    c. immunotherapy
    d. none of the above

12. A random genetic mutation can result in the loss of (choose all that apply):
    a. an oncogene
    b. killer T lymphocytes
    c. a tumor suppressor gene
    d. immune surveillance
    e. an anti-oncogene

SECTION ▶
6-45

III. FIGURES AND FACTS ABOUT CANCER

Now that you have learned about the general and clinical aspects of neoplasia, this section is presented to further your awareness about the epidemiology of cancer. As defined in Chapter 1, epidemiology is the field of medicine that examines the relationship of factors that determine the frequency and distribution of a disease.

▶ FREQUENCY OF THE TYPES OF CANCER BY SEX AND SITE OF ORIGIN

6-46

In today's society, the number one killer is heart disease. Malignancy is the second leading cause of death, striking about one out of three people. Although some malignancies affect the younger population, cancer is generally a disease of the older population. Peak ages for developing cancer vary slightly depending on the type of cancer, but the average age range is 50 to 70 years old. Breast cancer frequently strikes in the 50s. Lung cancer usually develops by the 60s. The majority of malignancy is seen in the 70s.

6-47

In men, the most common type of cancer is that of the prostate. Lung cancer is second, colorectal cancer is third, and cancer of the bladder is fourth. The number one cause of *death* is lung cancer, with prostate cancer coming in second. In men, both the incidence of cancer and the associated death rate are slightly higher than in women. For women, the most common malignancy is breast cancer. Colorectal cancer is second, lung cancer is third, and cancer of the uterus is fourth. The number one cause of *death* is lung cancer, and breast cancer is second. Lung cancer, the number one killer in both men and women, is largely preventable.

6-48

Considering the general population, the remaining types of cancer that are seen with the most frequency are:

1. Lymphoma (affecting the lymphoid tissue)
2. Malignant melanoma (affecting the skin)
3. Ovarian carcinoma
4. Renal carcinoma

5. Adenocarcinoma of the pancreas
6. Adenocarcinoma of the stomach
7. Leukemia (affecting the bone marrow)
8. Carcinoma of the mouth or larynx

Two fairly common skin cancers, basal cell and squamous cell carcinoma, may not be reflected in statistics acquired by the American Cancer Society. That is because these conditions usually are treated in a dermatologist's office and do not require hospitalization or major surgery. Primary malignancy of the liver and brain are not as common, but when they do occur there is a very high incidence of mortality. Most patients do not survive these types of cancer.

▶ SURVIVAL RATES

6-49

The overall survival rate for malignancy in the general population is slightly less than 50 percent. There are about 900,000 cases of cancer diagnosed yearly, with about 500,000 deaths. More than half of these deaths are due to the four most commonly seen cancers (prostate, lung, breast, colorectal). The success of treatment is measured by the number of years the patient is alive after diagnosis. This span of time is measured in 5-year increments, with a 5-year survival rate the most common way to gauge success.

6-50

The survival rate, or the prognosis, depends heavily on the stage in which the malignancy is diagnosed and treated. The best prognosis for survival is if the malignancy is still localized, or in the primary stage, even if some invasion has occurred. The worst prognosis is in cases of secondary metastases. This will also depend on the number of secondary growths and their locations. Other factors include the history of a specific type of cancer. The behavior of most malignancy is known, and these characteristics include the speed of growth or spread and response to treatment. Slow-growing tumors will have a higher survival rate than rapid-growing tumors. Some types of cancer respond well to current treatment, and others are resistant. For example, in carcinoma of the skin compared to carcinoma of the pancreas, pancreatic involvement is usually fatal while the skin malignancy is usually curable. The overall survival rates for the four common malignancies (assuming they are still in the primary stage, or have not metastasized) are prostate, 76 percent; lung, 13 percent; breast, 78 percent; and colorectal, 57 percent.

▶ PREVENTION OF CANCER

6-51

The most effective preventive measures against malignancy are to avoid known risk factors and to actively pursue lifestyle choices that may be protective. Risk factors to avoid include smoking, high-fat diet, known chemical carcinogens such as asbestos, heavy use of alcohol, and excessive sun exposure. Protective actions include a high-fiber diet, sufficient exercise, balanced nutrition (including vitamins, minerals, and anti-oxidants), and limited consumption of food preservatives.

6-52

Regular checkups are important, especially starting with middle age, and should include screening procedures such as a prostate exam, mammogram, Pap test, chest x-rays, and fecal occult blood. Self-examination of the breasts, testes, and skin should be practiced. It is also important to know the warning signs of cancer, as set forth by the American Cancer Society. These signs form the acronym "CAUTION," which means:

Change in bowel or bladder habits
A sore or ulcer that doesn't heal
Unusual bleeding or discharge
Thickening or lump in the breast or elsewhere
Indigestion or difficulty swallowing
Obvious change in a wart or mole
Nagging cough or hoarseness

CHAPTER ▶ SUMMARY

▶ SECTION I

As part of their normal functioning, the cells of the body constantly undergo reproduction, maturation, and, ultimately, differentiation into specific cell types. In some cases, differentiated cells may increase in number to aberrant levels (hyperplasia) or they may become abnormally large in size (hypertrophy). The opposite situation may likewise occur. Some differentiated cell populations may be markedly reduced in number and size in certain tissues (atrophy). Generally, when viewed under the microscope, cells exhibiting hyperplasia, hypertrophy, or atrophy are still easily recognizable as to their specific cell type.

In some tissues, however, one or more cells may remain nondifferentiated or may revert to the nondifferentiated state. They are, therefore, cells without specificity. Such cells microscopically appear abnormal and are referred to as dysplastic (bad form) or anaplastic (without form). Dysplastic cells that grow unrestrained and without control are characterized as neoplastic (new form) cells.

A localized mass of neoplastic cells is called a tumor and is defined as a space-occupying lesion. A tumor can also be unconfined to a localized mass, and would thus be characterized as diffuse. The disease leukemia is an example of a diffuse neoplasia.

A tumor that grows slowly, is encapsulated with normal cells, and does not invade other tissues or spread to other parts of the body is classified as benign. When surgically removed, a benign tumor, which is not life threatening unless it interferes with the activity of a vital physiologic function, does not recur. In contrast, a malignant tumor grows rapidly, is not encapsulated, invades local tissue, and is not easily removed surgically. A malignant tumor, also called a malignancy or a cancer, consists of dysplastic and anaplastic cells that can dissociate from the primary tumor, spread throughout the body (metastasize), and become established as secondary tumors.

Most neoplasias arise from either epithelial or connective tissue. Malignant tumors that arise from epithelial tissue (the tissue that gives rise to the internal organs) are called carcinomas. Those of connective tissue origin (bone, muscle, and blood) are called sarcomas. Cancers are named according to the tissue of origin and are designated either sarcoma or carcinoma.

The name carcinogen is applied to the many chemicals and environmental pollutants that are known to cause cancer. The latency period (the time from the initial exposure to the carcinogen to the clinical demonstration of the cancer) is often many years. A laboratory procedure called the Ames test is commonly used to identify carcinogens. Radiation from x-rays, nuclear power plants, the sun, and other sources can lead to certain types of malignancies.

A number of viruses, collectively called oncogenic viruses, have been implicated in the induction of different types of cancer. Oncogenic viruses are believed to work by incorporating their genetic material into the DNA of the infected host cell, causing abnormal host DNA and leading to mutated, or transformed, daughter cells. These in turn may replicate and grow in an uncontrolled fashion. Some viruses may act as promoters of cancer by initiating the proper conditions for later malignancy production by a carcinogen.

To date, statistical studies indicate that genetic inheritance probably does not play a major role in the tendency to develop cancer. Most likely, heredity predisposes a person to susceptibility by a cancer-causing agent. An individual's sex hormones, however, may be involved in certain malignancies. Certainly, a person's immune status is instrumental in determining propensity for tumor development.

Two theories have been proposed to explain the process of carcinogenesis. The epigenetic theory holds that in cancer cells normal DNA is expressed abnormally (e.g., inappropriate transcription or translation). The genetic theory states that the DNA itself undergoes mutation and therefore is expressed abnormally.

In either case, three distinct stages in cancer development are recognized. Initiation by one of many possible mechanisms begins the process of carcinogenesis, promotion enhances and expedites the journey to malignancy, and progression is the actual appearance of the malignancy. The fully developed cancer can then invade surrounding tissues with long "tentacles," and clumps of cells can break off and travel through the blood or lymph to other parts of the body (metastasize).

By examining tissue or cell samples removed from a cancer, pathologists can grade the degree of dysplasia and the growth rate of the tumor. Staging of the tumor involves determination of its size, the number of lymph nodes affected, and the extent of metastasis. Grading and staging are used to assist the physician in determining prognosis and an appropriate treatment regimen.

▶ SECTION II

Because it is a mass of rapidly growing cells, a tumor can lead to a situation called pressure necrosis, in which the normal tissue surrounding the tumor dies because of the mechanical pressure exerted by the tumor. The body's natural passageways (e.g., in the respiratory, circulatory, digestive, or urinary systems) can become obstructed by the tumor, creating a potentially life-threatening situation.

Several important clinical situations can occur as a result of a tumor. Bones housing a primary or secondary tumor can become extremely brittle. Unexplained hemorrhages, such as blood in the urine, stool, or sputum, is often the result of a malignancy, as are ulcerations in or on the body that do not heal. Microbial infection is a serious result of many malignant neoplasias. Often, passageway obstruction by a growing tumor leads to infection since one of the body's natural decontamination mechanisms is impaired. Anemia, recognized as a suppression in the amount of oxygen being delivered to the tissues by the blood, frequently is seen in victims of cancer. Most individuals with advanced malignancies exhibit cachexia (extreme emaciation) and anorexia (loss of appetite). If the malignancy is located in or affects a specific organ, physiological and biochemical activities conducted by that organ will naturally be affected. Occasionally, a malignancy will produce a compound that mimics one of the body's natural hormones.

To be sure, a person's own immune system, with its specialized antinonself, antineoplastic killer T lymphocytes, is normally the best defense against cancer. An individual's genetic constitution may likewise play a role in the occurrence of neoplasia. Researchers have found certain tumor suppressor genes, genetic units that may act to prevent the development of abnormal cells.

Genetic Diseases and Congenital Anomalies

▶ OBJECTIVES

SECTION II

Define all highlighted terms.

Define the difference between monogenic, polygenic, and sex-linked genetic diseases.

List examples of each type of abnormality and describe the phenotypic observations of each disease.

List several genetic diseases that involve chromosomal abnormalities, and describe the genotypic and phenotypic observations in these anomalies.

SECTION III

Define all highlighted terms.

List several factors that may lead to congenital anomalies.

Describe three congenital defects that involve the nervous system.

As they pertain to congenital defects of the cardiovascular system, distinguish between the terms "cyanotic" and "acyanotic."

Describe the tetralogy of Fallot and two other anomalies of the cardiovascular system.

Describe the congenital anomaly of pyloric stenosis.

List and describe several congenital anomalies involving the genitourinary system.

Describe two congenital anomalies involving the musculoskeletal system.

1. AN OVERVIEW OF GENETIC PRINCIPLES

◀ SECTION

▶ THE BASIS OF GENETIC OR INHERITED DISEASE

7-1

General principles of genetics, like other topics such as immunity and homeostasis, are presented in anatomy and physiology courses. We will briefly review some of those principles here, but they are not presented in the programmed format for retention learning.

7-2

The genetic makeup, or genetic constitution, of a person may contribute to a disease process. It may cause outright disease, or more commonly, cause someone to be predisposed to additional factors that cause disease. Gregor Mendel, the father of modern genetic principles, made discoveries that resulted in **Mendelian laws of inheritance.** His findings produced basic and simple explanations for genetic activities. These activities center around passing on traits to future generations. Distinct gene pairs and measurable traits formed the basis for these laws of inheritance. Genetic activity is much more complex than some of these simple laws, but Mendelian laws provide for initial understanding.

7-3

Genetic mechanisms can be best introduced by examining the terms associated with inheritance. You know that DNA, found in the nucleus of a cell, is composed of nucleotides or nucleic acids and carries all the genetic information for that individual. Normally, DNA is not visible with a light microscope because it is in fine strands and spread out, or dispersed, in the nucleus. In this fine state, it may be called **chromatin.** However, in preparation for cell division, or **mitosis,** the DNA begins to coil back and forth on itself. This results in a heavier or compact strand that is visible. In addition to condensing, the DNA has also made a copy of itself, or replicated itself. This copied, dense DNA is called a **chromosome.** The original strand of DNA is joined to its replication at a spot called the **centromere.** The two joined strands make up a pair that is called a **chromatid.** Therefore, a chromosome is two chromatids (original DNA and the copy) connected at the centromere. This is shown in Figure 7–1. The normal number of chromosomes for the human species is 46 (the number varies with different species).

7-4

Mitosis, or cell division, occurs with the **autosomal** cells of the body. Autosomal cells are *all* the cells of the body that are not sexually reproductive cells. The reproductive cells are the **germ cells** and are the ova and sperm. When germ cells divide, it is called **meiosis.** In meiosis, the chromosome splits into the two individual chromatids, and each goes to the new daughter cell, or **gamete.** Therefore, instead of 46 chromosomes, each gamete has only 23. This is necessary so that when the sperm and ova join, the total genetic material in the embryo is 46 chromosomes. This explains how each parent of a child contributes exactly half of the child's genes.

7-5

The chromosomes are the packaging for genes. **Genes** are specific nucleotides of the DNA that actually code or send a message for the cell to make a polypeptide out of a particular amino acid sequence. The polypeptide forms the basis for the remainder of the creation process. The gene is the blueprint and it dictates the resulting products. Genes determine a person's individual characteristics. Following the process of meiosis, genes are inherited in pairs, since they are on the chromosomes from each parent. The site on a chromosome where a particular gene is located is called the **loci.** Considering the pairs of chromosomes that exist, one from the mother and one from the father, the genes on the two different chromosomes that code for the same trait are called **alleles.** Consider, for example, the genes that

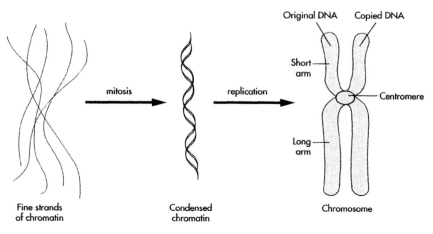

Figure 7–1. Chromosome formation.

control the color of your hair. If your parents had different hair color, you would have two different genes, but they are alleles because they both code for the same characteristic. Genes controlling eye color are *not* alleles of genes controlling hair color.

7-6

Two alleles that are the same are called **homozygous,** "homo" meaning the same. Two alleles that are not the same are called **heterozygous,** "hetero" meaning different. To illustrate this, consider again the example of hair color. Let us call the gene for brown hair "B" and the gene for blonde hair "b." Inheriting two B genes from two brown-haired parents results in the genotype BB. Since the alleles are the same, the individual is homozygous for the brown hair gene. One blonde parent would create a Bb genotype in the offspring, and they would be heterozygous for the hair gene. These alleles are different. These concepts are illustrated in Figure 7–2. A **genotype** is the literal genetic makeup of a person, or which genes are specifically present. In this example, a person may have either a BB makeup or a Bb makeup. A **phenotype** is the visible expression of the gene combination. It is what is seen in the person, or the physical effect of the gene combination. In this example, it is the hair color. Only in certain situations can the genotype be determined by the phenotype. We will discuss next why this is, but the phenotype of brown hair could be either the genotype BB or Bb.

7-7

Genes are either **dominant** or **recessive.** A dominant gene is strong. A recessive gene is weak. If a dominant gene is present, that trait is definitely expressed. With a recessive gene, the trait is only expressed if the dominant allele is absent. In the heterozygous state, a dominant allele will be seen in the phenotype. A recessive trait will only be seen if the alleles are homozygous (both genes in the pair are the same recessive genes). The gene B for brown hair is dominant so a genotype of either Bb (heterozygous) or BB (homozygous) will result in a phenotype of brown hair. The gene b for blonde hair is recessive. The phenotype of blonde hair will only result if the alleles are homozygous for the blonde gene, or if the genotype is bb. Another way to look at this is in terms of dosage. A dominant gene need only be present in a single dose (heterozygous) for expression, while a recessive gene requires a double dose (homozygous) to be expressed. The expression of a recessive gene is always masked by the presence of a dominant gene. Masked means it is not expressed or shown. This is an important concept to remember when we examine some genetic diseases. Examine Figure 7–3 to further your understanding before you proceed.

7-8

In disease states, a dominant gene that causes the disorder will be present in every generation. Of that particular gene pair, one allele is defective and one is normal in the heterozygous state. (Of course, the homozygous state also results in disease.) There are no carrier states. In other words, individuals that do not have the disease do not have the gene so it is impossible for them to pass it on to the next generation. Diseases caused by abnormal genes that are recessive tend to be more severe in their effects on the afflicted person. Carriers *do*

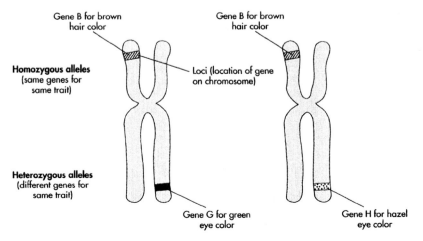

Figure 7–2. Homozygous and heterozygous alleles.

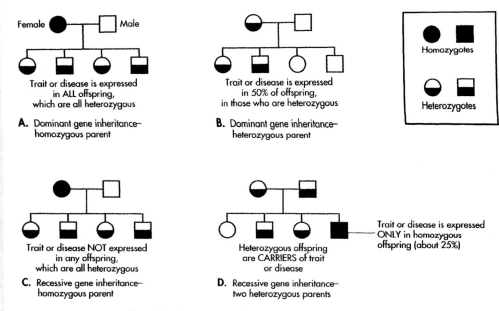

Figure 7–3. A comparison of dominant and recessive gene inheritance.

exist. Individuals who appear to be healthy may be heterozygous and harbor a hidden, recessive defective gene. A carrier of a genetic disease is heterozygous. If they should mate with another carrier, 25 percent of the offspring will be homozygous for the mutant recessive gene and therefore the disease will be expressed. Restated, in recessive genetic disease states, a heterozygous gene pair results in a carrier who can produce afflicted children, and a homozygous pair results in the disease (both alleles are mutant or defective).

7–9

In **sex-linked** or **X-linked** inheritance patterns, the abnormal gene is on one of the sex chromosomes (X or Y). Generally, it is on the X chromosome and is recessive. These characteristics mean sex-linked diseases are almost always seen as female carriers and afflicted males. Since females are XX, the recessive defective gene on one X chromosome is dominated by the normal allele on the other X chromosome. In males (XY), there is no corresponding X allele to repress the disease gene so the individual expresses the disease. This is illustrated in Figure 7–4.

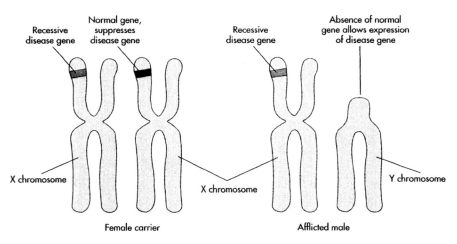

Figure 7–4. Sex- or X-linked inheritance.

II. SELECTED EXAMPLES OF GENETIC DISEASES ◄ SECTION

► MONOGENIC OR SINGLE-GENE DISORDERS

7-10

Relative to all of the other disease processes, genetic diseases are uncommon. Varying degrees of expression, or **penetrance,** means that even if a mutant gene is present in a person's genome (genetic makeup), it may not cause disease. Some genetic-based diseases are present at birth, or are congenital. Others may go undetected until the individual is older, or is an adults. This is known as adult onset. The first group of diseases you will learn about is classified as **monogenic,** which means there is primarily one defective gene responsible for the disorder. This is also called a **Mendelian** disorder, which means the inheritance of a single, mutant gene. Three categories of monogenic diseases are autosomal recessive, autosomal dominant, and sex- or X-linked. We will first consider the autosomal recessive category.

7-11

In an autosomal recessive disease, by definition, the patient has inherited a defective gene from both parents and that patient is homozygous for those alleles. Most of the time, the parents are heterozygous and appear healthy or normal. Therefore, they are carriers. Autosomal recessive diseases manifest when two carriers mate. Twenty-five percent of their offspring will develop the disease. (Refer back to Figure 7–3D.) Recessive diseases are more common than dominant diseases. Carriers can perpetuate a recessive disease gene through several generations. A dominant disease gene frequently prevents the affected person from reproducing and hence, eliminates the gene from that line. Disease caused by autosomal recessive genes is only seen if the individual is _____(1) for those genes. These diseases remain in the population because of the _____(2) state, which is undetected until carriers _____(3).

1. homozygous
2. carrier
3. mate

7-12

Cystic fibrosis is an autosomal recessive disease. This is a systemic abnormality of the exocrine glands. The interference in normal function of these glands is most frequently seen as disorders of the lungs, intestines, and pancreas. Sweat glands in the skin are also abnormal in the amount of sodium chloride, or salt, that is lost in the sweat. The mucous secretions from the exocrine glands associated with organs are extremely thick or viscous. In the intestines, this causes obstruction. In the lungs, it causes **dyspnea** (difficult breathing), **tachypnea** (increased rate of respiration), coughing, and frequent bouts of pneumonia. The pneumonia, a common cause of death, develops because of the inability of the lungs to expel the thick mucus. This allows bacteria to become trapped in the lungs and multiply. In the pancreas, the glands that normally secrete digestive enzymes become enlarged (cystic) and are replaced with scar tissue (fibrosis), hence the name. The lack of digestive enzymes leads to pancreatic insufficiency (see Chap. 12), and therefore poor digestion and poor absorption of nutrients. Diabetes mellitus may develop as the condition interferes with the secretion of insulin. Cystic fibrosis is a relatively common, fatal genetic disease. It is diagnosed partially by the **sweat test,** which measures the high concentration of salt on the skin. There is no specific treatment, but supportive measures may prolong life and increase comfort. These measures include management of diabetes, replacement of digestive enzymes, monitoring of sodium and hydration status, antibiotics, and physical techniques to help clear the lungs.

7-13

Cystic fibrosis is a condition that produces abnormal _____(1) throughout the body. Signs and symptoms of cystic fibrosis are due to abnormal function of the glands of certain _____(2). Two organs prominently affected are the _____(3) and _____(4). The secretion of these glands is a thick _____(5). In the lungs, trapped mucus and bacteria lead to _____(6), a common cause of _____(7). The name of this disease comes from its effect on the glands of the _____(8). Insufficiency of this organ

1. exocrine glands
2. organs
3. lungs
4. pancreas
5. mucus
6. pneumonia
7. death
8. pancreas

9. digest
10. absorb
11. diabetes mellitus

leads to interference with the ability to _____(9) and _____(10) food. Deficiency in insulin contributes to the development of _____(11).

Tay–Sachs disease primarily affects the Eastern Jewish population. The defect is a deficiency in an enzyme necessary for normal lipid metabolism in the brain. (Many genetic diseases manifest as a lack of a metabolic enzyme. Many of the proteins for which a gene codes are enzymes.) Because the lipids cannot be metabolized as they should, buildup causes destruction of the neurons. This nervous system disorder is seen as retardation, deafness, blindness, paralysis, and an early death by 4 years of age. The mental retardation begins in the womb and can usually be detected by 3 to 6 months of age. Tay–Sachs disease is one of the genetic defects that can be determined before birth by the process of amniocentesis. **Galactosemia** is another example of a deficiency of a metabolic enzyme. There is no enzyme for the conversion of galactose (the sugar from milk lactose) to glucose. Accumulation of galactose interferes with brain and liver development. Undiagnosed and untreated, galactosemia can lead to mental retardation and cirrhosis of the liver. Detection and early treatment (elimination of lactose from the diet) will allow normal development.

1. enzyme
2. metabolized
3. accumulate
4. brain

Tay–Sachs disease and galactosemia are examples of genetic diseases where an important _____(1) is missing. In the absence of an enzyme, a specific substance cannot be _____(2). Therefore, the substance will _____(3), or buildup, and interfere with normal function of some tissues or organs. Retardation and other neurologic defects result from accumulation in the _____(4).

1. phenylalanine
2. tyrosine
3. brain
4. mental retardation
5. tested
6. special diet
7. protein

A third metabolic disease produced by a genetic defect is **phenylketonuria,** or **PKU.** A missing enzyme means that a common amino acid, phenylalanine, cannot be converted to the harmless amino acid, tyrosine. Accumulation of phenylalanine is toxic to development of the brain and mental retardation will result. Diagnosis must be made early to prevent permanent brain damage. Due to the relative frequency of this condition, all newborns are routinely screened for PKU with a blood test that will detect high levels of phenylalanine. Treatment consists of a special diet of synthetic proteins to at least 6 years of age. All natural protein contains phenylalanine and must be strictly avoided. In infants with PKU, an enzyme deficiency causes _____(1) to build up because it cannot be converted to _____(2). This accumulation interferes with the development of the _____(3) and will be seen as _____(4). Newborns are routinely _____(5) for PKU. Diagnosed cases are treated with a _____(6) that has no natural _____(7).

1. hemoglobin
2. red blood cells
3. sickle
4. capillaries
5. blood
6. spleen
7. sickle cell trait

Sickle cell anemia (see Chap. 9) is a chronic, life-threatening condition affecting African and related populations. The hemoglobin in red blood cells is defective. In homozygous individuals, many of the RBCs are curved, or sickle-shaped. This abnormal shape causes the cells to block capillaries. These painful episodes impair circulation, damage blood vessels, and produce infarcts in vital organs. Because the RBCs are abnormal, they are continuously removed by the spleen. This leads to chronic anemia. In heterozygous individuals, the RBCs "sickle" under conditions of low oxygen or hypoxia. This forms the basis of a test for sickle cell anemia. Heterozygous individuals are characterized as having **sickle cell trait.** In sickle cell anemia, the defect is in the _____(1) inside the _____(2). It causes the cells to assume a _____(3) shape. The abnormal shape gets caught in _____(4) and can block _____(5) supply to various organs. Anemia is due to the destruction of the abnormal RBCs by the _____(6). People who are heterozygous for this gene are described as having _____(7).

7-18

Two other autosomal recessive conditions of which you should be aware are cretinism and albinism. Cretinism is an endocrine disease involving the thyroid glands. Abnormality of the tissue in these glands leads to inadequate amounts of thyroid hormone in the circulation. This defines hypothyroidism, which is discussed in Chapter 16 on endocrine diseases. Albinism is a defect in pigment-producing cells, and therefore is an absence of pigmentation. The skin is very white and translucent, the hair white, and the eyes very pale.

7-19

In autosomal dominant diseases, the afflicted individual inherits a defective gene from only one parent. The parent is most likely heterozygous for the mutant gene and offspring have a 50 percent chance of receiving the gene. The disease will be expressed whether the child is heterozygous or homozygous. There are no hidden carrier states so possession of the gene is easily recognized. In Chapter 3, you learned about a condition known as **diabetes insipidus.** Diabetes insipidus is an autosomal dominant disease in which inadequate amounts of antidiuretic hormone (ADH) are released by the pituitary gland. Since the role of ADH is to conserve water (antidiuretic), a deficiency results in polyuria, or excessive urination. Polyuria causes great losses of body water and electrolytes. This triggers extreme thirst, or polydipsia, and is seen as excessive fluid consumption. Dehydration and hypotension are constant threats so attention must be paid to the amount of water intake. ADH replacement is usually an effective treatment.

7-20

A patient with a genetic disease of the autosomal dominant type may be either _____(1) or _____(2) for the genes. There is no _____(3) state. An example of this category is a disorder that affects water and electrolyte balance, or _____(4). In this disorder, there is a deficiency of _____(5). The disease is seen as a copious amount of urine production, or _____(6), accompanied by increased thirst and drinking, or _____(7).

1. heterozygous
2. homozygous
3. carrier
4. diabetes insipidus
5. antidiuretic hormone
6. polyuria
7. polydipsia

7-21

A disease whose name literally means lack of formation of cartilage is **achondroplasia.** Cartilage is the tissue from which new bone can be formed. A defect in the development of enough cartilage means there will be little resource for bone development in the fetus. The result is **achondroplastic dwarfism.** Affected individuals have a trunk of normal length, but very short arms and legs because of lack of sufficient bone growth. Adults are generally of normal mental capacity and are sexually mature. Achondroplasia is a deficiency in the production of _____(1) in the fetus, from which _____(2) can be formed. This results in shortened _____(3) and _____(4) and the condition is called _____(5).

1. cartilage
2. bone
3. legs
4. arms
5. achondroplastic dwarfism

7-22

A common disorder is **familial hypercholesterolemia.** In spite of a low fat diet, these individuals have high levels of cholesterol circulating in the blood. This causes atherosclerosis, the accumulation of fatty plaques along the walls of blood vessels. This insoluble fatty lining increases blood pressure in the affected vessels and decreases circulation to the normally supplied area. Atherosclerosis is a common cause of myocardial infarction ("heart attack") and stroke. The defect is thought to be an abnormal receptor for the LDL type of cholesterol, or the "bad" fat. The defective receptor allows the LDL to remain in the circulation and attach to vessel walls. In addition to strict attention to diet, medications that interfere with fat absorption are used to manage this disorder. In familial hypercholesterolemia, the condition known as _____(1) is produced as fat builds up on vessel walls. The specific type of fat is _____(2) cholesterol and it is believed the _____(3) for this substance is defective. Atherosclerosis is a leading cause of _____(4) and _____(5).

1. atherosclerosis
2. LDL
3. receptor
4. myocardial infarction
5. stroke

7–23

1. degeneration
2. nervous
3. chorea
4. is

Huntington's chorea is a relentlessly progressive degeneration of the central nervous system. The onset is generally during middle age. The term "chorea" is descriptive of one of the effects of the disease, which is loss of voluntary control and replacement by involuntary jerky, fast movements. These bizarre movements are caused by rapid, random firing of nerve impulses that control skeletal muscle. Mental effects include impaired memory and dementia (complete mental incompetence). This nerve degeneration ends in death. There is no treatment for Huntington's chorea. Diagnosis of the condition is discussed in Frame 7–49, where it can be determined if offspring carry the gene. Huntington's chorea is a _____(1) of the _____(2) system. Rapid twitching motions that cannot be controlled are described by the term "_____(3)." Mental clarity and the ability to think coherently _____(4) is / is not (choose one) sacrificed during the course of this disease.

7–24

Other autosomal dominant genetic diseases of which you should be aware are retinoblastoma (congenital cancer of the retina), polydactyly (extra fingers or toes), and neurofibromatosis (multiple wart-like, benign skin nodules).

7–25

Genetic diseases attributed to a defective gene on the X chromosome are called **sex-linked** or **X-linked.** These diseases usually show only in males, who do not have a second normal X chromosome to dominate the recessive defective gene. (Refer back to Figure 7–4.) A female with a sex-linked genetic disease would have to be homozygous for the recessive disease gene, which is rare. The female, generally heterozygous, is a carrier and can pass the gene to a son. A male with the disease gene can pass it on to a daughter who then becomes a carrier. A famous X-linked disorder is **hemophilia,** made known in European history by royal female carriers and their afflicted sons. The literal interpretation of hemophilia is "blood loving" and it is often known as the "bleeding disease." In order for blood to clot, the complex interaction of many serum proteins is necessary. This series of events is referred to as a "cascade" because one stage leads into the next and all must be present and complete to reach the end product (a clot). In hemophilia, one of the proteins is missing. The proteins are called clotting factors, and the missing factor is Factor VIII (8). Hemophiliacs are subject to uncontrolled bleeding. Part of the management of the disease is to avoid even minimal trauma, such as any type of sport or physical activity. Cryoprecipitate is a product made from the blood of donors that contains Factor VIII and can be administered to a hemophiliac. However, the effect is temporary because the protein is used up, and the treatment is expensive.

7–26

1. X
2. Males
3. females
4. hemophilia
5. Factor VIII
6. clot
7. bleeding
8. physical

A sex-linked genetic disease has the defective gene on the _____(1) chromosome. _____(2) have the disease, while _____(3) are carriers. A genetic bleeding disorder is _____(4). The deficiency is an absence of the clotting protein, _____(5). Without this protein, the blood does not _____(6) and _____(7) can be uncontrolled. Management of the condition includes limiting _____(8) activity.

7–27

1. muscular dystrophy
2. sex- or X-linked
3. skeletal muscle
4. paresis
5. paralysis
6. respiration

Duchenne's muscular dystrophy is discussed at length in Chapter 17. Essentially, it is a wasting away of the skeletal muscle on both sides of the body (bilateral). Histologic examination of the muscle has shown defective structure of the muscle fibers. Effects of this X-linked disease begin in the legs, which become very weak, or **paretic.** Paralysis results by the early teen years, requiring the victim to use a wheelchair for mobility. Death occurs a few years later because of failure of the muscles involving respiration and the heart. Duchenne's _____(1) is a _____(2) genetic disease of the _____(3). Failure of the muscle fibers first begins as _____(4) and progresses to _____(5). Death is due to failure of the muscles of _____(6) and the heart.

TABLE 7–1. MENDELIAN OR MONOGENIC (SINGLE-GENE) DISORDERS

Autosomal Dominant	Autosomal Recessive	Sex- or X-Linked
Diabetes insipidus	Cystic fibrosis	Hemophilia
Achondroplasia	Tay–Sach's disease	Duchenne's muscular dystrophy
Familial hypercholesterolemia	Galactosemia	Color blindness
Huntington's chorea	Phenylketonuria	
Retinoblastoma	Sickle cell anemia	
Polydactyly	Cretinism	
Neurofibromatosis	Albinism	

7–28

The final monogenic disorder to be considered is **color blindness,** which is also sex-linked. Afflicted men cannot tell the difference between certain colors, usually red and green. There is a defect in the cones of the retina, the cones being the receptor cells that receive the wavelengths of light and color. The red and green primary wavelengths do not stimulate these abnormal cones, so the message is not passed to the brain for interpretation as vision. Table 7–1 summarizes the Mendelian, or monogenic (single-gene), disorders.

▶ POLYGENIC OR MULTIGENE DISORDERS

7–29

A polygenic or multigene disorder is one that is multifactorial. That is, there are several factors involved, not just a defective gene. "Risk genes" combine with specific environmental factors, lifestyle, and perhaps diet to place the individual at higher risk for a disease. This predisposition occurs in families but not with enough predictability to label it as a familial tendency. **Rheumatoid arthritis** (see Chap. 17) usually strikes females and is a chronic inflammatory condition of the joints with systemic effects. There appears to be a genetic predisposition for this disorder that is autoimmune in nature. The damage to joint tissues by autoantibodies causes continual inflammation, which destroys joint structures. Loss of mobility and stiffness of the joints is accompanied by permanent deformity of the joints. Generally, the hands and feet are affected. Treatment is palliative, or aimed at relieving the discomfort with steroids, other anti-inflammatories, physical therapy, and rest of the joints.

7–30

A polygenic disease results from the combination of _____(1) and certain _____(2) factors. A chronic inflammatory disorder of the joints is seen in _____(3). The destructive agent is thought to be a (an) _____(4). Joint destruction is due to continual _____(5), and leads to loss of _____(6) and deformity.

1. risk genes
2. environmental
3. rheumatoid arthritis
4. autoantibody
5. inflammation
6. mobility

7–31

In the disease known as **gout,** a biochemical defect causes overproduction and perhaps decreased excretion of the compound uric acid. Uric acid is a breakdown product of purines, which are the nucleotides of DNA. This abnormal metabolism of uric acid creates crystals of uric acid that deposit in joints, especially in the big toe. Chronic crystal deposits are seen as white plaques, known as tophi. Figure 7–5 shows urate deposits, or tophi, present in a knee joint (on the patella) and kidney. The presence of tophi causes a painful inflammation. Attacks of gout are sudden (acute) and very painful. Continued episodes of this destructive inflammation destroys joint surfaces and leads to some degree of disability and deformity of the affected joints. In Figure 7–6, severe deformity of the hands is seen in a patient with gout. Other effects include kidney stones and potentially serious dysfunction of the kidneys. Metabolic gout is an inherited condition that combines with lifestyle factors such as rich diet, insufficient water intake, and heavy alcohol intake. Management of the condition includes a

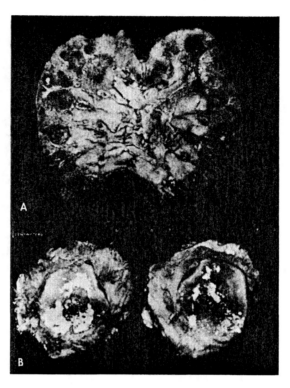

Figure 7–5. Urate deposits in gout. **A.** Several white urate deposits are seen within the opened kidney. **B.** White urate deposits (tophi) are seen on the surfaces of the patellae. *(From Kumar et al, Basic Pathology, 5th ed., Saunders.)*

low purine diet, adequate hydration, and avoidance of provoking lifestyle habits. Medication is available to decrease uric acid production and increase its excretion by the kidneys.

7–32

1. uric acid
2. purine
3. joints
4. inflammation
5. tophi
6. kidneys
7. lifestyle

In gout, there is abnormal metabolism of _____(1), which is an end product of _____(2) metabolism. This excess compound deposits in the _____(3) and causes painful and destructive _____(4). Visible chronic deposits are called _____(5). Vital organs that can be seriously affected are the _____(6). The gene that predisposes to gout combines with _____(7) factors to produce the condition.

7–33

Diabetes mellitus is a commonly known disorder that is presented at length in Chapter 8. It is an interference in normal carbohydrate metabolism because of lack of insulin from the pancreas, or because of decreased response by cells to insulin. Insulin is required for glucose to enter into cells for their use in creating the energy molecule ATP. Insufficient glucose inside cells leads to the abnormal metabolism of fat and proteins to replace glucose. The use of fats and proteins for energy is responsible for most of the signs, symptoms, and complications of diabetes. There are two major types of diabetes mellitus. Type I is called juvenile onset because it strikes before the age of 30. Type I is more severe and requires treatment with insulin injections, or is called insulin-dependent diabetes. A defective gene creates a susceptibility, so that some event triggers autoimmune destruction of the cells that manufacture insulin. Type II diabetes is referred to as adult onset because it develops slowly over the age of 40. It is milder and often insulin is not required, but instead is managed with diet, exercise, and other lifestyle factors. It is believed that there is also a gene that predisposes an individual to type II diabetes mellitus.

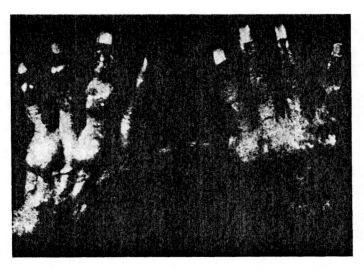

Figure 7–6. Severe formations of gouty tophi in the hands of a patient. *(From Sheldon, Boyd's Introduction to the Study of Disease, 11th ed., Lea & Febiger.)*

7–34

Abnormal carbohydrate metabolism in diabetes mellitus is because of insufficient
_____(1). This results in deficient amounts of _____(2) inside
the cells because _____(3) is required for glucose to enter cells. In place of
glucose, _____(4) and _____(5) are substituted for energy production. Type I is called _____(6) onset or _____(7) dependent
diabetes. Type II is called _____(8) onset and often does not require injections
of _____(9). In closing this topic, other multifactorial conditions in which
genetics probably play a role include hypertension, atherosclerotic heart disease, some cancers, and duodenal ulcer. A summary of polygenic or multigene disorders is presented in
Table 7–2.

1. insulin
2. glucose
3. insulin
4. fat
5. proteins
6. juvenile
7. insulin-
8. adult
9. insulin

▶ DISORDERS ASSOCIATED WITH ABNORMALITIES IN CHROMOSOMES

7–35

Abnormalities associated with defective genes lead to abnormal products from these genes,
such as enzymes or other proteins. Chromosomal aberrations mean that the products are normal, but there is an increase or decrease of the amount of product. Chromosomal abnormalities are divided into two categories. Either there is a change in the normal number that are
present, or there is a change in the normal structure. This might be a gene that is missing or
one that has translocated, or shifted, to another chromosome. Most chromosomal abnormalities are so severe the fetus is aborted, usually by 3 months of development. Decreased numbers of chromosomes, known as **monosomy,** is incompatible with life because the organism
cannot function without all of the necessary genes. Fetuses that live to term with abnormal
numbers of chromosomes usually have more than the normal 46 (or 23 pairs). Generally,
there is one extra chromosome and it is present in every cell of the body. This develops
because of an error during meiosis in which **nondisjunction** occurs. Nondisjunction is the
failure of the chromosomes to separate, or divide, properly before being transferred to the

TABLE 7–2. POLYGENIC (MULTIGENE) DISORDERS

Rheumatoid arthritis
Gout
Diabetes mellitus

daughter gamete cells. Instead of an even half going to each of two gametes, one will be deficient and one will have extra genetic material. This gamete, when combined with a normal gamete, produces a zygote with 47 chromosomes. This increase is known as **trisomy.**

Disorders of chromosomes are either an abnormality in _____(1) or in _____(2). Chromosomal abnormalities are responsible for spontaneous _____(3) by 3 months of term. A fetus with decreased numbers, or _____(4), does not survive. A fetus with increased numbers, or _____(5), may survive to term. Trisomy develops because of failure of chromosomal separation, or _____(6), during meiosis. A trisomy zygote will have _____(7) chromosomes.

The most common chromosomal aberration is **trisomy 21,** also known as **Down's syndrome,** or **mongolism.** Autosomal chromosome number 21 is present in triplicate instead of a pair. Figure 7–7 illustrates a karyotype, which is the arrangement of all the chromosomes as pairs. Look at chromosome number 21. You will see that there are three chromosomes instead of a pair. Down's syndrome is most commonly seen in pregnancies over the age of 40. Women are born with all of the ova they will ever produce, so the ova are the same age as the woman. These older ova are more likely to dysfunction during meiosis. Some cases of mongolism occur from pregnancies in younger women, or from extra chromosomes from the father. Children afflicted with trisomy 21 are easily recognized because of classic physical features. A skin fold at the medial canthus, or inner corner of the eye, gives the eyes a slanted appearance. The head may be enlarged, the nose is flattened, and an enlarged tongue protrudes from the slack mouth. Varying degrees of mental retardation are present. The severity or mildness of retardation dictates the amount of learning that is possible in these affectionate individuals. Internal organs are also affected by physical abnormalities. There is some malformation of the heart and dysfunction of the kidneys and intestines is present. Figure 7–8 shows some of the abnormalities in Down's syndrome. Patients with Down's syndrome have increased susceptibility to infections because of poor immune function. The incidence of leukemia is high in these patients and they often develop Alzheimer's-like lesions in the brain. All of these complications usually limit the life span to less than 30 or 40 years of age.

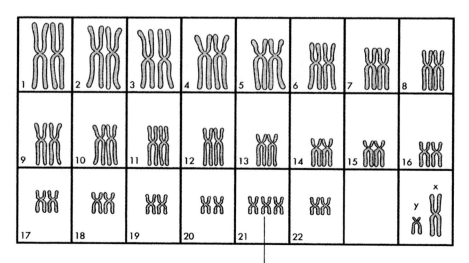

Chromosomes 21
present as three (trisomy 21)
instead of a pair

Figure 7–7. A karyotype of Down's syndrome or trisomy 21. Note the three chromosomes present at location 21.

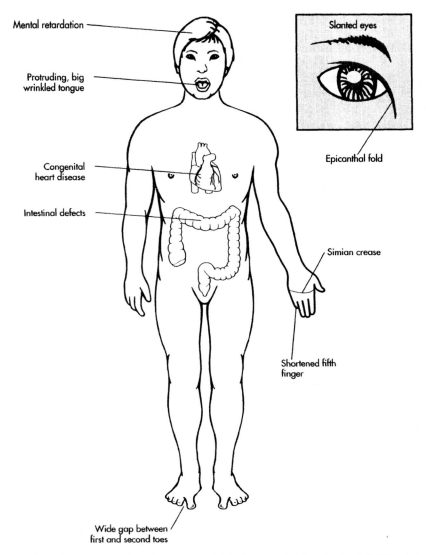

Slanted eyes

Mental retardation

Protruding, big
wrinkled tongue

Epicanthal fold

Congenital
heart disease

Intestinal defects

Simian crease

Shortened fifth
finger

Wide gap between
first and second toes

Figure 7–8. Typical features of Down's syndrome. *(Adapted from Damjanov, Pathology for the Health-Related Professions, Saunders.)*

7-38

A relatively common genetic disease in which there is an extra chromosome 21 is known as _____(1). It is also called _____(2) or _____(3). It is generally attributed to ova that are _____(4) and are more likely to err during _____(5). Children with Down's syndrome have recognizable _____(6) features, which involve the _____(7), head, and mouth. Mental _____(8) is always present to some degree. Other effects that shorten life span include malformation of the _____(9), predisposition to _____(10), and an increase in the likelihood of _____(11).

1. trisomy 21
2. Down's syndrome
3. mongolism
4. older
5. meiosis
6. physical
7. eyes
8. retardation
9. heart
10. infections
11. leukemia

7-39

A condition related to an abnormal X chromosome is **fragile X syndrome.** The end of the chromosome is fragile and breaks easily. This disruption causes the gene sequence to code for abnormal products. Because the sex chromosomes are involved, fragile X syndrome affects males while females are carriers. The particular product that is coded for by these genes are the neural connections in the brain. Since the neurons are not connected properly, a primary sign of the disorder is mental retardation. (After Down's syndrome, fragile X syndrome is the second most common cause of genetic-based retardation.) Another prominent characteristic is uncontrolled behavior that includes hyperactivity and temper tantrums. This behavior, which is difficult to manage, is due to an onslaught of overwhelming sensations that are weeded out and controlled in the normal brain. These patients react to every perceived sensation with no inhibitions. Treatment includes sensory integration therapy at an early age to teach the individual to sort out, ignore, or otherwise respond appropriately to sensory input. The true intelligence level of these individuals can only be accurately assessed after their behavior has been regulated.

7-40

1. X
2. breaks
3. products
4. gene
5. neuron
6. brain
7. retardation
8. behavior
9. sensations

Fragile X syndrome is so named because of the state of the _____(1) chromosome. The end of the chromosome _____(2) easily. This leads to abnormal _____(3) that are coded for by the disturbed _____(4) sequence. The products are the _____(5) connections in the _____(6). This results in mental _____(7) and unruly _____(8). The behavior pattern is due to a flooding of _____(9) that are normally controlled in healthy individuals.

7-41

Two sex-linked anomalies related to the X or Y chromosome are **Turner's syndrome** and **Klinefelter's syndrome.** These conditions are due to nondisjunction during meiosis that creates an abnormality in the number of sex chromosomes, resulting in greater or fewer than normal. Since the X or Y chromosome is not vital for survival, deletion in the numbers is still compatible with life. (This is in comparison to missing an autosome, which *is* required for life.) In Turner's syndrome, the patient appears female. This person is missing one of the sex chromosomes, and has only one X chromosome. There is no second X or a Y. The genotype is XO. There is no reproductive development of the ovaries and this is called **ovarian dysgenesis.** There is lack of ovulation and menstruation and this is called **amenorrhea.** These sterile individuals do not develop the secondary sex characteristics of a female. This state is usually diagnosed around puberty when there is an absence of reproductive development. In addition, there are heart abnormalities including coarctation, or misplacement, of the aorta, which creates hypertension. These abnormalities are represented for you in Figure 7–9.

7-42

1. dysjunction
2. greater
3. fewer
4. Turner's syndrome
5. reproductive
6. heart
7. X

Sex-linked abnormalities related to the X or Y chromosome occur because of failure of _____(1) during meiosis. This results in a person with _____(2) or _____(3) chromosomes than normal. The sex-linked anomaly in which the person looks female is _____(4). In this disease, there is complete lack of _____(5) development. The _____(6) is affected by a physical abnormality as well. The genotype is XO, which means the person has only the _____(7) sex chromosome.

7-43

In Klinefelter's syndrome, the person appears male. The genotype is XXY, so there is an extra X chromosome. These sterile individuals also do not mature sexually. The testes are very small and there is no production of sperm. Because of the influence of the extra X, they do develop some female secondary sex characteristics including female pubic hair distribution and slight enlargement of the breasts. This enlargement in men is called **gynecomastia,** regardless of the reason for the development. This condition is also suspected around

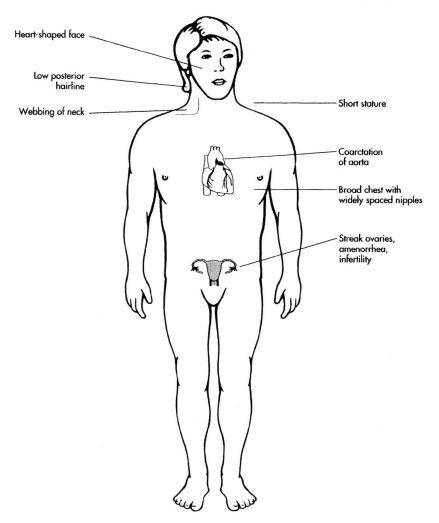

Figure 7–9. Typical features of Turner's syndrome. *(Adapted from Damjanov,* Pathology for the Health-Related Professions, *Saunders.)*

puberty. Some degree of mental retardation accompanies Klinefelter's syndrome, which is shown in Figure 7–10. Other unnamed sex-linked abnormalities include the genotype XXX (one extra X) in which the female develops normal secondary sex characteristics but has a slight mental disability. In the genotype XYY, these males develop relatively normally but studies have linked high levels of aggression to these men.

The genotype of XXY is seen in _____(1) syndrome and the person looks _____(2). There is lack of sexual maturity but these individuals do show some secondary characteristics of a _____(3). Laboratory diagnosis of sex-linked chromosomal irregularities is through the demonstration or absence of a **Barr body.** A Barr body is a visible sex chromatin in the nucleus of a cell. It is specifically the X chromosome because it condenses enough to be seen when stained. It appears as a dark mass and is present in the nucleus of every body cell in a normal female. A normal male never has a Barr body in his cells.

7–44

1. Klinefelter's
2. male
3. female

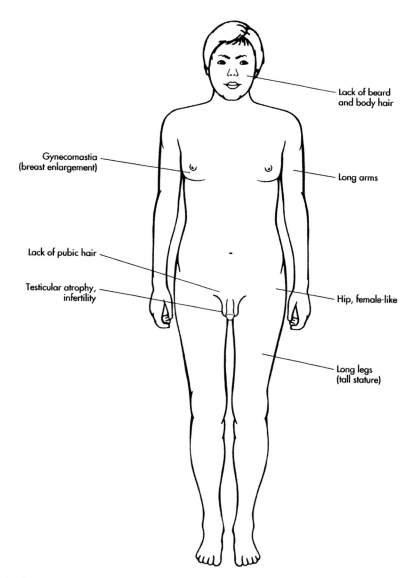

Figure 7–10. Typical features of Klinefelter's syndrome. *(Adapted from Damjanov,* Pathology for the Health-Related Professions, *Saunders.)*

II. REVIEW QUESTIONS

1. 1. c–monogenic
   2. a–chromosomal
   3. c–monogenic
   4. b–polygenic
   5. a–chromosomal
   6. c–monogenic
   7. a–chromosomal
   8. b–polygenic
   9. c–monogenic

1. Please match the categories of genetic disease in the left column with the correct descriptions in the right column. (You may use a category more than once.)

   a. chromosomal disorders
   b. polygenic disorders
   c. monogenic disorders

   1. _____ sex- or X-linked
   2. _____ monosomy (decreased numbers)
   3. _____ autosomal recessive
   4. _____ multifactorial
   5. _____ trisomy (increased numbers)
   6. _____ autosomal dominant
   7. _____ abnormal structure
   8. _____ risk genes/external factors
   9. _____ Mendelian disorder

2. Which of the following statements are true about autosomal recessive genetic disease? (Choose all that apply.)
   a. The parents are afflicted and produce children who are carriers.
   b. The parents are carriers and produce children who are afflicted.
   c. The affected individual is homozygous for the disease gene.
   d. The affected individual is heterozygous for the disease gene.
   e. A recessive gene frequently prevents the affected individual from reproducing.

3. Please match the categories of genetic disease in the left column with specific disease examples in the right column:
   a. monogenic—autosomal recessive
   b. monogenic—autosomal dominant
   c. monogenic—sex- or X-linked
   d. polygenic—multifactorial

   1. _____ cystic fibrosis
   2. _____ phenylketonuria
   3. _____ diabetes insipidus
   4. _____ Huntington's chorea
   5. _____ gout
   6. _____ sickle cell anemia
   7. _____ familial hypercholesterolemia
   8. _____ hemophilia
   9. _____ rheumatoid arthritis
   10. _____ Duchenne's muscular dystrophy
   11. _____ diabetes mellitus

4. Complete these sentences about cystic fibrosis using the terms listed below:
   The structures in the body affected by cystic fibrosis are the a. _____.
   They produce abnormally b. _____. This causes obstruction of the
   bronchi in the c. _____, and allows d. _____ to become
   trapped, leading to e. _____. Glands of the f. _____ become
   cystic and fibrotic. Dysfunction of this organ leads to g. _____,
   h. _____, and i. _____.

sweat glands	liver	pancreas	thick mucus
exocrine glands	salty fluid	lungs	bacteria
endocrine glands	insulin	viruses	tachypnea
thin mucus	kidneys	pneumonia	diabetes mellitus
poor absorption	polyuria	poor digestion	dyspnea

5. Tay–Sachs disease, galactosemia, and PKU are examples of:
   a. genetic disease in which hormones are missing
   b. genetic disease in which metabolic rates are greatly decreased
   c. genetic disease in which metabolic enzymes are missing
   d. genetic disease in which precursor substances are missing

6. The injury common to several metabolic genetic diseases is:
   a. insufficient development due to lack of precursor substances
   b. insufficient development due to lack of metabolic enzymes
   c. toxicity to the nervous system due to the accumulation of waste products
   d. toxicity to the nervous system due to the accumulation of precursor substances

7. Newborn babies are routinely tested for:
   a. Tay–Sachs disease, for lipid metabolism
   b. galactosemia, for conversion of galactose to glucose
   c. phenylketonuria, for conversion of phenylalanine to tyrosine
   d. familial hypercholesterolemia, for cholesterol levels

2. b–The parents are carriers and produce children who are afflicted. c–The affected individual is homozygous for the disease gene.

3. 1. a–monogenic—recessive
   2. a–monogenic—recessive
   3. b–monogenic—dominant
   4. b–monogenic—dominant
   5. d–polygenic—multifactorial
   6. a–monogenic—recessive
   7. b–monogenic—dominant
   8. c–monogenic—sex- or x-linked
   9. d–polygenic—multifactorial
   10. c–monogenic—sex- or x-linked
   11. d–polygenic—multifactorial

4. a–exocrine glands; b–thick mucus; c–lungs; d–bacteria; e–pneumonia; f–pancreas; g–poor digestion; h–poor absorption; i–diabetes

5. c–genetic disease in which metabolic enzymes are missing

6. d–toxicity to the nervous system due to the accumulation of precursor substances

7. c–phenylketonuria, for conversion of phenylalanine to tyrosine

8. a–sickle cell anemia
b–sickle cell trait

9. a–autosomal dominant disease

10. b–diabetes insipidus

11. a–familial hypercholesterolemia

12. d–degeneration of the nervous system with uncontrolled movements

13. d–a sex-linked genetic disease where lack of Factor VIII causes uncontrolled bleeding

14. a–a sex-linked genetic disease where skeletal muscle degeneration leads to death

15. False

16. b–Uric acid crystals build up as tophi and cause joint inflammation; d–Stones may develop in the kidneys and cause dysfunction; e–Lifestyle factors contribute

8. In people with the sickle cell gene, those who are homozygous have
a. _____ and those who are heterozygous have b. _____.

9. A heterozygous genotype and the absence of a carrier state is most characteristic of:
a. autosomal dominant disease
b. autosomal recessive disease
c. sex- or X-linked disease
d. polygenic disease

10. Polyuria and polydipsia are signs associated with the autosomal dominant disease:
a. diabetes mellitus
b. diabetes insipidus
c. pancreatic insufficiency
d. Huntington's chorea

11. Atherosclerosis is a result of the autosomal dominant disease:
a. familial hypercholesterolemia
b. achondroplasia
c. neurofibromatosis
d. retinoblastoma

12. Huntington's chorea is:
a. degeneration of skeletal muscle with fatal respiratory paralysis
b. mental retardation owing to chromosome abnormalities
c. degeneration of the nervous system with flaccid paralysis
d. degeneration of the nervous system with uncontrolled movements

13. Hemophilia is:
a. a sex-linked genetic disease where a deficiency of RBCs causes anemia
b. an autosomal dominant genetic disease where curved or bent RBCs block capillaries and blood flow
c. an autosomal recessive genetic disease where lack of Factor V causes uncontrolled bleeding
d. a sex-linked genetic disease where lack of Factor VIII causes uncontrolled bleeding

14. Duchenne's muscular dystrophy is:
a. a sex-linked genetic disease where skeletal muscle degeneration leads to death
b. an autosomal recessive genetic disease where nervous system degeneration ends with dementia
c. an autosomal dominant genetic disease where nervous system degeneration leads to retardation
d. a sex-linked genetic disease where skeletal muscle degeneration ends with paralysis

15. True or False: Polygenic diseases are due to more than one defective gene and they are inherited according to Mendelian laws. _____

16. Choose all the correct statements about gout:
a. Purine crystals build up as tophi and cause joint inflammation.
b. Uric acid crystals build up as tophi and cause joint inflammation.
c. Tophi crystals deposit in the liver and cause dysfunction.
d. Stones may develop in the kidneys and cause dysfunction.
e. Lifestyle factors contribute to abnormal uric acid metabolism.

17. Regarding diabetes mellitus:
    a. in type I, a defective gene may allow autoimmune destruction of insulin-producing cells
    b. in type II, a genetic predisposition combines with lifestyle factors to produce the disease
    c. type I requires treatment with insulin, while type II is often managed by diet and exercise
    d. all are correct
    e. none are correct

18. The presence of 45 chromosomes in a fetus would be called a. _____, while 47 would be called b. _____. This change from the normal 46 is because of c. _____ during meiosis.

19. Down's syndrome is also called (choose all that apply):
    a. monosomy 21
    b. trisomy 21
    c. mongolism
    d. trisomy 47
    e. monosomy 47

20. Down's syndrome is usually a product of:
    a. an abnormal X chromosome (sex-linked)
    b. nondisjunction by older ova
    c. an autosomal dominant disease gene
    d. an autosomal recessive disease gene

21. Down's syndrome affects (choose all that apply):
    a. the immune system
    b. the inflammatory response
    c. the liver
    d. facial features
    e. intelligence
    f. behavior
    g. the heart

22. Fragile X syndrome affects intelligence and behavior in:
    a. males only
    b. females only
    c. both males and females
    d. neither since afflicted fetuses are aborted

23. Please match the sex-linked disorder in the left column with the correct description in the right column:
    a. Turner's syndrome   1. _____genotype XXY
    b. Klinefelter's syndrome   2. _____genotype XO
                                  3. _____lack of reproductive development and sterility
                                  4. _____appears male
                                  5. _____appears female

to abnormal uric acid metabolism.

17. d–all are correct

18. a–monosomy; b–trisomy; c–nondisjunction

19. b–trisomy 21; c–mongolism

20. b–nondisjunction by older ova

21. a–the immune system; d–facial features; e–intelligence; g–the heart

22. a–males only

23. 1. b–Klinefelter's
    2. a–Turner's
    3. a–Turner's and b–Klinefelter's
    4. b–Klinefelter's
    5. a–Turner's

SECTION ▶ III. CONGENITAL ANOMALIES

1. congenital
2. genetics
3. teratogen

Congenital means present at birth. Some genetic diseases or defects are present at birth, such as cystic fibrosis and phenylketonuria. Some genetic diseases, like muscular dystrophy, do not develop until later so they are not congenital. However, a congenital disorder or problem may have nothing to do with genetics. An anomaly means an abnormality, an irregularity, or something that is aberrant. Therefore, a congenital anomaly means an irregularity that is present when a child is born. Some congenital disorders are commonly known as "birth defects." Birth defects that are not genetic usually represent a failure in the development of an embryo that may be a chance occurrence. It may also be due to the influence of a **teratogen,** which is an agent that causes a birth defect. A disorder that is present at birth is described as _____(1). A congenital anomaly may be due to heredity (_____) (2), or a spontaneous event, or a specific agent known as a _____(3).

1. hypoxia
2. birth
3. alcohol
4. rubella
5. syphilis

There are several factors that can lead to a congenital aberration. Hypoxia, or a decrease in the normal supply of oxygen to the embryo or fetus, can be very damaging. Maternal malnutrition can result in insufficient resources for development. Chemical teratogens, which cause birth defects, include maternal use of drugs or alcohol or exposure to some environmental chemicals. Infections in the mother can act as a teratogen. Rubella, which you learned about in Chapter 5, is able to cross the placental barrier and target the embryo to produce much damage. Other viruses have also been implicated in causing congenital defects. Syphilis is a potent teratogen and capable of causing multiple, severe defects. The pathogenesis of congenital anomalies is schematically shown in Figure 7–11. Lack of oxygen, or _____(1), or lack of proper nutrients can cause _____(2) defects. Chemical teratogens include drugs and _____(3). Biologic teratogens include the German measles virus or _____(4), and the venereal disease _____(5). In the remainder of this section, we will look at just a few examples of congenital anomalies of some body systems.

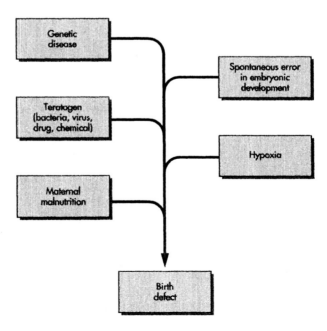

Figure 7–11. The pathogenesis of a congenital anomaly.

► THE NERVOUS SYSTEM

7-47

Damage to the central nervous system before or at birth can cause **cerebral palsy.** Cerebral palsy is a nonprogressive cause of paralysis. (Nonprogressive means it doesn't get worse.) Various etiologies have been identified as maternal rubella, diabetes, toxemia, hypoxia, or anoxia. A cause associated with birth is the asphyxiation of the newborn by the placement of the umbilical cord around the neck. An early postnatal cause is head trauma or meningitis. Premature babies are especially susceptible to brain damage. Cerebral palsy is the most common crippling disease of children. The legs are underdeveloped and there is extreme paresis with uncontrolled muscle contractions. Balance and coordination are affected in some types of cerebral palsy. Mental retardation and seizures are also present. Cerebral palsy is due to damage to the _____(1) at or close to _____(2). It is the most _____(3) reason for the crippling of children. It is frequently associated with anoxia or asphyxiation, which represents a lack of _____(4) to the brain.

1. brain
2. birth
3. common
4. oxygen

7-48

Spina bifida is a failure in fetal development where there is incomplete closure of the vertebrae, or the bones that enclose the spinal cord. The developing embryo is somewhat like a tubular organism with sections that grow toward each other to join at a midline. Several congenital abnormalities, such as cleft palate and spina bifida, represent a failure of this midline joining. There are three types of spina bifida, which are illustrated in Figure 7–12. The first is **occulta,** which means hidden. It is the least severe and the only sign is a dimple in the skin over the site. In the occult type, there is just a gap in the bone with no protrusion or herniation of any tissue. A **meningocele** occurs when part of the meninges and some spinal fluid escape out of the gap into a sac-like structure. This sac is visible externally at the site. The most severe form of spina bifida is a **myelomeningocele,** in which meninges, spinal fluid, and part of the spinal cord or a nerve root have herniated into the sac. This form can easily result in permanent neurologic deficits in sensation and motor ability. It must be corrected surgically. The prognosis depends on the amount of nervous tissue that has been pinched off during the protrusion.

Spina bifida is incomplete _____(1) of the _____(2). This leaves a hole in the bone. If no tissue sticks out through the hole, this is called the _____(3) form. Protrusion of meninges out of the hole and into a _____(4) is called a _____(5). If the spinal cord or a nerve _____(6) is involved, this is a _____(7). Impairment in perceiving sensation or in movement can result from the _____(8) type of spina bifida.

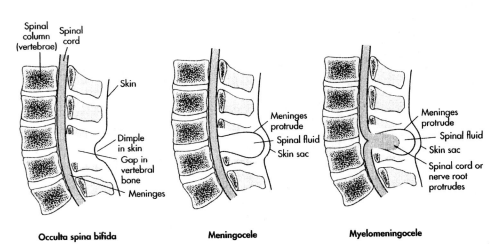

Figure 7–12. Manifestations of spina bifida.

7–50

1. ventricles
2. spinal fluid
3. obstruction or blockage
4. absorption
5. absorbed

Hydrocephalus can be loosely translated as "water on the brain." The ventricles, hollow spaces in the center of the brain, become overfilled with spinal fluid and enlarged. A developmental defect can block or obstruct the normal flow of spinal fluid or else poor absorption is the culprit. The physical finding of an enlarged head is fairly diagnostic. The enlarged ventricles apply pressure to parts of the brain so treatment is necessary. In a surgical procedure, a tube is inserted so that the excess fluid is diverted to a region such as the abdominal cavity. Here, the spinal fluid may be absorbed through the peritoneum and into the general circulation. Death is imminent without surgical correction. Even so, some degree of mental retardation and poor motor function will persist. Hollow spaces in the brain, called _____(1), will enlarge and cause pressure in the brain if they become overfilled with _____(2). This backup can be due to a physical _____(3) because of a defect, or because of poor _____(4). Treatment is to divert the fluid to another site where it can be _____(5).

▶ THE CARDIOVASCULAR SYSTEM

7–51

1. oxygen
2. lower, or less,
3. lungs
4. bluish

The heart is the target of many types of physical birth defects. They can be divided into two classifications, **cyanotic** and **acyanotic.** Cyanosis is a bluish discoloration of the skin and mucous membranes because of a decreased oxygen content in the blood (when hemoglobin is combined with oxygen it is red and is responsible for the pinkish tint to living tissue). Cyanosis occurs when there is inadequate function of oxygenation of the blood in the lungs. In some heart defects, there is poor oxygenation because some of the blood that should go to the lungs for oxygen ends up mixing with the blood bound for the systemic circulation. Therefore, the general circulation is partly composed of blood that still carries waste products like carbon dioxide, and is lacking in oxygen. In acyanotic defects, this mixing does not occur and the oxygenation of the general circulation approaches normal. Obviously, cyanotic conditions affect the patient more severely. A cyanotic heart anomaly is one in which the _____(1) levels in the blood are _____(2) than normal. This is because some blood that should have gone to the _____(3) for oxygen instead mixes with the systemic circulation. A cyanotic condition makes the patient look _____(4).

7–52

The most significant cyanotic defect is **tetralogy of Fallot.** This is actually a combination of four ("tetra") separate defects that occur together. The pulmonary artery, which runs from the right ventricle to the lungs for oxygen, is very narrow at the exit point from the ventricle. A narrowing, or stricture, is called a stenosis, so this condition is **pulmonary stenosis.** Pulmonary stenosis results in less blood to the lungs and increased pressure in the right ventricle. (In Chapter 10 on heart disease, you will learn in detail the various effects heart problems have on the body.) A **ventricular septal defect** or VSD is present. This is a gap or hole in the septum that is the dividing wall between the right and left atria and ventricles. The septum keeps the unoxygenated venous blood from the body separated from the oxygenated arterial blood from the lungs. A VSD allows these to mix so blood leaving the heart is not as well oxygenated as it should be. The aorta has experienced **dextroposition,** which is a change in its normal position from the exit port of the left ventricle. It now straddles the septum and so receives blood from both the right and left ventricles, further contributing to the mixing of blood. The last abnormality is enlargement, or **hypertrophy,** of the right ventricle. The enlargement of the muscular walls means that the ventricular chamber is smaller than normal and holds less blood.

7-53

Cyanosis in a newborn is a hallmark sign of tetralogy of Fallot. Dyspnea [difficult _____(1)] is present since the general circulation is crying for more oxygen. Tolerance for physical activity is greatly reduced. Tetralogy of Fallot is a combination of _____(2) individual abnormalities. The artery going to the lungs is pinched at the ventricular end and this is called _____(3). This means less _____(4) enters the lungs to receive _____(5). A hole is present in the _____(6) and this is known as a _____(7). This defect allows venous and arterial blood to _____(8). The aorta sits over both the right and left ventricles in a condition known as a _____(9). The right ventricular chamber is smaller than normal because of _____(10) of the muscle walls.

1. breathing
2. four
3. pulmonary stenosis
4. blood
5. oxygen
6. ventricular septum
7. ventricular septal defect, or VSD
8. mix
9. dextroposition
10. hypertrophy

7-54

Transposition of the aorta and pulmonary arteries is when these two great vessels have reversed positions. The aorta arises from the right ventricle instead of the left. The pulmonary artery emerges from the left ventricle. This results in two separate, closed-off circulatory systems. Blood circulates between the heart and lungs, and between the heart and body. This second system bypasses the lungs and oxygenation. Newborns experience severe cyanosis, cardiomegaly (enlargement of the heart), and congestive heart failure.

7-55

The following conditions are classified as acyanotic. A VSD can exist alone and this is commonly known as a "hole in the heart." The hole ranges from tiny to an entirely absent septum. A VSD is the most common acyanotic heart anomaly and is often seen in Down's syndrome. The same type of defect can exist in the septum dividing the atria and this is an **atrial septal defect** or **ASD**. In **coarctation of the aorta,** there is a narrowing of the lumen, or inside diameter, due to a defect in the aorta wall. This stricture increases blood pressure behind the flow of blood that is inside the heart. It also decreases blood pressure forward of the flow, which is the general circulation. An opening in the septum between the ventricles, called a _____(1), or an opening in the septum between the atria, called an _____(2) is classified as an _____(3) condition. A defect in the wall of the aorta that causes the lumen to be decreased in size is called _____(4). This condition results in abnormalities in _____(5).

1. ventricular septal defect
2. atrial septal defect
3. acyanotic
4. coarctation
5. blood pressure

7-56

Before birth, a vessel exists that is designed to bypass the lungs since the fetus does not breathe air. This vessel is called the **ductus arteriosus** and it runs in between the pulmonary artery and the aorta. Normally, this vessel closes at birth and disintegrates, allowing blood to enter the lungs. In a **patent ductus arteriosus** or **PDA,** this vessel remains open. This allows blood from the aorta, which is under greater pressure, to flow back into the pulmonary artery. This results in an overload in the circulation to the lungs. The increased amount of blood increases the pressure in the lungs and causes pulmonary edema and respiratory distress. A PDA, otherwise known as a _____(1), is a failure in the closure of the _____(2). This structure is designed to _____(3) the nonfunctioning _____(4) of the fetus. When it remains open, blood from the _____(5) flows back into the _____(6), causing them to be overloaded. You will see most of these heart defects illustrated in Chapter 10.

1. patent ductus arteriosus
2. ductus arteriosus
3. bypass
4. lungs
5. aorta
6. lungs

7-57

Diagnosis of congenital heart anomalies is through a careful history and physical exam, electrocardiogram (ECG), x-rays, heart catheterization and contrast dye studies, and echocardiogram (ultrasound of the heart). All of the defects presented here are corrected surgically.

▶ THE DIGESTIVE SYSTEM

A dramatic abnormality affecting the alimentary tract is **pyloric stenosis.** The pylorus is the distal, or exit end, of the stomach and it leads out into the duodenum, or first section of the small intestine. Pyloric *stenosis* would mean the pylorus is _____(1) than normal. This narrowing is due to the closure of the pyloric sphincter, a muscular ring controlled by nerves. This closure results in obstruction of the stomach. It is hallmarked by projectile vomiting by 2 to 4 weeks of age. The infant can eject stomach contents several feet. Dehydration and starvation accompany pyloric stenosis. It is easily diagnosed with a physical exam and x-rays. Treatment is a surgical procedure called a **pyloromyotomy** in which the muscles of the sphincter are incised (cut) and sutured open. This is very effective in returning function to normal.

_____(1) vomiting is a hallmark sign of _____(2). In this congenital anomaly, the pyloric _____(3) is closed down. This results in _____(4) to the passage of stomach contents. It must be repaired with a procedure called a _____(5) in which the _____(6) is opened.

▶ THE GENITOURINARY SYSTEM

Cryptorchidism is undescended testes, involving either one testicle or both. The testes are normally housed in the abdomen until about 8 months of gestation. They then move down into the scrotum. Retained testicles are seen more in premature infants. The signs are obvious. Treatment includes waiting to see if the cryptorchidism will correct itself with time by production of the hormone, human chorionic gonadotropin (HCG), that causes them to descend, or surgical correction. Retention inside the abdomen will cause the testicle to atrophy, or wither away, because of the higher temperature (relative to the scrotum). If both testicles are retained (bilateral cryptorchidism), this causes sterility. Testes or a testicle that is retained inside the _____(1) is called _____(2). Normally, the testes descend into the _____(3) by birth. Bilateral cryptorchidism causes _____(4).

There are several physical abnormalities that can involve the urinary tract. There may be **duplicated ureters,** in which there are two ureters associated with each kidney. A **retrocaval ureter** runs behind the inferior vena cava instead of in front of it. An **ectopic orifice** is an abnormal opening of the ureter into reproductive structures (vagina, prostate, or vas deferens), instead of into the bladder. A stricture, or **stenosis of the ureter,** will cause urine to back up into the kidney. In this potentially serious condition, the fluid overflow into the kidney can cause **hydronephrosis,** or degeneration of the kidney, due to fluid pressure. Surgical correction is necessary to prevent severe kidney damage. A **ureterocele** is the bulging or herniation of the ureter into the bladder. This abnormal mass of tissue in the bladder lumen can cause obstruction of the bladder and prevent urine flow.

The urinary bladder may contain a **diverticulum,** a pouching out of a portion of the wall. This small pocket in the wall leads to incomplete emptying of the bladder and susceptibility to urinary infections. The urethra may experience **hypospadias,** in which it opens on the underside of the penis or into the vagina. In **epispadias,** the urethra opens onto the upper surface of the penis or through an opening in the labia or clitoris.

Signs and symptoms of urinary anomalies may be obvious at birth or may not surface until later. Increased infections, difficulty urinating (**dysuria**), increased frequency of urination, decreased urine output, pain, and incontinence will be seen depending on the particular abnormality. Surgery to correct the defects is generally required. Congenital anomalies of the lower urinary tract can involve the _____(1), the _____(2), or the _____(3). Some are misplacements of the structures or their _____(4). A condition that immediately threatens the kidneys with degeneration or _____(5), is _____(6).

7-63

1. ureters
2. urinary bladder
3. urethra
4. openings
5. hydronephrosis
6. stenosis of the ureter

► THE MUSCULOSKELETAL SYSTEM

7-64

A **clubfoot** exists when the pull of ligaments causes the foot to be bent at various angles. It may be directed inward, outward, flexed upward, or extended downward. Sometimes a combination can exist such as bent inward and down. The condition can be corrected initially with surgery and casting, followed by night splints to train the ligaments and corrective shoes to maintain a normal position. When the foot of a baby is directed at abnormal _____(1), this is called a _____(2).

1. angles
2. clubfoot

7-65

Congenital hip dysplasia is an abnormal hip joint where there is some degree of dislocation between the head of the femur and the hip socket, or acetabulum. There are three manifestations. Dislocation of the femoral head can occur easily and it slides in and out of the acetabulum. There can be an incomplete dislocation, in which the femoral head rests on the edge of the bowl-like acetabulum. Or there can be complete dislocation, in which the femoral head remains outside of the acetabulum. Congenital hip dysplasia may go undiagnosed until the child attempts to walk. If diagnosed and treated before 3 months of age, hip dysplasia is managed with closed reduction and a brace. (Closed reduction means realigning bone by forceful manipulation from the outside and not through a surgical incision.) Cases in which the child is older requires open reduction (surgery) to replace the dislocation, followed by casting. Various degrees of _____(1) of the hip joint is called _____(2). There are _____(3) types. This condition may go unnoticed until the child tries to _____(4). Table 7–3 summarizes the congenital anomalies we have discussed according to the body system.

1. dislocation
2. congenital hip dysplasia
3. three
4. walk

TABLE 7–3. CONGENITAL ANOMALIES BY BODY SYSTEM

Nervous System	Genitourinary System
Cerebral palsy	Cryptorchidism
Spina bifida	Duplicated ureters
Hydrocephalus	Retrocaval ureters
	Ectopic orifice
Cardiovascular System	Stenosis of ureter
Tetralogy of Fallot (pulmonary stenosis,	Ureterocele
ventricular septal defect, aortic dextroposition,	Diverticulum
right ventricular hypertrophy)	Hypospadias
Transposition of aorta and pulmonary artery	Epispadias
Ventricular septal defect	
Atrial septal defect	**Musculoskeletal System**
Coarctation of aorta	Clubfoot
Patent ductus arteriosus	Congenital hip dysplasia
Digestive System	
Pyloric stenosis	

III. REVIEW QUESTIONS

1. c—one that is present at birth and is due to maternal factors, genetics, teratogens, or spontaneous events

2. d—cerebral palsy

3. d—Permanent damage to nerve function can occur if a myelomeningocele is not surgically repaired.

4. a—enlarged ventricles in the brain that are overfilled with spinal fluid and cause pressure in the brain

5. a—the mixing of venous and arterial blood, so that the general circulation contains less oxygen than normal

6. b—ventricular septal defect; f—pulmonary stenosis; g—hypertrophy of the right ventricle; h—dextroposition of the aorta

1. Choose the statement that BEST describes the meaning of a congenital disorder:
   a. one that is present at birth and is due to genetic causes
   b. one that develops shortly after birth and is due to maternal causes
   c. one that is present at birth and is due to maternal factors, genetics, teratogens, or spontaneous events
   d. one that develops shortly after birth and is due to teratogens

2. Lack of oxygen, or other factors, can cause brain damage in a newborn, with retardation, paresis, and paralysis. This describes:
   a. hydrocephalus
   b. spina bifida
   c. myelomeningocele
   d. cerebral palsy

3. Choose the correct statement about spina bifida:
   a. This disorder represents a failure in the closure of the meninges around the spinal cord.
   b. A meningocele is a hole in the vertebrae, through which no tissue or fluid escapes.
   c. Occulta spina bifida is identified by a small sac over the site where spinal fluid has leaked out of the vertebral gap.
   d. Permanent damage to nerve function can occur if a myelomeningocele is not surgically repaired.

4. Hydrocephalus is:
   a. enlarged ventricles in the brain that are overfilled with spinal fluid and cause pressure in the brain
   b. an enlarged head due to overgrowth of the cranium
   c. an enlarged head due to overfilling of the meningeal space with spinal fluid
   d. water buildup in the brain as edema, due to pressure and resulting inflammation

5. A cyanotic heart defect is an abnormality that leads to:
   a. the mixing of venous and arterial blood, so that the general circulation contains less oxygen than normal
   b. complete separation of the arterial and venous circulatory systems, so that the general circulation contains less oxygen than normal
   c. severe anemia, seen as a pale appearance of the patient
   d. oxygenation of the blood in a normal manner

6. Choose all of the defects that are present in tetralogy of Fallot:
   a. atrial septal defect
   b. ventricular septal defect
   c. hypertrophy of both atria
   d. dextroposition of the vena cave
   e. coarctation of the aorta
   f. pulmonary stenosis
   g. hypertrophy of the right ventricle
   h. dextroposition of the aorta
   i. patent ductus arteriosus

7. A patent ductus arteriosus is:
   a. an abnormal, extra vessel that diverts blood away from the lungs after birth
   b. a normal structure that is necessary after birth to send extra blood to the lungs
   c. a defect in the aorta wall that decreases the diameter of the lumen and adversely affects blood pressure
   d. failure of a normal pre-birth vessel to close, resulting in shunting of extra blood to the lungs

8. Pyloric stenosis results in:
   a. obstruction of the duodenum, or the first part of the small intestine
   b. severe diarrhea leading to dehydration and electrolyte imbalance
   c. obstruction of the stomach with vomiting, dehydration, and starvation
   d. obstruction of the stomach with severe diarrhea, dehydration, and electrolyte imbalance

9. Cryptorchidism is:
   a. retention of one or both testes inside the abdomen
   b. herniation of the ureter into the bladder
   c. stricture of the ureter leading to hydronephrosis
   d. rupture of one or both testes inside the scrotum

10. Hydronephrosis of the kidney (degeneration due to fluid pressure) may be the result of:
    a. a ureterocele
    b. a bladder diverticulum
    c. a retrocaval ureter
    d. stenosis of the ureter
    e. epispadias of the urethra

11. Congenital hip dysplasia results in:
    a. a loose hip joint where the femoral head slides in and out of the acetabulum
    b. an incomplete dislocation where the head of the femur sits on the edge of the acetabulum
    c. a complete dislocation where the femoral head remains outside of the acetabulum
    d. any of the above
    e. none of the above

CHAPTER SUMMARY ▶

▶ SECTION II

Monogenic diseases are genetic abnormalities in which one defective gene is responsible for the disorder. This group of diseases is further subclassified as autosomal recessive, autosomal dominant, or sex-linked.

In an autosomal recessive disease, the individual is homozygous for defective alleles. Individuals who inherit only one defective gene of an allelic pair are thus heterozygous for the trait and are generally phenotypically normal. They are, however, carriers of the defective trait. Cystic fibrosis, Tay–Sachs disease, galactosemia, phenylketonuria (PKU), and sickle cell anemia are examples of autosomal recessive diseases. In an autosomal dominant disease, only one defective gene, inherited from one parent, is needed for the individual to express the disease. There are, as such, no hidden carrier states. Diseases recognized as autosomal dominant include diabetes insipidus, achondroplasia, familial hypercholesterolemia, and Huntington's chorea. Sex-linked (or X-linked) diseases result from a defective gene on the X chromosome, and are therefore seen predominantly in males, who do not have a second, normal X chromosome to cover the defective gene. Sex-linked diseases are generally passed from mother to son, who in turn passes the abnormal gene to his daughter, who then becomes a carrier. Duchenne's muscular dystrophy and hemophilia are two examples of sex-linked disorders. Polygenic or multigene disorders involve several factors besides a defective gene. Lifestyle, diet, and perhaps other environmental factors combine with "risk genes" to place an individual at a higher risk for a specific disease. Rheumatoid arthritis, gout, diabetes mellitus, hypertension, atherosclerotic heart disease, and some cancers are thought to be this type of polygenic abnormality.

Some genetic disorders are due to changes, either in number or in structure, in the chromosomes themselves. Such conditions can result from errors during meiosis or from damage to a chromosome. Down's syndrome is a relatively common chromosomal aberration resulting from a chromosomal nondisjunction event during meiosis. Down's syndrome is medically termed trisomy 21, in which every cell in the individual contains three of chromosome 21. Fragile X syndrome, seen only in males, is a condition in which the X chromosome breaks easily. In Turner's syndrome, the affected individual has only one sex chromosome, an X. Individuals with Klinefelter's syndrome have one Y and two X chromosomes.

▶ SECTION III

A congenital disorder (a defect that is present at birth) may or may not be due to a genetic malfunction. Some birth defects may be due to a specific agent such as bacteria, a virus, or a chemical. Others may be the result of an embryonic developmental failure due, for example, to temporary oxygen deprivation (hypoxia) of the fetus or malnutrition during pregnancy.

Congenital abnormalities can involve any of the body's systems. Cerebral palsy is recognized as damage to the central nervous system due to fetal hypoxia or neonatal head trauma. Spina bifida and hydrocephaly are likewise congenital abnormalities of the nervous system, and are due to malfunctions during fetal development. The cardiovascular system is the target of many types of congenital anomalies. These defects are classified as cyanotic or acyanotic, and may involve the heart itself or the arteries exiting the heart. Birth defects can also be observed in other systems such as digestive (e.g., pyloric stenosis), genitourinary (e.g., cryptorchidism, ectopic orifice, duplicated ureters), and musculoskeletal (e.g., clubfoot, congenital hip dysplasia).

CHAPTER 8

Metabolic and Nutritional Disorders

▶ OBJECTIVES

SECTION II

Define all highlighted terms.

Characterize the biochemical defect and the symptoms involved in the diseases galactosemia, glucose-6-phosphate dehydrogenase deficiency, and phenylketonuria.

Define and characterize the symptoms associated with the lysosomal storage diseases. List four such diseases.

Define and characterize the symptoms associated with the condition of gout, and distinguish between primary and secondary gout.

SECTION III

Define all highlighted terms.

Distinguish between diabetes insipidus and diabetes mellitus.

Identify the symptoms and clinical observations associated with diabetes mellitus.

Describe the functions of the kidneys, the pancreas, and the hormone insulin as they pertain to the regulation of the amount of glucose in the blood.

Describe the developmental stages of diabetes mellitus.

Define and distinguish between types I and II diabetes mellitus.

Cite several conditions that could lead to abnormally high blood glucose levels.

Cite several factors that could lead to secondary diabetes.

Describe the pathogenesis associated with diabetes mellitus, including the conditions of polyuria, polydipsia, lipolysis, hyperketonemia, ketonuria, and ketoacidosis.

Describe the signs and symptoms of diabetes.

Describe the complications of diabetes mellitus.

Distinguish between and describe the conditions of diabetic coma and insulin shock and the treatment for each.

List and explain the reasons for hypoglycemia.

SECTION ▶ 1. REVIEW OF METABOLISM AND NUTRITION

▶ METABOLISM

8-1

Metabolism is defined as the sum of all the physical and chemical processes by which living substance is produced and maintained and also the transformation by which energy is made available for use by the organism. It is all of the biochemical reactions that continuously take place and allow us to live and prosper. Metabolism includes the building of substances **(anabolism)** and the breakdown of substances **(catabolism).** Many chemicals and active proteins are responsible for metabolism. These include some hormones and secretory products from cells, as well as enzymes. Enzymes are proteins and are vital in every biochemical reaction in the body. Their specific activities really form the basis for the biochemistry of metabolism.

8-2

The activity of enzymes includes the metabolism or processing of carbohydrates, fats, and proteins. The chemical reactions take place inside cells and include the Krebs cycle in the mitochondria. The Krebs cycle is a series of reactions that lead to the production of energy (ATP) from glucose. Chemical reactions in cells produce heat as well as energy, and they are responsible for the core body temperature. The **basal metabolic rate,** or **BMR,** is that amount of metabolism (energy production) that is required to maintain life for a body at rest. It is a baseline of energy that is needed to keep the body alive. A body performing work naturally needs more energy than that produced by the BMR. ("Work" in this instance means any kind of movement or activity.) People who have a high BMR use more energy, or burn more calories, just to stay alive than those with a low BMR. The basal metabolic rate heavily influences a person's body weight. Someone with a low BMR must eat less and exercise more to maintain proper weight compared to someone with a high BMR. The basal metabolic rate decreases with age so that fewer calories are needed to maintain life. Unfortunately, most of us don't cut down our food intake proportionately, so gaining weight with age is a common occurrence. Regular aerobic exercise is a good way to boost metabolism.

8-3

The metabolism of glucose, or processing and using of glucose, is the cornerstone of life. Glucose is the main fuel or energy for cells, especially in the brain. Cells of the body can turn to other food compounds for energy if necessary, but neurons are especially dependent on glucose and do not readily use other sources of energy. The amount of glucose at any given time in a healthy individual ranges from around 80 to 120 mg/dL. This range is important for normal physiologic functioning, especially for neurons. Maintaining this level, not too high or too low, is part of homeostasis. As you learned in Chapter 3, homeostasis is the maintenance of a balanced internal environment, and it has many aspects.

8—4

Normal glucose levels are maintained through several regulatory mechanisms. The pancreas secretes two hormones from clumps of cells called the **islets of Langerhans.** The islets are divided into **alpha** and **beta** cells. The hormone **insulin** from the beta cells lowers the amount of glucose in the blood. **Glucagon** is from the alpha cells, and it acts as an antagonist, or opposes insulin, by raising the blood glucose. It does so by stimulating the liver to release glucose from its storage form, **glycogen.** This is shown in Figure 8–1. The liver may lower blood glucose by storing it as glycogen. It may also raise blood glucose by breaking glycogen back down into glucose **(glycogenolysis)** or by making glucose from other sources such as fats or proteins **(gluconeogenesis).**

8—5

After being digested in the intestines, carbohydrates are absorbed in the form of glucose into the blood. This rise in blood glucose stimulates the release of insulin from the pancreas. Insulin causes glucose to move into cells and thereby lowers the blood glucose to normal again. Much of what is absorbed from the intestines is kept in the liver for conversion to glycogen for storage until it is needed. (Hepatocytes, or liver cells, do not require insulin for glucose to enter.)

8—6

Insulin lowers blood glucose levels by assisting molecules of glucose through the cell membrane. Tissues and cells that are classified as insulin-dependent need insulin to help transport glucose through the cell membrane to the inside of the cell. These tissues include muscle and adipose, or fat. Insulin-dependent cells have receptors on their membranes for insulin to lock onto and begin its activities. As previously mentioned, insulin is synthesized or made by the beta cells of the islets of Langerhans in the pancreas. Its release is directly stimulated by **hyperglycemia,** or an increased blood glucose. This hyperglycemia is physiologic or normal compared to the high levels seen in diabetes mellitus (see Frame 8–28). Physiologic hyperglycemia follows a meal and is produced by absorption of glucose from the intestines. So after eating, insulin will naturally be released from the pancreas in a healthy individual. The temporary hyperglycemia is resolved after insulin performs its work of assisting glucose into cells, and the level in the blood lowers once again to the normal range.

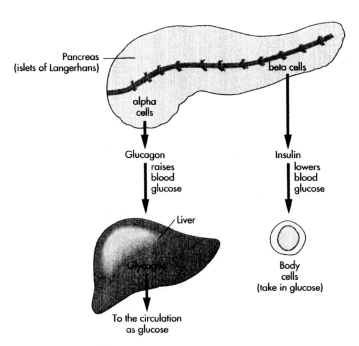

Figure 8–1. A simple representation of the maintenance of normal blood glucose levels.

Other functions of insulin are summarized in the following list.

1. Assisting the liver with glycogenesis, or the storing of glucose in the form of glycogen. This also lowers blood glucose.
2. Assisting protein synthesis from amino acids.
3. Inhibiting **lipolysis,** or fat breakdown. If insulin is present in working amounts in the blood, it follows that a meal was recently consumed so there is no need to break down fat.
4. Inhibiting glycogenolysis and gluconeogenesis by the liver. Again, there is no need to break down glycogen or make glucose from new sources after a meal.

An overview of the functions of insulin is presented in Figure 8–2.

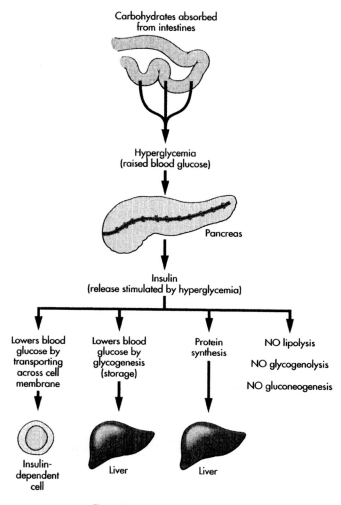

Figure 8–2. The main functions of insulin.

▶ NUTRITION

8–8

Proper nutrition is the basis for health, especially during the young, formative years and for newborns who have an increased need for calories, vitamins, and minerals. Other situations in which nutrition heavily influences health are pregnancy, lactation, and advanced age. Proper nutrition is the correct balance of carbohydrates, proteins, fats (lipids), vitamins, and minerals. A nutrient that is classified as **essential** is one that the body cannot manufacture and therefore must come from the diet. Of the amino acids, there are nine that are essential. Two of the lipids are essential, as are several vitamins and minerals. Vitamins and minerals are required for biochemical reactions and the integrity of some tissues. Proper hydration is vital since all biochemical reactions must take place in water. The energy the body gets from nutrients or food is in the form of calories. A **calorie** is the amount of heat needed to raise the temperature of a kilogram of water 1 degree Celsius. This heat energy, or calories, comes from the metabolism of carbohydrates, fats, and proteins.

8–9

The calories, or energy, in food are released through the process of oxidation, or "burning," that takes place in the mitochondria of cells. Carbohydrates and proteins produce about the same amount of calories. Fats produce about two and a half times as many calories. **Carbohydrates** (sugars and starches) are the main source of energy from food. Carbohydrates may be synthesized by the body from either proteins or fats. (That is why carbohydrates are not classified as essential.) **Proteins** are primarily used to form body structures, such as muscle, and substances, like enzymes and hormones. A diet lacking in the essential amino acids produces a disease called **kwashiorkor,** which is stunted growth in children. **Lipids,** or fats, can be used as a source of energy like carbohydrates, and they are important structural components of cell membranes. **Vitamins** act as coenzymes in the biochemistry of metabolism and are used in some tissue structure. **Minerals** have a variety of uses. Large amounts of calcium and phosphate are necessary for bone formation and calcification. Iron is the center molecule in hemoglobin. Magnesium is important for nerve and muscle function. Iodine is a component of the thyroid hormone, thyroxin. Minerals needed only in trace amounts include zinc for healthy skin and chromium for carbohydrate and fat metabolism. The ions, sodium and potassium (see Chap. 3), are considered by some to be minerals.

II. DISORDERS OF METABOLISM ◀ SECTION

8–10

Disorders involving the body's metabolism are historically called inborn errors of metabolism. This helps to characterize their nature. Inborn refers to both genetic and congenital. The error is abnormal metabolism. Metabolic disorders have as their basis a **biochemical lesion.** If you will recall from Chapter 1, a lesion is a pathological or traumatic discontinuity of the tissues. It is from the Latin meaning to hurt. Loosely translated, a lesion is an injury (which may or may not be traumatic) and is usually physical and localized. In a biochemical lesion, the "hurt" or injury is not a physical thing, but instead is a malfunctioning of the biochemical reactions of metabolism.

8–11

This section will examine just a few of the many known metabolic diseases. The disease, which shows itself in a variety of ways, begins at the biochemical level. This is even lower than the level of an individual cell. The "error" of Frame 8–10 is specifically the abnormal function of an enzyme or the absence of an enzyme. There are hundreds, even thousands, of enzymes that drive every reaction in the body. Their importance cannot be overstated. When there is some lack or deficiency of these proteins, disease will eventually result at some level. The malfunctioning or absence of a single type of enzyme will have far-reaching effects. In metabolic disorders, many of which are genetic in cause, the underlying defect lies with specific enzymes.

8-12

1. genetic
2. congenital
3. biochemical
4. biochemical
5. enzyme

An inborn error of metabolism refers to a condition that is both _____(1) and _____(2). The injury or "hurt" in this case is a _____(3) lesion. The start of disease begins at the _____(4) level. The specific lesion is a defect in, or an absence of, a particular _____(5).

▶ GALACTOSEMIA

8-13

This condition was mentioned in Chapter 7 on genetic diseases. Many disease processes can be categorized in more than one way because there are several aspects to them. Galactosemia is a genetic metabolic disorder, like others that belong to more than one category. In this disorder there is a deficiency of an enzyme from the liver known as *galactose-1-phosphate uridyl transferase*. This transferase enzyme is required to convert galactose to glucose. Milk contains the carbohydrate lactose, and galactose is derived from lactose. This unconverted galactose accumulates in the tissues. It is not especially toxic by itself, but its presence interferes in other metabolic processes. These processes include those responsible for normal development of a fetus and newborn. Abnormal development of the brain results in retardation, the liver is affected with cirrhosis or scarring from the buildup, and the eyes develop cataracts from the accumulation. The signs that are seen earliest are those associated with liver malfunction, and they are apparent by 6 months of age. The treatment for galactosemia is a galactose-free diet for life. If the condition is recognized early and treated before permanent brain and liver damage occur, the patient can improve greatly. However, impaired mental ability can be a sequela.

8-14

1. enzyme
2. liver
3. galactose
4. glucose
5. galactose
6. processes or development
7. brain
8. liver
9. eyes

Galactosemia is a metabolic disease due to lack of a (an) _____(1) from the _____(2). This enzyme is needed to change _____(3) to _____(4). Without this change, _____(5) builds up in the tissues. This accumulation will interfere with normal _____(6) in a fetus or newborn. Organs specifically affected include the _____(7), the _____(8), and the _____(9).

▶ GLUCOSE-6-PHOSPHATE DEHYDROGENASE DEFICIENCY

8-15

Glucose-6-phosphate dehydrogenase (G-6-PD) is an enzyme found inside red blood cells. Its important function is to protect cell membranes from the damaging effects of oxidation from compounds that are oxidants. (An oxidant is an unstable molecule that disrupts the electron balance of stable molecules. This causes the affected molecules to also become unstable and damaged.) G-6-PD deficiency is a sex- or X-linked genetic inheritance mainly affecting black males. (As a sex-linked condition, the affected males are homozygous, and females are heterozygous carriers.) Other populations such as Greek, Chinese, and Filipino can show this disorder. G-6-PD deficiency is asymptomatic most of the time. In this condition, the enzyme that is in older red blood cells loses its protective function. If the individual should take certain oxidizing drugs, an episode of hemolysis, or cell rupture, will result. These drugs include the antimalarial agent quinine, sulfonamide, and some analgesics. The hemolysis leads to **acute hemolytic anemia.** This is a sudden deficiency in red blood cells (acute anemia) due to rupture or hemolysis of the cells.

8-16

The hemolysis actually takes place in the spleen, not directly in the blood vessels, so it is called **extravascular hemolysis.** The spleen has a weeding-out function and removes old and damaged red blood cells. (This is normal, and a certain number of red blood cells are removed daily from the circulation.) The G-6-PD deficient cells that are damaged by oxidants are removed by the spleen. This number is far in excess of the normal, daily removal, so anemia results. A pregnant woman who had a G-6-PD deficient fetus, and who takes an oxidizing drug, could cause a hemolytic episode in the fetus. The anemia of G-6-PD deficiency is temporary and resolves when the drug is stopped. Occasionally, a transfusion may be necessary. Screening tests to detect those who are affected, combined with avoidance of certain drugs, is the best prevention.

8—17

G-6-PD, or _____(1), is an enzyme found inside _____(2). Its purpose is to preserve the integrity of the cell _____(3) that can be damaged by _____(4) compounds. In G-6-PD deficiency, which mainly affects _____(5), this enzyme in older red blood cells loses its ability to protect the cell. If certain oxidizing _____(6) are ingested, the red blood cells become damaged and therefore abnormal. Old, damaged, or otherwise abnormal red blood cells are normally removed by the _____(7). In G-6-PD deficiency, this removal takes place in greater numbers. This sudden loss of, and therefore deficiency in, red blood cells is called _____(8).

1. glucose-6-phosphate dehydrogenase
2. red blood cells
3. membranes
4. oxidizing
5. black males
6. drugs
7. spleen
8. anemia (in this case, acute hemolytic anemia)

▷ PHENYLKETONURIA

8—18

Lack of another liver enzyme, phenylalanine hydroxylase, causes accumulation of another substance, phenylalanine. Normally, phenylalanine is converted into tyrosine. Phenylalanine is found in the diet as part of most proteins. Phenylalanine buildup does have direct toxic effects and also disrupts normal development. This toxicity and abnormal development most dramatically affects the brain. Mental retardation is the result. Signs of untreated phenylketonuria, or PKU, can be detected at around 4 months of age. The baby exhibits abnormal behavior in the form of irritability, hyperactivity, and seizures. The urine and sweat have a musty odor due to the presence of phenylacetic acid in those body fluids.

8—19

PKU, or _____(1), is a metabolic defect, in which the enzyme for converting _____(2) to _____(3) is deficient. Phenylalanine is found in most _____(4). Its accumulation has direct toxic effects on the _____(5). Untreated PKU will result in mental _____(6). PKU may be prevented by testing all newborns for increased phenylalanine levels in the blood. Adults who are heterozygous carriers can also be detected during genetic screening and counseling. Treatment of babies affected with PKU centers around avoiding all phenylalanine in the diet. This means no meat or milk products, but instead, synthetic proteins in the diet. Blood levels of phenylalanine can be checked to determine the efficacy (effectiveness) of the treatment. Treatment must be initiated before permanent damage is done, since the retardation is irreversible after a time.

1. phenylketonuria
2. phenylalanine
3. tyrosine
4. proteins
5. brain
6. retardation

▷ LYSOSOMAL STORAGE DISEASES

8—20

A **lysosome** is a sac-like structure or vesicle in a cell's cytoplasm. A lysosome releases lytic enzymes to break down various substances in the cytoplasm. These substances are often the by-products or waste products of cellular metabolism. It is important that this "garbage" be disposed of properly so that it does not accumulate and damage the cell. It follows that if these lytic enzymes are missing, the waste products will build up and hurt the cell. (Keep in mind that for any of these disorders, when we talk of "an" enzyme and "a" cell, it is just to explain the mechanism. This damage occurs to millions of cells and therefore to tissues and organs.)

8—21

There are many different types of lysosomal storage diseases, because there are 25 to 30 different enzymes that could be involved. The common denominator is damage to a variety of organs including the brain, liver, spleen, and lungs. Treatment of lysosomal storage diseases has largely been unsuccessful to date. A lysosome is a vesicle in the cell's _____(1) that releases _____(2) that break down _____(3) products of metabo-

1. cytoplasm
2. enzymes

3. waste
4. accumulation
5. tissues
6. organs

lism. Failure to eliminate these waste products leads to their _____(4) inside the cell. This accumulation damages the cell and therefore the _____(5) and _____(6) that the cells form.

8-22

The following are examples of lysosomal storage diseases.

1. **Glycogenosis.** Glycogen accumulates inside cells.
2. **Lipidosis,** or **Gaucher's disease.** Lipid, or fat, builds up and is often manifest as an enlarged spleen, or splenomegaly.
3. **Mucopolysaccharidosis.** The abnormal metabolism of glucosaminoglycans in the extracellular matrix leads to defects in bone.

8-23

A disease we discussed in Chapter 7, **Tay–Sachs disease,** is a lysosomal storage disease. It is also known as **gangliosidosis.** The missing enzyme is hexosaminidase A. Ganglioside accumulates inside neurons, causing swelling and death of the neurons. This occurs in the central nervous system (brain and spinal cord), as well as in peripheral nerves. Mental and motor ability are greatly impaired in these affected babies. An early death is inevitable. The best "treatment" for Tay–Sachs disease is prevention through prenatal screening and identifying carriers of the gene for this disease.

8-24

A rare disorder involves the accumulation of glycogen inside cells due to either a defect in the synthesis or breakdown of glycogen. There are at least eight separate disorders corresponding to specific enzyme deficiencies, and they are collectively called **glycogen storage diseases.** One of them is glycogenosis, as mentioned in Frame 8–22.

► GOUT

8-25

1. purine
2. joints
3. tophi
4. inflammation
5. toe

Gout was presented to you under our study of genetic diseases, but it is also considered an inborn error of metabolism. It is another metabolic disease with a genetic basis. If you will recall, uric acid is the end product of _____(1) metabolism. Purines are the nucleic acids of DNA and RNA. In gout, there are episodes of increased levels of uric acid in the blood. This is called **hyperuricemia.** Along with hyperuricemia are attacks of arthritis. The arthritis is due to deposits of uric acid crystals in the _____(2). Visible deposits of uric acid seen as white plaques are called _____(3). Chronic tophus deposits cause chronic _____(4), a natural reaction to a foreign body. Chronic inflammation inside a joint will damage the surface and lead to pain, stiffness, and deformity. The joint most often affected is the great _____(5). It is unknown why urates tend to deposit in joints. But as they do, phagocytes are there to consume the crystals as foreign bodies. Lysosomal enzymes are naturally released as part of the protective response. These enzymes also contribute to the damage and pain of gouty arthritis.

8-26

In addition to the pain and inconvenience that accompanies gout, there are some serious side effects. The kidneys normally clear uric acid from the body, so it is not surprising that they can also become damaged from the abnormally high levels. About one third of gout cases will develop kidney stones made of urate. Other damage to the kidneys, or even renal failure, is not unheard of in gout. There are two categories of gout. The first is **primary gout,** and this is the inborn error of metabolism. It does tend to run in families, or be familial. There are more affected males than females. Because of a missing or defective enzyme, there is either an increase in the production of uric acid or a decrease in its excretion by the kidneys. Either case results in hyperuricemia. In **secondary gout,** again, there is either an increase in uric acid or a decrease in its excretion. However, the cause is due to either chronic renal failure or systemic disease that interferes with purine metabolism. Therefore, secondary gout is not an inborn error of metabolism.

TABLE 8–1. DISORDERS OF METABOLISM

Disorder	Biochemical Lesion	Manifestation
Galactosemia	Deficiency of galactose-1-phosphate uridyl transferase	Accumulation of galactose in tissues (retardation, cirrhosis, and cataracts)
Glucose-6-phosphate dehydrogenase deficiency	Deficiency of G-6-PD	Red blood cell hemolysis due to lack of protection from oxidation (anemia)
Phenylketonuria	Deficiency of phenylalanine hydroxylase	Accumulation of phenylalanine (retardation and abnormal behavior)
Lysosomal storage diseases	Deficiency of lysosome enzymes	Accumulation of waste products (damage to brain, liver, spleen, and lungs)
Tay–Sachs disease (gangliosidosis)	Deficiency of hexosaminidase A	Accumulation of ganglioside in neurons (retardation and early death)
Gout	Hyperuricemia	Chronic deforming arthritis, pain, kidney stones, and potential kidney failure

8–27

Increased levels of uric acid in the blood is called _____(1). The disease that accompanies this excess is called _____(2). It may be either primary or secondary. Primary gout is an inborn _____(3) of _____(4). Secondary gout is due to systemic disease or chronic _____(5) failure. In both cases, _____(6) production is increased, or uric acid _____(7) is decreased. To review the disorders of metabolism we have just discussed, refer to Table 8–1.

1. hyperuricemia
2. gout
3. error
4. metabolism
5. kidney
6. uric acid
7. excretion

II. REVIEW QUESTIONS

1. An inborn error of metabolism is:
    a. a birth defect in a newborn caused by abnormal maternal metabolism during pregnancy
    b. an excess of metabolic enzymes that creates toxic levels of by-products
    c. a biochemical lesion where the mitochondria does not function properly
    d. the absence of a biochemical enzyme

2. Inborn errors of metabolism produce disease by:
    a. creating abnormal conditions and damage in a cell, which translates through to the tissue and organ level
    b. creating physical lesions
    c. overactivity of enzymes
    d. halting metabolism in some tissues

3. Please match the metabolic disorders in the left column with their prominent features in the right column:
    a. phenylketonuria
    b. galactosemia
    c. Tay–Sachs disease
    d. glucose-6-phosphate dehydrogenase deficiency

    1. ____ oxidative damage to red blood cells leading to acute hemolytic anemia
    2. ____ insufficient tyrosine conversion leading to mental retardation
    3. ____ fatal lysosomal storage disease in the young
    4. ____ results from ingestion of lactose in milk

1. d–the absence of a biochemical enzyme

2. a–creating abnormal conditions and damage in a cell, which translates through to the tissue and organ level

3. 1. d–glucose-6-phosphate dehydrogenase deficiency
   2. a–phenylketonuria
   3. c–Tay–Sachs disease
   4. b–galactosemia

4. c–familial, more males
   affected, hyperuricemia,
   severe arthritis of the great
   toe, kidney damage

5. a–4; b–5; c–1; d–6;
   e–2; f–3

4. Which of the following features best describes primary gout?
   a. dietary related, more males affected, hypouricemia, generalized arthritis, existing renal failure
   b. genetic, more females affected, hyperuricemia, mild arthritis of the hands, kidney stones
   c. familial, more males affected, hyperuricemia, severe arthritis of the great toe, kidney damage
   d. congenital, more females affected, hypouricemia, arthritis of the spine, existing renal failure

5. Please *number in correct order* the events that lead to arthritis in gout:
   a. _____ phagocytes and lysosomal enzymes
   b. _____ damage to joint surfaces
   c. _____ hyperuricemia
   d. _____ pain, stiffness, deformity
   e. _____ tophus deposits
   f. _____ inflammation inside the joint

SECTION ▶ III. HYPERGLYCEMIA (DIABETES MELLITUS) AND HYPOGLYCEMIA

▶ DIABETES MELLITUS

····· 8–28 ·····

1. urine
2. glucose or sugar

Everyone is familiar with the common disorder diabetes mellitus, or "high blood sugar." If you remember from Chapter 3, a disorder of fluid and electrolyte imbalance occurs in diabetes insipidus. Compared with diabetes mellitus, diabetes insipidus is uncommon. Therefore, it is acceptable to refer to diabetes mellitus simply as diabetes, since most people will understand that to mean high blood sugar. The word **diabetes** is from the Greek and means "running through." This refers to the copious amount of urine that is produced and passed in this disease. Ancient diagnostic methods relied on the physical senses, which sometimes included taste. Physicians would taste the urine of those experiencing voluminous urine output, or **polyuria**. The glucose, or sugar, in the urine of a diabetic person would make it taste sweet, which is what the word **mellitus** means. In contrast, the urine of a person with diabetes insipidus would be tasteless, or insipid, hence the term **insipidus**. The term "diabetes mellitus" describes a condition in which there is a great amount of _____(1) produced, and the urine contains _____(2).

Definition

····· 8–29 ·····

The pathophysiology of diabetes is described in Frame 8–43. The definition of diabetes is that it is a chronic metabolic disorder of glucose metabolism that also affects protein and fat metabolism. (An abnormal carbohydrate metabolism leads to abnormal fat metabolism, which is responsible for many long-term complications and death.) The metabolic abnormality is due to an absolute or relative lack of insulin. Diabetes mellitus can also be classified as an endocrine disease because insulin is a hormone. Carbohydrates, specifically glucose, are used by cells as the principal source of fuel, or energy. Frame 8–6 explained that insulin is required for glucose to enter some cells. Insulin assists the transport of this molecule across the cell membrane and into the cytoplasm for use. In diabetes, the glucose cannot be used by insulin-dependent tissues because of insufficient or absent insulin from the beta cells of the islets of Langerhans in the pancreas. This is an absolute lack of insulin. A relative lack exists when there is poor or no response to insulin by the targeted cells. (This will be explained in Frame 8–38.) Diabetes is a disorder of _____(1) metabolism because of lack of enough _____(2) or because of poor _____(3) to insulin. Faulty response by cells to insulin is classified as a _____(4) lack of insulin.

8-30

1. carbohydrate
2. insulin
3. response
4. relative

Postprandial hyperglycemia stimulates the release of insulin from the pancreas. Postprandial means after a meal, and hyperglycemia means increased glucose in the bloodstream. After eating, carbohydrates are digested and absorbed in their simplest form, glucose. This elevated amount of "sugar" in the blood is the signal for insulin to be released and perform its work. Postprandial hyperglycemia is normal and temporary in a healthy person. Blood glucose returns to normal after insulin has caused glucose to enter target cells and to be stored in the liver as glycogen. This processing of glucose removes it from the circulation so that the hyperglycemia is resolved. When there is insufficient insulin, there is decreased entry of glucose into the cells that rely on insulin. (Recall from Frame 8–6 that insulin-dependent tissues include muscle and fat.) There is also decreased conversion into glycogen for storage in the liver. Therefore, much glucose remains in the circulation, producing the hyperglycemia, or high blood sugar, found in diabetes. A normal blood glucose value is about 80 to 120 mg/dL. In diabetes, this figure may hover around 600 or run as high as 1200 mg/dL. The stimulating factor for insulin release from the pancreas is _____(1). This is an increase in the blood _____(2) level that normally follows a _____(3). Return to a normal blood glucose value is a result of _____(4) entering _____(5)-dependent cells and of glucose being stored by the liver as _____(6). Hyperglycemia is not a temporary situation in a diabetic because _____(7) is not present in sufficient amounts, or else dependent cells do not _____(8) appropriately.

8-31

1. postprandial hyperglycemia
2. glucose
3. meal
4. glucose
5. insulin
6. glycogen
7. insulin
8. respond

The kidneys make urine by first producing a filtrate that has a composition similar to blood. Most of the substances in the filtrate are absorbed back into the circulation because they are not waste and are needed. The kidneys resorb, or reabsorb, glucose from the filtrate. The urine of a healthy individual contains no glucose. The amount of glucose that the kidneys are able to save from the filtrate is called the **renal threshold.** When the circulation is in a state of pathologic hyperglycemia, this threshold is surpassed. There is more glucose in the filtrate than the kidneys can retain, so the remainder passes out in the urine. This is also called "spilling over." The renal threshold for glucose is about 170 mg/dL. A blood glucose value exceeding that figure will result in the presence of glucose in the urine. Glucose in the urine is called **glucosuria.** This is very helpful in diagnosis and in monitoring the treatment of a diabetic. Glucose in the urine of a diabetic results from the amount of glucose in the _____(1), which is greater than the _____(2) can resorb. The excess glucose that is not returned to the blood "_____(3) over" into the urine. The point at which the kidneys cannot retain all of the glucose from the filtrate is called the _____(4). Glucose in the urine is called _____(5).

1. filtrate
2. kidneys
3. spills
4. renal threshold
5. glucosuria

Classifications

8-32

The development of diabetes has been theoretically proposed to consist of several stages. First is the **potential diabetic.** This is someone who is asymptomatic for any of the signs of diabetes, who has a normal fasting blood glucose value; a slightly abnormal glucose tolerance test, or GTT (Frame 8–61); and whose blood glucose is slow to return to normal after eating. The **latent diabetic** has a normal fasting blood glucose and a normal GTT but develops persistent hyperglycemia under physical stress. These stressors include illness and pregnancy. The hyperglycemia resolves with the removal of the stress, but these individuals should be monitored for clinical diabetes. The **prediabetic** has normal test values but is considered at risk genetically because a relative has diabetes. **Overt,** or **clinical diabetes,** is found in a person with an abnormally high fasting blood glucose, an abnormal GTT, glucosuria, and the signs presented in Frame 8–50.

8–33

Diabetes mellitus can be either a severe disorder or a mild one. It may or may not be associated with lifestyle. It can be primary or secondary. Primary diabetes is not caused by some additional disease but is the disease itself. Secondary diabetes *is* caused by another disease. Disorders of the pancreas or of the endocrine system can produce diabetes. Primary diabetes is divided into two types. **Type I diabetes mellitus** is also called **insulin-dependent diabetes mellitus (IDDM)** and **juvenile-onset diabetes mellitus.** IDDM has an acute or sudden onset and strikes people less than 30 years old. This type of diabetes is severe and may cause death directly. A fatal coma can develop rather quickly in those with IDDM who are not undergoing treatment. Coma and death result from ketoacidosis (Frame 8–52). IDDM requires daily injections of insulin and can be challenging to regulate.

8–34

Type II diabetes mellitus is also called **non–insulin-dependent diabetes mellitus (NIDDM)** and **adult-onset diabetes mellitus.** NIDDM has an insidious, or slow and unnoticed, onset. It affects those over 40 and is seen more often in women than in men. Adult-onset diabetes is much more common than juvenile-onset diabetes. NIDDM often has mild signs. Occasionally, it may be detected only during a routine physical exam and health screening. Only a few cases of NIDDM require insulin therapy. The majority are more easily managed with diet, exercise, and weight loss. It is interesting to note that obesity often accompanies NIDDM. It is thought that a diet high in calories for many years causes overstimulation of the pancreas and eventual "burnout." The two types of primary diabetes mellitus are compared in Table 8–2.

8–35

1. insulin-dependent diabetes mellitus
2. I
3. juvenile
4. severe
5. coma
6. death
7. insulin
8. suddenly
9. 30
10. non–insulin-dependent diabetes mellitus
11. not
12. mild
13. insidious or slow
14. 40
15. obesity

IDDM is an acronym for _____(1). It is also known as type _____(2) diabetes and _____(3)-onset diabetes. The signs and effects of this type are _____(4) and will lead to _____(5) and _____(6) if it is not treated. Treatment requires injections of _____(7). Type I diabetes develops _____(8) and affects those under _____(9) years of age. Type II is also called _____(10) or NIDDM. It usually does _____(11) require insulin because the signs are relatively _____(12) compared to IDDM. The onset of type II diabetes is _____(13), and it is seen in people over _____(14). Type II diabetes is associated with excess weight, or _____(15).

TABLE 8–2. A COMPARISON OF INSULIN-DEPENDENT DIABETES MELLITUS AND NON–INSULIN-DEPENDENT DIABETES MELLITUS

Insulin-Dependent Diabetes Mellitus (IDDM) (Type I or Juvenile Onset)	Non–insulin-Dependent Diabetes Mellitus (NIDDM) (Type II or Adult Onset)
Acute onset	Slow onset
Younger than 30 years	Older than 40 years
Less common	More common
Severe (ketoacidosis, coma, and death)	Mild to moderate
Requires insulin administration	Usually does not require insulin administration

Etiology

8-36

The causes of diabetes are varied and complex. They are not well understood. There are several factors involved, and the cause is not simply a deficiency of insulin or a lack of response to it. This is shown by the levels of insulin that can be present in a diabetic. Sometimes the levels are normal or even elevated. Also, the dosages of exogenous insulin that are needed in some treatment regimes support the concept of varied causes.

8-37

There are several activities that are responsible for creating normal amounts of insulin in the circulation. Insulin must first be synthesized or made by the beta cells in the islets of Langerhans. It must be properly stored and then released as needed. It must be taken up, or bound, by the cells that need insulin to obtain glucose, and it must be properly activated. High blood glucose can result from an abnormality in any of these activities. Such abnormalities could be decreased or no synthesis by injured beta cells, synthesis of faulty insulin, impairment of the secretion of insulin, or lack of response by target cells where the binding of insulin to receptors doesn't take place as it should. Diabetes can result from an abnormality in any of the activities that produce normal amounts of _____(1) in the _____(2). These activities include making insulin, or _____(3); its release, or _____(4); and cellular uptake, or _____(5), of insulin to _____(6).

1. insulin
2. beta cells
3. synthesis
4. secretion
5. binding
6. receptors

8-38

The lack of or poor response to insulin by target tissues is called **insulin resistance.** This is often the case in diabetes where a normal dose of insulin does not lower the blood glucose as expected. Higher doses are needed in these cases. The reasons for this may include defective cell membrane receptors or autoantibodies to insulin that render it ineffective. Autoantibodies to insulin are believed to have a genetic component. Tissues or cells that do not respond to insulin are also called **refractory,** or nonresponsive. Cells that do not bind and respond to insulin are described as having _____(1).

1. insulin resistance

8-39

Type I diabetes, or IDDM, is suspected to have a strong genetic link. Specific HLA haplotypes are present in affected individuals. (Recall from Chapter 4 that HLA are human leukocyte antigens, and a haplotype is the set of specific antigens that are present.) It is believed that the haplotypes may be coded for by the same genes that produce this disease. However, IDDM is not considered strictly hereditary because identical twins usually are not both affected. It could also be that this genetic makeup is very susceptible to certain viral infections that destroy the islet cells. Another theory is that individuals with these haplotypes are predisposed to form autoantibodies against the beta cells. In this case, certain viruses or other agents act as a triggering event to cause the production of anti-insulin antibodies. You can see then how the activities of insulin production may be normal, its amount in the blood may be normal, and target cell response may be normal. However, if the circulating insulin is destroyed by antibodies, diabetes will result. The genetic basis for IDDM lies in specific _____(1) of affected individuals. Because of genetics, these individuals may be predisposed to beta cell injury by some _____(2) infections. Also, they may form _____(3) against insulin following some viral infections.

1. HLA haplotypes
2. viral
3. autoantibodies

8-40

In IDDM, the histology of the pancreas, or microscopic picture of the tissue, reveals degeneration of the islet cells. This degeneration could be caused by viral injury or autoantibody destruction. Anti-insulin antibodies have been identified in the serum of IDDM patients. In addition to degeneration, there is infiltration by lymphocytes. Such an infiltration would accompany either a viral or antibody attack. Obviously, destruction of the cells results in decreased or no insulin, depending on the degree of injury. To summarize the potential causes of IDDM, there is an *absolute* deficiency of insulin because of a decrease in the number of beta cells. This decrease is most likely due to injury by a viral infection and subsequent attack by autoantibodies. Genetic makeup predisposes a person to a susceptibility to these injuries. In IDDM, microscopic examination shows _____(1) of the

1. degeneration

2. islet or beta
3. lymphocytes
4. virus
5. antibody or autoantibody

_____(2) cells. This injury is accompanied by an infiltration with _____(3). Such an infiltration is consistent with injury by either a _____(4) or a (an) _____(5).

8-41

Type II diabetes, or NIDDM, is familial, or tends to occur in families. It was presented in Chapter 7 as a multifactorial disease. It is believed to have a genetic predisposition, although no specific genes or antigen haplotypes have been associated with it. This predisposition likely combines with elements such as diet, weight, exercise, and other lifestyle or environmental factors. There is some debate as to whether NIDDM is an acquired condition or is genetically preprogrammed. Pancreatic histology in NIDDM is normal, and there is a normal number of beta cells. It stands to reason that there is normal production of insulin. Insulin levels in type II patients are often normal. Type II diabetes is likely due to a *relative* deficiency of insulin because of faulty secretion or insulin resistance by cells. Conditions such as obesity and pregnancy may stress glucose metabolism to the point of type II diabetes. Both types I and II have genetic and nongenetic factors. Neither is a simple Mendelian-type inheritance.

8-42

1. diet
2. weight
3. exercise
4. normal
5. normal
6. insulin resistance

In NIDDM, genetics may play a part, but other factors have a hand in its cause. These factors include _____(1), _____(2), and _____(3). The beta cells appear to be _____(4), so amounts of insulin may also be _____(5). Lack of cellular response or _____(6) is likely. Diabetes mellitus can also be a secondary condition. Anything that interferes with pancreatic function or glucose metabolism can lead to hyperglycemia, which partly defines diabetes. Disorders that can produce secondary diabetes are included in the following list.

1. Pancreatitis, in which inflammation destroys the glandular tissue, including the islet cells.
2. Pancreatic neoplasia, in which cancer destroys the tissue.
3. Cushing's disease, in which high levels of the steroid cortisol both raises blood glucose and lowers cellular response to insulin.
4. Drug therapy, in which steroids, diuretics, or antihypertensives interfere with glucose metabolism.
5. Genetic hyperlipidemia, in which abnormal lipid or fat metabolism is detrimental to glucose metabolism.

The possible causes of both IDDM and NIDDM are summarized in Table 8–3.

TABLE 8–3. POSSIBLE CAUSES OF DIABETES MELLITUS

Insulin-Dependent Diabetes Mellitus	Non–insulin-Dependent Diabetes Mellitus
Genetic predisposition	Genetic predisposition
Viral infection of pancreatic islet cells	Diet (high in calories)
Autoantibody against beta cells	Obesity
	Lack of exercise
	Insulin resistance (related to diet and obesity)
	Primary diseases
	Pancreatitis
	Pancreatic cancer
	Cushing's disease
	Hyperlipidemia

Pathogenesis

The deranged carbohydrate metabolism of diabetes is responsible for abnormal protein and fat metabolism. Proteins and fats are turned to for fuel, but with damaging effects. It is abnormality in fat metabolism that leads to many of the complications of diabetes, as well as the early demise of an untreated patient. Diabetes can be seen as a loss of glucose homeostasis. The pathogenesis we are about to discuss applies to type I diabetes, or IDDM, since this is the severe form of the disease. An overview is presented in Figure 8–3. In diabetes, abnormal carbohydrate metabolism also causes difficulty in _____(1) and _____(2) metabolism. The complications and possible death in diabetes are directly related to abnormal _____(3) metabolism.

8–43

1. protein
2. fat
3. fat

8–44

When insulin levels are low, there is low or decreased uptake of glucose by cells. There then becomes a deficiency of glucose inside cells. This occurs while there is hyperglycemia even in the fasting state. In other words, even when blood glucose is high, it is low inside the cells. In essence, the cells receive the message that the body is starving. If there is insufficient nutrition for the cells, in spite of hyperglycemia, then the body reacts accordingly. The cells don't "know" there is plenty of glucose or nutrition. The cells are starving in a sea of glucose. Since insulin also assists with glycogen storage in the liver, this process is also insufficient. This further contributes to glucose remaining in the circulation and being lost in

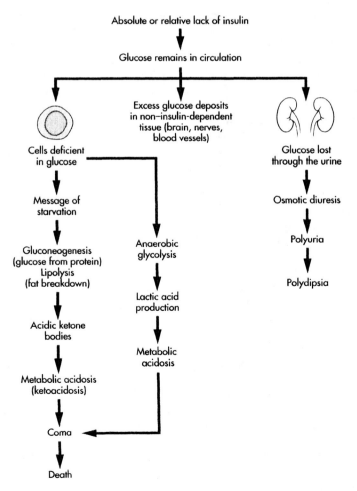

Figure 8–3. The pathogenesis of severe insulin-dependent diabetes mellitus.

1. glucose
2. cells
3. membranes
4. starving
5. glycogen
6. liver

the urine. In cases of insufficient insulin, there develops an insufficiency of _____(1) inside _____(2). [Remember, insulin is required for many cells to transport insulin through cell _____(3).] An intracellular deficiency of glucose sends the message that the body is _____(4). Hyperglycemia is further aggravated by the decrease in glucose storage in the form of _____(5) in the _____(6).

······ 8—45 ······

1. polyuria
2. diuresis
3. pull or attract
4. urine
5. thirst
6. polydipsia

Hyperglycemia causes osmotic diuresis. You learned the concepts of osmosis in Chapter 3. Diuresis is increased or excessive water loss in the form of urine. The many molecules of glucose in the kidney tubules pull water with them as the urine is formed. Increased loss of body water through the urine is **polyuria.** Polyuria naturally creates some degree of dehydration and therefore thirst. To relieve this thirst, the individual drinks more water than normal. Increased thirst is **polydipsia,** and excessive drinking is the visible result of polydipsia. A prominent manifestation of diabetes is excessive urination, or _____(1). This develops because hyperglycemia has an osmotic _____(2) effect on body water. This means that the glucose molecules _____(3) water with them as they pass from the body in the _____(4). Polyuria causes dehydration and _____(5). This is compensated for by drinking more, and this manifestation is called _____(6).

······ 8—46 ······

Because of the message of starvation, the body looks to other forms of nutrition for energy production. Protein is broken down and amino acids converted to glucose in the process gluconeogenesis. (Remember that "neo" means new and "genesis" is to create.) This use of proteins for food causes wasting of the skeletal muscle. A very significant result of the intracellular starvation is the onset of **lipolysis,** or fat breakdown. Normally, fat breakdown produces acetyl coenzyme A that enters the Krebs cycle. In IDDM, there is overwhelming lipolysis. Excessive fatty acids make their way through the liver and are eventually converted to **ketone bodies.** The ketones are beta hydroxybutyrate, acetoacetate, and acetone. Ketone bodies are very acidic compounds that represent a detour in normal fat conversion. The presence of excessive ketones in the blood is **hyperketonemia.** As in hyperglycemia, ketones are also lost in the urine, and this is known as **ketonuria.** Ketonuria is helpful in diagnosis and monitoring the treatment of a diabetic. Hyperketonemia causes the blood to be acidic. This acidosis is specifically known as **ketoacidosis,** or **ketosis.** This type of metabolic acidosis (see Chap. 3) can be directly responsible for coma and death.

······ 8—47 ······

1. gluconeogenesis
2. lipolysis
3. ketones
4. acidic or acids
5. ketoacidosis
6. ketosis
7. ketonuria
8. pH

Conversion of protein to glucose for use as food energy is called _____(1). Breakdown of fats for the same purpose is _____(2). Extreme lipolysis overwhelms normal metabolic pathways, and compounds called _____(3) are produced. The chemical characteristic of ketones is that they are _____(4). These acid compounds then cause acidosis of the blood, and this is described as _____(5), or _____(6). The presence of ketones in the urine is called _____(7). The metabolic acidosis of an IDDM diabetic is worsened by anaerobic glycolysis, to which the cells resort during periods of diabetic crisis. You know from physiology that anaerobic glycolysis creates lactic acid as a by-product. Lactic acid combines with the effects of ketones to result in life-threatening metabolic acidosis. Recall from Chapter 3 the direct toxic effects that acidosis has on the brain. Acidosis is the state of the _____(8) of the blood being lower than normal. Coma and death accompany untreated ketoacidosis.

······ 8—48 ······

Furthermore, the brain is non–insulin-dependent tissue, along with peripheral nerves, blood vessels, and the ocular lens. Insulin is not needed for glucose to enter the cells of these tissues. Hyperglycemia leads to excessive glucose deposits in these cells. The additional glucose is metabolized in an abnormal fashion into compounds with additional toxic effects. They are also osmotic and pull fluid into the cells, causing swelling and intracellular damage.

8-49

In type II diabetes, or NIDDM, insulin may be low or, more commonly, normal to increased. (The increase can be a result of attempted compensation.) Compared to the histologic picture of IDDM (islet destruction, fewer beta cells, fibrosis, and cellular infiltration), the pancreatic islets look fairly normal and healthy. Because of normal levels of insulin and normal-appearing islets, it appears that insulin resistance is a major factor in the development of NIDDM. This resistance by some tissues has been linked to obesity. There may be some genetic preprogramming, wherein the receptors on cell membranes become nonresponsive to insulin over time. An obese person has likely consumed many meals and calories, followed by postprandial hyperglycemia. Postprandial hyperglycemia is the stimulation for the release of _____(1). After a long while, the receptors may become "burned out" and less responsive to frequent and prolonged insulin secretion. Since there is little lipolysis that accompanies NIDDM, ketosis and coma do not occur. In NIDDM, insulin levels may be _____(2) or even _____(3). The islets of Langerhans in the pancreas appear _____(4). The defect is thought to be an insulin _____(5) exhibited by some tissues. A decreased response by cell membrane receptors may be linked to _____(6).

1. insulin
2. normal
3. increased
4. normal
5. resistance
6. obesity

Signs and Symptoms

8-50

NIDDM is often subclinical and may be found during a routine health screening. Even though it is not as severe, NIDDM is not to be taken lightly and should be managed well to avoid worsening of the disease. (You will understand the meaning of this when we discuss the complications of diabetes.) Since there is a cause-and-effect relationship among some of the signs and symptoms of diabetes, they are presented here in order of development.

1. urine

1. *Hypoinsulinemia* (inadequate insulin in the blood) or *insulin resistance* allows excessive glucose to remain in the circulation, which is the state of hyperglycemia.
2. *Hyperglycemia,* detectable by blood testing, is responsible for glycosuria.
3. *Glycosuria* means glucose in the _____(1). This makes the urine sticky, and the glucose, or "sugar," is easily demonstrated by a dipstick test. *Ketonuria,* or ketones in the urine, may be demonstrated in the case of IDDM. Passing glucose in the urine causes polyuria.
4. *Polyuria* is due to osmotic diuresis. The copious urine production of a diabetic is usually pale or like water. Polyuria leads to dehydration and therefore polydipsia.
5. *Polydipsia* causes increased drinking to relieve thirst. Polydipsia is a compensatory mechanism for polyuria.
6. Hypoinsulinemia and hyperglycemia are also responsible for *polyphagia,* which is increased appetite and food intake. Polyphagia develops because of the message of starvation the cells are receiving. A boost in caloric intake is the natural response. This is more often associated with IDDM. Along with polyphagia is weight loss.
7. *Weight loss* occurs in spite of accelerated eating. Unable to use glucose as fuel or nourishment, proteins and fats are broken down and used, causing weight loss. This also accompanies IDDM.
8. Hyperglycemia causes the tissue levels of glucose to be high, which greatly increases the incidence of *infections* in the diabetic. Bacteria thrive on the store of glucose in the tissues. These conditions make excellent culture media for bacterial growth. Abnormal protein metabolism in the diabetic creates *poor wound healing.*

8-51

1. increased appetite
2. glucose in the urine
3. excessive urination
4. decreased insulin in the blood
5. increased glucose in the blood
6. ketones in the urine
7. increased thirst and therefore drinking
8. weight loss
9. infection

Write the definitions for the signs and symptoms of diabetes mellitus.

1. Polyphagia _____
2. Glucosuria _____
3. Polyuria _____
4. Hypoinsulinemia _____
5. Hyperglycemia _____
6. Ketonuria _____
7. Polydipsia _____

Excessive protein and fat breakdown results in _____(8). High levels of glucose in the tissues increase the chances of _____(9).

8-52

1. type I
2. coma
3. Kussmaul breathing
4. deep

A crisis occurring in IDDM only is *ketoacidosis,* or *ketosis.* Ketoacidosis is a life-threatening event. It is the end result of continued lipolysis. Remember that fatty acids are converted to acidic ketone bodies. These acids lower the pH of the blood far below normal, to the point of death. If the pH of the circulation falls to 6.9 or less, coma will result and death ensue if the patient is not treated immediately and aggressively. A prominent sign that precedes a diabetic coma is **Kussmaul breathing,** which has been called air hunger. If you will remember from Chapter 3, the effect of acidosis on the brain is to stimulate the respiratory center to deepen respirations. This is a compensatory attempt to blow off some of the acid in the form of carbon dioxide. An IDDM diabetic exhibiting these deep respirations should be considered acidotic and treated immediately. Ketoacidosis occurs in _____(1) diabetes mellitus. Untreated, this condition results in _____(2). A visible warning sign of acidotic coma is air hunger, or _____(3). The patient's respirations will be _____(4).

Complications

8-53

The complications of diabetes may be seen in both types, but they are more serious and life threatening in IDDM because of the degree of pathology in that type. These secondary disorders are prominent in uncontrolled cases of diabetes or in those not controlled well enough. There are three important events to remember when considering these complications. They are summarized in the following list.

1. It all begins with **lipolysis,** which creates excessive fatty compounds, including cholesterol, that circulate in the blood.
2. High levels of fats in the blood lead to premature **atherosclerosis.** "Ather" refers to yellow, fatty plaques, and "sclerosis" is hardening. Circulating fat is deposited along vessel walls, causing buildup and hardening of the vessels. This damages the vessels. The deposits narrow the lumen of the vessel and interfere with the passage of blood.
3. Abnormality in carbohydrate metabolism causes swelling of the basement membrane of cells, including the endothelium of blood vessels. Combined with atherosclerosis, this results in pathology or disease of the blood vessels. The smaller vessels especially are injured. The term that describes the vessel damage is **microangiopathy.** Since all tissues and organs rely on the vessels to supply blood and oxygen, microangiopathy causes secondary injury to organs and tissues because of ischemia. Obstruction of vessels and ischemia produce tissue and organ necrosis. The signs of diabetic complications manifest when tissues and organs lose function because of ischemia and necrosis.

The basis for complications in diabetes begins with _____(1). This process creates high levels of _____(2) in the _____(3). These substances deposit along vessel walls, causing _____(4). This injures the vessels and interferes with _____(5) passage. The processes that lead to disease of the blood vessels, especially of the small ones, create a pathology called _____(6). Organs and tissues suffer inadequate blood supply, or _____(7), and necrosis because of microangiopathy. Ischemia and necrosis cause organs to cease their _____(8).

8-54

1. lipolysis
2. fatty acids
3. blood
4. atherosclerosis
5. blood
6. microangiopathy
7. ischemia
8. function

8-55

The *acute* complications of diabetes mellitus are the lethal wide swings in pH that accompany ketoacidosis in IDDM and produce coma and death. In NIDDM, **nonketogenic coma** is possible in cases of extreme osmotic diuresis. Loss of too much water, sodium, and other electrolytes produces hyponatremia and hypovolemic shock (see Chap. 3). Seizures, coma, and death are potential outcomes.

8-56

Keeping in mind the initiating factors of microangiopathy, ischemia, and necrosis, the *chronic* complications of diabetes mellitus affect the following body parts.

1. Brain, in which stroke or bleeding occurs when diseased vessels disintegrate.
2. Peripheral nerves, in which neuropathy causes loss of sensation and motor function.
3. Heart, in which atherosclerotic coronary artery disease causes myocardial infarction or heart attack. Occlusion or blockage of the coronary arteries is a common cause of death in diabetes.
4. Eyes, in which retinal hemorrhage and detachment lead to blindness. Diabetic retinopathy is the leading cause of blindness. Vision-obscuring cataracts are also formed because of abnormal carbohydrate metabolism. Unusual products of this metabolism include sorbitol and fructose that are deposited in the lens. They are osmotic compounds and cause swelling of the lens.
5. Kidneys, in which the glomeruli become sclerotic, or hardened (glomerulopathy), papillary tissue experiences necrosis, and renal failure results.
6. General tissues, in which infections and gangrene are common. Gangrene is the result of occlusion, or blockage, of blood flow to the extremities because of atherosclerosis. (Remember that atherosclerotic buildup narrows the lumens of vessels.)

The complications of diabetes mellitus are shown in Figure 8–4.

8-57

For each organ or tissue listed, cite the *end result* or sign of diabetic complication.

1. Heart _____
2. Eyes _____
3. Brain _____
4. Nerves _____
5. Kidneys _____
6. Tissues _____

1. heart attack
2. blindness
3. stroke
4. loss of sensation and motor function
5. renal failure
6. infections and gangrene

Diabetic Coma and Insulin Shock

8-58

The **diabetic coma** that is a result of ketotic acidosis can be triggered by skipping an insulin treatment, not taking enough insulin, too much food, or severe physical or emotional stress. In cases of extreme hyperglycemia, polyuria leads to dehydration, and lipolysis leads to acidosis. Intense polydipsia results to relieve the dehydration. The mouth and skin are very dry. Nausea, vomiting, and lethargy precede a lapse into a coma. The patient in a diabetic coma has a sweet or fruity odor to the breath because of the presence of the ketones. Respiratory compensation for acidosis causes deep respirations, or Kussmaul breathing. The emergency

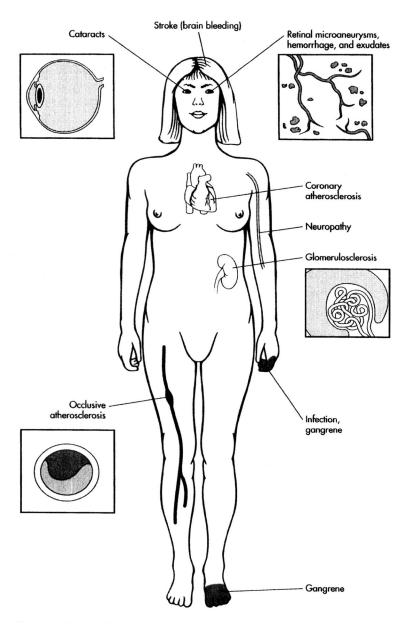

Figure 8–4. The complications of diabetes mellitus. *(Adapted from Damjanov,* Pathology for the Health-Related Professions, *Saunders.)*

treatment of the unconscious patient must include sufficient insulin to lower the blood glucose, IV fluids and electrolytes to combat the losses in polyuria, and sodium bicarbonate to correct the acidosis.

8–59

The *opposite* of diabetic coma is **insulin shock,** or **hypoglycemic shock.** This is caused by too much insulin, too little food, or extreme exercise. Since insulin lowers blood glucose, too much causes hypoglycemia. The central nervous system is as sensitive to hypoglycemia as it is to acidosis. (Remember that the brain relies primarily on glucose, not alternative nutrients, to function.) Patients going into insulin shock feel shaky and faint, sweat, and have slurred speech and blurred vision before they lose consciousness. Insulin shock looks like a diabetic coma. The important differences are that there is no ketotic breath; breathing is shallow, not deep; and the skin is sweaty instead of very dry. Glucose must be administered immediately. In early cases, ingestion of sugar in the form of candy or orange juice may be sufficient. Later cases require intravenous injection of glucose. In both cases, STAT, or immediate, blood glucose levels should be performed to determine the cause of unconsciousness. It is very important to distinguish the two because the treatments are exact opposites. Reversing the treatments will surely mean death.

8-60

An unconscious diabetic with dry skin, fruity breath, and deep respirations is most likely experiencing _____(1). This is caused by insufficient _____(2) or too much _____(3), which causes extreme _____(4). Polyuria produces _____(5), and lipolysis creates _____(6). The primary treatment is to give _____(7). An unconscious diabetic who is sweaty, with odorless and shallow breathing, is probably experiencing _____(8). The cause of this is too much _____(9) or not enough _____(10). This creates low blood sugar, or _____(11). The _____(12) cannot function during severe hypoglycemia. The treatment for this case is to administer _____(13) in some form.

1. diabetic coma
2. insulin
3. food
4. hyperglycemia
5. dehydration
6. acidosis
7. insulin
8. insulin or hypoglycemic shock
9. insulin
10. food
11. hypoglycemia
12. brain
13. glucose

▶ HYPOGLYCEMIA

8-61

Hypoglycemia is defined as low blood glucose, usually below 50 mg/dL. Its onset is usually sudden and it progresses rapidly. The central nervous system, especially the brain, relies acutely on glucose for energy. Inadequate glucose for brain use produces signs and symptoms that are associated with impaired brain function. The signs of this deranged cerebral function include headache, dizziness, weakness, confusion, strange behavior, and seizures. Coma and death result if a severe situation is not treated. The immediate and obvious treatment is to administer sugar in an appropriate form, as discussed in Frame 8–59.

8-62

The causes of hypoglycemia include the following.

1. Insulin shock or insulin overdose, as discussed in Frame 8–59.
2. Addison's disease, an endocrine disease in which there is hyposecretion of steroid hormones from the adrenal cortex. These glucocorticoid hormones assist glucose homeostasis by raising blood glucose when needed. Too little glucocorticoid can allow the glucose levels to fall too low. Addison's disease is treated by hormone replacement therapy.
3. An islet cell tumor, or tumor of the beta cells in particular. These uncommon tumors are generally of the benign type, or are an adenoma. As such, you should remember that they are still differentiated compared to the anaplastic, malignant neoplasia. Therefore, they are functional. They are hormonally active and secrete too much insulin. A benign beta cell tumor causes **hyperinsulinemia.** This would naturally result in a lowering of the blood glucose. This tumor that is composed of an increased number of beta cells may be called an **insulinoma.** The treatment for an insulinoma is effective and curative. Being benign and therefore encapsulated, this small, well-defined mass easily shells out during surgery.

8-63

Blood glucose less than 50 mg/dL defines _____(1). The signs and symptoms are all related to _____(2) function. Untreated severe hypoglycemia will result in _____(3). Causes of hypoglycemia include insulin _____(4) and the steroid insufficiency caused by _____(5). A tumor that occurs in the _____(6) cells of the pancreatic islets is usually the _____(7) type. Therefore, it is fairly differentiated and able to _____(8). This function is to secrete insulin, so the condition _____(9) results. This tumor is sometimes

1. hypoglycemia
2. brain or central nervous system
3. coma and death
4. overdose
5. Addison's disease
6. beta
7. benign
8. function
9. hyperinsulinemia

10. insulinoma
11. surgery

referred to as a (an) _____(10), and it is easily removed during _____(11).

III. REVIEW QUESTIONS

1. a–increased; b–sweet;
c–glucose or sugar

2. e–all of the above

3. d–any of the above

4. a–assist glucose through
cell membranes in insulin-
dependent tissues

5. b–return to normal glucose
levels; d–glycogen storage

6. d–postprandial hyper-
glycemia

7. a–the amount of glucose in
the blood is greater than the
renal threshold

1. The Greek term "diabetes mellitus" describes a. _____ urine output, and urine that is b. _____ tasting or has c. _____ in it.

2. Diabetes is a (an):
   a. endocrine disorder
   b. metabolic disorder
   c. carbohydrate metabolism disorder
   d. lipid metabolism disorder
   e. all of the above
   f. none of the above

3. The basis for diabetes mellitus is:
   a. relative lack of insulin
   b. absolute lack of insulin
   c. decreased tissue response to insulin
   d. any of the above
   e. none of the above

4. The function of insulin is to:
   a. assist glucose through cell membranes of insulin-dependent tissues
   b. assist glucose through the Krebs cycle for conversion to ATP
   c. assist glucose through cell membranes of non–insulin-dependent tissues
   d. assist lipolysis and the entry of fatty acids through cell membranes

5. The result of the function of insulin is (choose all that apply):
   a. hyperglycemia
   b. return to normal glucose levels
   c. hypoglycemia
   d. glycogen storage

6. Insulin release is stimulated by:
   a. hyperglycemia
   b. normal glucose levels
   c. hypoglycemia
   d. postprandial hyperglycemia
   e. lipolysis

7. Glucosuria occurs when:
   a. the amount of glucose in the blood is greater than the renal threshold
   b. the amount of ketones in the blood is greater than the renal threshold
   c. the amount of glucose in the blood is less than the renal threshold
   d. polyuria is present

8. Please match the types of diabetes mellitus listed in the left column with their characteristics in the right column:
   a. type I diabetes mellitus
   b. type II diabetes mellitus
   1. ____ adult onset (middle age or older)
   2. ____ insulin dependent (requires replacement therapy)
   3. ____ tissue resistance
   4. ____ treated with lifestyle management and hypoglycemic drugs
   5. ____ juvenile onset (less than 30)
   6. ____ non–insulin-dependent
   7. ____ ketosis and diabetic coma
   8. ____ less severe disease
   9. ____ IDDM
   10. ____ NIDDM
   11. ____ linked to obesity
   12. ____ relative deficiency of insulin
   13. ____ absolute deficiency of insulin

9. In IDDM, histology of the pancreas reveals (choose all that apply):
   a. degeneration of beta cells
   b. infiltration with macrophages
   c. degeneration of alpha cells
   d. infiltration with lymphocytes
   e. fibrosis
   f. granulomas

10. Lipolysis occurs in diabetes because:
    a. hypoglycemia necessitates the use of fats for alternate energy
    b. glucose is unable to enter insulin-dependent cells so the body reacts to starvation of the cells
    c. hyperglycemia is the stimulation for fat breakdown
    d. none of the above

11. Polyuria is produced because of 1. _____, and the visible response to polyuria is 2. _____.
    a. loss of renal concentration ability
    b. hyperglycemia greater than the renal threshold
    c. dehydration
    d. osmotic diuresis caused by glucose molecules in the pre-urine filtrate
    e. thirst
    f. polydipsia
    g. ketone bodies

12. Number in order the events that could end in diabetic coma:
    a. ____ lipolysis
    b. ____ production of ketone bodies
    c. ____ drop in blood pH
    d. ____ ketoacidosis

13. For the following signs and symptoms of diabetes, write the medical term:
    a. increased urine output _____
    b. increased appetite _____
    c. increased thirst and drinking _____
    d. glucose in the urine _____
    e. ketones in the urine _____

8. 1. b–type II; 2. a–type I; 3. b–type II; 4. b–type II; 5. a–type I; 6. b–type II; 7. a–type I; 8. b–type II; 9. a–type I; 10. b–type II; 11. b–type II; 12. b–type II; 13. a–type I

9. a–degeneration of beta cells; d–infiltration with lymphocytes; e–fibrosis

10. b–glucose is unable to enter insulin-dependent cells so the body reacts to starvation of the cells

11. a. 1–osmotic diuresis caused by glucose molecules in the pre-urine filtrate; 2. f–polydipsia

12. a–1; b–2; c–3; d–4

13. a–polyuria; b–polyphagia; c–polydipsia; d–glucosuria; e–ketonuria

14. b–repeated infection

15. c–a type I diabetic in ketoacidosis

16. a–lipolysis; b–atherosclerosis; c–microangiopathy; d–ischemia; e–necrosis

17. a–blindness; b–heart attack; c–stroke; d–gangrene; e–kidney failure

18. 1. b–insulin shock
    2. a–diabetic coma
    3. a–diabetic coma
    4. a–diabetic coma
    5. b–insulin shock
    6. a–diabetic shock
    7. b–insulin shock
    8. a–diabetic shock
    9. b–insulin shock

19. d–hypoglycemia

14. Increased glucose in the body tissues often results in:
    a. poor wound healing
    b. repeated infection
    c. immune suppression
    d. weight loss

15. Kussmual breathing is seen in:
    a. a type II diabetic in ketoacidosis
    b. a type II diabetic in insulin shock
    c. a type I diabetic in ketoacidosis
    d. a type I diabetic in insulin shock

16. The complications of diabetes are based on five conditions, which are:
    a. fat breakdown, or _____
    b. deposits of fatty plaques along vessel walls, or _____
    c. injury to or disease of the small blood vessels, or _____
    d. decreased blood flow to tissues, or _____
    e. tissue death, or _____

17. The complications of diabetes can produce:
    a. damage to the retina, therefore _____
    b. blockage of the coronary arteries, therefore _____
    c. bleeding in the brain or a _____
    d. blockage of blood flow to the extremities, therefore _____
    e. sclerosis and necrosis in the kidneys, therefore _____

18. Please match the acute complications of diabetes in the left column with their signs and treatments in the left column:
    a. diabetic coma
    b. insulin shock

    1. ____ shallow breathing
    2. ____ hyperglycemia
    3. ____ fruity breath
    4. ____ deep respirations or air hunger
    5. ____ sweaty skin
    6. ____ treat primarily with insulin
    7. ____ hypoglycemia
    8. ____ dry skin
    9. ____ treat with glucose

19. An insulinoma may result in:
    a. hyperglycemia
    b. an absolute lack of insulin
    c. metastasis to the liver
    d. hypoglycemia

IV. NUTRITIONAL DISORDERS ◀ SECTION

▶ MALNUTRITION

·· 8–64 ······

Malnutrition stems from the lack of required elements in the diet. Normal functions of the body suffer because of the insufficiency of resources, and body weight is less than normal. "Normal" is determined by standardized charts used by insurance companies. Normal body weight is determined after taking into account frame build, height, sex, and age. Malnutrition and weight loss will occur if a calorie deficit results from either too little food intake or excessive burning of calories. Some disease processes such as prolonged fever and neoplasia increase catabolism (break down processes) and may produce weight loss. Malnutrition is seen in this country but is a greater problem worldwide. Poverty is a major contributing factor in malnutrition, as are ignorance about proper nutrition and fad diets.

·· 8–65 ······

In children, two conditions of malnutrition may be seen. The first is **marasmus,** which is a total deficit of calories involving the carbohydrates, fats, and proteins. Marasmus is generalized undernourishment. **Kwashiorkor** is malnutrition specifically related to insufficient protein intake. Total caloric intake may be normal, but essential amino acids are missing from the diet. Most commonly, the signs of malnourishment in children manifest as developmental problems since children are in a period of growth. Growth is stunted, bone formation is poor, the onset of puberty is delayed, and mental retardation may be present. Diarrhea, with loss of body water and electrolytes, is a complicating factor. The severely undernourished child is debilitated and therefore very susceptible to infection. In fact, infection is a very common cause of death in these cases. Marasmus is an insufficient number of _____(1) in a child's diet. Kwashiorkor is a deficiency of _____(2). Either condition results in interference in a child's development or _____(3). Debilitation that accompanies malnutrition in children can easily result in death from _____(4).

1. calories
2. protein
3. growth
4. infection

·· 8–66 ······

A malnourished adult will be thin or, in severe cases, be **cachexic** or **emaciated** (extreme loss of weight and flesh to the point of wasting). There is loss of not only adipose tissue, but of muscle as well. Many derangements can stem from severe malnourishment including diarrhea, enlarged liver, polyneuropathy, hormone insufficiency, anemia, vitamin and mineral deficiencies, and infections, to name a few. The cause of *primary* malnutrition is improper intake of nourishment. This is most commonly seen in alcoholism, eating disorders, poverty, and fad diets. It is also seen in cases of increased need for calories because of catabolism associated with fevers and cancer. An adult who has lost so much weight and body tissue that he or she can be described as wasting is either _____(1) or _____(2). Insufficient intake of balanced nourishment is the cause of _____(3) malnutrition.

1. cachexic
2. emaciated
3. primary

·· 8–67 ······

Secondary malnutrition may be caused by a primary disease process. A painful lesion in the throat or esophagus may discourage eating and swallowing. More common are cases of **maldigestion** and **malabsorption** in gastrointestinal disturbances. In maldigestion, there is an error in the digestive process so that digestive enzymes are missing and food cannot be broken down for absorption. In malabsorption, the food has been digested normally but cannot traverse the intestinal lining or is otherwise unable to be consumed by the GI tract. Maldigestion may be due to:

1. A variety of conditions involving the stomach and intestinal tract where there is an insufficiency of digestive substances.
2. Pancreatitis (see Chap. 15), where inflammation of the pancreas interferes with its function of manufacturing and releasing digestive enzymes.

Malabsorption may be due to:

1. Bacterial or viral infection of the intestines, causing injury to the absorptive surfaces of the intestinal lining. The degree and depth of injury depends on the particular infectious agent.
2. Chronic vomiting and/or diarrhea, which do not allow the body time to assimilate nutrients before they are lost from the body.
3. Liver or biliary disease, in which there is insufficient bile present for fat assimilation.

8–68

1. maldigestion
2. malabsorption
3. maldigestion
4. malabsorption
5. maldigestion
6. malabsorption

Two conditions that lead to secondary malnutrition are _____(1) and _____(2). Lack of digestive enzymes causes _____(3). Interference in absorption causes _____(4). Pancreatitis can produce _____(5). Infection and diarrhea can lead to _____(6). The causes of primary and secondary malnutrition are listed in Table 8–4.

▶ STARVATION

8–69

As we talk about the events of starvation, keep in mind that the changes the body goes through are relatively gradual. In any chronic situation, the body adjusts or compensates for the changes up to a point. In an acute situation, there is no time for adjustment or compensation, so the effects are different. Slow changes are one reason why hypoglycemic shock or acute ketoacidosis are usually not features of starvation.

8–70

Starvation is an absolute lack of any type of nourishment. Blood glucose and glycogen stores from the liver last up to 48 hours. Theoretically, fat and protein stores could last about 2 months, but general debilitation or weakening causes many secondary problems that may result in death before these stores are exhausted. In starvation, the kidneys do not concentrate the urine very well, and polyuria results in loss of water and dehydration.

8–71

Early in starvation, after glucose and glycogen stores are gone, triglycerides in adipose tissue are broken down into glycerol and fatty acids. Fatty acids are converted to acetyl coenzyme A for use in the Krebs cycle for ATP or energy production. Ketones are also produced from fat. The liver uses amino acids from protein catabolism to form glucose in gluconeogenesis. This is necessary to provide the central nervous system with a supply of glucose to function. Since the nitrogen from amino acid conversion is not used, it is passed in the urine, causing a negative nitrogen balance, or deficit, in the body. Later, after about 7 to 10 days, the brain has changed its metabolism to be able to use the ketones from fat breakdown. Protein catabolism then slows until all fat stores are used. When these are all gone, the body turns to proteins once again. Muscle mass severely declines, internal organs waste away, and death is imminent.

TABLE 8–4. MALNUTRITION IN ADULTS

Primary Malnutrition	Secondary Malnutrition
Insufficient intake of nourishment	Primary or underlying disease process
Alcoholism	Maldigestion
Eating disorders	Gastric or intestinal disease
Poverty	Pancreatitis
Fad diets	Malabsorption
	Bacterial or viral enteritis
	Chronic vomiting and diarrhea
	Liver or biliary disease

8-72

The order of nutrient use in starvation is presented for review as follows.

1. Blood _____(1) and _____(2) from the liver.
2. Breakdown of adipose, or fat, to ultimately yield _____(3), which enter the Krebs cycle.
3. Catabolism of _____(4) for gluconeogenesis.
4. A decrease in protein breakdown when the brain has converted to using _____(5).
5. Use of the remainder of _____(6) in the body.
6. Use of the remainder of _____(7) in the body.

1. glucose
2. glycogen
3. fatty acids
4. protein
5. ketones
6. fat
7. protein

Lethargy is a feature of starvation because the body greatly decreases its energy output and conserves as much as possible. Loss of insulating fat makes hypothermia a great concern. Infections are prominent since there is decreased protein available for antibody production, and the function of lymphocytes, neutrophils, and macrophages is impaired.

► EATING DISORDERS

8-73

Anorexia nervosa is a disorder of psychogenic origin that creates an obsessive resistance to food. It results in malnutrition, cachexia, and starvation. The majority of cases occur in young females and stem from social pressure for thinness and an "acceptable" body image. The affected individual has an unrealistic view of herself and, in spite of extreme thinness, sees herself as overweight. This view is extremely real to the patient and strictly governs her eating habits. Anorexia nervosa begins as a weight loss diet and becomes a denial of malnutrition. The patient is literally starving but has lost the ability to eat. Related behavior changes include irritability, moderate to severe depression, and hostility toward those who would help her. This hostility is not unlike that seen with alcoholics and drug dependents who resist assistance. Anorexia nervosa is a disorder originating in the psyche, or _____(1), of a young female, and she strongly _____(2) food. The basis for the disorder is a body _____(3) that is unrealistic. The anorexic sees herself as _____(4) in spite of _____(5). Results of anorexia nervosa are _____(6) and _____(7). _____(8) changes also accompany this disorder.

1. mind
2. resists
3. image
4. overweight
5. extreme thinness
6. malnutrition
7. starvation
8. Behavior

8-74

The patterns of a patient with anorexia nervosa are to eat very few low-fat foods (mainly fruits and vegetables), to self-purge with vomiting and laxatives if she does give in to hunger or is forced to eat, and to exercise obsessively to increase weight loss. Her appearance becomes emaciated as she wastes away. An example of the emaciation is seen in Figure 8–5. **Amenorrhea,** or absence of menstruation, accompanies starvation. Physical examination will reveal low blood pressure and heart rate, anemia, dehydration, and electrolyte imbalances that can affect the heart. Debilitation and decreased resistance to infection pave the way for secondary disease. Getting the patient to break out of these patterns and eat well at home is almost impossible. Treatment usually requires hospitalization.

8-75

If a patient is hospitalized, **hyperalimentation,** or aggressive nutritional support, is required to prevent death. Feeding tubes are generally used, along with intravenous replacement of fluids and electrolytes. Of great importance is psychological therapy to address the compulsion for thinness. The prognosis for anorexia nervosa is guarded, as it has a significant mortality rate. An individual bent on starvation cannot be nutritionally forced for long. The origin of this aversion to food must be uncovered and resolved. Relapses after therapy are common. Death from starvation, or suicide because of depression, represent a common end to this disorder. Two treatment regimes for anorexia nervosa are _____(1) and _____(2). The probable outcome is _____(3) because many cases end in _____(4).

1. hyperalimentation
2. psychological therapy
3. guarded
4. death

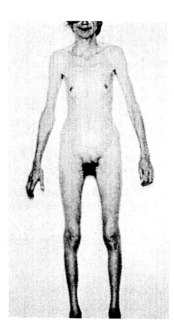

Figure 8–5. Anorexia nervosa. *(From Chandrasoma,* Concise Pathology, *2nd ed, Appleton & Lange.)*

8–76

1. psychogenic
2. weight
3. depressed
4. large
5. purge
6. calories

Bulimia is also an eating disorder affecting females, with psychogenic origins that stem from social pressure for a particular body image. It is similar to anorexia nervosa in that the goal is to avoid obesity and lose weight. Depression is also a feature of bulimia. It is unlike anorexia nervosa in that the individual goes through a binge-and-purge cycle. She will eat large quantities of food in a short period of time. A binge can be triggered by stress or have other emotional triggers. The bulimic will gorge on food to satisfy a variety of desires. But the binge is followed by self-induced vomiting and laxatives to purge, or rid, herself of the calories before they are absorbed. Diuretics are used to speed water loss and therefore some weight loss. Since the bulimic has periods of regular eating, she will have a relatively normal appearance, and the condition may go undetected until the effects of purging begin to surface. Bulimia is like anorexia nervosa because the origins are also _____(1), the goal is _____(2) loss, and the patient may be _____(3). However, the difference is that the bulimic will eat _____(4) amounts of food, then _____(5) herself through vomiting and laxatives. The purging techniques allow bingeing on food without absorbing the _____(6).

8–77

1. purging
2. teeth
3. esophagus
4. dehydration
5. electrolytes
6. acid–base
7. stomach
8. heart

The purging techniques have many ill and possibly fatal effects. Chronic vomiting, because of stomach hydrochloric acid, causes esophagitis and tooth decay. Loss of hydrogen, chloride, and sodium creates electrolyte and acid–base imbalance. Dehydration is also a feature. Violent contractions can cause rupture of the stomach, an immediate cause of death. Laxatives and diuretics contribute to dehydration and electrolyte imbalance. Upset in body water and electrolytes have detrimental effects on the heart, possibly leading to heart failure. In contrast to death by starvation in anorexia nervosa, bulimia can be fatal because of the effects of _____(1). Decay of the _____(2), inflammation of the _____(3), insufficient body water or _____(4), and imbalances in _____(5) and _____(6) are side effects of chronic vomiting, laxatives, and diuretics. Fatal results are rupture of the _____(7) and _____(8) failure. Treatment of the bulimic is mainly psychological therapy and antidepressants. This is a condition that often is not cured but must be managed over a lifetime.

▶ OBESITY

8-78

Obesity is defined as having a body weight greater than 20 percent above the average ideal weight, based on height, frame build, and age. These standards are usually set by life insurance companies who have tables of such statistics. It is estimated that in the United States about 20 percent of males and 40 percent of females are overweight to the point of being obese. Adipose tissue is located under the skin of most body parts, around organs, and in the omentum of the peritoneal cavity. It functions as an energy reserve that was vital to life in primitive times. Fat provides insulation and helps retain body heat. It also serves a protective function as padding.

8-79

The amount of adipose tissue in the body was designed to be regulated by the appetite center of the brain. The hypothalamus includes appetite regulation along with its many other homeostatic functions. The "on switch" that initiates eating is called the **feeding center.** Once genuine hunger has been relieved and the need for nourishment has been satisfied, the **satiety center** serves as the "off switch." However, food intake, as we all know, is motivated by many additional factors including stress, emotion, boredom, loneliness, and the sheer pleasure of enjoying good food. Also, today's lifestyle, filled with mechanical conveniences, removes the need for physical expenditure of energy. Life is literally not as hard as it used to be. Many people do not normally exert themselves during the course of the day, and so must make a conscious effort and schedule time to exercise. Combining a relatively sedentary lifestyle with external prompts to eat is a sure path to obesity.

8-80

People who are obese are at least _____(1) percent above the average ideal weight. Adipose tissue functions as a (an) _____(2) reserve, a heat _____(3), and protective _____(4). The urge to eat is under the control of the _____(5) center in the _____(6). The signal to stop eating when needs have been met comes from the _____(7) center.

1. 20
2. energy
3. insulator
4. padding
5. feeding
6. hypothalamus
7. satiety

8-81

There are two recognized types of obesity. In **lifelong obesity,** individuals are overweight as children and throughout puberty and adolescence. The fat is evenly distributed over the trunk and extremities. These individuals have the potential to become grossly overweight. The reason for this condition is **adipose hyperplasia.** The fat cells, or adipocytes, have undergone hyperplasia, or increased their numbers. Those with lifelong obesity have more fat cells than other people. These numbers increase throughout childhood. A genetic component is strongly suspected, since one or both parents may be obese. In addition, children who, for some reason, are always encouraged or prompted to eat may experience a "re-setting" of the hypothalamic satiety center. In lifelong obesity, the adipose tissue has undergone _____(1), which means there is an increase in the _____(2) of fat cells. The fat tends to be _____(3) distributed over the body. Lifelong obesity begins when the individual is still a _____(4).

1. hyperplasia
2. number
3. evenly
4. child

8-82

Adult-onset obesity is much more common and begins between the ages of 20 to 40, and steadily continues. The fat distribution tends to be in central regions. For men this is the upper abdomen, and for women the lower abdomen, hips, and thighs. The number of fat cells is normal, however, they are bulging with extra fat. Losing weight causes these cells to shrink. The reasons for adult-onset obesity include a slowing of metabolism with age. The same caloric intake from one's younger years is now too much and weight gain results. Fewer calories are needed to maintain the basal metabolic rate as we get older. If the physical level of exertion does not increase, weight gain results. Obesity depends on the basic equation of intake being greater then energy expenditure. Avoidance of obesity requires a decrease in intake or a sufficient increase in energy use. In adult-onset obesity, the number of fat cells is

1. normal
2. fat
3. centrally
4. basal metabolic rate
5. decreased
6. increased

_____(1). However, they are distended with _____(2). The fat tends to be _____(3) distributed. Weight gain associated with age is related to a slowing of the _____(4). To compensate, food intake must be _____(5), or physical exertion must be _____(6). The two types of obesity are compared in Table 8–5.

8-83

Hypothyroidism, or disease-based slow metabolism, is frequently blamed for obesity. However, it is not nearly as common as some would think. In addition to naturally slowing metabolism, psychological factors play a major role in obesity in today's society. Food is often used for comfort for a variety of mental stresses. High alcohol intake, another inappropriate coping mechanism, contributes to obesity because of its very high calorie content. Alcohol also decreases the ability to burn fat.

8-84

Listed below are the most significant effects of obesity on one's health. The result is that obesity shortens life expectancy, which is why life insurance companies take such an interest. Obesity can lead to the following physical states.

1. Type II diabetes, or NIDDM. Insulin resistance is a feature. Adipocytes have fewer insulin receptors.
2. Atherosclerosis. High levels of circulating cholesterol create fatty plaque deposits in vessel walls. This not only weakens the vessel, it decreases the lumen, possibly to the point of occlusion. This will result in tissue or organ ischemia and infarct in some cases.
3. Hypertension. The extra body mass increases the workload of the heart, and it must push the blood harder to overcome resistance. Combined with atherosclerosis, high blood pressure leads to stroke or heart disease.
4. Arthritis. Obesity affects the weight-bearing joints that are not designed to bear the additional mass.
5. Hypoventilation. The obese person can have difficulty breathing, and carbon dioxide retention causes lethargy (reluctance to move).
6. Hepatic lipidosis. Abnormal fat metabolism causes it to be deposited in hepatocytes, hence the phrase "fatty liver." This causes an infiltration degeneration that interferes with function.
7. Increased appetite. Adipose cells have a great need for glucose for their metabolism. The obese person truly becomes hypoglycemic and must eat to relieve the symptoms. The adipose tissue represents an extra hungry population of cells that cry to be fed. Satisfying this need creates larger adipocytes in a vicious cycle.

8-85

1. shorten
2. hypertension
3. hepatic lipidosis
4. non–insulin-dependent diabetes
5. atherosclerosis
6. heart

The complications of obesity serve to _____(1) one's life span. This is done through the following.

1. High blood pressure or _____(2).
2. Fatty liver or _____(3).
3. NIDDM or _____(4).
4. Fat deposits in vessels or _____(5).
5. Risk of stroke or _____(6) disease.

TABLE 8–5. A COMPARISON BETWEEN LIFELONG OBESITY AND ADULT-ONSET OBESITY

Lifelong Obesity	Adult-Onset Obesity
Cause	**Cause**
Possible genetic factor	Decrease in basal metabolic rate
Effects	**Effects**
Obesity begins in childhood	Obesity begins in adulthood
Fat evenly distributed over trunk and extremities	Fat centrally distributed
Adipose hyperplasia (increased *numbers* of fat cells)	Adipose hypertrophy (increased *size* of fat cells)

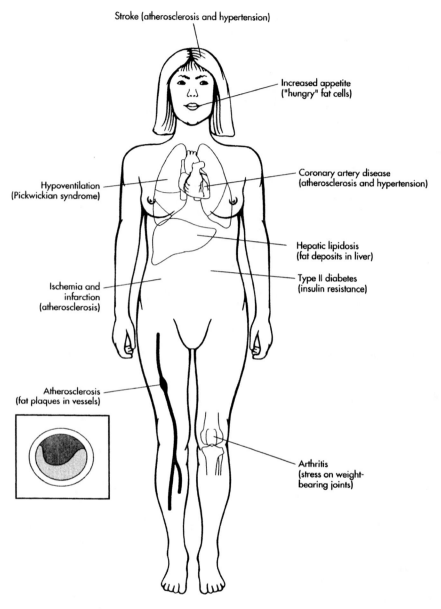

Stroke (atherosclerosis and hypertension)

Increased appetite
("hungry" fat cells)

Hypoventilation
(Pickwickian syndrome)

Coronary artery disease
(atherosclerosis and hypertension)

Hepatic lipidosis
(fat deposits in liver)

Type II diabetes
(insulin resistance)

Ischemia and
infarction
(atherosclerosis)

Atherosclerosis
(fat plaques in vessels)

Arthritis
(stress on weight-
bearing joints)

Figure 8–6. The complications of obesity.

The cycle of obesity is literally fed because _____(7) send strong signals for nourishment, and low blood glucose, or _____(8), can result. Examine Figure 8–6 to visualize the complications of obesity.

7. fat cells or adipocytes
8. hypoglycemia

IV. REVIEW QUESTIONS

1. A malnourished adult who has experienced weight loss to the point of wasting is described as (choose all that apply):
   a. emaciated
   b. anoretic
   c. bulimic
   d. cachexic

1. a–emaciated; d–cachexic

2. b–secondary malnutrition

3. d–ketones

4. a–obsessive resistance to food, depression, and behavior changes

5. b–a normal appearance with some depression

6. a–starvation; b–purging;

7. a–lifelong obesity

8. a–hypertension; e–atherosclerosis

2. Maldigestion and malabsorption cause:
   a. primary malnutrition
   b. secondary malnutrition
   c. starvation
   d. eating disorders

3. During starvation, brain metabolism changes to be able to use:
   a. fatty acids
   b. glucose
   c. proteins
   d. ketones

4. A patient with anorexia nervosa demonstrates:
   a. obsessive resistance to food, depression, and behavior changes
   b. mild resistance to food and normal behavior
   c. excessive intake of food followed by purging
   d. resistance only to high-fat foods, depression, and irritability

5. A patient with bulimia will most likely be seen as having:
   a. an emaciated appearance with some depression
   b. a normal appearance with some depression
   c. an obese appearance and a normal mental attitude
   d. a normal appearance and a normal mental attitude

6. Anorexia nervosa can easily end in death from a. _____, while bulimia is potentially fatal from the side effects of b. _____.

7. Adipose hyperplasia occurs in:
   a. lifelong obesity
   b. adult-onset obesity
   c. marasmus
   d. kwashiorkor

8. In obesity, two conditions that may directly cause a stroke or heart attack are (choose two):
   a. hypertension
   b. arthritis
   c. hypoventilation
   d. type II diabetes
   e. atherosclerosis
   f. hepatic lipidosis

CHAPTER SUMMARY ▶

▶ SECTION II

Inborn errors of metabolism are genetic or congenital disorders involving a specific aspect of the body's metabolic activity. Each such disorder has as its basis a malfunctioning metabolic reaction, referred to as a *biochemical lesion*.

Galactosemia is a condition that results from a deficiency of the enzyme that converts galactose to glucose. The accumulation of unconverted galactose interferes with other metabolic processes, some of which are responsible for normal fetal and neonatal development. *Glucose-6-phosphate dehydrogenase deficiency* is a sex-linked disease that results in an individual's red blood cells being highly susceptible to damage by the oxidizing effects of some drugs. *Phenylketonuria*, a condition in which affected individuals show abnormal brain development, is caused by the lack of the enzyme phenylanine hydroxylase.

Some inborn errors of metabolism are classified as *lysosomal storage diseases* and are characterized by the absence of one of the many lysosomal enzymes. In these diseases, accumulation of the products that would normally be metabolized by the missing enzyme leads to tissue damage. Glycogenosis, Gaucher's disease, mucopolysaccaridosis, and Tay–Sachs disease are examples of lysosomal storage diseases. Another category of disorders, collectively called *glycogen storage diseases,* involves a defect in either the synthesis or the breakdown of glycogen.

In the disease *gout,* excess levels of uric acid are found in the blood (hyperuricemia), leading to episodes of arthritis and possible kidney damage. Gout is classified as primary, which is the actual inborn error of metabolism, or secondary, which is the result of either chronic renal failure or a systemic disease that interferes with normal purine metabolism.

▶ SECTION III

In the nondiabetic individual, the hormone *insulin* is produced by the pancreas in response to an elevated level of glucose in the blood. The insulin then is responsible for the entry of glucose into cells. In individuals with the disease diabetes mellitus, insulin is either not produced or is ineffective, resulting in an elevated level of glucose in the blood (hyperglycemia) and, as the kidneys filter the blood, in the urine (glucosuria).

The development of diabetes may involve several stages. The *potential* diabetic is asymptomatic for the disease, but the blood glucose level is slow to return to normal after eating. The *latent* diabetic develops persistent hyperglycemia under physical stress such as illness or pregnancy. The *prediabetic* is at risk genetically because a relative has the disease. The *overt,* or *clinical,* diabetic shows all the signs and symptoms of the disease.

Diabetes may be classified as primary, where the condition is not caused by another disease, or secondary, in which the diabetes *is* caused by another disease. Primary diabetes is further classified as *type I* (also called insulin-dependent or juvenile-onset) or *type II* (non–insulin-dependent or adult-onset) *diabetes mellitus.* Type I, which has a sudden onset and strikes young people, is the most severe. Type II has a slow onset, generally affects those over 40, is seen more frequently in women, and in only a few cases requires insulin therapy.

The causes of diabetes mellitus are not well understood. Some factors responsible for the disease may be injured beta cells, synthesis of faulty insulin, impairment of the secretion of insulin, or nonresponsiveness of the target cells (insulin resistance). Type I diabetes is thought to have a genetic link that may involve susceptibility to certain viral infections or a predisposition to the production of autoantibodies to the beta cells. Type II diabetes is familial, and its occurrence may correlate to environmental factors or to an individual's lifestyle. Type II may be due to a faulty secretion of insulin or to insulin resistance of the target cells. Factors that can produce type II include pancreatitis, pancreatic neoplasia, Cushing's disease, genetic hyperlipidemia, and certain drugs. Neither type I nor type II diabetes is inherited in a simple Mendelian pattern.

The diabetic's defective carbohydrate metabolism leads to abnormal protein and fat metabolism. Because the cells are starving for glucose, the body catabolizes protein, and the amino acids are converted to glucose (gluconeogenesis). Stored fat is catabolized, leading to an excess of fatty acids in the blood. The fatty acids are converted by the liver to ketone bodies (hyperketonemia), which cause the blood to become acidic, often to the point of being life-threatening. Further, the excess glucose in the blood may lead to its deposition in specific tissues, such as the ocular lens. The kidneys attempt to remove the excess blood glucose. This process requires water. Thus, the diabetic produces copious quantities of urine (polyuria), leading to an increased sensation of thirst (polydipsia).

Symptoms of diabetes include, in their order of development, hypoinsulinemia or insulin resistance, hyperglycemia, glucosuria, polyuria, polydipsia, polyphagia (increased appetite and food intake), weight loss, increased incidence of infection, and poor wound healing. In both types I and II diabetes, the excess fatty acids in the blood can lead to atherosclerosis and microangiopathy. These conditions in turn can adversely affect the brain, peripheral nerves, heart, eyes, kidneys, and other tissues.

A *diabetic coma* is the result of ketoacidosis and can be caused by skipping an insulin treatment or not taking enough insulin, ingesting too much food, severe physical or emotional stress, or polyuria. *Insulin shock* is caused by too much insulin, too little food, or vigorous exercise. Both situations require treatment, and the treatment regimens are exactly the opposite of one another: the blood glucose must be lowered in diabetic coma, and raised in insulin shock.

Hypoglycemia is the condition of low blood glucose. Symptoms include headache, dizziness, weakness, confusion, strange behavior, and seizures. Hypoglycemia can result from insulin shock, Addison's disease, or a tumor of the pancreas, leading to an overproduction of insulin (hyperinsulinemia).

▶ SECTION IV

Malnutrition is the general term that describes an insufficient diet. Two components of malnutrition may be seen, especially in children. *Marasmus* is general undernourishment of carbohydrates, fats, and proteins. In *kwashiorkor*, only protein intake is insufficient. In cases of childhood malnutrition, numerous development and physiologic problems are seen. In severe cases, a malnourished adult will be cachexic (emaciated) and will show many physiologic dysfunctions. The condition of malnutrition may be classified as primary malnutrition, in which there is inadequate intake of nourishment, or secondary malnutrition, where food is improperly digested (maldigestion) or absorbed (malabsorption). Insufficient digestive enzymes, pancreatitis, infection of the intestine, chronic vomiting or diarrhea, and liver or biliary disease can all lead to maldigestion or malabsorption.

Starvation is the lack of any type of nutrient. In this condition, the body depletes its glucose and glycogen stores and then catabolizes stored fat, mobilizing triglycerides to use for energy production. Proteins are catabolized, and the amino acids are used to form glucose. Symptoms associated with starvation include lethargy, hypothermia, infections, and decreased immune function.

Anorexia nervosa is a psychogenic disorder characterized by a resistance to food, resulting in malnutrition, cachexia, and starvation. The affected individual (usually a young female) becomes emaciated and displays amenorrhea, low blood pressure and heart rate, anemia, dehydration, electrolyte imbalance, and decreased resistance to infection. Hyperalimentation, an aggressive nutritional approach, is used in extreme cases. *Bulimia,* also a psychogenic eating disorder affecting primarily females, is characterized by an eating pattern of bingeing and purging. The purging involves self-induced vomiting and the use of laxatives and diuretics. Esophagitis and tooth decay result from the chronic vomiting, as well as electrolyte and acid–base imbalance. Dehydration, stomach rupture, and heart failure can also occur in the bulimic person.

Obesity, defined as being greater than 20 percent above the ideal body weight, is of one of two types. In lifelong obesity, individuals are overweight throughout their entire lives. This condition is due to adipose hyperplasia, where the fat cells of the body have increased in number throughout childhood. Adult-onset obesity begins between the ages of 20 to 40, and body fat distribution is concentrated in central regions: the upper abdomen in men and the lower abdomen, hips, and thighs in women. In this condition, the number of fat cells is normal, but the cells contain excess fat. Adult-onset obesity is the result of the slowing of the body's metabolism with age.

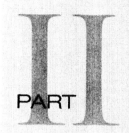

Major Diseases
of the Body Systems

CHAPTER

Blood and the Vascular System

▶ OBJECTIVES

SECTION II

Define all highlighted terms.

Characterize the different forms of anemia.

Characterize the different forms of leukemia.

Describe the forms of lymphoma.

Describe the disease multiple myeloma.

Describe the blood cell disorders polycythemia, leukocytosis (and its forms), leukopenia, and pancytopenia.

Characterize the pathologic conditions of vasculitis, platelet disorders, and clotting factor disorders.

SECTION III

Define all highlighted terms.

Characterize the clinical condition of edema and its forms.

Describe the forms of hemorrhage.

Describe the clinical condition of shock and its types, pathogenesis, and stages.

Define primary and secondary hypertension. Describe the causes, effects, and management of the condition.

Distinguish between the terms hypoxia, ischemia, anoxia, and infarction, and list reasons each occurs.

List and characterize the forms of emboli.

Define and describe the condition of thrombosis.

SECTION IV

Define all highlighted terms.

Characterize the clinical conditions of arteriosclerosis and atherosclerosis. Describe the causes, pathogenesis, effects, and therapeutic regimens.

Describe and characterize the conditions and forms of aneurysm, vasculitis, phlebitis, and varicose veins.

SECTION ▶ 1. ANATOMY AND PHYSIOLOGY IN REVIEW

▶ THE COMPONENTS OF BLOOD

9–1

Blood is sometimes referred to by the laboratory phrase **whole blood.** This is because much biochemical testing analyzes only portions of blood, such as the plasma or the cells. A laboratory procedure called centrifugation separates the components into the fluid part and the solid or cellular part. Whole blood, as is found in our circulatory system, is made of these two parts. The liquid portion is **plasma** and it is the medium in which the cells are suspended for circulation. Plasma carries many substances throughout the body. Just a few examples of these are nutrients, waste products, electrolytes, gases, antibodies, and proteins. Some of these proteins are albumin, fibrinogen and other clotting factors, antibodies, and enzymes. All of these substances in plasma are soluble, or are dissolved in this fluid. Plasma from a fasting patient, examined in the laboratory, appears clear. The **hematocrit** is a commonly performed laboratory test, and it is the ratio between the fluid portion and the solid portion of the blood. Normally, there should be about 55 percent plasma to 45 percent cells.

9–2

As just mentioned, plasma contains fibrinogen that ultimately causes blood to clot. Many laboratory tests need to avoid this protein because of the instruments used (fibrinogen can clog instrument parts). Blood that is outside of any vessel is designed to clot. The formation of a clot uses up fibrinogen; therefore, for many tests, blood is allowed to clot in a plain venipuncture (blood drawing) tube. After centrifugation, the fluid portion still contains all of its substances except fibrinogen. This fluid is now called **serum.** Tests that require whole blood, such as a complete blood count (CBC), are performed using venipuncture tubes that contain an anticoagulant. This is a substance that prevents the normal clotting mechanism and allows the blood to remain in the same state as in the circulation.

9–3

Suspended in blood are the cells, which are the solid portion. There are several types of blood cells that are presented in the following frames. The **bone marrow,** in the hollow center of many bones, is the primary site in an adult for the production of blood cells. Some cells also mature in the bone marrow as they go through several stages. Only mature cells are released from the marrow to enter the circulation. Occasionally, slightly younger cells may be found in the blood in significant numbers and this is very helpful in diagnosis. The presence of younger cells indicates some need the bone marrow is trying to meet by releasing these cells before they are ready. Two common examples are immature red blood cells called **reticulocytes,** which are needed to help combat anemia, and immature neutrophils called **bands** or **stabs.** Their presence indicates a fight against a bacterial invader. The blood cells can be thought of as an army for body defense. In times of "war," all the mature soldiers may be occupied with the fight but more resources are still needed. The bone marrow responds by sending the younger population before they are ready. The most important difference between these immature cells and the mature ones is function. The younger cells don't perform as well. That is why they go through the maturation process to become fully functional. But in times of need they are pressed into service.

9–4

Blood cells descend from a common precursor cell, the **pluripotent stem cell.** Pluripotent means it has many possibilities, or can differentiate into several different cell lines. Once this differentiation, or specialization, has begun, the stem cell becomes committed to that cell line. There are two major lines, the red blood cells and the white blood cells. The white cells continue to differentiate into five types. The first committed daughter cell of the stem cell is called a **blast.** This is like a newborn baby and, like a baby, passes through many stages before adulthood. Blasts are huge compared to the final small mature cell. The clinical significance of blast cells is that, if seen in the circulation, their presence signals serious disease. Blast cells are *never* seen in the blood of a healthy person.

▶ RED BLOOD CELLS

9–5

Red blood cells (RBCs) are called **erythrocytes.** "Erythro" means red, and you know "cyte" or "cyto" is cell. These cells (and therefore blood) get their color from the hemoglobin contained in them. This is especially true of hemoglobin that has oxygen bound to it. The production and development of RBCs is called **erythropoiesis.** Erythropoiesis is stimulated by the hormone **erythropoietin,** which is made by the kidneys. Key elements needed for erythropoiesis, especially hemoglobin synthesis, are iron, the B vitamin folic acid, and vitamins B_6 and B_{12}. The erythrocytes are unusual because the mature RBC does not have a nucleus. The cell is shaped like a biconcave disk. This shape increases its surface area to facilitate gas exchange. Figure 9–1 is an illustration of normal red blood cells. **Hemoglobin** is the major component of the RBC cytoplasm. It is made of globulin protein and a porphyrin ring with a molecule of iron in the center. Iron is an important part of hemoglobin, and hence the erythrocyte. The function of hemoglobin is to bind oxygen in the lungs. The function of the erythrocyte is to carry this complex to the cells. The oxygen is released at the cellular level, and the waste product carbon dioxide is picked up by hemoglobin. This is transported back to the lungs for release. More oxygen is picked up and the cycle is repeated. The amount of hemoglobin in RBCs that is considered healthy is about 15 or 16 mg/dL for males, and 12 to 14 mg/dL for females.

9–6

The red blood cell has a life span of about 120 days. When it is old it is removed by the spleen. This process of removing and destroying the RBCs is called **extravascular hemolysis.** Extravascular is outside the blood vessels, "hemo" refers to blood, and lysis is rupture or bursting. After hemolysis, most components are recycled. Globulin goes back to protein stores. Iron also goes back to storage until it is needed for new erythropoiesis. The remainder of hemoglobin (the porphyrin) eventually becomes the waste product bilirubin. Bilirubin must go to the liver for conjugation, a process that allows it to be excreted in the bile. Bilirubin must be excreted because in the unconjugated form it is toxic to brain cells. In Chapter 13 you will learn about the consequences of too much retained bilirubin when we study liver disease. Anemias that are due to abnormal excessive hemolysis also produce too much bilirubin.

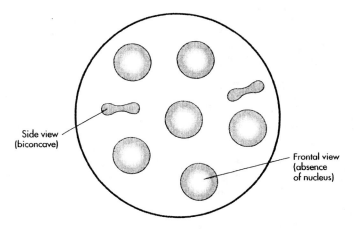

Side view
(biconcave)

Frontal view
(absence
of nucleus)

Figure 9–1. Normal red blood cells.

▶ RED BLOOD CELL ANTIGENS AND BLOOD GROUPS

9-7

The concept of antigens on cell surfaces was introduced in Chapter 4 when we discussed the HLA leukocyte antigens. Red blood cells also have antigens; in fact, they are covered with them. The most commonly known are the ABO blood group antigens and the D or Rh antigen. The antigens are groups of chemicals, mostly carbohydrates, on the cell membrane. The term "antigen" may be confusing since an antigen is a substance foreign to the body. The red cell membrane chemical groups are called antigens because, if those cells are introduced into the body of a person whose red cells do *not* have those antigens, then antibodies are formed against them and try to destroy them.

9-8

In the field of medical science known as blood banking, or transfusion services, there exists *Landsteiner's law.* This law states that for every ABO *antigen* that is *absent* on a person's RBCs, the corresponding *antibody* will be *present.* This means that a person who has the A antigen (and who is blood group A), naturally has anti-B antibody. A type B person has anti-A. Group O blood cells (which have neither A nor B antigens) have both anti-A and anti-B. Group AB blood cells have no antibody. These principles are used to find compatible (matching) blood for transfusion. In addition to being ABO compatible, the Rh or D antigen is matched as well. The presence or absence of the D antigen causes blood to be labeled as "positive" or "negative." Thus, A positive blood has the A of the ABO antigens and the D antigen. In addition to matching these major blood groups, a procedure called a crossmatch is used to find any incompatibility that might arise from the many minor antigen groups.

▶ WHITE BLOOD CELLS

9-9

White blood cells (WBCs) are also called **leukocytes.** "Leuko" means white. There are three lines of WBCs, the granulocytes, the lymphocytes, and the monocytes. The granulocytes (named for their grainy cytoplasm) are further divided into neutrophils, basophils, and eosinophils. The neutrophils are the phagocytes that were presented in Chapter 2 on inflammation. Neutrophils are of paramount importance in defense against bacterial infection. Properties that make them so well adapted for this function include great mobility or ability to migrate, chemotaxis or response to a signal, phagocytosis or ingestion of foreign particles, and lysis or destruction of phagocytized material.

9-10

Lymphocytes were discussed at length in Chapter 4 on immunity. Once they leave the bone marrow, lymphocytes further mature into T and B cells. T lymphocytes provide cell mediated immunity, while B lymphocytes are responsible for humoral immunity (antibodies). The monocytes are the most diverse of the leukocytes. Monocytes are found in the circulation and in the tissues and organs where they are known by several names. In the tissues they are macrophages or histiocytes. In the spleen they are reticuloendothelial cells. Liver monocytes are Kupffer cells. Monocytes in all their forms are vital in inflammation and immunity (see Chaps. 2 and 4). They make up the *mononuclear phagocytic system,* which was previously called the reticuloendothelial system.

▶ PLATELETS

9-11

Platelets are not really cells. They are fragments or pieces of the cytoplasm from the bone marrow cell, the megakaryocyte. They are also called **thrombocytes.** A thrombus is a clot, so the name indicates their function. Their activities help to form a blood clot to stop bleeding. When injury occurs, platelets gather at the site to help fill the gap created by the injury. Platelets demonstrate two properties that are suited for this purpose. One is **aggregation,** which means they stick to each other. The other is **adhesion,** which means they stick to *any*

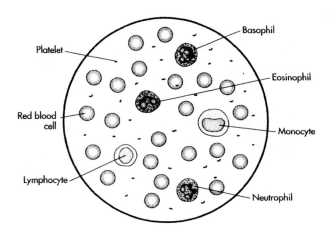

Figure 9–2. The cells of the blood.

surface *except* endothelial cells. This combination results in a **platelet plug,** which becomes part of a fibrin meshwork to create a clot (see Frame 9–14). Thrombocytes also release chemicals necessary for clot formation and aid in the healing process. The cells of the blood are shown in Figure 9–2.

► COAGULATION

9–12

Coagulation of the blood is the formation of a clot, or the transformation of a liquid substance (blood) into a solid. The process of coagulation is referred to as **hemostasis,** which literally means blood ("hemo") stop ("stasis"). The function of coagulation and hemostasis is to stop bleeding or minimize blood loss after an injury. Coagulation is a result of vessels, platelets, and plasma proteins called clotting factors working together. Coagulation is normally a highly regulated and rapid process. It is partly composed of a chain reaction that will be discussed shortly.

9–13

Hemostatis begins with the injury. Any break, or discontinuity, of the endothelial cells that line vessels acts as a signal that there has been some escape of blood from the vessel. Therefore, hemostasis is needed. The reaction by the injured vessel is vasoconstriction. This is a contraction of the vessel inward to decrease its diameter and size. Less blood passes through a smaller vessel, so vasoconstriction serves to decrease blood flow to the area and cut down on the amount lost.

9–14

Platelet aggregation and adhesion is activated to form a temporary plug. The coagulation process begins immediately. It is composed of a series of reactions by **clotting factors,** proteins (many of which are enzymes) that will ultimately lead to the formation of a clot. The interaction of these factors has been called the **coagulation cascade** because of their relationship with each other. The word cascade is very descriptive because one step of the process flows into the next like a row of dominoes knocking each other down. The product of one step acts as a catalyst for the next step, and so on. The purpose of the cascade is to turn soluble **fibrinogen,** a plasma protein, into insoluble or solid **fibrin.** The role of fibrin was mentioned in Chapter 2. If you will recall, fibrin is dense, stringy material that forms a web or scaffold that is the basis of the solid clot. A clot is medically known as a **thrombus.** Clot formation is also called **thrombosis.**

9–15

All clotting factors are vital in this chain reaction, but two are of more significance clinically because they are used in diagnostic tests. **Thrombin** is an enzyme at the end of the chain that catalyses the conversion of the dissolved fibrinogen into the solid fibrin. The precursor of this enzyme, which becomes thrombin, is **prothrombin.** It is activated or started in two different manners. The first manner is called the **extrinsic pathway,** extrinsic meaning by a stimulus outside of the blood. The stimulus is some type of injury to the tissues. During this injury, a chemical called **tissue factor** initiates the coagulation cascade. The second manner is the **intrinsic pathway,** and the stimulus is within the blood itself. These stimuli are certain disease states that cause factors in the circulation to activate the cascade. The cascade may be started by either of the two mechanisms, but after a few steps in the reactions, the remainder of the reactions are the same for either pathway. This remaining series of reactions is called the **common pathway.**

9–16

All of the enzymatic conversions in the cascade lead to the conversion of prothrombin into thrombin near the end of the chain. It is then that fibrinogen is converted by thrombin into fibrin. The final step is the stabilization of that fibrin. Fibrin acts as a net to capture the solid elements of the blood to create a clot. This fibrin net is pictured in Figure 9–3. An important coenzyme (enzyme helper) throughout the cascade is the mineral calcium. Coagulation and thrombus, or clot, formation is an important function of calcium. Within the blood are chemicals that act as inhibitors of hemostasis, so that spontaneous coagulation does not occur. Obviously, this is a process that must be carefully controlled. In this chapter we will a study a disease state in which this control is lost, to the severe detriment of the patient. The sequence of events that leads to hemostasis is reviewed in the following list.

1. Tissue injury.
2. Vasoconstriction to decrease blood flow to that area.
3. Platelet aggregation and adhesion (the platelet plug).
4. The coagulation cascade that forms fibrin.
5. Trapping of blood cells in the fibrin meshwork to form a thrombus.

9–17

Once hemostasis has occurred, healing begins to take place. For this to happen, the thrombus must be removed during repair. (Remember from Chapter 2 that demolition and removal of debris must precede healing.) The clot is considered debris because it is no longer needed. Removal of the clot is called **fibrinolysis,** or rupture of the fibrin. This is accomplished by the enzyme **plasmin,** which breaks the strands of fibrin into small pieces that dissolve in the blood. These soluble remains are called **fibrin split products** and are used in some diagnostic tests. During pathologic thrombosis, or clots formed because of a disease process, one

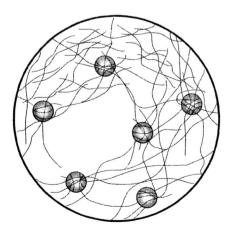

Figure 9–3. Net of fibrin capturing red blood cells to form a clot.

course of treatment is the drug streptokinase. This is an enzyme from the bacteria streptococci. It activates the plasmin precursor so that fibrinolysis may begin. This will be referred to when we study diseases that involve thrombosis.

▶ THE BLOOD VESSELS

9-18

The blood vessels serve as conduits of the blood supply, taking that vital material to all the tissues of the body. The circuit created by the vessels is summarized in the following list and shown in Figure 9-4.

1. The heart pumps oxygenated blood from the lungs into arteries.
2. Arteries, rich with oxygen, lead into arterioles (small arteries).
3. Arterioles lead into capillaries, the smallest vessels of the body.
4. Exchange of oxygen and nutrients, for carbon dioxide and waste, takes place in the capillaries. Here, the walls of the vessels are the thinnest and the flow of blood is the slowest.
5. Blood exits the capillaries to journey back to the heart by first entering venules (small veins).
6. Venules lead into veins, which carry the carbon dioxide and waste back to the heart.
7. Deoxygenated blood (low oxygen, high carbon dioxide) is moved from the heart and through the lungs to expire carbon dioxide and inspire oxygen.
8. Oxygenated blood returns to the heart to begin the cycle again.

9-19

Larger blood vessels are made of three layers, the adventitia on the outside, the media in the middle, and the intima on the inside. The intima is lined with endothelial cells. These cells control the exchanges in the capillaries. The media has elastic fibers and smooth muscle that work together to control the size of the vessel. The size may be increased (dilation), or decreased (contraction), according to need. The elastic fibers and muscle are in turn controlled by the sympathetic and parasympathetic nervous systems and various hormones.

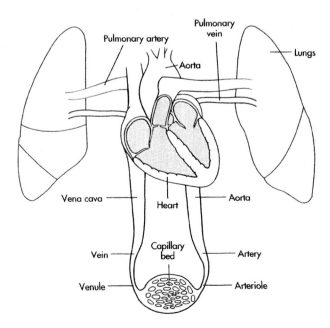

Figure 9-4. The systemic and pulmonary circulatory systems.

9-20

Arteries contain blood, which is under great pressure, having been forcibly pumped from the heart. This pressure runs around 100 mm Hg. To accommodate this pressure, the walls of arteries are very thick compared to veins. This thickness is a function of the amount of muscle present. Arteries keep their shape and do not collapse like veins because of this structure. The blood pressure contained in arteries is a direct function of the amount of blood present and resistance of the vessels. The amount of blood is governed by the rate of heart contractions and the volume of blood pumped by each contraction. Resistance by the vessels is a function of their size (in dilation there is less resistance, in contraction there is more resistance). A change in either the amount of blood or vessel size will change blood pressure. We will study more about this in Chapter 10 on the heart. Arteries are considered "active vessels" because they are the ones that respond to the nervous system and hormones to change size and to alter hemodynamics. **Hemodynamics** are the movements and forces associated with the circulation.

9-21

Veins are under low pressure (about 30 mm Hg) because the driving force from the heart has dissipated, or has spread out and been absorbed by the body. Blood moves in a relatively quiet manner back to the heart. The walls of veins are much thinner because they don't need the reinforcement to withstand high pressure. Veins are collapsible and flexible. They contain **valves** that close behind blood flow to keep it moving in one direction and prevent backflow. Since veins don't have the capacity to be involved in hemodynamics, they can be considered "passive vessels" that simply move blood back to the heart. The differences in structure between arteries and veins is illustrated in Figure 9–5.

9-22

Capillaries are the tiniest vessels of all, being only one layer thick. This layer is the intima lined with endothelial cells. Recall from Chapter 2 the active role endothelial cells play in inflammation as they create gaps or enlarged junctions through which phagocytes may pass. Their normal function is to allow and control the exchange of gases, nutrients, and waste products. Capillaries make up the largest volume of the blood vessels with miles of circuitry. Their configuration is designed to provide access to the blood's resources by almost every cell in the body.

9-23

The lymphatic system is an auxiliary vessel system designed to drain excess tissue fluid back into the general circulation. Vessels called lymphatics are dead-end, one-way, thin vessels that originate in the tissues. Tissue fluid seeps into them and starts through the system. The fluid, or lymph, passes through lymph nodes that filter and remove foreign material. The nodes also release lymphocytes as needed. The lymphatics eventually empty into the thoracic duct in the chest. The thoracic duct empties into the inferior vena cava (the largest vein, which enters directly into the heart).

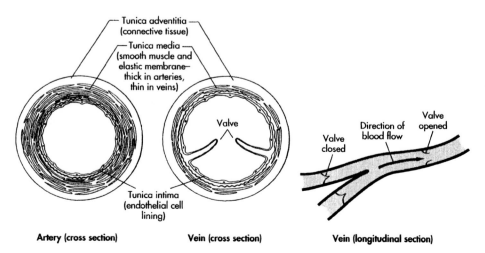

Figure 9–5. The structure of arteries and veins, which demonstrates the increased thickness of arteries and the valves of veins.

II. DISEASES OF THE BLOOD ◀ SECTION

▶ ANEMIA

Anemia is the state in which there is a deficiency of either red blood cells or hemoglobin. In either case, because of the function of RBCs and hemoglobin in providing oxygen, the result is hypoxia. You should know now that hypoxia is inadequate _____(1) to the tissues. Many of the signs of anemia are due to hypoxia, or a shortage of oxygen. These include fatigue and weakness, shortness of breath (dyspnea), and an increased heart rate (tachycardia). The patient exhibits **pallor,** or paleness. Remember that hemoglobin is responsible for the reddish color of blood and the pink color of healthy tissue. The signs of anemia are related to the state of _____(2), which results from insufficient numbers of _____(3) or insufficient _____(4).

9-24

1. oxygen
2. hypoxia
3. red blood cells
4. hemoglobin

The types of anemia may be grouped into two categories. First is the loss or destruction of red blood cells that is greater than the bone marrow's ability to replace them. Anemia due to bleeding or hemolysis is an example of this category. Second is decreased production of cells or hemoglobin (decreased erythropoiesis). An example is anemia due to states of deficiency in nutrients or failure of the bone marrow. Also, erythropoiesis or production may be abnormal, such as anemia seen in some genetic diseases. Anemia can be created by _____(1) of RBCs in excess of replacement capabilities. It can also result from _____(2) erythropoiesis, or _____(3) erythropoiesis.

9-25

1. destruction
2. decreased
3. abnormal

▶ BLOOD LOSS

Excessive bleeding and loss of RBCs creates hemorrhagic anemia. It develops rapidly. In order to maintain blood pressure, which is critical to avoid shock, plasma in vessels is quickly replaced to help normalize intravascular volume. However, this results in diluting the remaining red cell count. This state can also be called dilutional anemia. If the bleeding is stopped and the person is healthy, replacement of the RBCs by the bone marrow occurs in a few weeks without further treatment. Blood transfusion is usually necessary only in cases of shock or in a debilitated individual. Small amounts of blood lost over a longer period of time, or chronic hemorrhage, also leads to anemia. This state causes iron deficiency anemia and is also classified as secondary anemia, with the cause of bleeding being the primary disease. In anemia of chronic bleeding, the cells can be replaced, but iron stores may become depleted. This causes a deficiency in hemoglobin for the cells. Anemia due to acute hemorrhage is made worse by a homeostatic mechanism to maintain blood pressure. Plasma is replaced but it causes _____(1) of the remaining red cells. Hemorrhagic anemia is resolved by the bone _____(2). Chronic _____(3) also causes anemia that is categorized as a (an) _____(4) deficiency anemia or a _____(5) anemia.

9-26

1. dilution
2. marrow
3. hemorrhage
4. iron
5. secondary

▶ STATES OF DEFICIENCY

9-27

Production and proper maturation of red blood cells depends on specific nutrients. Cells or hemoglobin that is improperly formed will not function to full capacity, and so anemia is the result. The most common is **iron** deficiency. The numbers of red cells are normal, but hemoglobin is decreased. (Remember, iron is an essential molecule in hemoglobin.) Insufficient hemoglobin makes the cells look pale or **hypochromic** ("less color"). A dietary insufficiency will cause iron deficiency. A well-known example is "milk anemia," seen in babies kept on

1. nutrients
2. function
3. iron
4. pale
5. hemoglobin
6. bleeding

milk diets too long, without proper amounts of meat. Some states of gastrointestinal malabsorption, such as celiac and Crohn's disease, do not allow for absorption of iron and other nutrients. In pregnancy, the developing fetus may deplete the mother's iron stores. The most common reason for developing iron deficiency anemia is chronic blood loss and depletion of iron. This occurs in gastrointestinal ulcers, malignant neoplasia, and menorrhagia (heavy menstrual bleeding). Erythropoiesis will be decreased when the body is lacking certain _____(1). Red blood cells that are not formed properly will have impaired _____(2). The most common deficiency is of the nutrient _____(3). Red cells look hypochromic, or _____(4), because of insufficient _____(5). The most common reason for iron deficiency anemia is chronic _____(6).

------- 9-28 -------

1. vitamin B$_{12}$
2. maturation
3. intrinsic
4. mucosa

Folic acid is a nutrient also important for normal erythropoiesis. Malabsorption and dietary lack cause this anemia. Common reasons for a poor diet are alcoholism and poverty. Lack of **vitamin B$_{12}$** causes **pernicious anemia.** Maturation of the red blood cells requires an **extrinsic factor** (vitamin B$_{12}$) and an **intrinsic factor.** The extrinsic comes from the diet, and the intrinsic is manufactured by the cells of the gastric mucosa. Intrinsic factor is necessary for absorption of vitamin B$_{12}$. In pernicious anemia, intrinsic factor is not manufactured. This is thought to be due to atrophy of the mucosal cells with age. Another cause may be an autoantibody (anti-intrinsic factor) which damages the mucosal cells. The result is lack of absorption of vitamin B$_{12}$. Pernicious anemia results from a deficiency of _____(1), which is necessary for red cell _____(2). This deficiency most commonly results from an absence of _____(3) factor. Lack of intrinsic factor is due to disease of or injury to the gastric _____(4).

▶ HEMOLYTIC ANEMIA

------- 9-29 -------

1. hemolysis
2. extravascular hemolysis
3. intravascular hemolysis
4. intracorpuscular
5. extracorpuscular
6. bilirubin

Hemolysis ("blood-burst") is the rupture and destruction of red blood cells. It can be due to an *intracorpuscular defect* (inside the cell) or an *extracorpuscular defect* (outside the cell). An intracorpuscular defect is a structural abnormality in the cell, such as in sickle cell anemia, spherocytosis, or thalassemia. An extracorpuscular defect is an abnormality adhered to the cell membrane, such as in immune hemolysis or with infectious agents. Either way, an abnormal red blood cell is targeted by the spleen for removal. Destruction of abnormal or damaged cells by the spleen is called **extravascular hemolysis** (cells are destroyed outside the vessels). This is the most common form of hemolysis. **Intravascular hemolysis,** or destruction while still in the vessel, occurs because of the antibody–complement system. These two locations of red blood cell hemolysis are illustrated in Figure 9–6. Recall that red cell breakdown leads to the toxic waste product bilirubin, which must be eliminated from the body. Excessive red cell breakdown will overwhelm the liver's ability to conjugate the extra bilirubin for elimination. Unconjugated bilirubin will accumulate in the body. Bilirubin stains the tissues yellow and the visible result is **jaundice.** (Chapter 13 on liver disease will present more on jaundice.) Jaundice may be a feature of hemolytic anemia. Destruction of red blood cells is called _____(1). If it takes place in the spleen, it is called _____(2). If it occurs in the blood vessels, it is referred to as _____(3). Hemolysis can be because of a structural abnormality, or _____(4) defect, or because of an abnormality on the membrane, or _____(5) defect. Jaundice can occur in hemolytic anemia because of the build-up of _____(6).

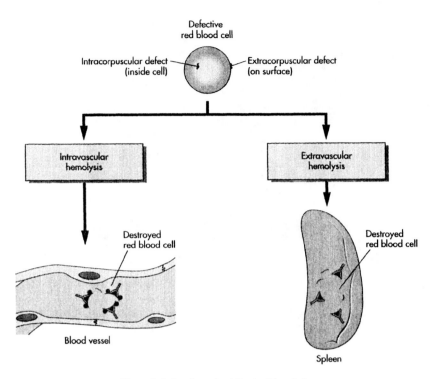

Figure 9–6. Locations of red blood cell hemolysis.

▶ GENETIC DISORDERS

9–30

In **hereditary spherocytosis,** the red cells are round like a sphere instead of being bicon-cave. This configuration makes them fragile and they rupture easily in capillaries. This com-bines with the fact that they are more rigid, or less flexible, than normal and so passage through the capillaries is more difficult. This mild anemia is generally due to extravascular hemolysis in which the spleen performs its function of removing abnormal RBCs. **Spleno-megaly,** or enlarged spleen, is usually a feature of hereditary spherocytosis. **Glucose-6-phosphate dehydrogenase deficiency,** as discussed in Chapter 8, is a defect in an enzyme inside the red cell. The normal function of this enzyme is to protect the cell membrane from the damaging effects of oxidizing compounds. G-6-PD in older cells lose this ability in this disorder. Hemolysis occurs only in the presence of oxidant drugs and resolves when the drug is stopped. Red blood cells that are rounded instead of biconcave are seen in _____(1). These cells are _____(2) and rupture easily. They are removed in great numbers by the _____(3), which becomes enlarged.

1. hereditary spherocytosis
2. fragile
3. spleen

9–31

Sickle cell anemia, presented in Chapter 7, is classified as a **hemoglobinopathy** (disorder of the hemoglobin). A defective gene called hemoglobin S codes for production of a hemo-globin that is abnormal. People who are homozygous for the S gene have clinical anemia. Heterozygotes, or carriers, have sickle cell trait, which means that even though they test pos-itive for the disease, they do not exhibit anemia. The hemoglobin S gene is confined mainly to the black population. The abnormal hemoglobin causes the cells to be abnormally shaped, like crescents or sickles. This configuration, which may be dramatic, is shown in Figure 9–7. This especially happens to the cells when they are under low oxygen tension. Abnormal hemoglobin decreases the life span of the RBCs and functions poorly. Sickled red cells are also easily ruptured in the capillaries and removed in great numbers by the spleen. Painful episodes, or crises, occur in sickle cell anemia, where the cells catch on each other and lodge in capillaries. This causes obstruction in the vessels and interrupts blood flow, causing ischemia and small infarcts. Conditions that cause the crisis, or periodic worsening, are any

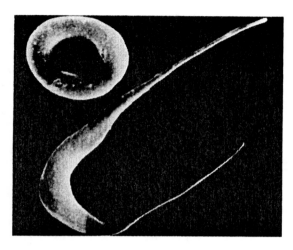

Figure 9–7. Scanning micrograph of a normal red blood cell and a sickled red blood cell in sickle cell anemia. *(From Porth,* Patho-physiology–Concepts of Altered Health States, *4th ed., JB Lippincott Co.)*

state of decreased oxygen supply (low oxygen tension precipitates sickling). Activities that produce exertion to the point of breathlessness and respiratory disease are two examples of inadequate oxygen in the body. Over time, these repeated attacks, which deprive organs of blood flow, cause severe damage to the organs. Patients with sickle cell anemia rarely live past 40 years of age.

9–32

1. crescents or sickles
2. sickle cell
3. hemoglobin
4. hemoglobinopathy
5. oxygen
6. capillaries
7. ischemia
8. infarcts

A genetic disease affecting blacks causes the red cells to be shaped like _____(1) in _____(2) anemia. The abnormal shape is linked to abnormal _____(3), which is coded for by a defective gene. Defective hemoglobin is classified as a _____(4). A condition that precipitates sickling by the cells is low _____(5). When sickled, the red cells obstruct _____(6), leading to _____(7) and _____(8) in the tissues and organs.

9–33

1. hemoglobinopathy
2. Mediterranean
3. fetal
4. poor
5. death

Thalassemia is another hemoglobinopathy affecting mainly the Mediterranean population. The abnormality lies in a lack of globulin production to be used in hemoglobin. The body tries to compensate by manufacturing fetal hemoglobin, or hemoglobin F. However, it functions poorly and produces a severe anemia. Ischemia and heart failure lead to death by adolescence. Individuals who are affected this way are homozygous for the disease, and the condition is named thalassemia major. Those who are heterozygous have a mild anemia, and this is called thalassemia minor. Thalassemia is a _____(1) affecting the _____(2) population. To make up for lack of normal hemoglobin, hemoglobin F, or _____(3) hemoglobin, is produced. The function of this hemoglobin is _____(4) and leads to early _____(5) in homozygous patients.

▶ IMMUNE-MEDIATED ANEMIA

9–34

In immune-mediated anemia, antibodies activate the complement system. The complement system is a series of plasma proteins that react together in cascade fashion to bring about rupture of a cell membrane. This cellular destruction is part of immune defense. The antibodies are directed toward any of the red cell surface antigens. Direct activation and destruction causes intravascular hemolysis. Extravascular hemolysis occurs when the antibodies do not activate complement, but instead just attach to the antigens. As these targeted

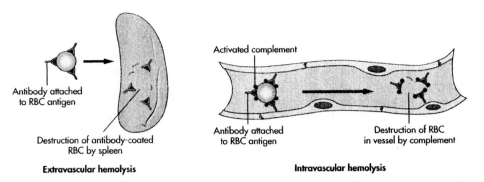

Figure 9–8. Mechanisms of hemolysis in immune-mediated anemia.

red cells circulate through the spleen, the coating of antibodies is interpreted as abnormal. The cells are then removed and destroyed. Figure 9–8 compares the mechanisms of extravascular and intravascular hemolysis. In **autoimmune hemolytic anemia,** the patient's immune system has lost some ability to recognize "self." **Autoantibodies** are then made against a particular antigen on the patient's red cell surface. "Auto" means self and designates that the antibodies in question are against the patient's own tissue or cells. The cause of autoimmune hemolytic anemia, or AIHA, is often idiopathic, which means _____(1). Rupture of red cells that is immune mediated is due to _____(2), which either directly activate the _____(3) system or attach and coat the red cell _____(4). Coated red cells removed by the spleen is _____(5) hemolysis. If the patient has made antibodies against their own tissue, the antibodies are called _____(6). Autoantibodies against red blood cells causes the disease _____(7).

1. unknown
2. antibodies
3. complement
4. membrane
5. extravascular
6. autoantibodies
7. autoimmune hemolytic anemia

9–35

A few types of drugs set off various immune reactions and cause hemolytic anemia through several mechanisms. Blood transfusions that are incompatible (not matched well enough) may cause intra- or extravascular hemolysis. The most severe reaction is seen in cases of ABO incompatibility. The naturally occurring ABO antibodies are very potent and cause immediate intravascular hemolysis. Other reactions involving the coagulation and kinin systems contribute to the development of shock. Kidney failure and death are possible in ABO incompatibility. Other types of incompatibility involving the other blood groups are usually confined to extravascular hemolysis with milder consequences. Receiving the wrong ABO blood type during a transfusion can cause death because of potent, naturally occurring _____(1). This reaction causes _____(2) hemolysis, the development of _____(3), and _____(4) failure prior to death.

1. antibodies
2. intravascular
3. shock
4. kidney

9–36

Another immune-mediated anemia is **hemolytic disease of the newborn (HDN),** also called **erythroblastosis fetalis.** If a mother is Rh negative (not having the D antigen) and the father is Rh positive, the fetus may inherit the D antigen from the father. The mother's immune system will detect this foreign antigen if the blood of the fetus mixes with hers. During delivery, upon placental separation, a **fetomaternal hemorrhage** often occurs. Fetal cells with the D antigen entering maternal circulation will cause the mother's immune system to create anti-D antibodies. She has now become sensitized. If a future fetus is also Rh positive, it is in danger from maternal anti-D. During pregnancy, very small amounts of fetal blood may enter maternal circulation. It is enough to cause an anamnestic response, and large amounts of anti-D will be produced and enter fetal circulation. Rh positive fetal red cells are targeted and destroyed by the antibody, causing anemia. The anemia of HDN varies greatly in severity, from subclinical to fatal. Fatal HDN is usually due to Rh incompatibility (anti-D is also potent). Antibodies to other blood group antigens cause milder forms of HDN. HDN due to ABO incompatibility is surprisingly common but is often subclinical.

9-37

Prior to birth, the greatest danger to the fetus is ongoing hemolysis by the ever present maternal anti-D. The anemia may become so severe that in attempt to compensate, the bone marrow kicks out immature erythroblasts. These can be seen on a blood smear from the fetus and are responsible for the name of this disease (erythroblastosis). The large amount of bilirubin that is produced from RBC destruction is conjugated by the mother's liver. Bilirubin toxicity is usually not a concern before birth. However, after birth, bilirubin toxicity is a major factor because the baby's immature liver cannot conjugate very well for a few weeks. Thus, any continuing hemolysis will lead to the accumulation of toxic unconjugated bilirubin. Clinically, this is seen as severe jaundice. Staining of the brain tissue with bilirubin is **kernicterus.** Kernicterus may lead to permanent brain damage.

9-38

1. hemolytic disease of the newborn
2. erythroblastosis fetalis
3. incompatibility
4. D or Rh
5. anti-D
6. mother
7. fetal
8. circulation
9. babies
10. blasts
11. anemia
12. anemia
13. bilirubin
14. brain damage
15. kernicterus

HDN stands for _____(1), and another name for this anemia is _____(2). The basis for this disease is _____(3) between maternal and fetal blood group antigens. The most severe form of HDN involves the _____(4) antigen and the corresponding antibody, _____(5). Anti-D is produced by the _____(6)'s immune system and it targets _____(7) red blood cells for destruction. The mother becomes sensitized when fetal red cells enter her _____(8) during pregnancy. Future _____(9) are in danger of this antibody-mediated hemolysis. Erythroblastosis fetalis is so named because of the presence of red cell _____(10) in the baby's circulation. The presence of blasts signals severe _____(11). The major concern for the baby before birth is _____(12). After birth, the presence of toxic _____(13) may stain brain tissue and cause _____(14). This neural staining is called _____(15).

▶ BONE MARROW FAILURE

9-39

1. aplastic
2. stem
3. erythropoiesis

Since the bone marrow is the primary site of red cell production, as well as other cells, failure of this organ is very serious. In these uncommon cases, the stem cells have been damaged beyond repair or have been replaced by metastatic cancer cells. Erythropoiesis comes to a halt. The disappearance of the stem cells can be caused by radiation, some drugs such as chloramphenicol, chemotherapy, or industrial toxins. The severe anemia produced is called **aplastic anemia.** Aplastic means "without form or development." Bone marrow atrophy and aplastic anemia caused by exogenous agents is considered a secondary condition. If the toxin is able to be removed, a response toward normal may be seen. Primary, or idiopathic, aplastic anemia has a poor prognosis, since the cause is unknown. Bone marrow damage to the point of failure causes _____(1) anemia. The _____(2) cells have been injured and are not replaced. There is a complete lack of red cell production, or _____(3).

▶ SECONDARY ANEMIA OF CHRONIC DISEASE

9-40

There are several disease states that adversely affect erythropoiesis. In chronic kidney failure, the hormone erythropoietin is not produced in sufficient quantities, and so stimulation of red cell production is decreased. Leukemia, cancer of white blood cells, crowds out the maturing erythrocytes and decreases their numbers. Other types of malignant neoplasia cause chronic bleeding, and metastases to the bone marrow interfere with its function. Table 9-1 summarizes the various types of anemia that you have just learned.

TABLE 9–1. TYPES OF ANEMIA

Destruction or Loss of Red Blood Cells	Decreased Erythropoiesis
Blood loss	Nutrient deficiency
Acute	Genetic disorders
Chronic	Spherocytosis
Hemolysis	G-6-PD deficiency
Structural abnormality (genetic disorder)	Sickle cell anemia
Immune mediated (destroyed by antibody)	Thalassemia
	Bone marrow failure
	Chronic disease
	Kidney failure
	Leukemia
	Bone marrow
	metastases

9–41

In the following frames we will study diseases of the white blood cells. Precursors of granulocytes and monocytes and lymphocytes are affected. We will examine some miscellaneous conditions of the blood cells at the end of this section, but the following diseases of white cells are all neoplastic. While deficiency is a hallmark of red blood cell disorders, excess is the rule in these white blood cell disorders. The principles of malignancy presented in Chapter 6 apply here as in any cancer. There is transformation of a cell line into a mutant with uncontrollable growth, much to the detriment of normal cells.

▶ LEUKEMIA

9–42

Leukemia is malignancy of the white blood cell precursors in the bone marrow. It is characterized by malignant cells spilling over into the circulation. Leukemia is an old term that means "white blood" because before early diagnosis and treatment, WBC counts in the circulation reached astronomical proportions. These excessive numbers could make the blood look milky. The transformed cells are actually the stem cells that produce malignant daughter blast cells. These blasts undergo little differentiation and maturation. There is no function with these cells because they don't mature. This is an important point because the demise of the patient is a result of a loss of this function. These huge, ineffective mutant cells make up a **diffuse** cancer. They are dispersed throughout the bone marrow of some bones and in the bloodstream. There is no localized solid mass or tumor. The pathogenesis of leukemia is really quite simple. Immature, nonfunctional, cancerous stem cells proliferate to the point where normal stem cells are replaced with them. Replacement or elimination of normal stem cells means a lack of normal cell line precursors and a lack of mature functional white blood cells. Production of red blood cells and platelets is also suppressed by the cancer cells. The severe deficiency of normal white cells leaves the body without their vital functions, and death results. Since white cells are normally released into the circulation, it follows that cancerous cells also make their way there.

9–43

The term leukemia comes from early cases where numbers of white cells in the _____(1) were very _____(2). Leukemia is _____(3) of the white blood cell precursors in the _____(4). The neoplasia begins with the _____(5) cell and it produces cancerous daughter _____(6) cells. The most significant aspect of malignant blast cells is they do not _____(7), and this is a direct cause of _____(8). Leukemia is characterized as a _____(9) cancer because it is not a localized mass or

1. blood
2. high
3. malignancy
4. bone marrow
5. stem
6. blast
7. function
8. death
9. diffuse

10. tumor
11. stem cells
12. replaced
13. function

_____(10). The basic pathogenesis of leukemia is that normal _____(11) are _____(12) by malignant cells, and the body loses all benefits of the _____(13) performed by mature white blood cells.

····· 9–44 ·····

The cause of leukemia is unknown, like most cancer. Viruses and oncogenes are suspected to play major roles. A virus in the same family as HIV, **human T-cell leukemia/lymphoma virus (HTLV-1),** has been proven in some cases. Epstein–Barr virus, or EBV, causes mild flu-like symptoms in most people as the causative agent of infectious mononucleosis. It has also been implicated in some cases of leukemia. Oncogenes may create a predisposition to malignancy, especially in the face of some viral infections. An oncogene, or cancer-promoting gene, may become activated if a chromosome breaks or if a translocation occurs. The **Philadelphia chromosome** (a shortened chromosome 22) is considered a marker for one type of leukemia because it is found in the majority of patients.

····· 9–45 ·····

1. cell line
2. timing
3. myeloid
4. lymphoid
5. acute
6. chronic
7. acute
8. chronic

There are four types of leukemia, as outlined in Table 9–2. Among these four types are two categories, which relate to the affected cell line. There are also two classifications, which relate to the timing or course of the disease. The two categories or cell lines are **myeloid** (granulocytes and monocytes) and **lymphoid** (lymphocytes). The two classifications, or course of disease, are **acute** (in children) and **chronic** (in adults). Therefore, leukemia may be acute myeloid, chronic myeloid, acute lymphoid, or chronic lymphoid. Acute leukemia is characterized by rapid proliferation of the cells. The cells are undifferentiated and primitive. Chronic leukemia moves at a slow pace, with relatively differentiated mature cells. Leukemia is categorized according to the _____(1) that is affected, and according to the _____(2) or course of disease. The cell lines are either _____(3) or _____(4). The timing is either _____(5) or _____(6). Explosive proliferation of very immature cells occurs in the _____(7) classification. The opposite is seen in _____(8) leukemia.

▶ ACUTE LYMPHOBLASTIC LEUKEMIA

····· 9–46 ·····

Acute lymphoblastic leukemia, or **ALL,** is generally seen in young children and is the most common form of leukemia in children. The bone marrow is infiltrated with neoplastic blasts of the B and T lymphocyte cell line. Poorly differentiated cells are present in the circulation. This disease has a very rapid course, and untreated cases result in fatality in 3 to 6 months. However, the acute nature of this cancer makes it responsive to antineoplastic drugs, and remissions are not hard to induce. (A remission is the diminishing of or absence of the symptoms of a disease, which may be temporary. It is not a cure.) The actual cure rate for ALL is about 50 percent.

TABLE 9–2. TYPES OF LEUKEMIA

Myeloid (Granulocytes and Monocytes)	Lymphoid (Lymphocytes)
Acute	**Acute**
Acute myelogenous leukemia (AML)	Acute lymphoblastic leukemia (ALL)
Chronic	**Chronic**
Chronic myelogenous leukemia (CML)	Chronic lymphocytic leukemia (CLL)

► ACUTE MYELOGENOUS LEUKEMIA

9-47

Acute myelogenous leukemia, or **AML,** is generally seen in adults and is the most common form of leukemia in adults. This malignant infiltration is by blasts of the granulocyte or monocyte cell line, or even by erythroblasts. It shares general characteristics with ALL, including fatality in 6 months without treatment. The difference is that the response to treatment is not as good with AML, with most cases experiencing relapse after remission. There is an overall 5-year survival rate in treated cases of AML. Figure 9–9 shows the presence of blast cells in the circulation in acute leukemia. Note the huge size of these cells in comparison to the red blood cells.

► CHRONIC MYELOGENOUS LEUKEMIA

9-48

Chronic myelogenous leukemia, or **CML,** also affects adults. The malignant stem cells produce myeloid precursors that have the ability to differentiate. Unlike just the presence of blasts in the acute forms of leukemia, various stages of maturation can be identified among the cells in CML. CML has a slow onset with mild to moderate nonspecific signs that can go undetected. The chronic phase lasts 2 to 3 years. Then, the patient abruptly enters an acute blast crisis similar to acute leukemia that precedes death. The long-term prognosis for CML is poor, with a 3- to 5-year survival rate. The Philadelphia chromosome is seen in 90 percent of these cases.

► CHRONIC LYMPHOCYTIC LEUKEMIA

9-49

Chronic lymphocytic leukemia, or **CLL,** is a disease of the older population and usually occurs in those older than 50 years. As the name implies, it is a cancer of the lymphocytes. CLL is different from the other leukemias because a specific gene bestows immortality upon a lymphocyte cell line. In other words, because of genetic programming, the cells don't die. Since they are continuously produced, eventually the circulation becomes overwhelmed with mature lymphocytes. The lymphocytes in circulation look normal, but the blood count is eas-

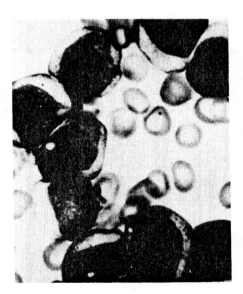

Figure 9–9. Blast cells in the peripheral blood in acute leukemia. *(From Kumar et al, Basic Pathology, 5th ed., Saunders.)*

ily four times normal. CLL has a slow progression with about a 7- to 9-year survival rate. The bad news is that it is not responsive to chemothera y because there is no uncontrolled proliferation. (Remember, chemotherapy targets fast growing cells, not slow growers.)

9-50

1. acute lymphoblastic leukemia
2. B and T lymphocyte
3. acute myelogenous leukemia
4. granulocyte or monocyte
5. rapid
6. months
7. chronic myelogenous leukemia
8. slow
9. Philadelphia
10. CML
11. chronic lymphocytic
12. lymphocytes
13. die
14. genetic
15. overwhelm
16. grow or proliferate

The most common leukemia in children is _____(1). It affects the _____(2) cell line. The most common leukemia in adults is _____(3). It affects the _____(4) cell lines. The course of acute leukemias is _____(5), with death in untreated cases occurring in several _____(6). A leukemia in adults that is characterized by different stages of maturing cells is _____(7). The course of CML is _____(8), but death is preceded by an acute crisis. The _____(9) chromosome is found in _____(10). The elderly are usually victims of _____(11) leukemia. In this case, the predominant cell population is mature _____(12) that do not _____(13). This immortality is because of _____(14) programming. The huge numbers of lymphocytes _____(15) the circulation. CLL is not responsive to chemotherapy because the cells _____(16) too slowly.

9-51

1. loss or crowding out
2. cell
3. anemia
4. bleeding
5. infection
6. immune
7. chronic

The signs and symptoms of acute leukemia (see Table 9–3) are related to the crowding out and loss of *all* cell lines in the malignant bone marrow. Red cells and platelets are also replaced by malignant white cells. There is just no room for the maturation and development of any normal blood cells. The deficiency in red blood cells causes anemia, and the signs of anemia accompany leukemia. Because platelets are necessary for blood clotting, their deficiency (thrombocytopenia) causes bleeding. As in other cancers, the excessive consumption of nutrients leads to weight loss and wasting. The most common cause of death in leukemia is infection because of suppression of cellular defense and the immune system. Adequate functional neutrophils are not available. The immune function of lymphocytes is greatly impaired. Chronic leukemia shows similar signs but with a gradual onset. Organs become infiltrated with the cancerous cells, causing enlargement of the spleen (splenomegaly), liver (hepatomegaly), and lymph nodes (lymphadenopathy). The signs and symptoms of leukemia are due to the _____(1) of the various _____(2) lines. Red cell deficiency leads to _____(3), and platelet deficiency causes _____(4). The most common cause of death is _____(5) because of impairment of the _____(6) system. Organ enlargement accompanies _____(7) leukemia.

TABLE 9–3. SIGNS AND SYMPTOMS OF LEUKEMIA

Anemia: Replacement of red blood cells by cancer cells
Bleeding: Replacement of platelets by cancer cells
Weight loss: Consumption of nutrients by cancer cells
Infection: Replacement of neutrophils by cancer cells, impaired lymphocyte function
Enlargement of spleen, liver, and lymph nodes

▶ LYMPHOMA

9–52

Lymphoma is neoplasia of the lymphocytes and their precursors. It generally originates in the lymph nodes. In contrast to leukemia, lymphoma does produce a mass lesion or solid tumor, usually in the lymph node. Also, in contrast to leukemia, the cancerous lymphocytes are not found in the circulation. There are several forms of lymphoma, and they are based on the specific cell type that has transformed. The etiology of lymphoma is as unclear as it is with leukemia. The same speculations about viruses and genes as causative factors apply. Patients with lymphoma are suspected to have an underlying problem with their immune system, which might allow a virus to cause a transformation. Lymphomas are less age related compared to leukemia. The pathogenesis is again uncomplicated, with malignant cells infiltrating lymph nodes, the spleen, bone marrow, or other organs. As always, massive infiltration destroys the fundamental function of the affected organ. Lymphoma is cancer of the _____(1) that begins in the _____(2). Two differences from leukemia are that lymphoma forms a solid _____(3) or _____(4), and malignant cells are not found in the _____(5). The pathogenesis of lymphoma relates to _____(6) of various organs with cancer cells, which seriously interferes with _____(7).

1. lymphocytes
2. lymph nodes
3. mass
4. tumor
5. circulation
6. infiltration
7. function

▶ HODGKIN'S DISEASE

9–53

Hodgkin's disease is the most common type of lymphoma. It can strike at any age but usually develops between the ages of 25 and 55. Hodgkin's disease is further subdivided into four more types, based on characteristics of the lymphocytes. In examining biopsy specimens of a lymph node, liver, spleen, or bone marrow, a pathologist can also stage this disease. This is very helpful in determining a treatment regime and in setting forth a prognosis. The determination of stage is based on which organs have been infiltrated with the malignant lymphocytes. Also seen on biopsy will be the presence of the **Reed–Sternberg cell.** This particular cell defines this disease. That is, it is only found in Hodgkin's disease-type lymphoma. This is a multinucleated, abnormal lymphocyte, with a clear halo around the nucleoli, as shown in Figure 9–10.

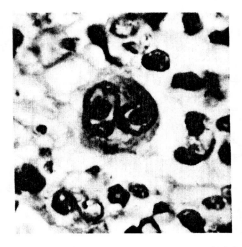

Figure 9–10. The Reed–Sternberg cell in Hodgkin's disease. Note the double nucleus with halos around the large nucleoli. *(From Chandrasoma and Taylor, Concise Pathology, 2nd ed., Appleton & Lange.)*

Hodgkin's disease in **stage I** shows involvement of a single lymph node or of nodes in the same group. **Stage II** is defined by two or more lymph nodes, or different groups, on the same side of the diaphragm (above in the chest, or below in the abdomen.) **Stage III** reveals malignancy on both sides of the diaphragm (chest and abdomen). There may or may not be **extranodal spread** in stage III. Extranodal spread is movement of the cancer outside of lymph nodes to organs such as the spleen, liver, or bone marrow. **Stage IV** is most severe with widespread dissemination and extranodal involvement of nonlymphoid organs, including the lungs. Stage I has an excellent prognosis, and stage II is good also, with close to a 100 percent cure rate with treatment. By stage IV, only half of the cases with Hodgkin's survive 5 years with treatment. The most common form of lymphoma is _____(1). A lymphoma may be diagnosed as Hodgkin's disease only if the _____(2) cell is found on biopsy. A biopsy examination allows this disease to be _____(3), which is helpful for _____(4) and treatment. The determination of stage is based on how many _____(5) are affected, on which side of the _____(6) the malignancy is located, and if there is spread outside of the lymph node system, called _____(7) spread.

The signs of Hodgkin's disease begin with **lymphadenopathy,** which are enlarged lymph nodes. This may originate in the neck, chest, or abdomen. "Systemic constitutional symptoms" accompany Hodgkin's. This phrase means generalized symptoms. This reference is used frequently to describe the clinical features of many diseases. It means nonspecific signs, or a general feeling of illness. These are signs and symptoms that could be caused by any number of diseases, and so are not very helpful in the diagnosis. These signs include fatigue (tiredness), lethargy (listlessness), anorexia (loss of appetite), fever, and weight loss. (Sometimes nausea and diarrhea are considered a generalized symptom and sign.) Be certain you remember what "generalized signs and symptoms" mean, since you will see this reference often in this book. The predominant signs of early Hodgkin's disease are enlarged lymph nodes, or _____(1), and general feelings of _____(2).

▶ NON-HODGKIN'S LYMPHOMA

Non-Hodgkin's lymphoma (NHL) is often referred to as just "lymphoma." The Reed–Sternberg cell is absent on a biopsy; therefore, it is non-Hodgkin's. NHL is classified according to histologic findings that correlate with the clinical outcome. These classifications are arrived at by looking at the nuclei of the lymphocytes and at the overall structure of the lymph node. The purpose of the classification is like staging, in that it is useful in guiding treatment and estimating the prognosis. The invasion by neoplastic cells will be either **follicular** or **diffuse.** In follicular invasion, the structure of the lymph node follicle will be preserved. Follicular lymphoma is less serious and carries a better prognosis. Diffuse lymphoma destroys the architecture of the follicles and therefore the lymph node. This destruction correlates with the deadly nature of the disease, and diffuse lymphoma carries a poor prognosis. The difference between Hodgkin's disease and non-Hodgkin's lymphoma is that in NHL, the _____(1) cell is absent. In classifying NHL, malignant invasion is described as either _____(2) or _____(3). In follicular lymphoma, the structure of the _____(4) is preserved. In _____(5) lymphoma, it is destroyed. _____(6) carries the worst prognosis.

NHL is further divided into grades, based on the classifications of follicular or diffuse. **Low grade** is most common, is of the follicular type, and has a 7- to 9-year survival rate. The slow growth of the cancerous cells does not make this disease very responsive to chemotherapy. **Intermediate grade** and **high grade** are predominantly diffuse lymphomas, with survival rates of 3 and 2 years, respectively. Extranodal spread is common, with resulting organ failure. The prognosis for intermediate and high grade is variable. Chemotherapy can induce remission in about 75 percent of the cases. The most common type of non-Hodgkin's lymphoma is graded as _____(1). It is of the _____(2) type of lymphoma. _____(3) grade and _____(4) grade, which are _____(5) lymphomas, respond better to chemotherapy.

1. low
2. follicular
3. Intermediate
4. high
5. diffuse

9–58

An unusual lymphoma is Burkitt's lymphoma, which seems confined to children in some parts of Africa. There is a very high association of the Epstein–Barr virus and the development of Burkitt's lymphoma in these children. This is a highly malignant tumor of the lymphoid stem cells either in the bone marrow or lymph nodes. The nodes around the jaw and face are frequently affected, making the tumors visible in a characteristic manner. Extranodal spread is common in this fatal malignancy.

9–59

The clinical features, or signs and symptoms, of non-Hodgkin's lymphoma vary according to the invaded organs. Lymphadenopathy is accompanied by generalized symptoms, splenomegaly, and lymphocytosis (increased numbers of mature-looking lymphocytes in the blood). Extranodal tumor spread is common in diffuse NHL, where the neoplastic cells enter an organ and interfere with their function. Since NHL develops a solid tumor, it is a space-occupying lesion. Depending on the location of extranodal spread, the tumor may cause pressure necrosis. This is most commonly seen in lymphoma of the brain and spinal cord, in which the vertebrae and skull leave little room for a space-occupying lesion. In addition to interference with organ function, diffuse NHL further contributes to the disease process by causing _____(1) necrosis, by nature of its presence as a solid _____(2).

1. pressure
2. mass or tumor

▶ MULTIPLE MYELOMA

9–60

Multiple myeloma is cancer of the plasma cells in the bone marrow. If you will recall from Chapter 4 on the immune system, B lymphocytes turn into plasma cells when they contact an antigen, or are activated. Plasma cells produce antibodies. Multiple myeloma begins with the malignant transformation of only one cell. If you remember the nature of plasma cells, they make tremendous numbers of clones of themselves, so that there are adequate amounts of antibody that can be made. Since the daughter cells are clones, the antibodies are exactly alike. Since the daughters all come from one cell, they are called **monoclonal,** and the antibodies are also considered monoclonal. The amounts and types of antibody in the circulation are helpful in diagnosis of multiple myeloma.

9–61

The descendants of this malignant clonal expansion overrun the bone marrow. They crowd out other cell lines as in leukemia. Multiple myeloma is very destructive to the bone that surrounds the cancerous marrow. Cellular proliferation causes "punched out" lesions, or holes in the bone, that can be seen on x-ray. Bone destruction causes release of stored calcium and leads to **hypercalcemia,** or excessive calcium in the blood. Excessive calcium tends to be deposited in the soft tissue of some organs, especially the kidneys. This calcification of the parenchyma, or functional tissue, leads to kidney failure. The increased amounts of antibody also tend to precipitate in the kidney tubules, contributing to organ failure. The replacement of other cell lines causes anemia and **leukopenia** (decreased white blood cells in the circulation), and therefore infection. **Pathologic fractures** (a break in the bone because it is weakened by disease) are common. The signs and symptoms of multiple myeloma are reviewed in Table 9–4. Multiple myeloma has a poor prognosis, with death in 3 to 4 years from kidney failure and infection.

TABLE 9–4. SIGNS AND SYMPTOMS OF MULTIPLE MYELOMA

Bone destruction

Hypercalcemia

Calcification of organ parenchyma (especially kidney)

Kidney failure

Anemia

Bleeding

Infection

Pathologic fracture

.... 9–62 ....

1. plasma cells
2. marrow
3. B lymphocyte
4. antibodies
5. monoclonal
6. cell lines
7. anemia
8. infection
9. holes
10. hypercalcemia
11. kidney
12. pathologic fractures
13. kidney failure
14. infection

Multiple myeloma is neoplasia of _____(1) in the bone _____(2). The precursor of the plasma cell is the _____(3). The function of the plasma cell is to make _____(4). Malignant daughter cells and their antibodies are characterized as _____(5) because they clone or descend from a single transformed cell. The effects of plasma cell proliferation are squeezing out other _____(6), resulting in _____(7) and _____(8), destruction of surrounding bone, which appear as _____(9) on an x-ray, and increased blood calcium or _____(10), which can cause _____(11) failure. Also seen are breaks in the diseased bone, known as _____(12). Death is due to _____(13) and _____(14).

▶ OTHER DISORDERS OF BLOOD CELLS

.... 9–63 ....

1. red blood cells
2. blood
3. erythrocytosis
4. hypoxia
5. oxygen

Polycythemia is a significant increase in the red blood cells in the circulation. The word literally means many cells in the blood. There is an increase in the other cells from the bone marrow as well. This increase is because of hyperactivity of the bone marrow, to be explained shortly. Polycythemia specifically referring to red cells is also called **erythrocytosis.** The suffix "cytosis" means an increased cell count in the blood. Excessive RBCs in the circulation also means an increased hematocrit, with the cellular elements now consisting of up to 70 percent of the whole blood. **Primary polycythemia,** or **polycythemia vera,** is similar to leukemia in that there are neoplastic erythroblasts in the bone marrow. **Secondary polycythemia** is more common and is a compensatory hyperplasia by the bone marrow to make up for chronic hypoxia. Conditions that create hypoxia include heart or lung disease and living at high altitudes where there is less oxygen in the air. In these conditions, the kidney hormone erythropoietin stimulates more erythropoiesis. Increased numbers of red blood cells are able to carry more oxygen to try to correct the hypoxia. Polycythemia most specifically refers to increased numbers of _____(1) in the _____(2). It may also be called _____(3). The secondary condition is a response to chronic _____(4). An increase in red blood cells means an increased capacity to carry _____(5).

.... 9–64 ....

Erythrocytosis causes the blood to become thick or viscous, and the flow becomes sluggish. The signs and symptoms of polycythemia are related to this. Hypertension, or high blood pressure, is created by the extra resistance, and all the signs of hypertension are present. Hypertension also creates resistance, and so this leads to an increased workload for the heart. The thickened blood also has a tendency to clot, or form thrombi, which further decreases flow and causes ischemia and infarcts. Polycythemia is easily diagnosed by a CBC, particularly by the red cell count and the hematocrit. Primary polycythemia must be ruled out with a bone marrow biopsy. **Phlebotomy,** or the removal of blood, immediately helps to decrease blood volume and pressure. It is a palliative treatment for secondary polycythemia, and the primary cause must be addressed. Primary polycythemia is treated with chemotherapy and radiation. The signs and symptoms of polycythemia are due to the _____(1) of the blood. Increased resistance leads to _____(2), and the signs of high blood _____(3) are seen in polycythemia.

1. thickness or viscosity
2. hypertension
3. pressure

_____ 9-65 _____

Leukocytosis is an increase in the white blood cell count greater than the normal 10,000/µL (10,000 per microliter). Leukocytosis is a reaction to a disease, rather than a disease itself that requires treatment. It may be broken down into the specific type of WBC that is increased. This is very helpful in diagnostics. **Granulocytosis** is increased neutrophils and is also called **neutrophilia.** This is most commonly caused by bacterial infection and inflammation. Stress and steroids also lead to slight neutrophilia. **Eosinophilia** involves the eosinophils and is seen in allergic states or in parasitic infections. **Lymphocytosis,** or increased lymphocytes, signals viral infection, some chronic bacterial infections, or autoimmune disease. Lymphadenopathy may accompany lymphocytosis, especially in upper respiratory infection and in infectious mononucleosis. **Monocytosis** is usually the hallmark of chronic inflammation. If leukocytosis is persistent, and no cause can be found for it, it may reflect an early state of leukemia. Regarding the same for lymphadenopathy, lymphoma may be developing. Leukocytosis is an increase in the _____(1) in the blood. It is a _____(2) to disease. Neutrophilia is most commonly associated with _____(3) and _____(4). Lymphocytosis accompanies _____(5) infection, some _____(6) bacterial infection, and _____(7) disease.

1. white blood cells
2. reaction
3. bacterial infection
4. inflammation
5. viral
6. chronic
7. autoimmune

_____ 9-66 _____

Leukopenia is the opposite condition, that is, a decrease in the WBC count below 5000/µL. The suffix "penia" means a lack or decrease. Leukopenia is most often caused by suppression of the bone marrow production of cells. Toxicities to the bone marrow are produced by industrial and environmental chemicals, and especially by chemotherapy. Chemotherapy is a leading cause of suppressed WBC counts, and this side effect must be carefully monitored during treatment. Radiation is another leading cause, either through accidental exposure or cancer therapy. The idiopathic bone marrow failure that creates aplastic anemia naturally creates leukopenia as well. Leukopenia due to bone marrow aplasia or to cytotoxic cancer drugs creates a deficiency in neutrophils. This is called **neutropenia** or **agranulocytosis.** (The prefix "a" meaning without granulocytes.) Some diseases may target specific cells and cause selective leukopenia. An example of this is the AIDS virus that destroys helper T lymphocytes. This leukopenia would be subclassified as lymphopenia.

_____ 9-67 _____

The signs of leukopenia, and possible demise of the patient, are because of the impaired defense against infection. Neutropenia leaves one vulnerable to bacterial infection. A severe deficiency, such as is seen in agranulocytosis, can lead to death from overwhelming infection. Decreased numbers of lymphocytes creates susceptibility to some bacteria, to viruses, and to fungi. Treatment for leukopenia is temporary and aimed at artificially controlling infection with antibiotics for bacteria, or antiviral or antifungal agents. Treatment is effective only if the bone marrow is healthy enough to eventually regenerate the cell lines.

_____ 9-68 _____

In true bone marrow aplasia, the depletion of all cell lines is called **pancytopenia,** "pan" referring to "all." This hypocellular condition of the marrow has a poor prognosis, and the signs of anemia, leukopenia, and thrombocytopenia are seen. Leukopenia means a _____(1) in the _____(2) blood cells. It may result from suppression of the _____(3). A common cause of this is _____(4) to treat cancer. Signs and death in these cases are because of _____(5). Significant lack of all the cell lines is called _____(6).

1. decrease
2. white
3. bone marrow
4. chemotherapy
5. infection
6. pancytopenia

▶ BLEEDING DISORDERS

A disease characterized by bleeding represents a pathologic change in the normal process of hemostasis. Hemorrhage, or blood loss, may be external (loss from the body), or internal (into tissues or a body cavity). Some disorders are a combination of pathology involving the vessels, platelets, and clotting factors. The disorders which can lead to bleeding are presented in the following frames.

▶ VASCULAR DISORDERS

1. injury
2. weak
3. Immune
4. vasculitis
5. autoantibodies
6. hypersensitivity

The most common problem affecting the blood vessels is injury. Trauma can range from bruising (escape of blood under intact skin) to an open wound. Other causes of vessel pathology are weaknesses in the walls and immune-mediated injury. Vessel wall weakness seems inherent in some people who tend to bruise easily. Aging leads to fragility of the vessels, and a deficiency in vitamin C (scurvy) also causes fragility. Vitamin C is needed to create a strong matrix in the vessel walls. The immune system can damage vessel walls and cause inflammation, or **vasculitis.** This erosive type of damage can be caused by autoantibodies or during type III hypersensitivity (see Chap. 4). The most common reason for a breach in the integrity of a vessel wall is _____(1). Also, the walls may be _____(2) for various reasons. _____(3)-mediated injury causes inflammation, or _____(4). The antibodies in question may be _____(5) or be part of a _____(6) reaction.

▶ PLATELET DISORDERS

An abnormality with platelets or thrombocytes is characterized as qualitative or quantitative. A qualitative disorder is decreased or abnormal function, while a quantitative one is decreased numbers of these cell fragments. A platelet count of less than 70,000/μL defines **thrombocytopenia** (remember that "penia" means lack). If the count should fall to about 20,000/μL, spontaneous hemorrhage occurs. This condition is also called **purpura.** There are several reasons for the development of thrombocytopenia. There may be *decreased production* by the bone marrow, such as that which occurs in bone marrow aplasia or aplastic anemia. In leukemia, platelets and red cells are replaced by malignant white cells. Platelets can be *destroyed* by the immune system in some autoimmune disorders. A condition of unknown cause where there are autoantibodies targeting platelets is **idiopathic thrombocytopenia purpura,** or **ITP.** Autoimmune hemolytic anemia can also involve the platelets. Platelet destruction is seen in systemic lupus erythematosus. A blood transfusion may be compatible as far as the red cell antigens go, but be incompatible regarding the platelets. Finally, fetomaternal incompatibility, such as is seen in HDN, may exist. Increased use or *consumption* of platelets leads to a deficiency. This is most often seen in cases of DIC (see Frame 9–75).

1. thrombocytopenia
2. hemorrhage
3. production
4. immune system
5. consumption or use
6. ITP or idiopathic thrombocytopenia purpura

A deficiency in platelets, reflected in a count of about 70,000, is called _____(1). Sudden or unprovoked _____(2) can occur if the count falls to less than 20,000. Thrombocytopenia can develop through decreased _____(3), destruction by the _____(4), or through _____(5). Autoantibodies specifically directed against platelets are seen in the disease _____(6). Conditions of abnormal function are less common and usually not so severe that spontaneous bleeding develops. In **von Willebrand's disease,** there is absence of one of the clotting factors (von Willebrand's factor). The lack of this protein decreases platelet adhesion, which is so important in clot formation. Aspirin decreases platelet function also by interfering with release of clotting chemicals. This is generally not a problem, but individuals with bleeding tendencies should be careful in their use of aspirin. Also, blood donors who have taken aspirin recently should not have their platelets used for transfusion.

► CLOTTING FACTOR DISORDERS

9–73

Deficiencies in the coagulation cascade are suspected if there is excessive bleeding after injury or in cases of spontaneous hemorrhage. These are generally congenital genetic defects where an abnormal or missing gene cannot code for the specific factor. The most common genetic factor disorder is **hemophilia.** Hemophilia is a sex-linked genetic disease. The particular factor gene is located on the X chromosome. Therefore, females are carriers and males are affected. There are two types of hemophilia, A and B. A is more common and severe. It is the absence of Factor VIII. In type B there is a lack of Factor IX. Missing just one of these proteins in the cascade makes the whole process ineffective. The result of hemophilia is uncontrolled bleeding after injury, no matter how mild. Affected boys and men experience tremendous amounts of bruising. Any surgical procedure, even a tooth extraction, puts the patient at serious risk of fatal hemorrhage. Degenerative arthritis often develops in these cases because of chronic bleeding into the joints. Historically, the life span of hemophiliacs has been relatively short. The most common genetic clotting factor disorder is _____(1). It is a _____(2) linked disease. Type _____(3) is more common and significant. The result is _____(4) that is uncontrolled after any _____(5).

1. hemophilia
2. sex- or X-
3. A
4. bleeding or hemorrhage
5. injury

9–74

A decrease in production of the clotting factors leads to their deficiency. This may be seen in chronic liver disease. The liver makes all but one of these proteins. This condition is sometimes called **hypofibrinogenemia** because fibrinogen is the most abundant and measurable of the factors. This term literally reads as _____(1) fibrinogen in the _____(2). A deficiency of vitamin K will cause a lack of clotting factors. The liver uses vitamin K to manufacture four of the factors. Vitamin K is produced by intestinal bacteria, or commensals. It is also fat soluble, or requires fat for absorption from the intestines into the portal circulation. Antibiotic therapy that is prolonged can kill the normal intestinal bacteria, and vitamin K is not produced. Any malabsorption syndrome involving fat absorption will also not allow vitamin K to be available for the liver. In pancreatic disease there may be inadequate amounts of lipase (an enzyme for fat absorption), or in biliary disease, inadequate bile. Clotting factors may not be produced sufficiently in chronic _____(3) disease. Or there may not be enough vitamin _____(4) for use in their production.

1. decreased
2. blood
3. liver
4. K

9–75

Clotting factors can be excessively consumed or used up in a condition known as **disseminated intravascular coagulation,** or **DIC.** DIC is the spontaneous formation of multiple clots, or thrombi. In the state of shock (see Frame 9–87), the integrity of the endothelial cells becomes compromised. The now abnormal surface of the vessels leads to clot formation. (Remember, any change from the normal is interpreted as an injury and so hemostasis begins.) The injured ischemic endothelial cells allow leakage of the tissue factor thromboplastin, which initiates clotting. Massive release of tissue thromboplastin underlies DIC. Other conditions that lead to this state are infection, which may injure the vessels, or bacteria that initiate the process. So then, severe septicemia may be a precursor to DIC. Massive soft tissue injury can release enough thromboplastin to create DIC. Widespread metastasis of cancer can lead to DIC as the neoplastic cells create sufficient injury to tissues. The process of DIC is known as a **consumptive coagulopathy,** which describes the pathogenesis very well. Spontaneous formation of multiple clots is known as the condition _____(1). The underlying cause is sufficient release of tissue _____(2). Any abnormality of the vessel wall initiates _____(3). The pathogenesis of DIC is described as a _____(4).

1. disseminated intravascular coagulation
2. thromboplastin
3. hemostasis or clotting
4. consumptive coagulopathy

The steps of DIC, shown in Figure 9–11, are as follows.

1. Massive or widespread thrombi formation uses up all of the available fibrin, clotting factors, and platelets.
2. The enzyme plasmin begins fibrinolysis to dissolve the clots.
3. Blood starts to flow again through the vessel, but will escape from the injured areas.
4. The escape (hemorrhage) cannot be stopped now by hemostasis because there are no clotting resources left.
5. Death from exsanguination (massive bleeding to the point of death) is the most common end.

DIC is a paradox of bleeding on top of excessive coagulation. It also causes hypofibrinogenemia, which is detected by blood tests.

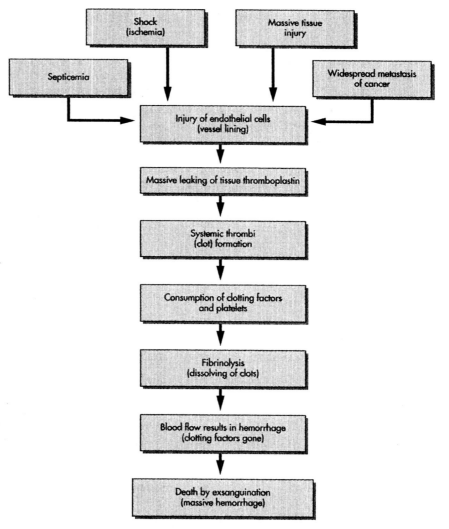

Figure 9–11. Pathogenesis of disseminated intravascular coagulation.

TABLE 9–5. CATEGORIES AND CAUSES OF BLEEDING DISORDERS

Blood Vessel Disorders
Trauma

Wall weakness

Immune-mediated vasculitis

Platelet Disorders
Thrombocytopenia
  Bone marrow aplasia, aplastic anemia
  Leukemia
  Idiopathic thrombocytopenia purpura
  Autoimmune hemolytic anemia
  Systemic lupus erythematosus
  Transfusion incompatibility
  Disseminated intravascular coagulation

von Willebrand's disease

Clotting Factor Disorders
Hemophilia A and B

Hypofibrinogenemia (chronic liver disease)

Vitamin K deficiency

Disseminated intravascular coagulation (consumptive coagulopathy)

9–77

In the process of DIC, excessive _____(1) occurs first. This _____(2) all of the elements needed for further clotting. After clot breakdown, or _____(3), hemostasis is unable to stop the often fatal _____(4). Other causes of uncontrolled bleeding may be iatrogenic, or treatment induced. Anticoagulant drugs used to prevent pathologic thrombosis can cause hemorrhage at doses higher than the therapeutic dose (i.e., at a toxic dose). Examples of these drugs are Coumadin and heparin. The categories and causes of bleeding disorders presented in the preceding frames are reviewed in Table 9–5.

1. clotting
2. uses or consumes
3. fibrinolysis
4. bleeding

9–78

Some of the less obvious signs of bleeding disorders include the following.

1. **Petechiae,** which are pinpoint hemorrhages under the skin seen in cases of thrombocytopenia. Petechiae look like little red dots.
2. **Hematuria,** which is blood in the urine.
3. **Fecal occult blood,** which is unnoticed blood in the stool.

The localized bleeding under the skin, commonly called a bruise, is medically termed a **hematoma,** or an **ecchymosis.**

II. REVIEW QUESTIONS

1. Anemia is defined by (choose all that apply):
   a. a deficiency in white blood cells
   b. a deficiency in hemoglobin
   c. an excess of red blood cells
   d. an excess of white blood cells
   e. a deficiency in red blood cells
   f. an excess of hemoglobin

1. b–a deficiency in hemoglobin; e–a deficiency in red blood cells

2. b–hypoxia

3. a–loss of red blood cells in excess of the bone marrow's ability to replace them; c–decreased erythropoiesis

4. b–iron for hemoglobin

5. d–both a and b are correct

6. a–spleen

7. b–hereditary spherocytosis; d–sickle cell anemia

8. b–sickle cell anemia; c–thalassemia major

9. a–true; b–false; c–true; d–false

2. The end result of anemia is:
   a. anoxia
   b. hypoxia
   c. infection
   d. bleeding

3. Anemia may be caused by (choose all that apply):
   a. loss of red blood cells in excess of the bone marrow's ability to replace them
   b. excessive erythropoiesis
   c. decreased erythropoiesis
   d. malignant transformation of erythroblasts in the bone marrow

4. Anemia due to chronic hemorrhage leads to a deficiency in:
   a. globulin protein for hemoglobin
   b. iron for hemoglobin
   c. vitamin B_{12} for hemoglobin
   d. folic acid for hemoglobin

5. Hemolytic anemia can be caused by:
   a. an intracorpuscular defect where a structural abnormality signals the spleen to remove the defective RBC
   b. an extracorpuscular defect where an antibody adhered to the surface signals the spleen to remove the defective RBC
   c. neither a nor b is correct
   d. both a and b are correct

6. Extravascular hemolysis takes place in the:
   a. spleen
   b. liver
   c. blood vessels
   d. bone marrow

7. Extravascular hemolytic anemia is seen in (choose all that apply):
   a. thalassemia major
   b. hereditary spherocytosis
   c. pernicious anemia
   d. sickle cell anemia

8. Which of the following are hemoglobinopathies (choose all that apply)?
   a. immune-mediated anemia
   b. sickle cell anemia
   c. thalassemia major
   d. hereditary spherocytosis
   e. aplastic anemia

9. Mark each statement about immune-mediated anemia as true or false:
   a. _____ Antibodies are directed against antigens on red cell membranes.
   b. _____ Antibodies always activate complement to produce hemolysis.
   c. _____ Hemolysis may be intravascular or extravascular.
   d. _____ An ABO incompatible blood transfusion causes autoimmune hemolytic anemia (AIHA).

10. Hemolytic disease of the newborn occurs because of (choose all that are correct):
    a. incompatibility of the D antigen between a mother and fetus
    b. incompatibility of the D antigen between a father and fetus
    c. sensitization of the fetal immune system against the mother's D antigen
    d. sensitization of the maternal immune system against the fetal D antigen

11. Severe erythroblastosis fetalis results in (choose all that are correct):
    a. anemia in the mother after birth of the fetus
    b. anemia in the fetus after birth
    c. kernicterus in the fetus after birth
    d. anemia in the fetus before birth
    e. kernicterus in the fetus before birth

12. Failure of the bone marrow produces:
    a. aplastic anemia
    b. secondary anemia
    c. iron deficiency anemia
    d. hemolytic anemia
    e. blood loss anemia

13. Please match the characteristics of leukemia and lymphoma:
    a. leukemia   1. _____ diffuse malignancy
    b. lymphoma   2. _____ cancer of white blood cell lines in the bone marrow
                       3. _____ neoplastic cells found in the circulation
                       4. _____ solid tumor
                       5. _____ cancer of lymphocytes in the lymph nodes

14. The pathogenesis of leukemia is described as:
    a. a severe wasting and starvation as the cancerous cells use all available nutrients
    b. an infiltration of vital organs and resulting pressure necrosis
    c. the loss of WBC, RBC, and platelet cell lines that are replaced with nonfunctioning malignant cells
    d. an overproduction of all bone marrow cell lines, which overloads the circulation and produces sluggish blood flow and ischemia

15. The two broad cell lines that categorize leukemia are a. _____ and b. _____. The two classifications that describe the course of disease are c. _____ and d. _____.

16. Please match the types of leukemia with their prominent characteristic:
    a. acute lymphoblastic leukemia   1. _____ presence of Philadelphia chromosome
    b. acute myelogenous leukemia   2. _____ immortal mature lymphocytes in the circulation
    c. chronic myelogenous leukemia   3. _____ most common type in children
    d. chronic lymphocytic leukemia   4. _____ most common type in adults

17. Please indicate the clinical result of these effects of leukemia.
    a. loss of functional neutrophils and lymphocytes lead to fatal _____
    b. decrease in red blood cells leads to _____
    c. decrease in platelets leads to _____

10. a—incompatibility of the D antigen between a mother and fetus; d—sensitization of the maternal immune system against the fetal D antigen

11. c—kernicterus in the fetus after birth; d—anemia in the fetus before birth

12. a—aplastic anemia

13. 1. a—leukemia
    2. a—leukemia
    3. a—leukemia
    4. b—lymphoma
    5. b—lymphoma

14. c—the loss of WBC, RBC, and platelet cell lines that are replaced with nonfunctioning malignant cells

15. a—myeloid; b—lymphoid; c—acute; d—chronic

16. 1. c—CML
    2. d—CLL
    3. a—ALL
    4. b—AML

17. a—infection; b—anemia; c—hemorrhage or bleeding

18. d–a lymphoma where the Reed–Sternberg cell is present on biopsy

19. d–stage IV

20. a–follicular; b–diffuse

21. a–plasma cells in the bone marrow

22. a–infection; d–kidney failure

18. Hodgkin's disease is:
    a. an unusual leukemia seen in children in Africa
    b. a lymphoma in which the Reed–Sternberg cell is absent on biopsy
    c. a high-grade follicular lymphoma
    d. a lymphoma in which the Reed–Sternberg cell is present on biopsy

19. In Hodgkin's disease, malignancy of lymph nodes on both sides of the diaphragm and extranodal spread is seen in:
    a. stage I
    b. stage II
    c. stage III
    d. stage IV

20. In non-Hodgkin's lymphoma, the low-grade classification tends to be of the
    a. _____ type, while intermediate and high-grade tend to be of the
    b. _____ type.

21. Multiple myeloma is cancer of the:
    a. T lymphocytes in lymph nodes
    b. B lymphocytes in the bone marrow
    c. plasma cells in the bone marrow
    d. plasma cells in the lymph nodes

22. Death in multiple myeloma is most commonly due to (choose all that apply):
    a. infection
    b. hypercalcemia
    c. pathologic fractures
    d. kidney failure
    e. anemia

SECTION ▶ 9-79   III. DISTURBANCES IN HEMODYNAMICS

Hemodynamics are all of the forces and movements that make up the circulatory system. In this section, we will consider some states that cause a disturbance in these forces and movements, and examine some of the consequences. Hemodynamics is closely linked to the state of health or disease of blood vessels. Pathology of the vessels will cause some of the conditions in this section, and some of those same conditions will result in pathology of the vessels. Please keep this two-way communication in mind so that you do not become confused by the relationship. The separation of hemodynamics and disease of the blood vessels is arbitrary in these frames. This is done to break this information into more manageable sections.

▶ EDEMA

9-80

Edema was discussed at length in Chapter 3. It is the leakage of plasma or fluid from the vessels into the tissues or a body space. The identifiable accumulation of this fluid is edema. To review, there are three main causes for edema.

1. An increase in venous pressure, which causes blood to back up and pressure to increase to the point where fluid is squeezed out. An increase in pressure in veins that makes them distend or bulge is called **congestion.** Congestion, or the backup of venous blood, is often

due to an obstruction in flow. (It is helpful to think of a vessel as being a garden hose with water running through, and an obstruction as being a kink in the hose.) In addition to veins distending, some "spongy" organs, like the liver and spleen, can become distended and filled with blood. When the liver leaks fluid into the abdomen, this edema is specifically called **ascites.**

2. An increase in vessel wall permeability, such as in inflammation.
3. A decrease in plasma albumin (hypoalbuminemia), and therefore a decrease in oncotic pressure. Recall that oncotic pressure is the force that holds molecules of fluids inside vessels. Edema may result from an upset between the forces that retain fluid in the vessels and the mechanisms for release.

9–81

A buildup of fluid from vessels in tissues or spaces is called _____(1). It results when fluid _____(2) from vessels. Edema may result from an increased venous _____(3). This pressure is from a backup of blood, and this condition is called _____(4). Congestion results from a (an) _____(5) in blood flow. Edema can also result from an increase in vessel wall _____(6), or a decrease in _____(7) pressure. Decreased oncotic pressure is created by too little albumin in the blood, and this is called _____(8). Please recall from Chapters 2 and 3 the difference between edema that is characterized as a transudate or an exudate. An exudate contains moderate to high levels of protein and inflammatory cells. A transudate does not. Edema is both an important sign and a pathology. As a sign, it is a signal of disturbed function of organs such as the heart, liver, or kidney. As a pathology, its presence can be a space-occupying lesion that interferes with function. Edema or fluid in the lungs can make breathing difficult. Pericardial edema (in the sac surrounding the heart) will prevent maximum expansion of the heart. In the skull or vertebral column, edema can create enough pressure on the brain or spinal cord that serious injury results.

1. edema
2. leaks
3. pressure
4. congestion
5. obstruction
6. permeability
7. oncotic
8. hypoalbuminemia

9–82

There are two broad types of edema. Localized edema is confined to whatever organ is experiencing disease. Examples of this are pulmonary edema (fluid in the lungs), cerebral edema (fluid in the brain), and hydrothorax (fluid in the chest or pleural cavity). Generalized edema is widespread and is often due to hypoalbuminemia. Generalized edema may be called **anasarca.** Hypoalbuminemia can result from its decreased production in chronic liver disease, or from increased loss in kidney disease, or in some intestinal diseases. Edema confined to a particular organ is _____(1) edema. Hypoalbuminemia can cause _____(2) edema, which is also called _____(3).

1. localized
2. generalized
3. anasarca

9–83

There are several forms of edema. It is not uncommon to have more than one form at a time, depending on the cause. Where specifically in the body these forms occur will be presented with the disorders of the body systems. These forms are presented in the following list.

1. *Hydrostatic edema*—due to increased arterial or venous pressure, such as is seen in hypertension or congestive heart failure, respectively.
2. *Inflammatory edema*—due to increased vessel wall permeability, such as is seen in inflammation. Inflammation of the vessels themselves (vasculitis) can create anasarca.
3. *Oncotic edema*—due to hypoalbuminemia, such as is seen in liver, kidney, or some intestinal disease (a protein-losing enteropathy).
4. *Hypervolemic edema*—due to retention of sodium, such as is seen in kidney disease or Cushing's disease.
5. *Obstructive edema*—due to obstruction of vessels, especially lymphatics, such as is seen with a tumor or thrombus.

Note the relationships between the forms of edema in this frame and the general causes in Frame 9–80. The relationships are demonstrated in Table 9–6.

TABLE 9–6. FORMS OF EDEMA AND THEIR CAUSES

Form of Edema	Cause
Hydrostatic	Increased arterial or venous pressure Hypertension Congestive heart failure
Inflammatory	Increased vessel permeability
Oncotic	Hypoalbuminemia (decreased albumin) Chronic liver disease Kidney disease Intestinal disease (protein-losing enteropathy)
Hypervolemic	Sodium retention Kidney disease Cushing's disease
Obstructive	Obstruction of vessels Thrombi Tumor

1. inflammatory
2. hydrostatic
3. hypervolemic
4. oncotic
5. obstructive

An increase in vessel permeability causes _____(1) edema. An increase in arterial or venous pressure causes _____(2) edema. Sodium retention causes _____(3) edema. Hypoalbuminemia causes _____(4) edema. Lymphatic blockage causes _____(5) edema.

▶ HEMORRHAGE

9–84

1. hemorrhage
2. externally
3. internally
4. intravascular
5. blood pressure
6. perfusion

Everyone is familiar with **hemorrhage,** or bleeding. (In practice, the term "hemorrhage" is generally reserved for greater blood loss, rather than minor bleeding.) Hemorrhage is the disruption of a blood vessel which leads to the loss of blood from the *intravascular space.* This blood loss may be external and therefore gone from the body. Or it may be internal and technically still be within the body. However, internal bleeding can have the same devastating results as an external bleed, because it is the amount of blood *within* the *vessels* that carries significance. This *intravascular volume* is responsible for normal blood pressure and normal perfusion or supply of blood to the tissues. And, of course, blood carries oxygen and nutrients and rids waste products. Hemodynamics and homeostasis are very dependent on intravascular blood volume. Therefore, internal hemorrhage has the same effects as external hemorrhage. Two examples of internal hemorrhage are blood in the chest (hemothorax) and blood in the abdomen (hemoperitoneum). A relatively large bleed is called a _____(1). Blood may be lost _____(2), outside of the body, or _____(3), into a body cavity. Either location has the same result because it is the _____(4) blood volume that is responsible for normal _____(5) and _____(6).

9–85

Minor bleeding that is not due to trauma occurs in a variety of forms. These forms are called "hemorrhages" by some sources. You learned about **petechiae** (tiny red dots of bleeding) as a consequence of thrombocytopenia. An **ecchymosis** is a larger bleed under the skin and is commonly called a bruise. **Purpura** is also bleeding under the skin, somewhere in size between petechiae and ecchymosis.

9–86

There are several causes of hemorrhage. First, and most obvious, is trauma or injury. Other causes are the bleeding diseases discussed in the last section and disease of the blood vessels presented in the next section. Pathology of the organ systems can result in bleeding into these systems. Blood from the renal system appearing in the urine is **hematuria.** Coughing up blood from the lungs is **hemoptysis.** Vomiting blood from the stomach is **hematemesis,** and partially digested blood in the stool is **melena.** Chronic blood loss because of a body system pathology occurs in small amounts, but over time can result in _____(1) anemia. This is most commonly seen in gastric or duodenal ulcers, or with malignancies. Death from external hemorrhage itself is confined to acute and severe bleeding from trauma. Massive blood loss (greater than 1500 to 2000 mL) creates hypovolemia and shock, leading to death. Internal hemorrhage, if in critical amounts, can also lead to death in the same manner. In addition, internal hemorrhage can act as a space-occupying lesion and interfere with organ function through pressure or compression, like edema.

1. iron deficiency

▶ SHOCK

Shock is a vascular change resulting from several kinds of injury in which there is hypo-perfusion of the tissues with blood. In shock, the cardiovascular system fails to maintain adequate blood pressure. The result of irreversible shock is system-wide **anoxia** (no oxygen), organ failure, and death. Perfusion is the adequate supply of blood and oxygen to all tissues of the body. It is made possible primarily through the blood pressure, which is the driving force behind perfusion. Blood pressure is a function of blood volume, vascular resistance, and cardiac output. Therefore, inadequate blood volume, loss of vessel tone, and failure of cardiac output will lead to hypoperfusion and shock. All of these cause decreased blood pressure, or **hypotension.** Hypotension is a feature of shock. Hypotension results in hypoperfusion. The underlying pathology in shock is inadequate _____(1) of tissues with _____(2). This is called _____(3)perfusion. Decreased blood pressure, or _____(4), causes hypoperfusion. Hypotension develops if there is not enough _____(5) volume, decreased vascular _____(6), or a failure of _____(7). Because the pathogenesis of shock can be difficult to grasp, information in the following frames is in list format to increase your understanding.

9-87

1. perfusion
2. blood
3. hypo
4. hypotension
5. blood
6. tone
7. cardiac output

The following list presents examples of the events that lead to hypotension and hypoperfusion.

1. Decreased blood volume due to hemorrhage or other types of fluid loss (extreme dehydration, too much urine loss, severe burns).
2. Decreased vessel tone due to generalized vasodilation seen in anaphylaxis, sepsis with bacterial endotoxins, and reactions by the autonomic nervous system.
3. Decreased cardiac output due to heart failure, or as a consequence of decreased blood volume.

Widespread vasodilation _____(1) vessel tone, which decreases blood _____(2). Hemorrhage or extremes of other fluid loss decreases blood _____(3), which also decreases blood _____(4). Heart failure results in inadequate _____(5).

9-88

1. decreases
2. pressure
3. volume
4. pressure
5. cardiac output

The types of shock are given in the following list.

9-89

1. *Hypovolemic*—due to decreased blood volume for the reasons stated in the previous frame.
2. *Neurogenic or hypotonic*—due to decreased vascular resistance in vasodilation. An example of mild neurogenic shock is fainting, or **syncope,** which is seen in some people in an extreme emotional state. In this case the sudden loss of pressure and perfusion to the brain causes ischemia and loss of consciousness.
3. *Anaphylactic*—due to severe antigen–antibody reactions seen in type I hypersensitivity and incompatible blood transfusions.
4. *Cardiogenic*—secondary shock due to massive infarction of the myocardium (heart muscle) and failure to pump blood.

9-90

The pathogenesis of shock is a series of events or cycles that feed into each other, creating a spiral that worsens with every turn. Moderate to severe shock will result in death if the events are not interrupted. These events are presented in the following list in order of their occurrence.

1. Hypoperfusion is created by one of the causative agents listed in the previous frame. The vessels react or try to *compensate* by constricting and redirecting peripheral blood to vital organs, leaving the skin cool and clammy.
2. Despite compensatory peripheral vasoconstriction, the kidneys become hypoperfused and glomerular filtration rates decrease, causing little or no urine output.
3. The tissues experience anoxia from lack of blood. This causes metabolism to switch over to anaerobic ("without oxygen") pathways. Generalized anaerobic metabolism produces large amounts of lactic acid, so metabolic acidosis results.
4. Acidosis further decreases cardiac output because it depresses contraction of heart muscle. Acidosis also causes vasodilation, which further decreases blood pressure.
5. Pooling of blood in the lungs creates pulmonary edema and respiratory distress. This worsens anoxia because less oxygen is inspired. It also leads to the development of respiratory acidosis because less carbon dioxide can be expired.
6. Anoxia causes chemical mediators to be released, which further increases vasodilation and fluid loss into the tissues, lowering blood pressure even further. This especially occurs in septic shock.
7. DIC develops because endothelial cells are damaged and blood flow is sluggish. Normal inhibition of hemostasis is removed so generalized thrombosis, then uncontrollable bleeding results.
8. Death is imminent.

The pathogenesis of shock is schematically represented in Figure 9–12.

9-91

1. anoxia
2. hypoperfusion
3. anaerobic
4. lactic acid
5. metabolic acidosis
6. vasodilation
7. cardiac output
8. edema
9. anoxia
10. respiratory
11. disseminated intra-
    vascular coagulation

Lack of oxygen in the tissues is called _____(1). It results from inadequate perfusion, or _____(2). Anoxia leads to _____(3) metabolism. This pathway produces _____(4). This compound causes the body to experience _____(5). Acidosis further decreases blood pressure by causing _____(6) and depressing _____(7). Respiratory distress results from pulmonary _____(8). This makes _____(9) worse and creates _____(10) acidosis. Loss of control of hemostasis develops into _____(11), and death follows.

9-92

The three stages of shock that can be clinically identified by their signs are summarized in the following list.

1. Compensated or early shock is characterized by tachycardia (increased heart rate) to increase cardiac output, constriction of arterioles in the extremities to shunt blood to organs (which leaves the skin with a pallor), and decreased urine output to conserve fluid. For a limited time, these compensatory reactions are able to maintain adequate blood pressure for vital organs.
2. Decompensated or later shock develops when compensatory mechanisms give out. Hypotension (inadequate blood pressure), respiratory distress with anoxia, anuria (no urine output), and metabolic and respiratory acidosis characterize decompensated shock. Decompensated shock is reversible only if treated aggressively. Treatment must reverse both the cause and effects of shock. It includes intravenous replacement of fluids, transfusion with plasma or whole blood if indicated, epinephrine or steroids given IV, bicar-

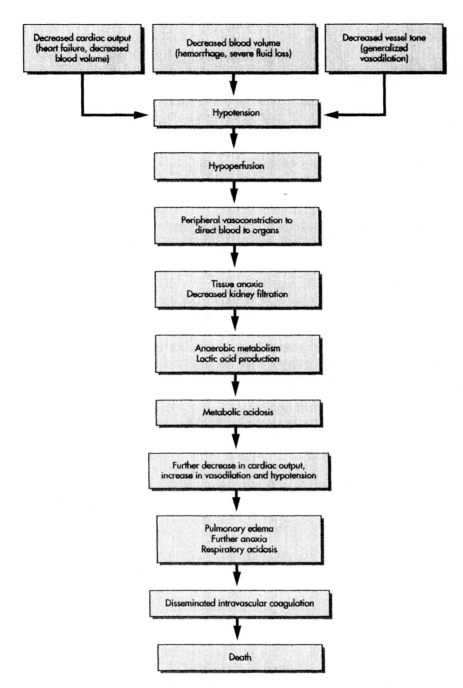

Figure 9–12. Pathogenesis of shock.

bonate to combat acidosis, and medications that cause vasoconstriction to increase blood pressure.

3. Irreversible shock is untreated decompensated shock. It marks the collapse of the circulatory system. Hypoperfusion and anoxia are severe, DIC ensues, and all organs fail. Death is likely even if treated at this end stage.

▶ HYPERTENSION

9-93

1. hypertension

Hypertension is the state of consistently elevated blood pressure, with pressure readings measuring greater than 160 mm Hg systolic, or 90 mm Hg diastolic. Normal blood pressure is approximately 140 over 90. The systolic measurement represents pressure when the heart is pumping blood (force of expulsion). The diastolic reading is the pressure when the heart is resting in between contractions. The elasticity of healthy arteries allows them to expand and absorb some of the pressure, therefore dissipating it. Blood pressure is determined by the amount of blood in circulation (blood volume), the amount that is pumped by each heart contraction (cardiac output), and the resistance by arterial walls. Changing any of these parameters changes blood pressure. An increased diastolic pressure is more significant in terms of potential injury to the body because it represents residual pressure. This means pressure is always too high, never allowing the vessels a brief respite in between heart contractions. Blood pressure that persistently reads greater than 160 mm Hg systolic, or 90 mm Hg diastolic, defines _____(1).

9-94

Primary or essential hypertension is largely idiopathic. A single causative factor has not been positively identified. It is believed to be multifactorial, with genetics, lifestyle, and stress playing major roles. Primary hypertension is by far the most common. An important factor is the state of health or disease of the arteries. We will soon be discussing arteriosclerosis and atherosclerosis, diseases of arteries. In these states, arteries lose much of their elasticity. They become rigid and do not expand as they should. Expansion is a major part of dissipating the pressure from the expulsion force of blood. Since this force is not dampened as it should be, pressure remains high. This sclerosis (hardening) of the arteries creates a persistent increased resistance to blood circulation. The left ventricle senses the increased resistance and pumps harder to overcome it. This further increases blood pressure and feeds the hypertension. Vessel size is also important in determining the amount of resistance to blood flow. In atherosclerosis, deposits of fat narrow the vessel lumen and make the internal diameter smaller. This increases resistance and pressure. Two mechanisms of primary hypertension are shown in Figure 9–13.

9-95

1. idiopathic
2. common
3. arteries
4. expand
5. dissipate
6. resistance
7. left ventricle or heart

Primary hypertension is _____(1) in cause. Its occurrence is the most _____(2). The condition of the _____(3) plays an important role. If they are rigid, they cannot _____(4) as they should. This expansion helps to absorb or _____(5) some of the pressure to create normal levels. Vascular _____(6) to blood flow is increased. Hypertension is made worse by the reaction of the _____(7) to increased resistance. Secondary hypertension is a direct

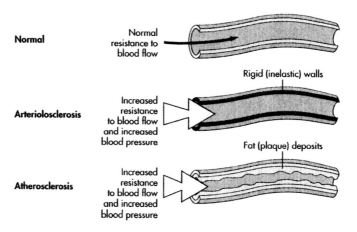

Figure 9–13. Two mechanisms of primary hypertension.

result of a primary or initial disease. Secondary hypertension can occur in some kidney diseases, some hormonal disease states, and in toxemia of pregnancy.

9–96

The effects of hypertension, as shown in Figure 9–14, develop over several years. Sustained high blood pressure causes injury to the cardiovascular system. Some diseases of the vessels can in turn cause hypertension. This relationship is seen in the following example. Hypertension will cause the arteries to harden over time because of the increased pressure. This partly defines arteriosclerosis. Arteriosclerosis itself will cause hypertension because of the increased resistance of the vessels. Returning to the effects of hypertension on the vessels, the high pressure leads to thickening of the walls and a decrease in elasticity, especially of the smaller arteries and arterioles. The increased vascular resistance signals the heart to work harder to pump blood that is now more difficult to move. Anytime a muscle is worked hard, it enlarges or hypertrophies. The left ventricle, which pushes directly against the resistance, enlarges and creates a cardiomyopathy. The hypertrophy decreases the size of the lumen in the ventricle so that it holds less blood. Therefore, cardiac output is decreased. The increased muscle mass is *not* supplied with more vessels to service the muscle, so some degree of ischemia develops in the heart muscle. The coronary arteries, which supply the heart itself, undergo arteriosclerosis like the other vessels. This causes serious ischemia and fibrosis of damaged heart muscle. Heart failure because of ischemic heart disease is the most common cause of death due to hypertension.

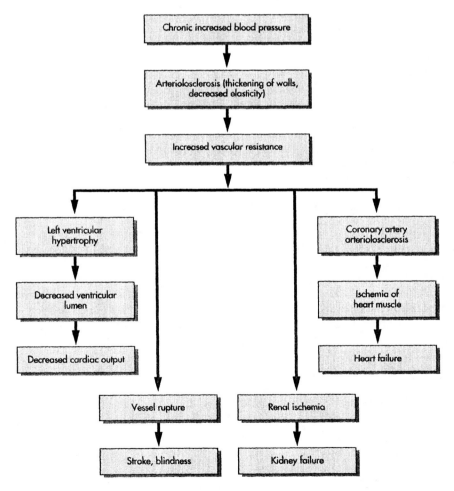

Figure 9–14. Effects of hypertension.

1. cardiovascular
2. hard or thick
3. elasticity
4. sclerosis
5. resistance
6. left ventricle or heart
7. hypertrophies
8. ischemia
9. Heart failure

The primary injury caused by hypertension is to the _____(1) system. Continued high blood pressure causes the arterial walls to become _____(2) and lose their _____(3). Hypertension is one cause of arterio_____(4). Arteriosclerosis increases the _____(5) of vessels to blood flow. This resistance is interpreted by the _____(6) as a need to work harder. The muscle of the left ventricle becomes enlarged, or _____(7). The need for more blood supply to enlarged muscle is combined with arteriosclerosis of the coronary arteries, and the result is _____(8) of the heart. _____(9) is the most common cause of death in hypertension.

In addition to hardening the arteries, hypertension can cause a vessel to burst. This makes stroke the second most common cause of death. A stroke results when small vessels rupture in the brain. This leads to cerebral hemorrhage and infarct in areas of the brain. Areas of infarction heal with fibrosis, leaving permanent loss of function provided by those areas. Small arteries in the retina are also susceptible to rupture and bleeding. This can create permanent blind spots where the retinal tissue has been damaged by infarction. Complete blindness is also a possibility. Rupture of other vessels might cause visible signs such as epistaxis (nosebleed) or hemoptysis (coughing up blood). Renal ischemia because of arteriosclerosis of renal arteries can become severe enough that kidney failure ensues. Hypertension is called the "silent killer" because most cases are asymptomatic for up to 15 years while the damage is slowly being done. This is why screening for high blood pressure is so important. Once severe arterial pathology has developed, life span is not expected to be longer than 5 years, especially if the condition is untreated.

1. stroke
2. brain
3. retina
4. blindness
5. silent killer
6. 15

Another common reason for death due to hypertension is _____(1). This is rupture and bleeding of vessels in the _____(2). The same can occur with vessels in the _____(3), possibly leading to _____(4). Hypertension is called the "_____(5)" because the condition may show no signs for as long as _____(6) years. The prognosis for hypertension is extremely variable, depending on the severity, duration, and manageability of the case. Hypertension is easily diagnosed with blood pressure readings using a sphygmomanometer. Examination of the retina during an ophthalmic exam is very helpful in assessing the state of the arteries, since these arteries are easily visible.

Treatment or management of hypertension follows three premises in this list.

1. Diagnosing it as early as possible with regular health screenings.
2. Ruling out secondary hypertension by looking for a primary cause which may be treatable.
3. Managing current cases with medications to decrease blood volume and promote excess fluid loss through the urine (diuretics) and medications to decrease blood pressure. A restricted sodium diet decreases fluid retention, and a low-calorie diet promotes weight loss to ease the burden on the heart. Exercise is needed to promote weight loss and improve circulation. Lifestyle changes such as cessation of smoking, avoidance of excessive alcohol consumption, and stress management are required.

▶ DISRUPTION IN BLOOD SUPPLY AND OXYGEN

Some of the terms in the next frames have been used frequently to this point and their definitions already presented. We will redefine them here for the sake of completeness. **Hypoxia** is decreased or inadequate oxygenation of cells or tissues. Insufficient oxygen supply, or hypoxia, may arise through several mechanisms. *Hypoxic hypoxia* means that the Po_2 (partial pressure of oxygen in the blood) is decreased because of lung disease. The lungs are not able to deliver enough oxygen to the blood passing through them. *Anemic hypoxia* develops if there are not enough red blood cells or hemoglobin to carry a normal amount of oxygen to the tissues. *Ischemic hypoxia* is a result of inadequate blood supply to the tissues, perhaps because of heart failure or obstruction of a vessel. In understanding hypoxia and its mechanisms of development, remember the following simple premises.

1. Oxygen must move from the atmosphere, through the lungs, and into the blood vessels.
2. Hemoglobin inside red blood cells must pick up oxygen for transportation to the cells and tissues.
3. Hemoglobin-bound oxygen must then be provided to all parts of the body by the circulatory system, which includes the heart as well as the vessels.

Disruption in any of the above mechanisms will cause disruption in oxygen supply. _____(1) is the state of insufficient oxygen reaching tissues. It may develop because of low _____(2) during lung disease, because of _____(3), or because of poor _____(4) supply.

9–102

1. Hypoxia
2. Po$_2$
3. anemia
4. blood

Ischemia is decreased or inadequate blood supply to an area. Its most important consequence is hypoxia, for reason number 3 in Frame 9–101. Ischemic hypoxia results in immediate harm to cells by depriving them of oxygen. Waste products are also not removed. The accumulation of waste products causes pain at an ischemic site. There are many specific causes of ischemia. As we study each body system, reference will be made to the disease process that causes ischemia. In Chapter 2 you learned that ischemia is the most common cause of general injury to the body. We can divide ischemia into two types, generalized and localized. Generalized ischemia is a consequence of poor cardiac output, or of cardiac arrest. In cardiac arrest, the brain is the most immediately sensitive organ to hypoxia. Lack of oxygen to the brain that lasts longer than 3 minutes will cause some degree of permanent damage. Hypoxia or anoxia (complete lack of oxygen) produces brain death after 8 minutes. These facts provide the guidelines for length of time in cardiopulmonary resuscitation efforts. Localized ischemia is more common and affects specific areas, defined by the vessels that serve them. Localized ischemia is due to partial arterial obstruction. These obstructions include embolism, thrombosis, or atherosclerosis (to be discussed soon).

9–103

Decreased blood supply to a site is _____(1), and the immediate injury caused by ischemia is _____(2). The most common cause of injury in the body is hypoxia because of _____(3). Cardiac arrest causes _____(4) ischemia, which most adversely affects the _____(5). Partial loss of function occurs after _____(6) minutes, with irreversible damage and death after _____(7) minutes. _____(8) ischemia is more common. It is usually because of partial arterial _____(9).

1. ischemia
2. hypoxia
3. ischemia
4. generalized
5. brain
6. 3
7. 8
8. Localized
9. obstruction

9–104

Complete and sudden lack of oxygen in the tissues is **anoxia,** with the prefix "a" meaning _____(1). Hypoxia and anoxia are differences in degree of the same problem. So it is with ischemia and infarction. While ischemia represents inadequate circulation, **infarction,** or an **infarct,** is tissue death because of complete absence of blood supply and oxygen. The area that is normally supplied will die. There develops a circumscribed or specifically defined area of necrosis, termed *ischemic necrosis.* Unfortunately, the long-term consequences of infarction are that the necrotic tissue may be replaced with nonfunctional scar tissue, which is significant in a vital organ. During an infarct, individual cells first die, then coalesce into a larger visible site of death. After necrosis sets in, autolysis, or breakdown, begins, and surrounding healthy tissue reacts with a wide ring of inflammation. (Remember, necrotic tissue is interpreted as foreign and so inflammation will be the response.) Complete lack of blood supply causes a (an) _____(2). This is _____(3) of tissue normally supplied with blood. This death is specifically called _____(4). The normal reaction by healthy tissue to necrosis is _____(5).

1. without
2. infarction
3. death
4. necrosis
5. inflammation

1. regeneration
2. function
3. fibrosis or scar tissue
4. function
5. fibrosis
6. obstruction or occlusion

The fate of the necrotic area depends on the organ or tissue in which it is found. In epithelial-based organs (liver or kidney), regeneration is the primary resolution effort. (Remember that regenerated tissue is truly reproduced, with its function returning.) Of course, regeneration has its limits, so severe acute injury or chronic injury will result in scar tissue instead. Some tissues, like heart muscle and nerve, have almost no regenerative capabilities. In these cases the necrotic tissue is replaced with granulation tissue that later matures into scar or fibrotic tissue (see Chap. 2). Obviously, function is lost in a directly proportional manner. The size of an infarct and its location determine the ultimate results (healing versus loss of vital function). The cause of infarction is complete arterial or venous obstruction. (Occlusion is a word often used in place of obstruction.) The mechanisms for obstruction are the same as in ischemia, that is, thrombosis, embolism, or atherosclerosis. Epithelial-based organs respond to infarction and necrosis with the healing process of _____(1), within limits. In regeneration, restoration of _____(2) is possible. In other vital organs, regeneration is very poor and most repair is by replacement with _____(3). The amount of _____(4) that is lost is directly proportional to the amount of _____(5) present. Complete arterial or venous _____(6) produces infarction.

An **embolus** is a freely traveling mass in the circulatory system, like a foreign body. It is visible and has significant mass, unlike cellular elements or dissolved substances in the blood. An embolus has the potential to cause ischemia or infarction through degrees of obstruction of vessels. (Embolic ischemia or infarction is like a clogged drain.) The following list presents potential elements that could become an embolus.

1. A thrombus (see Frame 9-109) may break off or detach from a vessel wall. Thrombi from veins, for instance, in the legs, enter easily into the heart. From there they pass through the lungs and become trapped in small pulmonary vessels, creating a *pulmonary embolism.* Thrombi from arteries enter arteries of the vital organs, creating, for instance, a *cerebral embolism.* A thrombus is the most common embolus.
2. Fat may be liberated into the bloodstream from the bone marrow after a fracture of a long bone.
3. A mass of neoplastic cells occurs during metastasis.
4. A mass of bacteria may be created during septicemia, called a *septic embolism.*
5. A part of a fat plaque may break off from a site of atherosclerosis.
6. Air may be introduced iatrogenically, that is, through a treatment technique such as IV catheterization.

1. embolus
2. thrombus
3. broken
4. vessel

A freely traveling mass in the circulatory system is a (an) _____(1). The most common is a _____(2). A thrombotic embolus has _____(3) off from the wall of a _____(4). The most clinically significant result of an embolus is the production of an **embolism.** An embolism is the partial or complete occlusion of a vessel by an embolus. Thromboembolism is most common. An embolism that partly obstructs a vessel causes ischemia to the normally supplied area. An embolism that completely obstructs a vessel causes infarction in the area. Because of the route of circulation, an embolus in the veins ends up in the lungs, causing pulmonary embolism and possible pulmonary infarction. An embolus in the arterial system will enter organs and the extremities. Emboli from the heart are frequently associated with bacterial endocarditis. Those originating from the aorta are often bits of atherosclerotic plaque. The danger of infarction of areas of the heart or in the brain are very great and often result in death. A **saddle embolus** is particularly dangerous because it lodges at a bifurcation, or fork, in a major artery. By straddling this area, it effectively cuts off both branches of circulation. Involvement of the bifurcations of pulmonary arteries causes death due to acute anoxia.

An embolus causes a (an) _____(1), which is the partial or complete _____(2) of a _____(3). Partial occlusion causes _____(4), while complete occlusion causes _____(5). Death frequently occurs from infarction in the _____(6) or _____(7). The plugging of both routes of circulation is done by a _____(8), which gets caught at the _____(9) of a major artery.

1. embolism
2. obstruction
3. vessel
4. ischemia
5. infarction
6. heart
7. brain
8. saddle embolus
9. fork, or bifurcation

A **thrombus** is a blood clot. In Figure 9–15 you can see several thrombi that were present in a vein. Their formation is called **thrombosis.** Thrombosis develops when the mechanisms of hemostasis are activated inside an intact vessel that has not suffered grossly visible injury. There are three initiating factors of thrombosis, microscopic endothelial cell injury, changes in normal blood flow (sluggish or turbulent), and hypercoagulability of the blood (involving platelets and the clotting factors). The clots are at first adhered, or stuck, to the wall of the vessel because coagulation factors interact with the cells when the thrombus is formed, thus causing the clot to be developed at this site. A major reason for thrombosis is the loss of antithrombotic, or anticoagulative properties of the endothelial cells. In even microscopic trauma, blood is exposed to tissue, which precipitates clotting. In widespread vasculitis, some chemical mediators of inflammation initiate clotting by damaging endothelium. A blood clot is a _____(1). The formation of one is _____(2). This occurs when _____(3) is activated inside vessels. Changes in _____(4) flow and injury to _____(5) cells are reasons for thrombosis. Injury causes endothelial cells to lose their _____(6) properties.

1. thrombus
2. thrombosis
3. hemostasis
4. blood
5. endothelial
6. antithrombotic or anticoagulant

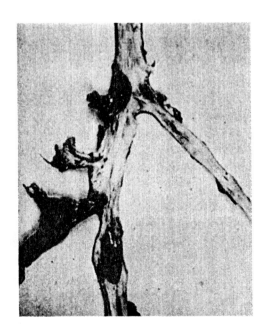

Figure 9–15. Several thrombi in a vein. *(From McCance and Huether,* Pathophysiology–The Biologic Basis for Disease in Adults and Children, *1st ed., Mosby.)*

9–110

1. injury
2. blood flow
3. turbulent

Examples of conditions that favor thrombosis, and sites of formation include the following.

1. Veins where blood flow is relatively slow and the thrombus has a chance to form before being swept away.
2. Areas of turbulence that separate the cellular elements, mechanically stimulate platelets, and allow them exposure to endothelium. Turbulence also damages the endothelium.
3. Diseased heart valves.
4. Existing lesions in vessels, which cause platelets to adhere and begin the process. The best example of this is in atherosclerosis (see Frame 9–115).
5. Areas where blood flow is slow or sluggish, as in poor circulation of the legs (dilated varicose veins), and in viscous conditions (polycythemia).
6. On the inner heart wall overlying an area of myocardial infarction.

Considering all the vessels in the body that could experience thrombosis, the coronary vessels of the heart, and the cerebral vessels of the brain are over-represented. To review, conditions most favoring thrombosis are a (an) _____(1) to the lining of vessels, sluggish _____(2), or _____(3) blood flow.

9–111

The end result or clinical significance of thrombosis is very similar to embolism. (A thrombus can become an embolus, but remember an embolus can be other things. A thrombus is adhered to its site of formation, but if it breaks off it is then an embolus.) Like embolism, thrombosis causes varying degrees of occlusion of vessels, leading to ischemia or infarction. Once a thrombus is formed, there are several mechanisms that attempt to resolve or remove it, such as breaking it down or tunneling through it. A thrombus that remains will narrow the lumen of the vessel and restrict blood flow. This restriction by definition is ischemia. The result of ischemia is hypoxia. Complete blockage is possible and is a very common cause of myocardial infarction when the coronary arteries are occluded. (It is sadly ironic that survival of a myocardial infarction can later cause thrombosis at the injured site and re-injury.) Blockage of cerebral arteries and brain infarction is also a leading cause of death. At any time, a thrombus can break off and travel as an embolus to cause deficiency in blood supply at a distant site.

9–112

1. occlusion
2. ischemia
3. infarction
4. narrowing
5. heart
6. brain
7. embolus

The clinical significance of thrombosis is _____(1) of vessels, leading to _____(2) or _____(3), depending on the amount of obstruction. A thrombus restricts blood flow by _____(4) the lumen of the vessel. Complete occlusion often results in death when the vessels of the _____(5) or _____(6) are affected. A thrombus can interrupt blood supply elsewhere in the body if it breaks from its site of formation and travels as a (an) _____(7).

III. REVIEW QUESTIONS

1. b–all of the movements and forces behind the circulatory system

2. a–hypoalbuminemia; 2–pressure; 3–permeability

1. Hemodynamics is:
   a. the process through which the heart pumps blood
   b. all of the movements and forces behind the circulatory system
   c. the state of health or disease of blood vessels
   d. the maintenance of normal blood pressure

2. Edema may be caused by any of the following mechanisms:
   a. a decrease in plasma albumin, or _____
   b. squeezing out of fluid because of increased venous _____
   c. an increase in the _____ of vessel walls

3. Please match the forms of edema in the left column with their cause in the right column:

   a. hypervolemic   _____ 1.   increased arterial or venous pressure
   b. inflammatory   _____ 2.   sodium retention
   c. oncotic   _____ 3.   hypoalbuminemia
   d. hydrostatic   _____ 4.   increased vessel wall permeability

4. Significant hemorrhage can result in (choose all that apply):
   a. hypertension
   b. hypotension
   c. hypervolemia
   d. hypovolemia
   e. hyperperfusion
   f. hypoperfusion
   g. hypoxia

5. Choose the correct statement about hemorrhage:
   a. external blood loss is more significant because it decreases intravascular volume
   b. internal blood loss is more significant because it decreases intravascular volume
   c. both external and internal loss are equally significant
   d. neither type of loss significantly affects intravascular volume because the bone marrow and kidneys immediately provide replacement cells and fluid

6. The features of shock that can lead to organ failure and death include (choose all that apply):
   a. hypotension
   b. hypoperfusion
   c. anoxia
   d. all of the above

7. Additional features in the pathogenesis of shock include (choose all that apply):
   a. metabolic acidosis
   b. metabolic alkalosis
   c. respiratory alkalosis
   d. respiratory acidosis
   e. pulmonary edema
   f. pulmonary embolism
   g. disseminated intravascular coagulation
   h. thrombosis

8. During the early stages of shock, tachycardia, arteriole constriction, and decreased urine production represent:
   a. attempts at compensation to maintain perfusion to vital organs
   b. attempts at decompensation to maintain perfusion to vital organs
   c. the only stage in which treatment is possible
   d. changes that immediately precede death

9. Factors that influence blood pressure include (choose all that apply):
   a. expansion of arterial walls
   b. expansion of venous walls
   c. the amount of resistance by the blood vessels
   d. heart rate
   e. the size of the vessel lumen

3. 1. d–hydrostatic; 2. a–hypervolemic; 3. c–oncotic; 4. b–inflammatory

4. b–hypotension; d–hypovolemia; f–hypoperfusion; g–hypoxia

5. c–both external and internal loss are equally significant

6. d–all of the above

7. a–metabolic acidosis; d–respiratory acidosis; e–pulmonary edema; g–disseminated intravascular coagulation

8. a–attempts at compensation to maintain perfusion to vital organs

9. a–expansion of arterial walls; c–the amount of resistance by the blood vessels; e–the size of vessel lumen

10. a–1; b–5; c–2; d–6; e–4; f–3; g–7

11. a. 1–rupture; 2–infarction; b. 1–rupture; 2–retina; c. 1–ischemia; 2–arteriosclerosis

12. 1. c–infarction
    2. b–hypoxia
    3. a–ischemia
    4. d–anoxia

13. a. 1–red blood cells; 2–hemoglobin; b. 1–oxygen; c. 1–insufficient or inadequate; 2–obstruction

14. d–repair by fibrosis in which organ function is decreased

15. b–thrombi

16. 1–ischemia; 2–infarction

17. a–injury to endothelial cells; c–abnormalities in blood flow

18. a–heart; d–brain

10. List the following effects of hypertension in order of occurrence:
    a. _____ thickening of arterial walls and decreased elasticity
    b. _____ decreased cardiac output
    c. _____ arteriosclerosis
    d. _____ heart muscle ischemia
    e. _____ left ventricular hypertrophy
    f. _____ increased vascular resistance
    g. _____ heart failure

11. Additional effects of hypertension can be:
    a. stroke, because of 1. _____ of vessels in the brain, causing loss of blood supply and tissue death or 2. _____
    b. blindness, because of 1. _____ of vessels in the 2. _____
    c. renal failure, because of decreased blood supply or 1. _____ caused by 2. _____ of renal arteries

12. Please match the terms in the left column with the definitions in the right column:
    a. ischemia   1. _____ tissue death due to absence of blood supply
    b. hypoxia   2. _____ inadequate oxygenation of cells
    c. infarction   3. _____ inadequate blood supply
    d. anoxia   4. _____ absence of oxygenation of cells

13. Hypoxia can develop due to any of the following mechanisms:
    a. anemia, which is insufficient 1. _____ or 2. _____
    b. lung disease, which can lower amounts of 1. _____ in the blood
    c. ischemia, which is 1. _____ blood supply due to partial 2. _____ of the vessels

14. The most significant consequence of infarction is:
    a. repair by regeneration in which organ function is maintained
    b. repair by fibrosis in which organ function is maintained
    c. repair by regeneration in which organ function is decreased
    d. repair by fibrosis in which organ function is decreased

15. The most common emboli are:
    a. clumps of bacteria
    b. thrombi
    c. masses of malignant cells
    d. fat globules

16. The clinical significance of an embolism is that it may produce 1. _____ or 2. _____ depending of the degree of vessel occlusion.

17. Thrombosis is most often associated with (choose all that apply):
    a. injury to endothelial cells
    b. hypertension
    c. abnormalities in blood flow
    d. hypoxia

18. Thrombosis of which two organs produces significant death rate?
    a. heart
    b. liver
    c. kidneys
    d. brain
    e. lungs

IV. DISEASE OF THE BLOOD VESSELS ◀ SECTION

▶ ARTERIOSCLEROSIS AND ATHEROSCLEROSIS

9–113

Everyone is familiar with the phrase "hardening of the arteries." This describes **arteriosclerosis.** The word root "sclerosis" means hardening, and tissue that is sclerotic is hard. Therefore, arteriosclerosis means hardening of the arteries. This is a condition directly related to age and it represents a degeneration. This degenerative change consists of loss of elasticity of the arteries and a thickening of the intima over time. This causes the affected vessels to become relatively brittle and they are somewhat susceptible to rupture. Almost every geriatric adult has some degree of arteriosclerosis. It is the degree or severity that dictates the onset of clinical problems. Arteriosclerosis means _____(1) of the _____(2). This disorder is classified as a _____(3) change, related to _____(4). The arteries lose some _____(5) and become _____(6).

1. hardening
2. arteries
3. degenerative
4. age
5. elasticity
6. thickened

9–114

There are two forms of arteriosclerosis. The first is **arteriolosclerosis,** and it consists of generalized thickening of small arteries and arterioles. It is a common reaction to systemic hypertension. The high pressure causes the muscular layer of the vessels to enlarge through hypertrophy, and the intima layer to undergo fibrous thickening. As the wall then becomes thicker, this decreases the size of the vessel lumen, or internal diameter. The narrowed lumen creates increased resistance to blood flow, which worsens hypertension. (Arteriosclerosis and hypertension are two states that have a "two-way street" type of relationship.) In addition to increased resistance and pressure, less blood can pass through, creating some degree of ischemia depending on the amount of narrowing. This consequence is especially seen when the renal arteries are affected. Here, ischemia leads to degeneration and scarring of the renal parenchyma. The end-stage hardened condition is called nephrosclerosis. Widespread thickening of the smaller arteries and arterioles is a form of arteriosclerosis known as _____(1). It develops in response to _____(2). The high pressure causes parts of the vessel wall to become _____(3). This _____(4) the size of the lumen, which _____(5) resistance to blood flow even more. The smaller lumen allows less _____(6) to flow through and can lead to _____(7) of the supplied tissues or organs.

1. arteriolosclerosis
2. systemic hypertension
3. enlarged or hypertrophied
4. decreases
5. increases
6. blood
7. ischemia

9–115

The second form of arteriosclerosis is prevalent and well known. It is **atherosclerosis.** You know what sclerotic means. "Athero" is from the Greek and it means soft, specifically porridgy. Therefore, atherosclerosis is a condition that combines both softness and hardness in the same lesion. This is a very significant form of arteriosclerosis and is directly responsible for many deaths. The lesion itself is a fatty **plaque,** sometimes called an **atheroma** (soft lump). Almost all adults have atheromas to some degree. The plaque is formed on the surface of the intima. The center, being composed of fat (specifically *cholesterol*), is soft and yellow, or porridgy. The fat becomes covered with a hard cap of fibrous tissue. This is the sclerotic portion. Figure 9–16 shows the components and result of a significant fatty plaque. Atherosclerosis is a disease of the arteries in which the lesions are a combination of _____(1) and _____(2). The soft portion is predominantly _____(3), especially _____(4). The hard part is a covering of _____(5) tissue. The lesion is commonly referred to as a _____(6), or might be called a (an) _____(7).

1. softness
2. hardness
3. fat or lipids
4. cholesterol
5. fibrous
6. plaque
7. atheroma

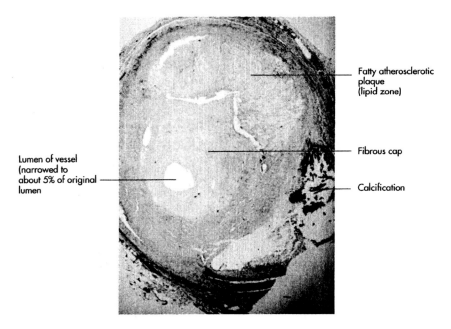

Figure 9-16. Atherosclerosis producing significant narrowing of a coronary artery. *(From Chandrasoma and Taylor,* Concise Pathology, *2nd ed. Appleton & Lange.)*

9-116

1. injury
2. lipids
3. smooth muscle
4. LDL cholesterol
5. foam cells
6. sclerotic
7. repair
8. fibrous tissue
9. fat

The pathogenesis or development of atherosclerosis is unclear, but is believed to have its basis in injury to the endothelial lining of the intima. This injury could be due to a wide range of causes, including certain risk factors, vasculitis, turbulence, or any hemodynamic stress. The microscopic injury leaves exposed areas of intima where lipid, or fat in the blood, and macrophages enter. Platelets are deposited at the site. The proliferation of smooth muscle cells is stimulated by these changes. The muscle cells appear to act as receptors for LDL cholesterol. (LDL cholesterol is a lipid that is relatively insoluble and has the potential to build up.) The muscle cells become engorged and laden with fat. Their yellow appearance has earned them the label **foam cells.** Around these soft lipid deposits on and in the intima, attempts at repair are made. These attempts leave typical scar tissue or fibrosis. The tough, fibrous tissue over the soft, fatty pocket comprises the sclerotic portion of the plaque. Atherosclerosis probably begins with _____(1) of endothelial lining. Exposed intima serves as a gathering site for _____(2) in the blood. This, along with deposits of macrophages and platelets, stimulates an increase in the number of _____(3) cells. These act as receptors for _____(4), and their enlargement with this fat causes them to be called _____(5). The hard, or _____(6), part of the plaque stems from attempts at _____(7) of the lesion. The activity leaves tough _____(8), which overlays the soft _____(9) center.

9-117

Atherosclerosis is seen in the aorta and major arteries, especially at points of branching where some turbulence exists. It is also well represented in the medium-sized arteries of the heart and brain. In fact, the coronary and cerebral arteries are often most severely affected. The involvement of these arteries is responsible for most atherosclerotic-related deaths. Myocardial infarction and stroke (cerebral vascular accident, or CVA) make up the majority of deaths. Atherosclerosis of arteries supplying the extremities is called **peripheral vascular disease.** In this state, most clinical difficulties are due to atherosclerosis of the renal and intestinal arteries. Atherosclerosis of arteries in the legs can become an obstruction and cause gangrene. Atherosclerosis often is localized and may affect one organ much more than others. The most common clinical forms of atherosclerosis are in the following list.

1. Coronary heart disease, which affects the coronary arteries and leads to myocardial infarction.
2. Cerebral vascular disease, which affects arteries of the brain and leads to stroke or CVA.
3. Aortic aneurysm, which affects the abdominal aorta and leads to fatal rupture.
4. Peripheral vascular disease, which affects arteries of extremities and organs and leads to gangrene or abdominal organ failure.

9–118

There are many ill effects of atherosclerosis, which are summarized in Table 9–7. The bulging of the intima as the plaque is formed, and its continued growth, causes gradual *obstruction* of the vessel lumen (refer back to Fig. 9–16). As this narrowing occurs in the medium-sized and small arteries, ischemia can easily develop in the supplied area. Should the plaque grow to completely block the vessel, this occlusion causes infarction and necrosis of the supplied area. This is the mechanism behind gangrene of the legs and kidney failure in peripheral vascular disease, myocardial infarction, and stroke. Also, the increased vascularity around the plaque (an inflammatory response) can lead to bleeding at the site and acute obstruction in that manner. *Thrombosis* can develop from several causes. The plaque can rupture from the internal pressure, releasing material that is very thrombogenic. This leaves an ulcer over the surface of the fibrous cap. This injury stimulates clotting at the site. Also, the turbulence surrounding a plaque may stimulate clot formation. The presence of thrombi further decreases the lumen and contributes to ischemia or infarction. Thrombosis seems prone to occur in the cerebral and coronary arteries. The thrombus may break off and become an *embolus*. The clot and atheromatous material then travel to the vessels of the nearest organs, where obstruction and infarction are great dangers.

9–119

Weakening of the vessel wall in response to the plaque lesion can develop into a bulge, or an *aneurysm*. This seems to appear most often in portions of the abdominal aorta, where atherosclerosis can be at its worst. Rupture of the aneurysm generally results in death due to exsanguination (bleeding to death). Another reaction to the presence of the plaque is *calcification*. As the local tissue degenerates, calcium salts from the blood can deposit there. This causes a rigidity or hardening of the entire wall, making it brittle and susceptible to rupture. The effects of atherosclerosis include those presented in the following list.

1. obstruction
2. ischemia
3. infarction
4. thrombosis
5. ulcer
6. ischemia
7. infarction

1. Occupation of space in the vessel lumen, causing _____(1). The consequences are decreased blood supply [_____(2)] or absence of blood supply [_____(3)].
2. Clot formation or _____(4), which develops at the site of an _____(5) in the cap of the plaque. Thrombosis worsens _____(6) or _____(7).

TABLE 9–7. EFFECTS OF ATHEROSCLEROSIS

Partial obstruction of vessel lumen
  Ischemia
Complete obstruction (occlusion) of vessel lumen
  Infarction
  Necrosis
Thrombosis
Embolism
  Obstruction
  Infarction (heart, brain)
Aneurysm
  Rupture
  Exsanguination
Vessel calcification
  Rigidity
  Rupture

8. embolus
9. aneurysm
10. brittle

3. Loss of a thrombus into the bloodstream, creating an _____(8).
4. Weakening of the wall, which may lead to _____(9) formation and rupture. Rupture can also occur if the wall becomes _____(10).

9–120

The exact cause of atherosclerosis is unknown. Almost all adults have some degree of it. Atherosclerosis is a multifactorial disease, with injury to vessels combining with various risk factors. There are many factors that have been identified as predisposing to atherosclerosis, as summarized in the following list.

1. Smoking, in which the tar and nicotine injure vessels.
2. Hypertension, in which physical force injures vessels.
3. Family history, in which atherosclerosis or diabetes has been prominent.
4. Hypercholesterolemia, in which a genetic defect in LDL receptors allows its build-up in the circulation.
5. High-fat diet, in which levels of LDL cholesterol, triglycerides, and lipoproteins are increased. Evaluation of serum cholesterol level is a useful screening tool for atherosclerosis. A protective level is 200 mg/dL or less. A result of greater than 260 mg/dL indicates five times the risk for atherosclerosis.
6. Age, in which time allows the build up of plaques.
7. Sex, in which men are over-represented. Premenopausal women benefit from the protective effects of estrogen.
8. Hyperlipidemia, in which circulating amounts of fats are increased. This can be a primary familial disease, or more commonly, a secondary condition associated with obesity. A genetic predisposition to obesity combined with overeating creates excess body fat, and blood lipids increase proportionately. Therefore, there is more fat present to become deposited in the intima. Obese subjects develop atherosclerosis earlier and to a worse degree than normal subjects. In addition, the complicating presence of diabetes, with its abnormal fat metabolism, is an important contributing factor. If you will recall, atherosclerosis is a significant complication of diabetes.

9–121

1. fat or lipids
2. diet
3. obese
4. diabetes
5. injury

A very common predisposing factor in the development of atherosclerosis is the presence of high amounts of _____(1) in the blood. This can result from a high-fat _____(2), being overweight or _____(3), or having _____(4) mellitus. Smoking and hypertension set the stage for atherosclerosis by causing _____(5) to the vessel lining. Prevention of atherosclerosis is far more important than treatment. To diminish risk, protective factors such as exercise and a low fat diet, must be combined with avoidance of the known contributing factors listed in previous frames. In other words, attention to lifestyle habits is of paramount importance. It is interesting to note that management of atherosclerosis is very much like managing hypertension. Treatment consists of repairing the damage caused by the effects of atherosclerosis. It includes bypass grafts of occluded arteries, plaque removal, and grafting of aneurysms.

9–122

An **aneurysm** is a localized dilatation, or bulging out, of the wall of an artery. The three basic configurations of an aneurysm are illustrated in Figure 9–17. This protrusion, or sac-like formation, is because of weakness there in the wall. One cause of an aneurysm is congenital weakness. This is most often seen in the circle of Willis in the brain. Atherosclerosis of the large arteries, especially the aorta, is a major cause of aneurysm. Because of hardening, the artery cannot expand during systole as it should. This leads to hypertension. Also, the atherosclerotic vessel is narrowed so pressure at that site is further increased. The pathology of the vessel combined with increased pressure pushes the wall outward. Atherosclerotic aneurysm is most common in the abdominal aorta. Another cause of aneurysm is inflammation of the vessel in some infections. This is demonstrated in the case of syphilitic aortic aneurysm. The degeneration of arteriosclerosis can also create aneurysm.

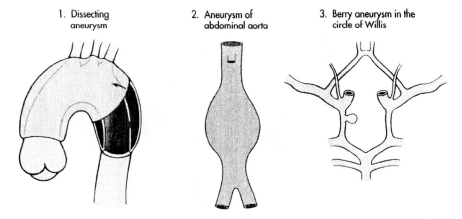

1. Dissecting aneurysm   2. Aneurysm of abdominal aorta   3. Berry aneurysm in the circle of Willis

Figure 9–17. Three forms of aneurysms. *(Adapted from Porth,* Pathophysiology–Concepts of Altered Health States, *4th ed., JB Lippincott Co.)*

9–123

A _____(1) in a vessel wall can cause it to protrude outward in pouch-like fashion. This bulge is called a (an) _____ (2). Causes of aneurysm include weakness present at birth, or _____(3) aneurysm, plaque formation and hardening of arteries in _____(4), degenerative hardening in _____(5), and some infections. The great vessel most often affected by aneurysm is the _____(6). The clinical effects of aneurysm include the following.

1. Thrombosis at the site.
2. External pressure on surrounding vessels, especially at a point of branching, which can create blockage and ischemia.
3. Sudden rupture and death by exsanguination.

An aneurysm is most often silent until it reaches a critical point. Its rupture is a significant cause of sudden death.

1. dilatation
2. aneurysm
3. congenital
4. atherosclerosis
5. arteriosclerosis
6. aorta

9–124

Sudden death due to an aneurysm occurs because of _____(1) and subsequent _____(2). A different form of an aneurysm is the *aortic dissecting aneurysm.* In this condition, instead of a localized bulge, blood leaks into and along the interior of the wall. The blood dissects, or cuts through, the planes of tissue within the wall. A tear in the intima because of high blood pressure allows blood to pass into the media of the wall, where it may travel quite a distance. The force of the hypertension inside the aorta can push the blood along the entire length of the aorta. The resulting swelling of the aorta can put external pressure on branches running off to vital organs. This includes the coronary arteries of the heart, leading to myocardial infarction. Other organs can also undergo infarction if their vessels are occluded. Another consequence of a dissecting aneurysm is compression of the vessel lumen, as shown in Figure 9–18. A dissecting aortic aneurysm can also rupture, with exsanguination. The aortic dissection aneurysm is different from a localized aneurysm because there is no _____(3) formation. Instead, _____(4) leaks into the interior of the _____(5) because of a tear in the lining. The aorta swells, which can lead to _____(6) of its branches because of external _____(7). This occlusion can cause _____(8) in the associated organ. A dissecting aortic aneurysm may _____(9), resulting in fatal hemorrhage. An aneurysm diagnosed early enough may be repaired by removing the affected area and replacing it with a graft made of a plastic like Dacron.

1. rupture
2. exsanguination
3. bulge
4. blood
5. wall
6. occlusion
7. pressure
8. infarction
9. rupture

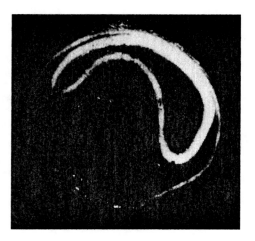

Figure 9–18. Cross-section of the aorta with a dissecting aneurysm showing the aortic lumen squeezed by the column of blood. *(From McCance and Huether,* Pathophysiology–The Biologic Basis for Disease in Adults and Children, *1st ed., Mosby.)*

▶ OTHER DISORDERS OF BLOOD VESSELS

9–125

1. antibodies
2. vasculitis
3. immune
4. edema
5. thrombi
6. atherosclerotic plaque
7. Narrowing
8. ischemia

Vasculitis is inflammation of blood vessels. This inflammatory disease is generally immune-mediated, as in the case of type II hypersensitivity (see Chap. 4). It may also be an autoimmune disease, exemplified by systemic lupus erythematosus (see Chap. 4). In SLE, vasculitis is widespread. An immune-mediated disease is one in which damage is done to tissue as a result of the interactions of _____(1) and antigens. The inflammation or vasculitis produced during the immune reactions can lead to edema because of increased permeability, thrombus formation because of endothelial damage, or the development of an atherosclerotic plaque in response to endothelial injury. Infiltration of the walls of the vessels can produce narrowing of the vessel lumen and subsequent ischemia to supplied areas. In one type of vasculitis, **polyarteritis nodosa,** the infiltration can be massive to the point of obliteration of the lumen and infarction. An inflammatory condition of blood vessels is called _____(2). The injury is usually _____(3)-mediated. The infiltration can result in the following.

1. Fluid leakage, or _____(4).
2. Formation of _____(5) or _____(6).
3. _____(7) of the lumen and subsequent _____(8).

9–126

1. embolus
2. vein
3. inflammation of a vein
4. thrombophlebitis
5. sluggish
6. turbulent
7. phlebothrombosis
8. embolism

Phlebitis is inflammation of veins. It most commonly occurs in the legs. ("Phleb" refers to vein.) Phlebitis of the superficial veins is usually of little consequence. Phlebitis of the deep veins often creates thrombi in reaction to the wall injury. If this does develop, the condition is called **thrombophlebitis.** Thrombosis *not* related to inflammation, but to sluggish or turbulent blood flow, is called **phlebothrombosis.** Note that the word part "itis" is not included. The thrombus may occlude the vessel if it is large enough, or it may break off and become a (an) _____(1) and travel to the lungs. Pulmonary embolism and possible pulmonary infarction are important concerns in cases of thrombophlebitis. A localized thrombus may need to be removed surgically. A more common treatment is to administer anticoagulant medications to prevent the development of more thrombi. "Phleb" means _____(2), so phlebitis means _____(3). If during the inflammation a clot should develop, the condition is called _____(4). If inflammation is absent and clot formation is because of _____(5) or _____(6) blood flow, it is called _____(7). An important clinical concern in these conditions is the production of a pulmonary _____(8).

Varicose veins are dilated veins containing stagnant blood, with incompetent valves. They most likely occur in the superficial veins of the lower legs. A small amount of pooling of blood causes a normal vein to become slightly distended. This dilation does not allow the valves to properly meet and close. They remain open. Therefore, more blood pools there because it is not pushed forward then stopped by closed valves. This causes more distention to the point of defining a varicose vein. Venous valvular insufficiency, caused by an initial slight distension, is the root cause of this chronic state. The now-sluggish circulation through the varicose area is susceptible to thrombi formation and possible emboli formation. Inadequate drainage of blood from the legs may lead to ischemia, skin ulcers, and necrosis through mechanisms not discussed here. A varicose vein is one which is _____(1), and whose _____(2) do not work properly. This valvular insufficiency is because initial distention does not permit them to _____(3). Therefore, the _____(4) becomes worse and enters the chronic state. Two consequences of varicose veins can be the formation of _____(5) or _____(6).

1. distended or dilated
2. valves
3. close
4. distention or dilation
5. thrombi
6. emboli

The causative factors of varicose veins are included in the following list.

1. Genetically weak connective tissue that allows the wall to distend easily.
2. Standing still for long periods of time. This does not permit blood to be pumped up out of the legs as it is during the muscle contractions of exercise, such as walking. Venous blood can easily pool in this condition.
3. Pregnancy, where compression of the large veins in the abdomen by the gravid uterus prevents proper return.
4. Thrombophlebitis, which can contribute to pooling behind the site.

Two specific types of varicose veins are **hemorrhoids** that develop because of rectal pressure and **esophageal varices.** Esophageal varices are dilated veins along the esophagus that develop in cirrhosis of the liver (see Chapter 13). Esophageal varices are prone to rupture and fatal hemorrhage is not uncommon.

Noninvasive management of varicose veins includes wearing external support to prevent further distention, in the form of elastic bandages or heavy support hose. Surgical correction uses a procedure called "stripping," where the distended veins are completely removed and are naturally replaced by the collateral circulation. In compression sclerotherapy, injections of strong saline into the vein cause enough scarring that they fuse shut and blood is shunted around them. The same principle is used to treat esophageal varices, except it is called endoscopic sclerotherapy because it requires an endoscope.

IV. REVIEW QUESTIONS

1. Define the term arteriosclerosis: _____

2. A common reaction to hypertension by the arteries is:
   a. atheroma formation
   b. plaque formation
   c. atherosclerosis
   d. arteriosclerosis

3. In atherosclerosis, the lesion on the vessel wall is called a a. _____, or sometimes a (an) b. _____.

1. hardening of the arteries

2. d–arteriosclerosis

3. a–plaque; b–atheroma

4. b–cholesterol; c–hyperplastic smooth muscle cells; e–foam cells; g–fibrosis

5. b–aorta; c–cerebral arteries; e–coronary arteries

6. a–myocardial infarction; b–stroke

7. a–obstruction; b–thrombosis; c–embolism; d–aneurysm

8. a–weakness

9. c–exsanguination

10. b–pulmonary embolism

11. a–thrombosis; b–embolism

4. An atherosclerotic plaque is composed of (choose all that apply):
   a. calcium
   b. cholesterol
   c. hyperplastic smooth muscle cells
   d. atrophied smooth muscle cells
   e. foam cells
   f. injured endothelial cells
   g. fibrosis

5. Arteries *most often* affected by atherosclerosis include (choose all that apply):
   a. pulmonary artery
   b. aorta
   c. cerebral arteries
   d. renal arteries
   e. coronary arteries
   f. hepatic arteries

6. In atherosclerosis, death due to heart involvement is usually from
   a. _____, while death due to brain involvement is usually from
   b. _____.

7. In atherosclerosis, ischemia and infarction develop because of these effects:
   a. narrowing of vessel lumens or _____
   b. development of blood clots or _____
   c. obstruction of vessels by a traveling thrombi or _____
   d. localized bulging of large arteries or _____

8. In an aneurysm, the protruding sac or pouch in the wall of the artery develops because of:
   a. weakness
   b. obstruction
   c. hypertension
   d. infarction

9. Death due directly to an aneurysm is from:
   a. infarction
   b. embolism
   c. exsanguination
   d. stroke

10. An important consequence of thrombophlebitis, or phlebothrombosis of the deep leg veins, is:
    a. myocardial infarction
    b. pulmonary embolism
    c. stroke
    d. aneurysm

11. Important consequences of varicose veins are (choose all that apply):
    a. thrombosis
    b. embolism
    c. aneurysm
    d. myocardial infarction
    e. stroke

▶ **SECTION II**

Anemia is the condition marked by a deficiency in erythrocytes (red blood cells, RBCs) or hemoglobin, resulting in inadequate oxygen delivery to the tissues (hypoxia). The condition may result from one of several clinical situations, hemorrhagia, nutrient deficiency (iron, folic acid, vitamin B_{12}), hemolysis of the RBCs, or from certain genetic abnormalities (spherocytosis, sickle cell anemia, thalassemia). In some cases, the anemia may be due to autoimmune destruction of the RBCs (autoimmune hemolytic anemia, hemolytic disease of the newborn). Anemia can also result from chemical toxicity or radiation damage to the bone marrow, from cancer of the bone marrow, or from chronic disease. Anemia is diagnosed by microscopic study of the morphology and the number of RBCs. Other tests are performed to determine the specific cause of the anemia. The condition may be treated in several different ways, administration of a specific nutrient, splenectomy, blood transfusions, or bone marrow transplants.

Leukemia ("white blood"), a condition classified as a diffuse cancer, is characterized by the appearance in the blood of malignant, immature, nonfunctional white blood cells (WBCs). Leukemia causes disease and death through the loss of function of WBCs and the crowding out of other cell lines (RBCs and platelets). The cause of leukemia is unknown, but viruses and oncogenes may play significant roles. Leukemias are classified into four types: acute lymphoblastic, acute myelogenous, chronic myelogenous, and chronic lymphocytic. These forms differ in the specific leukocyte types involved and in the age at which individuals become affected. The leukemias are diagnosed by microscopic observation of the WBCs. Confirmation is made with a bone marrow biopsy. The treatment for all forms of leukemia is chemotherapy.

Lymphoma, which generally arises in the lymph nodes and produces a solid tumor, is neoplasia of the lymphocytes and their precursors. A biopsy is required for the diagnosis of lymphoma. Therapeutic regimens involve, as with malignancies in general, chemotherapy or radiation. Like leukemia, the causes of the condition are unclear, but viruses and oncogenes are suspected. The most common type of lymphoma is *Hodgkin's disease,* a condition that progresses through four stages, each with defined characteristics. A specific cancerous cell type, the Reed–Sternberg cell, is diagnostic of Hodgkin's disease. In *non-Hodgkin's lymphoma* (NHL), Reed–Sternberg cells are not present. Diagnosis of NHL is by examination of the lymphocytes and the structure of the involved lymph node. NHL is divided into grades, based on classification of follicular (lymph node structure is preserved) or diffuse (lymph node structure is destroyed). Follicular invasion is less serious and has a better prognosis. *Burkitt's lymphoma,* a malignancy of lymphoid stem cells apparently confined to children in certain parts of Africa, is thought to be due to the Epstein–Barr virus.

Multiple myeloma is malignancy of the antibody-producing B cells (plasma cells) in the blood. Because plasma cells reproduce to high numbers, the transformation of only one cell is necessary for oncogenesis. Eventually, the rapid proliferation of the transformed cell leads, as in leukemia, to a "crowding out" of other cells in the marrow. Bone destruction, hypercalcemia, kidney failure, leukopenia, and anemia result. Diagnosis of multiple myeloma involves detection of high levels of a single kind of antibody ("monoclonal") in the blood, and of the unique Bence Jones protein in the urine. While bone marrow transplants may offer some hope in the treatment of this fatal disease, drugs or radiation are currently the therapeutic regimens of choice.

Many other disorders of blood cells are known. In *polycythemia* (or erythrocytosis), a marked increase in circulating RBCs causes the blood to become viscous, resulting in hypertension, increased cardiac workload, and the formation of clots within the vessels (thrombi). *Leukocytosis* is characterized by a significant increase in the circulating WBCs, and is generally the result of a reaction to a disease. Leukocytosis may be of several different types, granulocytosis or neutrophilia (increased neutrophils due to bacterial infection or inflammation), eosinophilia (increased eosinophils due to an allergic state or a parasitic infection), lymphocytosis (increased lymphocytes due to a viral or bacterial infection), and monocytosis (increased monocytes due to chronic infection). *Leukopenia,* the condition of decreased numbers of WBCs in circulation, may be caused by chemical or radiation toxicity to the bone marrow or by bone marrow aplasia.

A number of blood-related diseases are classified as bleeding disorders. *Vascular disorders,* leading to internal or external hemorrhagia, may be due to trauma of the blood vessels, to immune-mediated damage to the vessel walls (vasculitis), or to a vitamin C deficiency. *Thrombocytopenia,* the condition of an abnormally low number of platelets, may be due to a decrease in the bone marrow's production of platelets, to leukemia, to immune destruction, or to fetomaternal incompatability. *Hemophilia* is the most common of the genetic defects known as clotting factor disorders. The condition results from the absence of one of the factors in the blood clotting cascade. Liver disease or a vitamin K deficiency may lead to a deficiency in one or more of the clotting factors. In the condition of *disseminated intravascular coagulation* (DIC), the clotting factors are consumed in the formation of multiple thrombi. Signs of bleeding disorders include petechiae (pinpoint hemorrhages under the skin), hematuria (blood in the urine), and fecal occult blood (blood in the stool). Bleeding disorders are diagnosed by several tests, including platelet count, bleeding time, activated partial prothrombin time, prothrombin time, fibrinogen assay, and the fibrin split products test. Depending on the nature of the disorder, treatment regimens may involve transfusion, bone marrow transplant, steroid medication, or infusions of clotting factors.

▶ SECTION III

All the forces and movements of the circulatory system are collectively called *hemodynamics.* One form of disturbance in hemodynamic equilibrium is *edema,* a leakage of plasma or fluid from the vessels into the tissues. Edema may be localized (confined to a single organ) or generalized (affecting the entire body), and it may be of several forms. Hemorrhage, which may be external or internal, is the disruption of a blood vessel leading to the loss of blood from the intravascular space. Internal hemorrhage has the same adverse effect on blood pressure and perfusion as external hemorrhage. Some bleeding conditions (petechiea, ecchymosis, purpura) are not due to trauma.

Shock results from a hypoperfusion of the tissues with blood, which may be due to inadequate blood volume, loss of vessel tone, or marked decrease in cardiac output. Several different types of shock are recognized: hypovolemic, neurogenic, anaphylactic, and cardiogenic. Three distinct stages of shock can be clinically defined. *Hypertension,* defined as a consistently elevated blood pressure, may be primary (with many causative factors) or secondary (the result of a disease). The condition can lead to hardening of the arteries, cardiomyopathy, a decrease in cardiac output, cardiac ischemia, cardiac fibrosis, blindness, kidney failure, and stroke. Early diagnosis and, often, a change in one's lifestyle are essential in managing hypertension.

Inadequate oxygen supply to cells (hypoxia) may arise through several mechanisms: lung disease, an insufficient number of RBCs, or inadequate blood supply to the tissues. *Ischemia* is a decreased blood supply to an area of the body, resulting in inadequate oxygen delivery to that area and to the nonremoval of metabolic wastes. Ischemia is classified as generalized (due to poor cardiac output) or localized (due to an obstruction in the vessels of a specific anatomical area). *Anoxia* is the complete lack of oxygen supply to an area of the body, leading to an *infarction* (tissue death).

A freely traveling mass in the circulatory system is an *embolus,* which could be a thrombus (blood clot), a globule of fat, a mass of neoplastic cells or bacteria, or air. An embolism occurs when the embolus, whatever its nature, occludes a blood vessel. *Thrombosis* is described as the formation of a blood clot inside a vessel, a situation that can lead to ischemia or infarction. Thrombus formation, which may occur for several different reasons in any of a number of anatomical sites, is the most common cause of embolism.

▶ SECTION IV

Arteriosclerosis (literally, "hardening of the arteries), a degenerative loss of elasticity of the vessels, causes the vessels to be susceptible to rupture. The condition may be due to chronic hypertension or to the deposition of a hardened, fatty plaque on the surface of the intima. This latter situation is defined as *atherosclerosis,* and is believed to be caused by injury to the endothelial lining of the vessels. The coronary and cerebral arteries are often the most seriously affected. The condition can cause an infarction in the tissue supplied by the obstructed vessel, or it can lead to an aneurysm (a weakening of the vessel wall which can rupture) or to calcification of the site of plaque deposit. Many factors have been identified as predisposing a person to atherosclerosis.

Inflammation of the blood vessels, generally immune mediated, is termed *vasculitis.* Phlebitis is inflammation of the veins specifically, and can lead to thrombi generation in deep veins. Varicose veins are dilated veins containing stagnant blood, usually in the lower extremities. Several factors may account for the development of varicose veins. Hemmorhoids and esophageal varices are two specific types of varicose veins.

The Heart

► OBJECTIVES

SECTION II

Define all highlighted terms.

Distinguish between exogenous and endogenous congenital heart defects.

Define and characterize the types of shunts that can occur, and list their clinical consequences.

Define and characterize the septal defects, and list their clinical consequences.

Define the four abnormalities associated with tetralogy of Fallot, and characterize their clinical consequences.

SECTION III

Define all highlighted terms.

Characterize the clinical observations of hypertensive heart disease.

Describe the effects, etiology, and clinical observations of atherosclerotic coronary artery disease.

List the causes, symptoms, clinical observations, and complications of myocardial infarction.

Define and describe the symptoms, clinical presentation, and causes of congestive, right-sided, and left-sided heart failure.

Define and characterize the three forms of cardiomyopathy.

SECTION IV

Define all highlighted terms.

List and define the clinical observations associated with rheumatic heart disease.

List and define Jones' major criteria for rheumatic fever.

Define and characterize the causes and clinical observations of endocarditis, infectious endocarditis, myocarditis, and pericarditis.

SECTION V

Define all highlighted terms.

Define and characterize the causes and clinical observations of valvular insufficiency and valvular stenosis.

Define and characterize the observations associated with the types of cardiac dysrhythmias.

Define and characterize the clinical observations associated with atrial and ventricular fibrillation.

List and characterize the types of heart blocks.

SECTION ▶ 10-1

1. ANATOMY AND PHYSIOLOGY IN REVIEW

The heart is composed of two separate pumping chambers working in perfect rhythm with each other to receive and then move blood to the entire body. It is divided into right and left sides. Each side has an upper *receiving* chamber (the **atrium**), and a lower *pumping* chamber (the **ventricle**). The right and left sides of the heart are separated by a common wall, or **septum.** The upper portion of this partition is the **interatrial septum,** and the lower portion is the **interventricular septum.** The septum keeps the venous and arterial circulation separated from each other. A defect or hole in the septum allows mixing of oxygenated and deoxygenated blood, which causes imbalance in the body. The atria and ventricles are connected by valves. The **tricuspid valve** is in between the right atrium and ventricle, while the **mitral valve** is in between the left atrium and ventricle. The powerful muscle of the heart is called the **myocardium.** The inner lining of all four chambers is called the **endocardium.** The heart lies within a sac called the **pericardium,** or the **pericardial sac.** The major structures of the heart are shown in Figure 10–1.

10-2

The right side of the heart receives blood from the veins, or venous blood, by way of the inferior and superior vena cava, which empty into the right atria. Venous blood carries little pressure, since it is more or less a passive return from the tissues, compared to arterial blood, which is forcibly pumped into arteries. Venous blood is relatively **deoxygenated,** or contains a lower PO_2 than arterial blood. Much of the oxygen has been released at the cellular level. Venous blood carries waste products and is relatively high in **carbon dioxide,** a gaseous waste product of cellular respiration.

10-3

Because venous blood contains less pressure, the walls of the right side of the heart are less muscular, or not as thick as the left side. Venous blood is received into the atrium, falls down through the tricuspid valve into the ventricle, and is squeezed up and out through the **pulmonary valve** into the **pulmonary artery** and then into the lungs. The hemoglobin in the red blood cells releases carbon dioxide and picks up oxygen. As this happens, the blood becomes **oxygenated** arterial blood. From the lungs, arterial blood returns to the heart and enters the left atrium by way of the **pulmonary vein.** It passes down through the mitral valve into the thick-

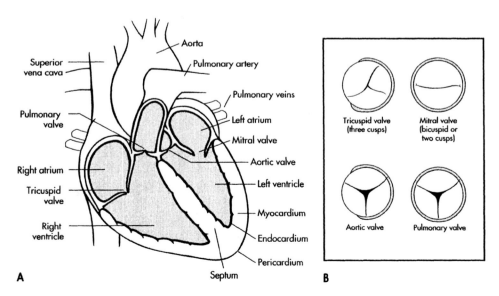

Figure 10–1. Structure of the heart. **A.** Structure of the heart and great vessels. **B.** Valves of the heart.

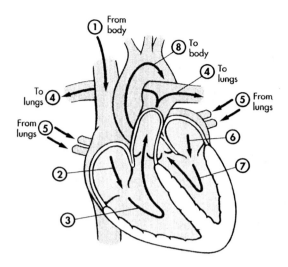

Figure 10–2. The pathways of blood through the heart.

walled left ventricle. The thicker myocardium is able to contract powerfully enough to propel blood out through the aorta with enough force or pressure that it lasts down to the smallest arterioles in order to perfuse all tissues. It is important to realize that the activities of the right and left sides happen simultaneously—that is, blood enters and exits the right side while blood also enters and exits the left side. Figure 10–2 demonstrates the pathways of blood entering and exiting the heart. Each step in the pathway is numbered in order of occurrence.

10–4

The valves of the heart are like doors opening and closing to keep blood moving in a forward direction at all times. The valves open to let blood pass through, then close behind the flow to prevent blood from flowing backwards. Closing tightly and properly is very important during contractions by the ventricles so that blood is not pushed backwards into the atria. Incompetency by the valves allows backup of blood in the circuit and the development of some abnormal states that we will be discussing.

10–5

The myocardium is composed of **cardiac muscle** fibers. They resemble skeletal muscle fibers but include branching for efficient conduction of nerve impulses. These fibers also contain inherent contraction ability and depend less on nerve impulse than does skeletal muscle. The myocardium uses tremendous amounts of energy to contract at the normal heart rate of about 60 to 90 times a minute. Therefore, its oxygen requirements are accelerated. The great demand for oxygen is supplied by the right and left **coronary arteries,** which branch directly off the aorta. This assures that the myocardium has all the oxygenated blood it needs. The coronary arteries are illustrated in Figure 10–3. It is easy to see why disease of these arteries is life threatening. Ischemia of the myocardium causes heart disease, and significant infarction causes death.

10–6

The perfect rhythmical contractions of the heart are due to an intricate, highly coordinated electrical conduction system. The **sinoatrial node** (sometimes called the **natural pacemaker)** initiates pulses of electrical current to which the muscle responds by contracting. From the sinoatrial node, impulses jump down to the **atrioventricular node,** and from there spread over the ventricles through the **bundle of His.** The bundle of His splits into right and left bundle branches. The electrical pattern causes the muscle contraction to begin at the *bottom* of the ventricles and roll upwards. In this manner, blood is efficiently moved upward and out of the heart. The contractions of the heart, or its beats, are also influenced by the autonomic nervous system. The vagus nerve of the parasympathetic system slows the rate, while the sympathetic system speeds up the rate.

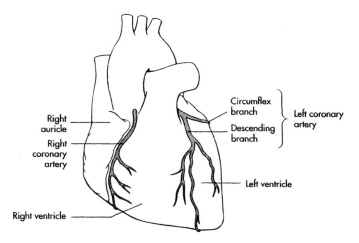

Figure 10–3. Supply of heart muscle by the right and left coronary arteries.

10-7

The cycle of heartbeats is divided into two phases. The phase of contraction is **systole,** or the work period. Systole is responsible for ejecting blood from the heart into the lungs and aorta. The rest period in between contractions is **diastole.** Diastole is important because it allows the chambers to relax and expand for adequate filling with blood. This readies the heart for the next contraction. The amount of blood that is pumped out with each systole is the **cardiac output.** A shortened period of diastole leads to inadequate filling of the chambers because of lack of time. This decreases cardiac output. The atria are in diastole while the ventricles are in systole, and the ventricles are in diastole while the atria are in systole. In other words, the atria relax and receive blood from the body and lungs, while the ventricles squeeze blood out to the body. The ventricles relax and receive blood from the atria when the atria contract.

► CATEGORIES OF HEART DISEASE

10-8

Before we study specific diseases of the heart, let us examine some general facts about heart disease and some categories. The incidence of cardiovascular disease is very high and is responsible for more than half of deaths in industrialized countries. Much of this is related to diet, stress, and other lifestyle factors. Many deaths are preventable through a healthy lifestyle. The major contributing factors are atherosclerosis of the coronary arteries, hypertension, and thrombosis of the coronary arteries leading to myocardial infarction.

10-9

The largest category of cardiac pathology is **ischemic heart disease.** It represents over 80 percent of the cases. The ischemia develops because of narrowing of the coronary artery lumen. This narrowing is a result of atherosclerosis (the most common cause of cardiac-induced death), hypertension, and thrombosis. The second largest category is **compensatory overload,** where the heart is overworked to make up for increased vascular resistance. This resistance is usually due to hypertension. Increased workload represents about 5 percent of the cases. **Immune-mediated injury** occurs in about 2 percent of the cases. The antigen–antibody reactions in some hypersensitivities and in rheumatic fever can damage the heart valves or endocardium. The same is true in the autoimmune disease systemic lupus erythematosus.

10-10

Infectious heart disease makes up about 1 percent of cardiac pathology. During bacteremia, the heart is a major target because all of the body's blood volume passes through it. The endocardium is most frequently infected by the passing bacteria because it is the surface in contact with the blood. This produces bacterial endocarditis. The valves are also frequent sites of colonization by the organisms. Any existing injury, especially of the valves, predisposes the interior of the heart to growth at the site by bacteria. In about 1 percent of heart disease, **congenital defects** are responsible. Malformation of the vessels or structure of the heart is relatively common in newborns. These malformations cause an abnormal pathway of blood flow and increased workload for the heart. **Electrolyte imbalance** can cause heart disease or even death. This is usually due to hyperkalemia, or excessive potassium in the blood. Elevated potassium interferes with conduction of nerve impulses, creating disturbances and abnormal rhythms. **Malignancy** of the heart is rare and will not be discussed.

II. CONGENITAL HEART DEFECTS ◀ SECTION

▶ CONGENITAL HEART DISEASE

10-11

Congenital heart disease is a defect or defects of the heart present at birth. Of all the internal organs, the heart is most often affected by abnormal development. We will discuss the specific effects of these disorders, but, in general, the abnormalities place cardiac muscle under stress as the heart tries to compensate for the abnormalities. Minor defects produce mild signs that may not appear until later in life. Major defects can produce severe signs and death if not treated. In general, congenital heart disease requires surgical correction in about 40 percent of cases to prevent an early death. Advancements in open heart surgery have greatly decreased the mortality rate of children born with heart defects.

10-12

The etiology of congenital heart disease in many cases is idiopathic. Spontaneous malformation may not be traceable to its cause. Of known causes, they are either exogenous or endogenous. Exogenous causes include **teratogens.** You know from Chapter 7 that a teratogen is an agent capable of causing _____(1) defects. These teratogens include drugs, chemicals, viruses, and x-rays. A widely used drug that causes birth defects is alcohol. In **fetal alcohol syndrome,** a variety of anomalies may be present. Alcohol has been proven to directly interfere with the development of the heart. The best-known viral cardiac teratogen is the rubella virus, the agent of German measles (see Chap. 5). If this virus is contracted by a woman during the first trimester of pregnancy, the virus is able to cross the placental barrier, enter fetal circulation, and damage the developing heart. This is an important reason for the continuation of immunization practices against rubella. An endogenous cause of congenial heart disease is genetics. Chromosomal aberrations can lead to abnormal formation. A well-known example is trisomy 21, or _____(2) syndrome (see Chap. 7).

1. birth
2. Down's

10-13

An external cause of congenital heart disease is labeled _____(1), while an internal cause is called _____(2). An exogenous agent is also called a (an) _____(3). Examples of teratogens include the drug _____(4) and the virus _____(5). An endogenous cause is due to an abnormality with a _____(6). Congenital heart defects, depending on severity, lead to a disturbance in blood flow. The most significant consequence is a mixing of blood of the pulmonary circulation with the general circulation. This is most often associated with a **shunt.** A shunt is an abnormal pathway. It may be thought of as a detour. The normal circuit of blood

1. exogenous
2. endogenous
3. teratogen
4. alcohol
5. rubella
6. chromosome

flow must be observed for the body to be in a state of health. As blood enters the heart from the general circulation, this normal circuit is:

1. Into the right atrium.
2. Down into the right ventricle.
3. Up and out through the pulmonary artery.
4. Through the lungs.
5. Into the left atrium through the pulmonary vein.
6. Down into the left ventricle.
7. Up and out through the aorta.

Refer back to Figure 10–2 to review these steps.

10–14

In the case of a shunt, blood does not follow this route. A **left-to-right shunt** is the passage of blood from the left side of the heart back into the right side, when it should be exiting the heart. This is often of minor consequence because the blood passes through the lungs a second time. However, a **right-to-left shunt** is of clinical significance. Blood passes from the right side to the left side *before* it has gone to the lungs for oxygen. Because of this, various degrees of **cyanosis** develop. Cyanosis is a bluish discoloration of the skin because of inadequate oxygenation of the blood. Blood that is normally oxygenated (arterial blood) is a bright red because of the bonding of oxygen to hemoglobin. The color of arterial blood gives tissues their pink tint. Deoxygenated blood, represented by the venous circulation, is much darker. In cyanosis, deoxygenated blood mixes with oxygenated blood because some defect has prevented passage through the lungs. (Keep in mind that we are not talking about the body's entire blood volume experiencing abnormal flow all at the same time. Rather, it is a combination of normal and abnormal flow that yields the sum total of a less-than-normal systemic circulation.) In right-to-left shunts, some amount of blood is pushed from the right heart out to the systemic circulation instead of the lungs.

10–15

1. shunt
2. lungs
3. right
4. cyanosis
5. lungs
6. oxygen

A detour in normal blood flow is termed a _____(1). In a left-to-right shunt, blood goes through the _____(2) twice, so the effects on the body are minor. In a _____(3)-to-left shunt, bluish discoloration of the skin [called _____(4)] indicates that some amount of blood has bypassed the _____(5). Because of this, that blood contains less than normal amounts of _____(6).

▶ SEPTAL DEFECTS

10–16

1. septal defect

A **septal defect** is a failure of complete formation of the septum that divides the two sides of the heart. It is commonly known as a "hole in the heart." This failure leaves a gap or hole in the dividing wall. A septal defect may also be due to lack of closure by the foramen ovale, a small normal hole in the septum before birth. The size of the hole left by malformation ranges from a pinhole to an entire section of the wall missing. The most common septal defects are small holes. They usually occur alone but may be present with other defects. Septal imperfections are the most common congenital heart defects found in adults. A gap or hole in the dividing wall of the heart is called a _____(1).

10–17

1. left-to-right
2. right

An **atrial septal defect (ASD),** or interatrial septal defect, allows a communication between the upper two chambers. Blood passes from the left atria to the right atria through the space. (Under normal circumstances, blood will always flow from the left side to the right side because the pressure is much higher on the left side.) This left-to-right shunt results in more blood present in the right heart and in the lungs than is normal. While cyanosis is not a problem, the workload of the right side is increased. Clinically, a **murmur** can be heard with a stethoscope. A murmur is a collection of abnormal heart sounds created by turbulent blood flow. An atrial septal defect results in a _____(1) shunt and increased workload for the _____(2) side.

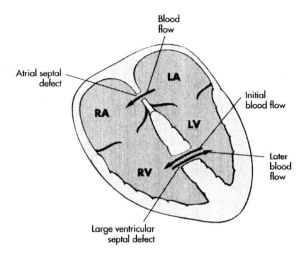

Figure 10–4. Atrial and ventricular septal defects.

10–18

A **ventricular septal defect (VSD),** or interventricular septal defect, allows a communication between the lower two chambers. Atrial and ventricular septal defects are illustrated in Figure 10–4. A small VSD may not present with much in the way of clinical signs. But a larger VSD produces a large left-to-right shunt. This shunt increases the workload for the left ventricle because the shunted blood coming through again from the right side must be moved along with the normal cardiac output. The workload of the right ventricle is also increased by the extra blood from the left side. The circulation to the lungs is increased, which increases pulmonary pressure. This creates pulmonary hypertension. In response, you know that the vessels will react by getting thicker, which _____(1) the lumen. As the lumens narrow, this further increases vascular resistance to blood flow. In time, because of pushing against pulmonary resistance and hypertension, the pressure on the right side becomes *greater* than the pressure on the left side. There is now a *right-to-left* shunt. Cyanosis develops as blood bypasses the lungs. Blood always takes the path of least resistance. In this case, it is into the left ventricle and out into the systemic circulation. The systemic circulation will contain less oxygen than normal. Heart failure due to increased work is a possibility. Any symptoms of a large VSD are due to cyanosis and hypoxia. Clinically, a distinct murmur can be **auscultated,** or heard through a stethoscope. Treatment must take place before the right-to-left shunt develops, in order to restore normal balance. It consists of surgically patching the defect with a synthetic material.

1. narrows or decreases

10–19

Initially, a large ventricular septal defect produces a _____(1) shunt. The results of the extra blood entering the _____(2) ventricle are:

1. Increased work for the right _____(3).
2. Increased blood through the _____(4).
3. Increased pulmonary _____(5) and the development of pulmonary _____(6).
4. Decreased size of the _____(7) of pulmonary vessels, which increases vascular _____(8) to blood flow.
5. A reversal in the pressure differences between the right and left sides, with the right side now _____(9) than the left.
6. The creation of a _____(10) shunt, which results in _____(11).

1. left-to-right
2. right
3. ventricle
4. lungs
5. pressure
6. hypertension
7. lumen
8. resistance
9. greater
10. right-to-left
11. cyanosis

▶ PATENT DUCTUS ARTERIOSUS

······ 10–20 ······

Normally, before birth, blood bypasses the lungs because the lungs have not expanded and the extreme resistance by the collapsed tissue prevents any circulation through the tissue. The cells of the fetus receive oxygen from the mother's circulation. The normal circuit of blood flow is from the right ventricle, through the pulmonary artery, and *to the aorta (not the lungs)*. This passage is made possible by the **ductus arteriosus,** a small connecting vessel that runs between the pulmonary artery and the aorta. The ductus is normally present only in the fetus or youngest newborn. After birth, the lungs expand, the resistance is gone, and blood circulates through the lungs. The ductus arteriosus is no longer needed and it soon closes off.

······ 10–21 ······

1. patent ductus arteriosus
2. fetal
3. pulmonary artery
4. aorta
5. close
6. left-to-right
7. ventricles
8. hypertension

If the ductus arteriosus fails to close and remains open, it is called a **patent ductus arteriosus,** or **PDA.** Patent means open. A PDA is the continued existence of this detour vessel. Because of the pressure differences between the aorta (high) and the pulmonary artery (low), a left-to-right shunt is created. This causes increased workloads for both ventricles, increased pulmonary circulation, and pulmonary hypertension. The flow of blood in a PDA can be seen in Figure 10–5. Working against the high pulmonary resistance can lead to failure of the right side of the heart. Clinically, a classic "machinery" murmur can be heard. Also, a **thrill** may be present. A thrill is the vibration that can be felt on the outside of the chest by palpating the precordial area. Treatment consists of surgically closing off the PDA. PDA stands for _____(1). It is the continued presence of the _____(2) vessel that runs between the _____(3) and the _____(4). It is supposed to _____(5) after birth. A PDA causes a _____(6) shunt. This shunt places strain on both _____(7) and leads to pulmonary _____(8).

▶ TETRALOGY OF FALLOT

······ 10–22 ······

Tetralogy of Fallot is made up of multiple heart defects. It always consists of the same four abnormalities, namely:

1. Ventricular septal defect
2. Dextroposition of the aorta
3. Pulmonary stenosis
4. Right ventricular hypertrophy

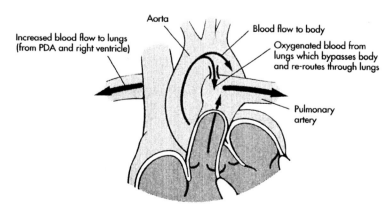

Figure 10–5. Blood flow in a patent ductus arteriosus.

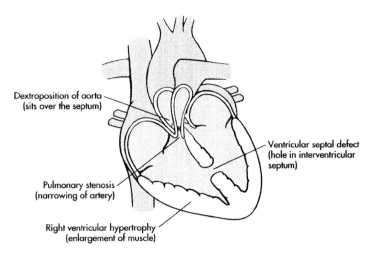

Figure 10–6. Defects in tetralogy of Fallot.

These defects are presented in Figure 10–6. While ASD, VSD, and PDA are all **acyanotic** defects [_____(1) cyanosis], tetralogy of Fallot is a cyanotic condition. It is the most common reason for cyanosis of newborns. The general circulation is a mixture of oxygenated and deoxygenated blood. Tetralogy of Fallot develops when the base of the heart is twisted too far to the right. This causes misplacement of the aorta, so that it straddles or sits over the septum and the VSD. Because of this, the aorta receives blood from *both* the left and right ventricles. Therefore, cardiac output consists of both arterial and venous blood. Venous blood from the right ventricle has not entered the lungs for oxygenation.

1. without

.... 10-23 ......

The misplacement, or dextroposition, of the aorta puts pressure on the pulmonary artery. This external pressure causes narrowing of the artery, and this is called pulmonary **stenosis.** ("Stenotic" means narrowed.) Pulmonary stenosis is probably the most clinically significant defect in tetralogy of Fallot. Blood trying to exit the right ventricle for the lungs meets the resistance of the stenosis. The resistance increases pressure on the right side, and the VSD allows the blood that can't get through the pulmonary valve to enter the left ventricle and then the systemic circulation. Therefore, a right-to-left shunt is created and cyanosis develops. The excessive work performed by the right ventricle in trying to get blood through the pulmonary stenosis causes hypertrophy or enlargement of the myocardium. Therefore, right ventricular hypertrophy is not really a defect but a compensatory reaction.

.... 10-24 ......

Tetralogy of Fallot is made up of _____(1) (how many?) actual defect(s), and _____(2) (how many?) compensatory reaction(s). Because the heart is twisted too far to the right, the _____(3) sits over the septum and a VSD, so it receives _____(4) from both the right and left _____(5). Aortic dextroposition also presses on the _____(6) artery and causes it to become narrowed. The term that describes narrowing or constriction is _____(7). Pulmonary stenosis creates such resistance to blood flow that the right ventricle enlarges in response to the extra work. This enlargement is called _____(8). Blood that can't get through the stenosis passes through the septal gap or _____(9), into the left ventricle, and out the aorta. This is a _____(10) shunt and is accompanied by poorly oxygenated blood, which is visible as _____(11). The systemic circulation is therefore composed of percentages of blood with these properties:

1. three
2. one
3. aorta
4. blood
5. ventricles
6. pulmonary
7. stenosis
8. hypertrophy
9. VSD
10. right-to-left
11. cyanosis
12. oxygenated
13. lungs

1. Blood from the left ventricle, which has been oxygenated in the lungs.
2. Blood from the right ventricle, passing directly into the aorta, which has not been _____(12) in the lungs.
3. Blood from the right ventricle, passing into the left side through the VSD, which has not been oxygenated in the _____(13).

1. hypoxia
2. hypoxia

Clinically, tetralogy of Fallot produces the typical murmur of abnormal blood flow. More significantly, it causes cyanosis and hypoxia early in the life of the patient. Pulmonary stenosis causes a major right-to-left shunt, and the oxygen content of the general circulation is decreased overall. Babies born with this condition are often so cyanotic that the phrase "blue baby" has been coined to describe it. Generalized hypoxia develops quickly. Signs of this condition include tachypnea (fast breathing), tachycardia (fast heart rate), breathlessness, and lack of ability to exert oneself. Syncope or fainting occurs during cerebral hypoxia. Polycythemia develops as a response to hypoxia, so that more red blood cells and hemoglobin are present in the blood that does pass through the lungs. Tetralogy of Fallot must be surgically corrected to prevent early death from heart failure. The prognosis depends on the extent or severity of the defects. Most importantly, the obstruction at the pulmonary artery must be bypassed. Cyanosis indicates that a patient is in a state of inadequate oxygen to the tissues, or _____(1). Signs and compensatory reactions are because of this _____(2).

II. REVIEW QUESTIONS

1. b–a teratogen

2. d–a shunt

3. a–cyanosis; b–right-to-left; c–lungs

4. a–which side of the heart contains the greater pressure; d–which side of the heart meets with the greater resistance

5. c–a septal defect

6. a–5; b–1; c–3; d–4; e–2

1. A congenital heart defect in fetal alcohol syndrome is a result of a drug classified as:
   a. hereditary
   b. a teratogen
   c. an endogenous cause
   d. idiopathic

2. An abnormal pathway of blood flow similar to a detour is:
   a. a septal defect
   b. cyanosis
   c. a ductus arteriosus
   d. a shunt

3. Insufficient oxygen, which causes bluish discoloration of the skin is called
   a. _____. This is caused by a b. _____shunt. The reason insufficient oxygenation develops is because some blood bypasses the
   c. _____.

4. The direction of a shunt is determined by (choose all that are correct):
   a. which side of the heart contains the greater pressure
   b. which artery is abnormally placed
   c. where a septal defect is located
   d. which side of the heart meets with the greater resistance

5. A "hole in the heart" is medically termed:
   a. a patent ductus arteriosus
   b. tetralogy of Fallot
   c. a septal defect
   d. cyanosis

6. List *in order of occurrence* the events of a large ventricular septal defect:
   a. _____ cyanosis
   b. _____ left-to-right shunt
   c. _____ pulmonary hypertension
   d. _____ right-to-left shunt
   e. _____ increased pulmonary circulation

7. A patent ductus arteriosus is:
   a. the shunt created by an atrial septal defect, which can cause left-sided heart failure
   b. dextroposition of the aorta, which can cause right-sided heart failure
   c. the continued presence of a fetal vessel, which can cause left-sided heart failure
   d. the continues presence of a fetal vessel, which can cause right-sided heart failure

8. Choose all of the defects that are present in tetralogy of Fallot:
   a. aortic stenosis
   b. dextroposition of the aorta
   c. atrial septal defect
   d. ventricular septal defect
   e. pulmonary stenosis
   f. patent ductus arteriosus
   g. right ventricular hypertrophy
   h. left ventricular hypertrophy

9. Which of the following congenital heart defects cause cyanosis?
   a. patent ductus arteriosus
   b. tetralogy of Fallot
   c. ventricular septal defect
   d. atrial septal defect

10. Regarding tetralogy of Fallot, which relationship is correct?
    a. Dextroposition of the aorta creates so much resistance that blood is shunted from right to left through the VSD.
    b. Pulmonary stenosis creates so much resistance that blood is shunted from right to left through the VSD.
    c. Dextroposition of the aorta creates so much resistance that blood is shunted from left to right through the VSD.
    d. Pulmonary stenosis creates so much resistance that blood is shunted from left to right through the VSD.

7. d–the continued presence of a fetal vessel, which can cause right-sided heart failure

8. b–dextroposition of the aorta
   d–ventricular septal defect
   e–pulmonary stenosis
   g–right ventricular hypertrophy

9. b–tetralogy of Fallot

10. b–Pulmonary stenosis creates so much resistance that blood is shunted from right to left through the VSD.

III. DEGENERATIVE STATES AND HEART FAILURE ◀ SECTION
10-26

Degeneration is disease produced by loss of function. In heart disease, this is primarily due to ischemia. Of all diseases common in the United States, ischemic heart disease is of extreme significance. What is commonly known as a "heart attack" is a result of ischemia and hypoxia, infarction, and anoxia. These states are caused by pathology of the two coronary arteries that supply the myocardium. They are very susceptible to atherosclerosis, which narrows their lumens and decreases blood flow to heart muscle. Ischemic heart disease results from energy requirements greater than available blood flow and oxygen. It is the most common cause of heart failure. Some of the causes and effects of ischemic heart disease are outlined in Table 10–1. Loss of function causes the disease state known as _____(1). In the heart this is because of _____(2). Inadequate blood flow, and therefore _____(3), is caused by disease of the two _____(4).

1. degeneration
2. ischemia
3. ischemia
4. coronary arteries

▶ HYPERTENSIVE HEART DISEASE

10–27

1. hypertensive heart disease
2. hypertrophy
3. left ventricle
4. smaller
5. blood
6. cardiac output
7. atherosclerotic plaques
8. coronary arteries

Hypertensive heart disease is a secondary disorder in response to systemic hypertension. Increased vascular resistance of the arteries increases the workload of the heart, particularly the left ventricle. It is this chamber that pushes directly against the arterial resistance. Excessive work by a muscle causes enlargement or **hypertrophy.** Therefore, left ventricular hypertrophy is a feature of hypertensive heart disease. The end result is heart failure. In ventricular hypertrophy, the walls enlarge in both an outward and inward direction (concentric hypertrophy). This decreases the size of the inside of the chamber and it holds less blood. It then pumps less blood out to the body and cardiac output is decreased. Enlargement of the left ventricle causes the heart to be enlarged overall, and this is known as **cardiomegaly.** In addition to decreased cardiac output for the general circulation, systemic hypertension greatly increases the production of atherosclerotic plaques in the coronary arteries. Atherosclerotic coronary artery disease is discussed in Frame 10–29. Ischemia and infarction follow coronary artery disease. In response to systemic hypertension, the secondary disorder _____(1) is produced. The most prominent feature is enlargement or _____(2) of the _____(3). The inside of the left ventricular chamber becomes _____(4) and it holds less _____(5). This decreases _____(6). Systemic hypertension also increases the formation of _____(7) in the _____(8).

10–28

1. oxygen
2. vessels
3. die
4. scar tissue
5. function
6. failure

The consequence of hypertrophy in the heart is that the larger muscle fibers need more oxygen. This is not supplied, because the vascularization does not increase proportionately. In other words, there are no new vessels created to supply the larger muscle. Some fibers die because of the ischemia, and they are replaced by scar tissue, creating some degree of myocardial fibrosis. A significant amount of fibrosis will result in myocardial failure since scar tissue has no function. Later in hypertensive heart disease, the right ventricle also hypertrophies. Inadequate cardiac output causes blood to back up in the lungs, increasing pulmonary resistance and increasing the workload of the right ventricle. The effects of right ventricular hypertrophy are described under the topic of cor pulmonale. In hypertrophy, larger muscle fibers need more _____(1). This would require more _____(2) to carry the oxygen, which does not occur. The ischemia causes some fibers to _____(3) and be replaced with _____(4). The result of excessive fibrosis in heart muscle is loss of _____(5), leading to heart _____(6).

▶ ATHEROSCLEROTIC CORONARY ARTERY DISEASE

10–29

In general, **coronary artery disease (CAD)** may be caused by any compromise in the size of the lumen. If a clot forms on the walls, it may cause CAD, and this is specifically known as **coronary thrombosis.** Systemic hypertension can cause narrowing of the lumen. It also contributes to the formation of atherosclerotic plaques. Atherosclerosis of the coronary arteries represents the most common form of CAD. Coronary thrombosis can be a complication of atherosclerotic CAD, since ulcerated sites of the plaques are a prime target for thrombi formation. The risk factors for atherosclerotic CAD are those that were presented in Chapter 9 under atherosclerosis.

10–30

In atherosclerotic CAD, plaque builds up on the intima or inside walls of the right and left coronary arteries. As a space-occupying lesion, the presence of plaque narrows the vessel lumen and decreases blood flow to heart muscle, which defines ischemia. In addition to ischemia of the myocardium, the electrical conduction system also suffers from hypoxia. Symptoms and signs of atherosclerotic CAD may result from affected myocardium or the conduction system. This is an important factor in ischemic heart disease. Any narrowing of the lumen of a coronary artery produces the general state of _____(1), or CAD. Clot formation, or _____(2), and plaque buildup, or _____(3), represent the majority of cases of CAD. CAD causes decreased blood flow or _____(4) of both the _____(5) and the _____(6).

1. coronary artery disease
2. thrombosis
3. atherosclerosis
4. ischemia
5. myocardium
6. electrical conduction system

10–31

The effects of atherosclerotic coronary artery disease depend on several factors. These are:

1. The degree of obstruction or occlusion caused by the presence of the plaques. This is shown in Figure 10–7.
2. The location in the vessels of this occlusion (either up high in a main trunk or down lower in a smaller side branch—occlusion of the main trunk obviously injures more tissue than one in a side branch, which supplies less tissue).
3. How widespread the plaques are.
4. Acute complete blockage versus chronic interference with blood flow.

1. obstruction or occlusion
2. located
3. widespread
4. acute
5. chronic

The location of the plaques determines the specific areas of myocardium and the conduction system that suffer ischemic injury. These injured areas correspond to the diseased branch of the vessels that supply them. Clinical signs depend on the amount of obstruction. Up to 25 percent obstruction may be asymptomatic or cause slight angina pectoris (chest pain). Up to 70 percent causes chest pain and eventual heart failure. A 100 percent or complete blockage causes a myocardial infarction (see Frame 10–36). The effects of atherosclerotic CAD depend on: a) the amount of _____(1) in the vessels caused by the plaques; b) where the plaques are _____(2) in the vessels; c) how _____(3) the plaques are; and d) whether the situation is _____(4) or _____(5).

10–32

An acute clinical situation may develop when mild ischemia becomes severe when great demands are placed on the heart, such as during strenuous exercise or extreme stress. If coronary thrombosis develops on the plaques (a common occurrence), this may complete an obstruction, or a piece of plaque may break off and lodge in the middle of the lumen. The acute or sudden blockage of blood flow to heart muscle causes an infarct in the area corresponding to that vessel's territory. Or a severe arrhythmia can occur. An arrhythmia is abnormal timing in the conduction system causing abnormal contraction rhythms. This arrhythmia is usually ventricular fibrillation or a heart block. The classic "heart attack" is often a combination of severe arrhythmia initially, with myocardial infarction developing in survivors.

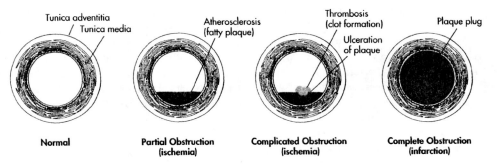

Figure 10–7. Vessel occlusion in coronary artery disease.

1. infarction
2. arrhythmia
3. acute
4. stress
5. thrombosis
6. plaque
7. fibrosis
8. heart failure

Chronic ischemia because of partial or slow occlusion leads to hypoperfusion of the myocardium, patches of atrophy of this muscle, fibrosis, and a progression to heart failure. Myocardium that suffers chronic insufficiency of coronary artery flow becomes painful if it is exerted. Ischemia directly causes pain and produces the familiar chest pain in persons with "heart conditions." Again, the name of this pain is **angina pectoris.** Myocardial death or _____(1), and abnormal timing of the conduction system, or _____(2), is caused by a (an) _____(3) clinical situation. An acute situation develops in times of great _____(4) or exertion, in cases of clots or _____(5), or if a piece of _____(6) breaks off and barricades the lumen against blood flow. Chronic insufficiency in blood flow leads to scarring or _____(7), and eventually _____(8).

1. angina pectoris

Clinically, symptomatic atherosclerotic coronary artery disease most often presents in three ways. First is chest pain or angina pectoris. This pain comes on suddenly and can be severe and stabbing. The pain is a result of ischemia and hypoxia of cardiac muscle. The pain may be referred, or felt elsewhere, in the shoulder or radiating down the left arm. Angina pectoris can accompany any condition where muscular exertion is greater than oxygen supply. Symptomatic relief of angina is possible with the administration of nitroglycerin, which dilates the arteries to increase blood flow. This works in mild to moderate cases. Angina pectoris is often present in cases of myocardial infarction, but may also be absent. The feeling in these cases has been described as a "crushing" sensation along with the pain. Loss of consciousness, or fainting, can accompany myocardial infarction. In atherosclerotic CAD, pain may be felt in the chest or other areas, and this is called _____(1).

The constant hypoxia that results from CAD can eventually lead to a second presentation, failure of the muscle. This is discussed in Frame 10–43 on heart failure. The third manifestation is myocardial infarction, caused by severe interference with blood flow. This will be discussed next. Obstruction of the coronary arteries may be diagnosed through a procedure called an arteriogram. Radiopaque dye is injected and x-rays are taken to allow visualization of the obstruction. An electrocardiogram taken during exercise may reveal ischemic-induced arrhythmias. Early or mild CAD may respond to vasodilators, medications that help open the vessels to increase blood flow. Moderate cases may be candidates for angioplasty. In this procedure, a catheter with a balloon tip is inserted into the vessels, and the tip is expanded like a balloon. This crushes and breaks down plaque build up. Severe occlusion usually requires surgical bypass, where the blocked section of artery is removed and replaced with a graft from a vein.

▶ MYOCARDIAL INFARCTION

1. myocardial infarction
2. ischemic

A **myocardial infarct** is an area of dead muscle, and the process is called **myocardial infarction.** It is often abbreviated as an **MI.** An MI, or a heart attack, is the worst consequence of ischemic heart disease, and is brought on by coronary artery disease. A severe decrease in blood flow through the coronary arteries causes hypoperfusion to the point of anoxia. The muscle fibers then die from lack of oxygen. The symptoms and signs of an MI range from none to various degrees of pain or sudden death. The section of heart most commonly affected is the left ventricle. An example of left ventricular MI is shown in Figure 10–8. Myocardium, or heart muscle, ranks low, along with nerve tissue, in regeneration after injury. Fibrosis is the rule in healing. After an MI, inflammation develops surrounding the necrotic tissue. Granulation tissue forms and collagen is produced. This matures into tough, dense scar tissue or fibrosis. The significance of this type of healing is that there is loss of function directly proportional to the amount of necrosis and fibrosis. This "healed" tissue will never function again as heart muscle. Death of muscle in the heart is called a an) _____(1). It is a result of _____(2) heart disease, which is due to

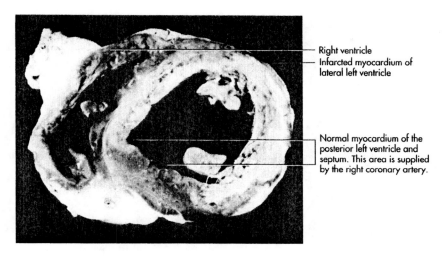

Right ventricle
Infarcted myocardium of
lateral left ventricle

Normal myocardium of the
posterior left ventricle and
septum. This area is supplied
by the right coronary artery.

Figure 10–8. Cross-section of a heart showing myocardial infarction. The infarcted zone is pale. This infarct was associated with thrombotic occlusion of the main left coronary artery. *(From Chandrasoma and Taylor, Concise Pathology, 2nd ed., Appleton & Lange.)*

_____(3) disease. Cardiac muscle heals primarily with scar tissue, or _____(4), instead of regeneration. The significance of this is that _____(5) is permanently lost in the infarcted area.

3. coronary artery
4. fibrosis
5. function

10–37

Myocardium is not the only tissue injured by anoxia. The conduction system also suffers. For this reason, arrhythmia accompanies an MI. Ventricular fibrillation is the complete loss of the coordination of contractions that produce the cardiac output. In ventricular fibrillation, the cardiac output approaches zero. Death is rapid if this arrhythmia is not treated *immediately.* About 25 percent of MI cases die suddenly because of either a major arrhythmia or because of asystole. Asystole means "without contraction," and is the feature of cardiac arrest, which is discussed in Frame 10–42. Immediate death in myocardial infarct is because of injury to the _____(1) system. Abnormal rhythm, or _____(2), is the result. The most life-threatening arrhythmia is _____(3) where cardiac output may cease. Another cause of immediate death in an MI is cardiac arrest because of _____(4).

1. conduction
2. arrhythmia
3. ventricular fibrillation
4. asystole

10–38

Survival of a myocardial infarct depends on the amount of heart muscle that was lost. About 75 percent of cases in a first MI do survive, but with many complications. These include:

1. Eventual heart failure, depending on the amount of dead myocardium. Pulmonary edema, dyspnea, and cardiogenic shock accompany heart failure. This most often develops in cases where previous MIs have lost a large percentage of function already. Other organs begin to fail as poor cardiac output causes systemic hypoperfusion. The kidneys are usually the organs that fail first. The combination of heart and kidney failure leads to a rapid demise.
2. If the patient experienced cardiac arrest, the complete absence of cardiac output injures brain tissue. Extended arrest before being revived causes permanent damage in the brain because of anoxia.
3. The original infarcted area may enlarge if the heart is not rested properly.
4. The remaining myocardium enlarges, or undergoes hypertrophy, to take over function of the lost tissue. This is another road to eventual heart failure.
5. Other complications, which will not be discussed, include rupture of the infarcted area, ventricular aneurysm, endocardial thrombosis, and cerebral embolism with stroke.

TABLE 10–1. CAUSES AND EFFECTS OF ISCHEMIC HEART DISEASE

Cause	Effects
Hypertensive heart disease (secondary to systemic hypertension)	Left ventricular hypertrophy Decreased cardiac output Cardiomegaly Increased atherosclerosis of coronary arteries Myocardial ischemia Myocardial fibrosis Heart failure
Atherosclerotic coronary artery disease	Narrowing of coronary artery lumen due to hypertension, fatty plaques, or thrombosis Myocardial ischemia Arrhythmia Chest pain Heart failure Myocardial infarction
Myocardial infarction	Necrosis of areas of heart muscle Fibrosis Arrhythmia Ventricular fibrillation Near zero cardiac output Cardiac arrest Heart failure

10–39

1. heart
2. kidneys
3. infarct
4. hypertrophy

After surviving a myocardial infarction, the patient is at risk for _____(1) failure; failure of other organs, especially the _____(2); enlargement of the original _____(3); and cardiac enlargement, or _____(4). A few diagnostic techniques specific for myocardial infarction follow. An **electrocardiogram** measures the electrical activity of the heart and produces a tracing that is evaluated for abnormalities. A very good idea of the site of the damage and the extent of the damage is gleaned by examining these tracings. Laboratory tests on the blood are invaluable. Levels of **cardiac enzymes** are measured. Most enzymes are inside cells with only a small amount normally in the blood. When cells are injured, these enzymes are released into the circulation. Particular enzymes are tested for that correspond to the suspected necrotic tissue.

10–40

There are three enzymes that are associated with myocardium. They are **creatine phosphokinase (CK), aspartate aminotransferase (AST),** and **lactic dehydrogenase (LDH).** The timing of the peak elevations of these enzymes in the blood after an MI is extremely helpful in diagnosis. CK rises first and rapidly, within 6 hours after an MI. It peaks at around 24 hours and returns to normal shortly thereafter. Because CK is also found in skeletal muscle and brain, the **isoenzyme CK-MB** is part of the evaluation because it is specific for the heart. AST rises second, peaks at around 48 hours, and remains elevated longer than CK. LDH doesn't elevate until around 72 hours or more and remains high for quite some time. Usually, these enzyme levels are evaluated every 8 to 12 hours for the first few days after an MI.

10–41

Treatment for an MI depends on the presentation of the case. In asystole or cardiac arrest, cardiopulmonary resuscitation (CPR) is designed to support general circulation and respiration until the heart can be started again. Electrical shock is helpful to re-establish the conduction system. In arrhythmias, electrical shock can also be used to stop the abnormal contractions and re-establish normal conduction. Medications for an MI include a thrombolytic agent (a clot dissolver) to remove thrombosis from coronary arteries. Two examples are tissue plasminogen activator and streptokinase. Anticoagulants like heparin and aspirin help prevent future thrombosis. Since the cause of an MI is coronary artery disease, angioplasty and coronary artery bypass may also be used to manage MI survivors.

► CARDIAC ARREST

Cardiac arrest occurs when **asystole** is present. Asystole means _____(1) contractions. It is the sudden and complete stopping of all electrical activity and myocardial contraction. Needless to say, cardiac output during asystole and arrest is zero. Clinically, cardiac arrest presents as an absence of the pulse and respiration. Asystole and arrest are caused by anoxia of the conduction system. It simply stops the electrical circuitry of the heart. Some causes of cardiac arrest are myocardial infarction, major arrhythmia, electrocution, drug overdose, drowning or other types of respiratory arrest, and massive hemorrhage. An electrocardiogram (ECG) will characteristically show ventricular fibrillation. (The result of ventricular fibrillation is asystole, as described in Frame 10–76.) CPR must be successful within 4 to 6 minutes to prevent permanent brain damage. Defibrillation (stopping and restarting the impulses with electric shock) is required. Drugs to stimulate the heart are administered, and these include epinephrine and isoproterenol. Lidocaine is a drug that helps regulate arrhythmia.

1. without

► HEART FAILURE

Normally, the heart copes with the usual load of blood volume even during strenuous exercise. During times of increased metabolism, which require a greater cardiac output, there are reserve mechanisms that enable the heart to meet the accelerated demands. The mechanisms are increased force of contraction, when muscle fibers are stretched to the limit by increased filling with blood; increased muscle tone stimulated by the sympathetic nervous system; and increased heart rate. **Heart failure** is defined as an inability to meet the body's needs through adequate cardiac output, even though the venous return is normal. (This is saying there is enough blood entering the heart from the body, but there is not enough being pumped back out.) Heart failure is first noticed during exercise, when demands are greater. Eventually, the effects are seen even when resting because failure of the myocardium is progressive and only gets worse as time passes. If the muscle of the heart cannot contract effectively enough to move a sufficient amount of blood out to the body, this is defined as _____(1).

1. heart failure

The right ventricle or the left ventricle may each fail individually. If both sides of the heart fail together, this is called **congestive heart failure (CHF). Congestion** is the distention or swelling of veins because of increased pressure within them. The increased pressure is because of increased blood that is present. In CHF, insufficient output causes blood to back up *behind* the site of failure in the circulatory circuit. Therefore, there is more blood present in the veins than normal. The clinical presentation of right or left or congestive heart failure is directly related to this backing up of blood prior to or behind the site of failure. In this respect, heart failure is like obstruction of blood flow and several effects are the same. Since the signs of heart failure are directly related to the path of blood flow, keep the normal circuitry in mind to understand what a backup of blood and pressure causes. Failure of both sides of the heart is called _____(1). Congestion means that the veins are _____(2) because of increased _____(3) and therefore increased _____(4). The signs of CHF are related to the _____(5) of blood _____(6) the site of failure. The effects of CHF are similar to what is seen in other types of _____(7) in blood flow.

1. congestive heart failure
2. distended
3. blood
4. pressure
5. backup
6. behind
7. obstruction

There are several major causes of heart failure. The minor causes will not be discussed. The major causes are:

1. Ischemic heart disease or myocardial ischemia. Coronary artery disease and myocardial infarct are leading causes of ischemic myocardial disease.
2. Myocarditis and cardiomyopathy. These are diseases of the myocardium not caused by ischemia.
3. Excessive burdens placed on the heart that cannot be sustained. The burdens include too much resistance encountered by the ventricle (systemic or pulmonary hypertension, pul-

monary or aortic stenosis); excessive cardiac output (heart valve regurgitation); and systemic disease (anemia, hyperthyroidism).

4. Arrhythmias.

5. Hypertrophy.

10-46

In right ventricular failure, if the right ventricle can't eject all of its blood volume, the right atrium (the structure immediately behind) distends. Then the pressure continues to rise in all structures behind the right side. The large veins expand. *Distention of the jugular vein* in the neck becomes visible. Cardiac output decreases because the left ventricle isn't receiving its normal volume from the lungs. The right ventricle is not able to move a normal amount of blood through the lungs, so oxygenation is also affected. The visceral organs become distended with backed-up blood, so the organs become *congested.* The swollen liver leaks fluid into the abdomen, and this type of edema is ascites. *Peripheral cyanosis* develops in the extremities because of sluggish circulation. In response to hypoxia, the bone marrow creates the state of *polycythemia. Edema* develops in dependent areas of the body such as the lower legs in a patient who is ambulatory. Fluid is squeezed out by the high venous pressure, and also more water has been retained because the kidneys increase their retention of sodium. (This effect is thought to be due to a redistribution of blood and response by the kidneys.) Edema that occurs *around* the lungs (not in them) in the pleural space is called **pleural effusion.** Pleural effusion interferes with the ability of the lungs to expand, so respiration may be difficult.

10-47

1. ventricle
2. blood
3. behind
4. distend
5. pressure
6. jugular vein
7. congested
8. ascites
9. edema
10. pleural effusion
11. expansion
12. breathing

In right-sided heart failure, the right _____(1) cannot pump out a normal amount of _____(2). This makes all of the structures located _____(3) the right ventricle swell or _____(4) with extra blood. This also makes the _____(5) increase in these structures. A visible sign in the neck is distension of the _____(6). Other effects of right-sided failure are the swelling of organs with blood, causing them to be called _____(7). A congested liver weeps fluid into the abdomen, creating _____(8). Excess fluid in the peripheral tissue is called _____(9), and this is also present in right-sided heart failure. Edema in the pleural space is called _____(10). This may interfere with _____(11) of the lungs, making _____(12) difficult.

10-48

In left-sided heart failure, the left atrium distends behind the failing left ventricle. Therefore, blood emptying into the left side from the lungs begins to back up. Pressure rises in these structures since they are behind the obstruction. The increased pressure in the pulmonary circulation squeezes fluid *into* the lungs, causing **pulmonary edema.** While right-sided failure causes edema of the organs and extremities, left-sided failure causes edema of the lungs. A small amount of fluid in the lungs causes coughing. A significant amount interferes with breathing. Difficulty in breathing is called **dyspnea.** While lying down, fluid easily accumulates in the lungs. For this reason, severe acute episodes of dyspnea often happen at night, and this is called **paroxysmal nocturnal dyspnea.** This is a potentially life-threatening situation. *Hypoxia* develops if the edema is severe enough to interfere with oxygen exchange. Small capillaries in the lungs may rupture from the high pressure. The fluid coughed up will then be bloody, and this is **hemoptysis.** The increased pulmonary pressure and resistance leads to pulmonary hypertension. This increases the workload for the right ventricle. Eventually, the right ventricle fails also and congestive heart failure is the result.

10-49

1. pulmonary
2. pulmonary edema
3. breathing
4. dyspnea
5. paroxysmal nocturnal dyspnea

Failure of the left ventricle causes increased pressure in the _____(1) circulation. This causes fluid to leak out of the vessels into the lungs and creates _____(2). The significance of pulmonary edema is that it interferes with _____(3). Difficulty breathing is called _____(4). The worst episodes can happen at night when lying down, and this is known as _____(5). The presence of fluid in the lungs decreases oxygenation of the blood, creating

_____(6). Coughing up blood, or _____(7), may also occur. Sooner or later, the _____(8) fails also because of increased work caused by pulmonary _____(9).

10-50

In congestive heart failure, dyspnea is a prominent feature because of both pulmonary edema and pleural effusion. CHF combines all the clinical features of both right- and left-sided failure. All organ functions are affected because of hypoperfusion and poor oxygenation. Hypoxia becomes chronic since cardiac output is poor and venous return is impeded by resistance in the backed-up cardiac chambers. Liver and kidney failure follow congestive heart failure. The entrance into the terminal stage is signaled by loss of consciousness as the brain becomes anoxic. Advanced cases of CHF are fatal. While there is no cure short of a transplant, milder cases can be managed for quite a while with rest, a low-salt diet (to decrease water retention and edema), and medications. Digitalis is a drug that increases the strength of myocardial contractions to make the most of every pump cycle. Diuretics promote excess water loss to minimize edema. A very visible sign of CHF is _____(1). Generalized hypoperfusion and insufficient oxygen or _____(2) eventually lead all organs into _____(3). A review of the pathogenesis of heart failure is presented in Figure 10–9.

1. dyspnea
2. hypoxia
3. failure

► CARDIOMYOPATHY

10-51

Cardiomyopathy literally means heart muscle disease. This term is reserved for disease *not* associated with ischemia or inflammation. Cardiomyopathy is not well understood, especially its causes. The condition presents itself, causes may be guessed at, and the only cure is a heart transplant. Cardiomyopathy, or **CMP,** has been identified in three different forms.

1. Dilated CMP. The heart chambers are enlarged, but they are thin and flabby with a significant amount of fibrosis. Muscle contraction is inefficient. Dilated CMP has been associated with alcoholism, viral myocarditis, and some chemotherapy drugs. Many cases are idiopathic.
2. Hypertrophic CMP. The muscle of the left ventricle is enlarged and the walls of the chamber are very thick. Figure 10–10 pictures hypertrophic cardiomyopathy. The size of the interior of the chamber is reduced by the thickening, so it holds less blood, reducing output. While most cases are idiopathic, others seem to have a genetic component. Familial hypertrophic CMP is found in some family lines. Recently, a gene has been isolated that is associated with this form of CMP.
3. Restrictive CMP. The myocardium is unable to expand because it has been infiltrated with a foreign substance. Most often this is amyloid, the abnormal protein produced in amyloidosis (see Chap. 2). Rarely, the infiltration may be by metastasis or spreading cancer. Cardiomyopathy leads to congestive heart failure with all its clinical presentations. As mentioned, heart transplant is the only true treatment.

10-52

Disease of the myocardium not caused by ischemia or inflammation is called _____(1). Very often, the cause of CMP is _____(2). In the first form, the heart is enlarged but is _____(3) and flabby. This is called _____(4) CMP. In the second form, the enlargement is from _____(5), which makes the walls very _____(6). It also makes the inner chamber _____(7) in size. This is called _____(8) CMP. Infiltration by foreign substances interferes with _____(9), and this is _____(10) CMP. CMP leads to _____(11).

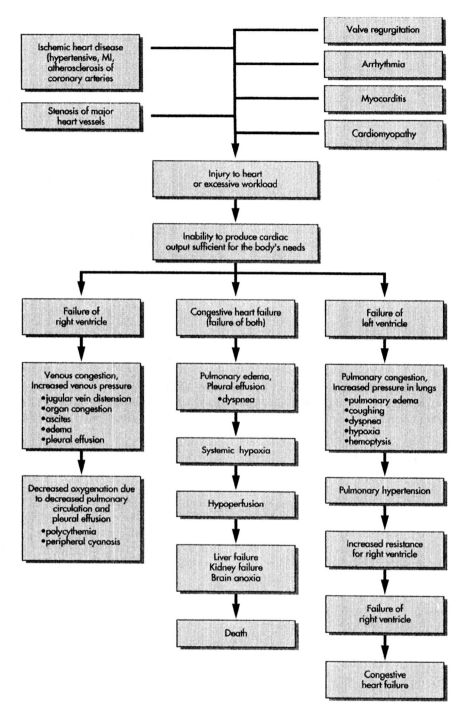

Figure 10–9. The pathogenesis of heart failure.

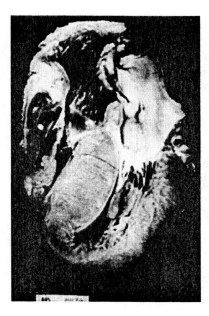

Figure 10–10. Hypertrophic cardiomyopathy with extreme thickening of the left ventricular wall, and especially of the interventricular septum. The banana-shaped left ventricular lumen is very reduced in size, and the bulging interventricular septum interferes with the outflow tract. *(From Kumar et al, Basic Pathology, 5th ed., Saunders.)*

III. REVIEW QUESTIONS

1. Hypertensive heart disease is a reaction to:
   a. systemic hypertension
   b. pulmonary hypertension
   c. coronary artery hypertension
   d. hypertrophy of heart muscle

2. Hypertensive heart disease causes:
   a. hypertrophy of the right ventricle only and cardiomegaly
   b. hypertrophy of the left ventricle and heart failure
   c. atherosclerosis of the coronary arteries
   d. increased cardiac output

3. The most common form of coronary artery disease is:
   a. coronary thrombosis
   b. arteriosclerosis
   c. systemic hypertension
   d. atherosclerosis

4. Atherosclerotic coronary artery disease causes decreased blood flow or
   a. _____, and therefore decreased oxygen supply or
   b. _____. This causes ischemic disease of the heart muscle or
   c. _____, and of the electrical d. _____ system.

1. a–systemic hypertension

2. b–hypertrophy of the left ventricle and heart failure

3. d–atherosclerosis

4. a–ischemia; b–hypoxia; c–myocardium; d–conduction

5. c–chest pain caused by ischemia of the myocardium

6. b–myocardial infarction; d–heart failure

7. 1. a–fibrosis
   2. e–function

8. c–arrhythmia

9. (Any two of these in any order) heart failure; brain damage; enlargement of the infarct; hypertrophy leading to heart failure

10. a–without contraction e–cardiac arrest

11. 1. c–myocardial contractions
    2. e–cardiac output

12. congestive heart failure

13. c–Veins and organs become congested; e–Blood backs up behind the site of failure.

5. Angina pectoris is:
   a. the medical term for a heart attack
   b. chest pain caused by ischemia of the heart's conduction system
   c. chest pain caused by ischemia of the myocardium
   d. chest pain caused by spasm of the coronary arteries

6. Life-threatening consequences of atherosclerotic coronary artery disease include (choose all that apply):
   a. angina pectoris
   b. myocardial infarction
   c. hypertensive heart disease
   d. heart failure
   e. cardiomegaly

7. A myocardial infarct heals by 1. _____, and the result is loss of 2. _____.
   a. fibrosis
   b. blood supply
   c. regeneration
   d. oxygen
   e. function

8. Which of the following *disorders* accompanies an MI?
   a. loss of consciousness
   b. angina pectoris
   c. arrhythmia
   d. left ventricular hypertrophy

9. List two of the four complications of MI that were discussed:
   a. _____
   b. _____

10. Asystole means _____, and this is the main feature of (choose all that apply):
    a. without contraction
    b. coronary artery disease
    c. hypertensive heart disease
    d. heart failure
    e. cardiac arrest
    f. cardiomyopathy

11. In heart failure, 1. _____ are inefficient and therefore 2. _____ is insufficient for the body's needs.
    a. electrical impulses
    b. venous return
    c. myocardial contractions
    d. heart rate
    e. cardiac output
    f. oxygen

12. Failure of both the right and left sides of the heart is called _____.

13. The effects of heart failure are (choose all that apply):
    a. Venous return from the body is inadequate.
    b. Blood backs up in front of the site of failure.
    c. Veins and organs become congested.
    d. Arrhythmia decreases cardiac output.
    e. Blood backs up behind the site of failure.

14. Please match the forms of heart failure in the left column with the signs listed in the right column:

a. right-sided heart failure
b. left-sided heart failure
c. congestive heart failure

1. _____ all of the signs listed here
2. _____ pulmonary edema
3. _____ vein distention
4. _____ organ congestion
5. _____ paroxysmal nocturnal dyspnea
6. _____ peripheral edema
7. _____ ascites
8. _____ hemoptysis
9. _____ pleural effusion

15. Please match the terms in the left column with the statements in the right column:

a. cardiomyopathy
b. dilated CMP
c. hypertrophic CMP
d. restrictive CMP

1. _____ thin and flabby walls
2. _____ interference by infiltration
3. _____ nonischemic, noninflammatory disease of the heart muscle
4. _____ thick walls with decreased lumen of the left ventricle

14. 1. c–CHF
2. b–LHF
3. a–RHF
4. a–RHF
5. b–LHF
6. a–RHF
7. a–RHF
8. b–LHF
9. a–RHF

15. 1 b–dilated CMP
2. d–restrictive CMP
3. a–cardiomyopathy
4. c–hypertrophic CMP

IV. INFECTIOUS AND INFLAMMATORY HEART DISEASE ◄ SECTION

► RHEUMATIC HEART DISEASE

10-53

Rheumatic heart disease is a consequence of rheumatic fever. This is a systemic disease that may follow a group A hemolytic streptococcal infection in some people. The most commonly associated streptococcal infection is the familiar "strep throat," although other respiratory strep infections may precipitate rheumatic fever. In this hypersensitivity reaction, some tissues of the body "get in the way" of the immune attack against the organisms. In particular, these tissues are connective tissue of the skin, the joint surfaces, the central nervous system, and the heart. Rheumatic fever and rheumatic heart disease are much less common than they used to be because of effective antibiotic treatment that contains and cures the infection.

10-54

Rheumatic fever is a disease of children and young adults. There are five important manifestations, called **Jones' major criteria,** which define this disorder. They are:

1. Polyarthritis—inflammation of many joints.
2. Carditis—inflammation of structures of the heart.
3. Chorea—brain inflammation that causes involuntary movements.
4. Inflammation of the connective tissue of the skin.
5. Nodules in the skin.

The **minor criteria** include joint pain (arthralgia), a previous infection with group A hemolytic streptococci, and an abnormal ECG. These criteria are used in diagnosing rheumatic fever and rheumatic heart disease. Rheumatic heart disease is a complication of _____(1). This is a disorder in which some tissue is damaged by the action of the _____(2) system against group A hemolytic _____(3). In diagnosing rheumatic fever and associated heart disease, important signs have been identified, and they are called _____(4).

1. rheumatic fever
2. immune
3. streptococci
4. Jones' major and minor criteria

After a strep throat or other streptococcal respiratory infection, the subsequent antigen–antibody reactions can damage certain tissues. This is thought to be because of a cross-reaction that may occur. It seems that some tissues, such as the heart and joints, have antigens that are remarkably similar to the antigens on the bacteria. Therefore, anti-streptococcal antibodies target these tissues as well. There has also been shown to be damage from cell-mediated activity of lymphocytes and macrophages. In the heart, the three types of tissue that can be mistaken for foreign bacterial antigens are the endocardium, myocardium, and pericardium. The underlying pathogenesis of rheumatic heart disease is the mistaken identity of structures in the _____(1) being taken for _____(2) antigens. This cross-reaction occurs in antigen–_____(3) reactions, as well as in _____(4)-mediated immune reactions.

Endocarditis is inflammation of the inner lining of the heart chambers and valves. In rheumatic heart disease, the most common site for damage and subsequent inflammation is on the valves in the left side. The immune activity that causes the inflammation leaves ulcers or erosions on valve surfaces. The ulcers become covered with fibrin, a normal reaction, and with thrombi. Altogether, this forms small nodules on the valves known as **vegetations.** The damage from inflammation is followed by attempts at healing, which of course lead to scarring. Since scar tissue contracts, the valves suffer structural deformity. The once thin and delicate valve leaflets become thickened and sticky and covered with vegetations. Thin strands of connective tissue that anchor the valves (the chordae tendineae) shorten with the constriction and may fuse together. The effects of rheumatic heart disease are pictured in Figure 10–11. The deformity of the valves and the cords causes valvular insufficiency (see Frame 10–67). The valves are incompetent because they cannot close efficiently and blood flow becomes abnormal. The fibrotic contraction and adhesions can also cause valvular stenosis, thereby narrowing the passageway for blood flow. In rheumatic heart disease, the most common site of injury is the endocardium of the _____(1) on the _____(2) side. Nodules called _____(3) form on the valves, and these are a combination of _____(4) and _____(5) that form over erosions or _____(6). Structural deformity of the valves and anchoring cords occurs because of the attempts at _____(7). After fibrosis, shrinking or _____(8) of the structure follows. The two results of this contractual deformity are inability of the valves to _____(9) as they should [known as valvular _____(10)] and narrowing of the passageway for blood, called valvular _____(11).

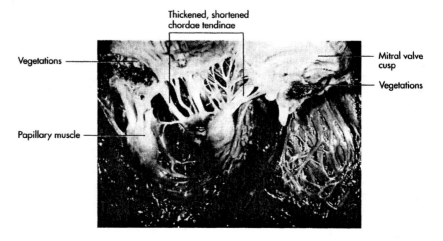

Figure 10–11. Rheumatic heart disease, showing small vegetations typical of acute rheumatic fever. Note that the chordae tendineae are thickened and shortened, suggesting chronic rheumatic heart disease. This patient gave a history of recurrent attacks of acute rheumatic fever over several years. *(From Chandrasoma and Taylor,* Concise Pathology, *2nd ed., Appleton & Lange.)*

10-57

1. workload
2. heart failure
3. infection
4. break off

The effects of valvular insufficiency and stenosis are presented in the next section. The end result is a backflow or reflux of blood into the previous chamber or vessel, and increased workload for the heart. Or in the case of stenosis, increased resistance when pushing blood through the narrowed valve, also increases cardiac work. The excessive burden borne by the heart causes hypertrophy and can lead to heart failure. Remember that in rheumatic heart disease, the most common result is mitral valve fibrosis and eventual left-sided heart failure. Also, an injured valve is susceptible to infection, so bacterial endocarditis (see Frame 10-59) is the most common complicating factor in rheumatic heart disease. Should bacterial endocarditis develop, a further complication is possible septic emboli, since the infected thrombotic vegetations can easily break off. These emboli commonly travel to the brain or kidneys. The pathogenesis and complications of rheumatic heart disease are outlined in Figure 10-12. Two other manifestations of rheumatic heart disease are inflammation of the muscle (myocarditis) or the pericardium (pericarditis). In rheumatic myocarditis, the necrosis and fibrosis that destroy muscle fibers typically affect only a small area and are not problematic unless in direct line of the conduction system. Rheumatic pericarditis occurs only in the most severe cases. The bottom line of valvular insufficiency or stenosis is abnormal blood flow and an increased _____(1) for the heart. Eventually, this can lead to _____(2). The damaged valves are also susceptible to _____(3), and this itself can have complications if bits of the infected vegetations _____(4) and travel to other organs.

10-58

The diagnosis of rheumatic fever and rheumatic heart disease requires the presence of at least two of the major Jones' criteria, or one major criterion and two minor ones. Also, the ASO test is employed. The antigens on the group A streptococci are called O antigens. The antibodies against them are called anti-streptolysin O, or ASO. An elevated titer of these antibodies is highly suspicious for rheumatic fever or heart disease. The best treatment for the rheumatic disorders is their prevention by treating streptococcal infections with effective antibiotics for at least 10 days. Untreated rheumatic disease creates damage in the heart that is permanent because it is structural. The only treatment is surgical replacement of the ravaged valves with artificial ones. If this is not done, death due to heart failure is inevitable.

▶ INFECTIOUS ENDOCARDITIS

10-59

1. bacteremia
2. pus producing
3. infectious endocarditis

Infectious endocarditis is inflammation of the endocardium caused specifically by infection with a microorganism. While viruses and fungi occasionally cause infectious endocarditis, the vast majority of cases are due to bacteria. Therefore, **bacterial endocarditis** is the phrase often used to describe this disorder. Since the heart is in direct contact with the entire blood volume of the body, this organ is very susceptible to blood-borne infection. The term you learned in Chapter 5 that describes the presence of bacteria in the blood is _____(1). The bacteria most often responsible for bacterial or infectious endocarditis are the pyogenic microorganisms. Pyogenic means _____(2) (see Chap. 5). These are the staphylococcal and streptococcal organisms. Other microorganisms may cause infectious endocarditis in immunosuppressed patients (AIDS patients and those receiving chemotherapy). An inflammatory condition affecting the endocardium caused by microorganisms is called _____(3).

10-60

The endocardium of the valves on the left side of the heart are the usual targets of pyogenic microorganisms. The sources of the bacteria include tooth abscess, skin infection, urinary tract infection, and pulmonary or respiratory infection. Infection of the valves is predisposed to occur if there has been previous injury of the valves. The most common predisposing injuries are rheumatic heart disease and congenital heart disease affecting the valves and making them abnormal. As the organisms settle on the valves and begin to colonize there, this causes ulcerations or erosions. The bacteria release lytic enzymes that eat away at the endocardium of the valves. An inflammatory reaction follows this colonization. As always,

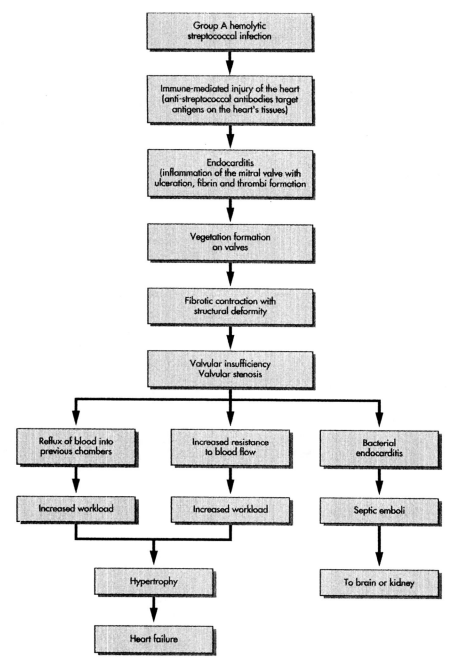

Figure 10–12. The pathogenesis and complications of rheumatic heart disease.

the injured surface is a prime site for thrombi formation (the interior of the heart can be thought of as a continuation of the blood vessels). Fibrosis follows inflammation as the only way of attempted healing. These reactions occur continuously (growth of the bacterial colony, inflammation, thrombi formation, fibrosis), until bumps or nodules are formed on the surface. These growths are also called vegetations, as they are in noninfectious endocarditis of rheumatic heart disease. However, there are more of them and they are more severe because the presence of the bacterial colonies adds to the vegetations. These vegetations are infected compared to the sterile ones of rheumatic heart disease. The infection, inflammation

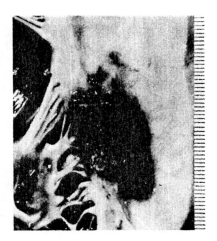

Figure 10–13. Bacterial endocarditis of the mitral valve. *(From McCance and Huether,* Pathophysiology: The Biologic Basis for Disease in Adults and Children, *Mosby.)*

with its production of debris, and fibrosis cause structural deformity of the valves and chordae tendineae. Bacterial endocarditis of the mitral valve can be seen in Figure 10–13.

10–61

In bacterial endocarditis, the sites most often attacked and colonized are the _____(1) of the _____(2) side of the heart. The pyogenic organisms usually responsible are _____(3) and _____(4). The lesion this infection produces is a combination of growths or _____(5) by the bacteria, an _____(6) reaction; formation of clots, or _____(7); and scarring, or _____(8). The nodules formed by these activities are called _____(9). The result of these processes is _____(10) of the valves and their anchoring cords.

1. valves
2. left
3. staphylococci
4. streptococci
5. colonies
6. inflammatory
7. thrombosis
8. fibrosis
9. vegetations
10. deformity

10–62

Structural deformity of the valves and associated structures causes the same effects we discussed in rheumatic heart disease. Valvular insufficiency causes reflux of blood back into the previous chamber or vessel. Abnormal blood flow puts a strain on the heart as workload is increased. Hypertrophy and heart failure follow continued incompetency of the valves. A very serious complication of bacterial endocarditis is the formation of **septic emboli.** This is a mass of bacteria that has broken off from the valve vegetation and is traveling through the circulation. The infected vegetations are friable, or fragile, and can fracture easily. These septic emboli, or infected foreign bodies in the blood, travel to other sites, especially the kidneys, brain, and extremities. There they cause septic infarcts as well as new areas of infections. The new pocket of infection is called a **microabscess.** The signs that develop depend on the organ that is assaulted by infarct and infection. Examples are stroke (brain), arthritis (joints), lung infarction or infection, gangrene (extremities), osteomyelitis (bone), kidney infarction or infection, and myocardial infarction. The most important complication of bacterial endocarditis is the formation of _____(1). These are masses of _____(2) traveling through the _____(3). They land and infect other _____(4), causing _____(5) and/or _____(6).

1. septic emboli
2. bacteria
3. circulation
4. organs
5. infarction
6. microabscesses

10–63

Bacterial endocarditis is partly diagnosed by its clinical presentation. As in many bacterial infections, fever is present. A CBC reveals leukocytosis as neutrophils rally to the defense. Chills and shaking occur when bacteria are released from the valvular colonies back into the circulation. The abnormality of blood flow, or its turbulence, creates audible murmurs. Disorders of organs other than the heart support the suspicion of septic emboli. A **blood culture** is used to confirm the differential diagnosis of bacterial endocarditis. A sample of venous blood is injected into a liquid growth media, and any growth of a pathogen is a positive result. Treatment is aggressive antibiotic therapy. Aggressive means a potent antibiotic, a substantial dose, and a prolonged course of treatment. Since rheumatic fever is a closely related disorder and the most common predisposing factor for bacterial endocarditis, proper antibiotic treatment of pyogenic infections serve better to prevent infectious endocarditis. Deformed and incompetent valves require surgical replacement to prevent heart failure.

▶ MYOCARDITIS

10-64

1. infectious inflammation
2. myocardium
3. virus
4. heart failure

Myocarditis is infectious inflammation of the myocardium. It is most often caused by a viral infection, and often known as viral myocarditis. Since a virus is an intracellular organism, it enters into the muscle cells instead of colonizing a surface like bacteria. Inside the cells, it kills them. Severe cases that produce widespread permanent damage can lead to dilated CMP and heart failure. Cell-mediated immunity is the defense against viruses, and the activity of T cells contributes to the injury. Anti-viral lymphokines from the T cells are also toxic to myocardial cells. The signs of myocarditis vary considerably and range from infection to eventual heart failure. The only way to positively diagnose myocarditis is to perform a biopsy and examine the parasitized muscle cells microscopically. Myocarditis is _____(1) of the _____(2), most often caused by a _____(3). Severe and permanent injury eventually causes _____(4).

▶ PERICARDITIS

10-65

Infection or inflammation of the epicardium and the pericardium is called **pericarditis.** It most often follows infection or inflammation of the myocardium. Severe rheumatic heart disease is one example of cause. Occasionally, inflammatory conditions of other structures in the chest may spread to the pericardium, causing pericarditis. Systemic disorders such as the autoimmune disease SLE, and uremic poisoning can inflame the pericardium. Normally, a small amount of serous fluid is present in the pericardial sac to prevent painful friction as the heart moves within its covering. As you know, inflammation produces exudate, and so it is in pericarditis. The composition of the exudate depends on its cause. Viral infection creates clear, serous exudate; rheumatic heart disease and bacterial infection create fibrinous (high in sticky fibrin) exudate; and pyogenic bacteria cause purulent exudate. The presence of exudate in the pericardial sac causes pain as friction is increased when the heart beats. The most dangerous consequence occurs in situations of voluminous exudate production. The excessive amount of material in the sac prevents the heart from expanding as it needs to in order to fill with enough blood for sufficient cardiac output. The effect of this restriction of heart expansion is called **pericardial tamponade.**

10-66

1. myocarditis
2. exudate
3. purulent
4. fibrinous
5. serous
6. expansion
7. pericardial tamponade

Pericarditis usually is associated with _____(1), although other inflammatory conditions may spread to the pericardium. The inflammation produces a (an) _____(2), and its content depends on its cause. The presence of pus is a _____(3) exudate, fibrin creates a _____(4) exudate, and a virus causes a _____(5) exudate. The most serious consequence is prevention of heart _____(6), and this restriction is called _____(7).

IV. REVIEW QUESTIONS

1. Choose the *incorrect* statement about rheumatic heart disease:
   a. It is a disorder that may follow rheumatic fever.
   b. It is a disorder that may follow group A streptococcal infection.
   c. It is a disorder that is immune mediated.
   d. It is a disorder affecting the elderly.

2. The most common structure of the heart that is damaged in rheumatic heart disease is:
   a. the endocardium
   b. the pericardium
   c. the endocardium of the valves on the left side
   d. the myocardium
   e. the endocardium of the valves on the right side

3. The mechanism of injury in rheumatic heart disease is:
   a. autoantibodies produced against cardiac tissue
   b. infection by group A streptococci through bacteremia
   c. antibodies produced against group A streptococci that react with similar antigens in the heart
   d. inflammation in rheumatic fever that spreads to the heart

4. A vegetation in rheumatic heart disease is:
   a. a bacterial growth on valve leaflets
   b. deforming scar tissue of the valves
   c. nodules on valve leaflets made of fibrin and thrombi that form in response to erosion
   d. nodules on valve leaflets made of fibrin and thrombi that form to protect the tissue from antibodies

5. Valvular stenosis and/or insufficiency is a result of:
   a. contraction following fibrosis
   b. erosions that leave holes in the valve leaflets
   c. vegetations on the valve leaflets
   d. abnormal blood flow

6. In infectious endocarditis, the most common manifestation is:
   a. bacterial endocarditis
   b. viral endocarditis
   c. fungal endocarditis
   d. all are equally common

7. Infectious endocarditis most often develops as a result of:
   a. a direct, penetrating wound of the heart
   b. bacteremia
   c. spread of infection from the lungs
   d. inhalation of staphylococcal or streptococcal organisms

8. Characteristics of vegetations in infectious endocarditis that differ from vegetations in rheumatic heart disease include:
   a. the presence of multiplying bacterial colonies
   b. increased severity
   c. increased numbers
   d. all of the above

1. d–It is a disorder affecting the elderly.

2. c–the endocardium of the valves on the left side

3. c–antibodies produced against group A streptococci that react with similar antigens in the heart

4. c–nodules on valve leaflets made of fibrin and thrombi that form in response to erosion

5. a–contraction following fibrosis

6. a–bacterial endocarditis

7. b–bacteremia

8. d–all of the above

9. The most serious *complication* of infectious or bacterial endocarditis is:
   a. valvular deformity
   b. septic emboli
   c. reflux of blood in heart chambers
   d. myocardial hypertrophy and heart failure

10. In severe pericarditis, excessive exudate in the pericardial sac causes (choose all that are correct):
    a. infection in adjacent structures in the chest
    b. interference with expansion of the heart
    c. infection of the myocardium
    d. pericardial tamponade

SECTION ▶ V. OTHER DISORDERS OF THE HEART

▶ DISEASE OF THE VALVES

10–67

In the previous section, you were introduced to valvular disease as a consequence of a primary disorder. The end results of injury or disease of the valves are either **insufficiency** or **stenosis**. Insufficiency, sometimes called incompetency, is the case when the valve opening is too wide. The leaflets, or individual flaps of the valve, do not meet and close the opening entirely. Since their function is to close tightly, when this does not occur, the effort is insufficient or incompetent. This allows blood to fall or flow backward instead of forward. This movement in reverse is described as **reflux, or regurgitation.** In stenosis, the opening is too narrow so it does not allow a normal amount of blood to pass through, and it also increases resistance for blood that does pass through. Figure 10–14

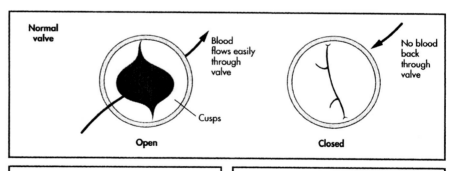
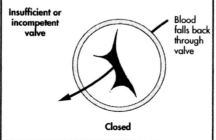
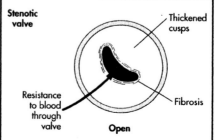

Figure 10–14. Valvular insufficiency and valvular stenosis.

compares a normal valve with valves that are incompetent and stenotic. A valve opening that is too wide is described as _____(1) or _____(2). This means that the leaflets do not _____(3) completely, and so do not sufficiently _____(4) the opening. This allows blood to flow in reverse, called _____(5) or _____(6). A valve opening that is too narrow is described as _____(7). This increases _____(8) to blood flow through the smaller opening.

1. insufficiency
2. incompetency
3. meet
4. close
5. reflux
6. regurgitation
7. stenotic
8. resistance

10-68

Regurgitation of blood volume and resistance to blood flow are the underlying basis for the effects of valvular disease on the rest of the heart and body. In stenosis, the increased resistance works the myocardium to excess and so it hypertrophies. In insufficiency, the reflux into the previous chamber overloads that chamber, since it also contains the normal amount of forward-moving blood. This also increases the workload of that chamber, and the muscle responds with enlargement, or _____(1). As you know from Section III, hypertrophy eventually leads to heart _____(2). To review the causes of valvular disease, they are rheumatic heart disease and infectious endocarditis, which both create vegetations on the valve leaflets and fibrotic shrinking; formation of thrombi on otherwise injured valve endocardium, which thickens the leaflets; and congenital defects of the leaflets.

1. hypertrophy
2. failure

10-69

On the right side of the heart, the **tricuspid valve** is between the right atrium and ventricle. Rarely, rheumatic heart disease may cause stenosis. More often, failure of the right heart causes dilation of the chamber and valve area, resulting in insufficiency and reflux. The **pulmonary valve** is the passageway from the right ventricle into the pulmonary artery and lungs. While rheumatic endocarditis may affect this valve on rare occasions, more often there are congenital malformations that produce stenosis.

10-70

The valves of the left side of the heart are more commonly damaged, and of the two, disease of the **mitral valve** (between the left atrium and ventricle) is the most common valvular disorder. Chronic rheumatic endocarditis causes stenosis with some degree of regurgitation also. The opening becomes quite small and rigid, as seen in Figure 10–15. This obstruction leads to dilation of the left atrium in response to the resistance. Blood then backs up through the pulmonary circulation, and the resistance of pulmonary hypertension causes right-sided heart enlargement. Thrombi formation in the left atrium poses the danger of cerebral embolism. Systemically, venous congestion is present. Insufficiency occurs in left-sided heart failure when the chamber and valve become dilated, preventing closure of the valve. Rheumatic endocarditis and infectious endocarditis also cause this reflux because of contractual deformity. The most common valvular disorders affect the _____(1).

1. mitral valve

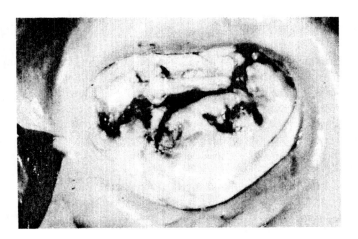

Figure 10–15. Mitral valve stenosis. The mitral valve opening shows the typical "fishmouth" appearance. *(From Chandrasoma and Taylor, Concise Pathology, 2nd ed., Appleton & Lange.)*

10-71

The **aortic valve** is the entrance into the aorta from the left ventricle. Congenital deformities and chronic rheumatic endocarditis cause stenosis. Insufficiency and reflux develop when the elastic tissue of the aorta and valve area break down in the face of systemic hypertension. Incompetency is also a feature following rheumatic and infectious endocarditis. Aortic valve disease causes hypertrophy of the left ventricle, dilation of the chamber, and eventual left-sided failure. Valvular disorders are suspected when murmers are heard upon auscultation of the heart. The murmurs are due to turbulent blood flow and vibrations of the walls of the heart. It may be possible to palpate a thrill, depending on the extent of the damage. Abnormalities of the pulse may also be palpated. For a damaged valve, the only curative treatment is replacement with an artificial valve.

► CARDIAC ARRHYTHMIA

10-72

1. diastole
2. systole

It is important to understand the precise coordination that exists among the chambers of the heart so that they can work together to produce normal cardiac output. At the start of each cycle, both the right and left atria are relaxed, or in _____ _____(1), so that they may fill with blood from the systemic venous return on the right, and from the pulmonary circulation on the left. At the *same time,* both the right and left ventricles are contracting, or are in _____(2). They move blood into the lungs from the right, and into the aorta and systemic circulation from the left. Then, the opposite occurs. The right and left atria contract during systole and push blood into the relaxed diastolic ventricles to fill them. The heart is now ready to begin the next cycle, commonly called the heartbeat. The contractions are initiated and precisely controlled by the electrical conduction system. It is this system that is responsible for the coordination. The critical result is a sufficient cardiac output.

10-73

1. dysrhythmia
2. bradycardia
3. tachycardia
4. arrhythmia

A variety of pathologies can interrupt or interfere with the pathway of the spread of impulses over the myocardium. **Dysrhythmia** is a deviation from the normal cardiac cycle. A cycle or beat that is too slow is **bradycardia.** It may cause the body to suffer from delayed reception of blood supply. A cycle that is too fast is **tachycardia.** If the heart beats too quickly, there is not enough time for diastole when the chambers relax to be filled. Inadequate filling leads to inadequate output. A beat or rhythm that is irregular is **arrhythmia.** It causes inefficient contractions and a compromised output. Any change from the normal in the cardiac cycle is called _____(1). A beat that is too slow is _____(2), while one that is too fast is _____(3). Abnormal rhythm of contraction is _____(4).

10-74

1. ectopic beat
2. paroxysmal tachycardia
3. filling

The remainder of this topic will deal with arrhythmia. An **ectopic beat** is stimulated by an impulse that originates or begins at a site other than the sinoatrial node. (Ectopic means outside of where something is supposed to be.) An ectopic beat "confuses" the myocardium, and it will pause before beginning a normal contraction. A single or few ectopic beats are of little consequence. Many ectopic beats can cause some of the other arrhythmias we are about to discuss. Ectopic beats are due to tissue damage in ischemic myocardial disease. **Paroxysmal tachycardia** is an episode of rapid, closely spaced beats. (Paroxysmal means in a fit, or in quick succession.) This prolonged tachycardia occurs after stimulation by several ectopic beats. Paroxysmal tachycardia interferes with the normal filling of the chambers by not allowing enough rest time in between contractions. It is also associated with ischemic myocardial disease and may precede ventricular fibrillation in myocardial infarction. Stimulation of contraction by an impulse that comes from outside of the SA node causes a (an) _____(1). Many ectopic beats can cause the heart to beat too quickly for several cycles, and this is termed _____(2). Sustained tachycardia interferes with _____(3) of the chambers with blood.

Atrial fibrillation is a fairly common and significant arrhythmia. It is a quivering of the atrium caused by multiple ectopic stimuli. While these discharges may occur at various rates, they may approach up to 600 per minute. Instead of a single solid contraction, there are waves of incomplete contractions. When the uncontrolled electrical stimuli reach the ventricles, the ventricles can respond only to about 100 to 160 of these irregular rhythms. The contractions of the lower chambers are also incomplete and much too fast. The contractions are not strong enough to propel enough blood out of the ventricles, and this is combined with the fact there has been less time for filling. The inadequate cardiac output can lead to systemic ischemia and hypoxia. Atrial fibrillation can be precipitated by injury received during rheumatic heart disease, ischemic heart disease, systemic hypertension, and hyperthyroidism. Immediate treatment of atrial fibrillation is administration of anti-arrhythmic drugs such as verapamil or procainamide. Long-term management is regular administration of digitalis, a drug that decreases conduction of the excessive impulses and therefore decreases the stimulation of the ventricles. Digitalis slows the contractions and strengthens them, making them more effective.

Incomplete contractions of the atria that can be described as quivering is called _____(1). The significance is the number of ectopic _____(2) that are spreading through the muscle. When they reach the _____(3), these chambers respond as often as they can, which is about _____(4) times per minute. The ventricles are contracting too _____(5), and the contractions are weak. This greatly compromises the normal _____(6).

When **ventricular fibrillation** occurs, it is even more significant. Random multiple impulses make these chambers quiver uncontrollably. Whereas atrial fibrillation led to inefficient ventricular contraction, ventricular fibrillation leads to an *absence* of contractions (asystole). The myocardium twitches helplessly, expulsing no blood, and yielding zero cardiac output. This arrhythmia occurs during myocardial infarction and is fatal if not treated immediately. The treatment is defibrillation, which is stopping the heart and restarting it with external electrical shock. When beating resumes, it is hoped that the impulses have been normalized. A fatal arrhythmia is _____(7), because the cardiac output is _____(8). Contractions are _____(9) because the chambers only twitch and quiver. The types of arrhythmia are summarized in Table 10–2.

1. atrial fibrillation
2. impulses
3. ventricles
4. 100 to 160
5. fast or quickly
6. cardiac output
7. ventricular fibrillation
8. zero
9. absent

TABLE 10–2. TYPES OF ARRHYTHMIA

Arrhythmia	Manifestation	Cause
Ectopic beat	Electrical impulse originating outside of sinoatrial node	Ischemic heart disease
Paroxysmal tachycardia	Quick succession of rapid, closely spaced beats	Multiple ectopic beats Ischemic heart disease
Atrial fibrillation	Extremely rapid waves of incomplete contractions (quivering)	Multiple ectopic beats Ischemic heart disease Rheumatic heart disease
	Excessive stimulation of ventricles	Systemic hypertension
	Inadequate cardiac output with possible systemic ischemia and hypoxia	
Ventricular fibrillation	Extremely rapid waves of incomplete contractions (quivering)	Myocardial infarction
	Asystole (absence of contractions)	
	Zero cardiac output	
	Fatality	

10-77

A **heart block** is interference with impulse conduction along the path that connects the atria and ventricles. As an impulse fails to reach the ventricles, the heart misses or skips a beat. A **complete block** is when no impulses get through to the lower chambers. After a time, the ventricles will begin to beat on their own, since spontaneous contraction is a characteristic specific to cardiac muscle fiber. Even so, the contraction rate is only about 40 beats per minute, which is not adequate for an extended time. The lapse of time in between the block and the start of spontaneous beats can easily cause loss of consciousness. Heart block is caused by ischemic heart disease and an overdose of digitalis. Complete heart block requires the surgical insertion of an artificial pacemaker for long-term management. This blockage is also called **third-degree block,** because other degrees of impulse obstruction exist. In a **first-degree block,** impulses are delayed but are eventually conducted normally. In a **second-degree block,** the impulses are completely obstructed, but only on an intermittent basis.

10-78

1. impulses
2. conduction
3. ventricles
4. complete
5. artificial pacemaker

A heart block exists when _____(1) are prevented from moving through the _____(2) system. For every impulse that does not reach its destination, the _____(3) do not contract. In _____(4) block, the lower chambers beat on their own after a while, but this is inadequate. This condition must be corrected with the implantation of a (an) _____(5).

10-79

1. heart
2. ischemia
3. arrhythmia

The decreased cardiac output that occurs during significant arrhythmia has a cyclic effect on the heart. Even though myocardial contractions are ineffective, they use more energy than a normal contraction. Therefore, the struggling muscle needs more blood and oxygen than normal. However, the supply through the cardiac arteries is diminished because of diminished output. This worsens the ischemia that caused the arrhythmia in the first place, leading to a worsening of the arrhythmia and potential heart failure. All arrhythmias are diagnosed by examining the tracing produced during an electrocardiogram. Each arrhythmia has a characteristic pattern. The inadequate cardiac output during arrhythmia may decrease blood supply to the _____(1) itself, increasing the amount of _____(2) that is present, and causing further _____(3).

▶ **COR PULMONALE**

10-80

We have already examined the effects of increased resistance in the pulmonary circulation, due to either volume overload or stenotic obstruction. Both situations increase pressure and create pulmonary hypertension. Frequent cardiac causes of pulmonary hypertension are left-sided heart failure and mitral valve stenosis. And you know that the effects of pulmonary hypertension are manifested in the right side of the heart, with right ventricular hypertrophy. However, lung disease can create the same resistance, pulmonary hypertension, and right ventricular enlargement. When right ventricular hypertrophy is secondary to lung disease, this is called **cor pulmonale.** Cor pulmonale can also end in right-sided heart failure.

▶ **CLINICAL PRESENTATION IN HEART DISEASE**

10-81

The signs and symptoms in heart disease depend on what the particular ailment is. Some of these have already been described for you. In general, the signs and symptoms most commonly associated with heart disease are:

1. Cyanosis—associated with some congenital heart defects and with significant interference in oxygenation of the blood.
2. Chest pain or angina pectoris—associated with ischemic heart disease (therefore coronary artery disease) and with myocardial infarction.

3. Palpitation—described as a conscious awareness of the force of one's heartbeat, may be caused by heart disease or by extreme emotions (stress, anxiety).
4. Dyspnea—associated with left-sided and congestive heart failure, where shortness of breath is a prominent feature.
5. Irregular beats—due to various arrhythmias.
6. Murmurs—created by some congenital defects and valvular disease.
7. Syncope or fainting—in the case of cerebral ischemia or hypoxia, induced by a general ischemic or hypoxic state.
8. Distention of peripheral veins, peripheral edema, and abdominal swelling (ascites)—due to right-sided or congestive heart failure.
9. Coughing (pulmonary edema)—in cases of left-sided congestive heart failure.

V. REVIEW QUESTIONS

1. A diseased heart valve that is too wide to close properly is described as valvular
   a. _____. A diseased valve that is too narrow is described as valvular
   b. _____.

2. Choose the correct statement about the effects of valvular disease:
   a. Stenosis allows blood flow to fall backwards, or reflux in the previous chamber.
   b. Insufficiency creates increased resistance to the passage of blood.
   c. Both conditions increase cardiac workload, leading to myocardial hypertrophy and potential heart failure.
   d. All of the above are correct.

3. The heart valve that most often becomes injured or diseased is the:
   a. tricuspid
   b. pulmonary
   c. mitral
   d. aortic

4. Sufficient cardiac output requires:
   a. effective contractions by the myocardium
   b. coordination of contractions between the atria and ventricles
   c. proper control of contractions by the electrical conduction system
   d. an absence of dysrhythmia
   e. all of the above

5. Please match the arrhythmias in the left column with their descriptions in the right column:
   a. heart block
   b. paroxysmal tachycardia
   c. ventricular fibrillation
   d. ectopic beat
   e. atrial fibrillation

   1. _____ rapid succession of heartbeats
   2. _____ multiple ectopic stimuli of the upper chambers at a rate of up to 600 per minute
   3. _____ impulse originating outside of the SA node
   4. _____ interference with the conduction pathway between the atria and ventricles
   5. _____ lack of contractions caused by twitching of the lower chambers

1. a–insufficiency or incompetency; b–stenosis

2. c–Both conditions increase cardiac workload, leading to myocardial hypertrophy and potential heart failure.

3. c–mitral

4. e–all of the above

5. 1. b–paroxysmal tachycardia; 2. e–atrial fibrillation; 3. d–ectopic beat; 4. a–heart block; 5. c–ventricular fibrillation

6. d–sending far too much stimuli to the ventricles, resulting in incomplete ventricular contractions

7. a–ventricular fibrillation

8. c–complete heart block

9. d–all of the above

6. Atrial fibrillation can cause insufficient cardiac output by:
   a. an absence of electrical stimuli to the ventricles
   b. lack of atrial contraction which does not fill the ventricles
   c. stimulating ectopic beats in the ventricles
   d. sending far too much stimuli to the ventricles, resulting in incomplete ventricular contractions

7. The arrhythmia that is associated with myocardial infarction and is responsible for absence of cardiac output is:
   a. ventricular fibrillation
   b. atrial fibrillation
   c. complete heart block
   d. paroxysmal tachycardia

8. An artificial pacemaker may be necessary in cases of:
   a. ventricular fibrillation
   b. atrial fibrillation
   c. complete heart block
   d. paroxysmal tachycardia

9. Inadequate cardiac output caused by arrhythmia may:
   a. decrease blood supply to the heart itself
   b. worsen ischemia already present
   c. worsen the arrhythmia
   d. all of the above

CHAPTER ► SUMMARY

► SECTION II

The etiology of *congenital heart disease* (a defect or defects of the heart present at birth) is, in many cases, idiopathic. Known causes include teratogens such as drugs (e.g., alcohol interferes with embryonic development of the heart), chemicals, viruses (such as rubella), and x-rays. Certain congenital heart defects may lead to a "shunting" of the blood, or an abnormal pathway in the blood's normal route. Blood may flow from the left side of the heart to the right, or from the right to the left. The direction of the shunt is determined by which side of the heart contains the greater pressure. The latter situation is of serious clinical consequence because deoxygenated blood is not routed to the lungs.

A *septal defect,* commonly known as a "hole in the heart," may occur between the atria or between the ventricles. Because blood is shunted from the left side of the heart to the right, both atrial and ventricular septal defects lead to an increase in the workload of the right side of the heart. Septal defects can lead to pulmonary hypertension, hypoxia, and heart failure. In the condition of *patent ductus arteriosus,* the ductus arteriosus, a vessel that connects the aorta to the pulmonary artery in the fetus (in order to bypass circulation to the fetus' incompletely developed lungs), fails to close after birth. This situation can lead to right-sided heart failure. In *tetralogy of Fallot,* which occurs when the base of the heart is twisted too far to the right, four abnormalities occur: ventricular septal defect, dextroposition (displacement) of the aorta, pulmonary stenosis (narrowing of the pulmonary artery), and right ventricular hypertrophy (enlargement of the myocardium of the right ventricle). Tetratology of Fallot causes hypoxia, cyanosis, tachypnea, tachycardia, breathlessness, syncope, polycythemia, and early death if not surgically corrected.

▶ SECTION III

Degeneration (disease produced by loss of function) in the heart is due primarily to cardiac ischemia and hypoxia. *Hypertensive heart disease,* manifested as left ventricular hypertrophy, results from systemic hypertension. The ventricular enlargement decreases the volume of blood pumped to the body, increases the development of atherosclerotic plaques in the coronary arteries, and leads to an overall enlargement of the heart (cardiomegaly). *Coronary artery disease* is caused by a decrease in the size of the vessel lumen, and may be due to blood clots on the vessel walls (coronary thrombosis), systemic hypertension, or atherosclerotic plaques. The effects of coronary artery disease, the severity and progression of which depend on several factors, include ischemia, angina pectoris, arrhythmia, fibrosis, and myocardial infarction.

Individuals who survive a *myocardial infarction* (manifested as an area of dead myocardial tissue) often have many long-lasting complications, including pulmonary edema, dyspnea, kidney failure, injury of brain tissue, ventricular aneurysm, and stroke. An electrocardiogram measures the electrical activity of the heart and is used to diagnose cardiac abnormalities associated with infarctions. The measurement of the levels of specific myocardium-associated enzymes (creatine phosphokinase, aspartate aminotransferase, lactic dehydrogenase) are used to determine the severity of and recovery time from the infarction.

Cardiac arrest occurs when the heart suddenly and completely stops all electrical activity and myocardial contraction (asystole), causing an absence of the pulse and respiration. Causes of cardiac arrest include myocardial infarction, arrhythmia, electrocution, drug overdose, respiratory arrest, and massive hemorrhage. *Heart failure* is defined as the inability of the heart to meet the body's demand for blood, such as during periods of intense exercise. Causes of heart failure include ischemic heart disease, myocarditis, excessive burdens on the heart, arrhythmia, and hypertrophy. Failure of only the right ventricle leads to distention of the large veins and organs, edema, decreased cardiac output, and decreased oxygenation of the blood. Left ventricle failure leads to pulmonary edema, dyspnea, and hypoxia. *Congestive heart failure* (CHF) is the simultaneous failure of both the left and right sides of the heart, causing an increase in blood volume within the veins. CHF combines all the clinical features of both left- and right-sided heart failure.

Cardiomyopathy (literally, "heart muscle disease") that is not associated with ischemia or inflammation occurs in three different forms: dilated (the enlarged heart chambers are thin and flabby), hypertrophic (the myocardial tissue of the left ventricle is thickened), and restrictive (the myocardium is unable to expand due to the presence of a foreign substance). Cardiomyopathy leads to congestive heart failure, and the only true treatment is a heart transplant.

▶ SECTION IV

Rheumatic fever, a disease of children and young adults, is caused by a group A hemolytic streptococcal infection. The disease is characterized by five manifestations (Jones' major criteria), and in some people can result in *rheumatic heart disease.* Damage to cardiac tissue, and to other tissues in the body, occurs when the infected individual reacts immunologically to the streptococcal bacteria; the antibodies thus produced react with and cause damage to specific tissues, including the endocardium, myocardium, and pericardium. The most common site of damage in rheumatic heart disease are the valves in the left side, leading to a backflow of blood and increased workload for the heart. Bacterial endocarditis, resulting in septic emboli, is a consequence of valvular insufficiency.

Infectious endocarditis, which is usually caused by a bacterium, is inflammation of the endocardium due to microbial infection. The valves on the left side are the most frequently infected sites in the heart, and infection leads to ulceration, erosion, inflammation, and structural deformity of the valves. Serious complications can subsequently occur, including hypertrophy, heart failure, formation of septic emboli, and microabscesses. *Myocarditis,* or infectious inflammation of the myocardium, is most often caused by a virus. The myocardium is damaged by the infecting virus itself, as well as by the immune reactivity against the virus. *Pericarditis* (inflammation of the epicardium and pericardium), which often follows an infection of the myocardium, occurs when exudate enters the pericardial sac. At high enough volume, the exudate may prevent the heart from properly expanding (pericardial tamponade).

▶ SECTION V

The two major forms of *valvular disorders* are insufficiency (the valve opening is too wide) and stenosis (the valve opening is too narrow). Insufficiency of a valve allows for blood to flow backward, a process called reflux or regurgitation. Stenosis of a valve does not allow a normal amount of blood to pass. While the valves on the right side of the heart can show insufficiency or stenosis, the valves on the left side (especially the mitral valve) are the most commonly affected. Rheumatic endocarditis and infectious endocarditis can affect the mitral valve; congenital deformities as well as endocarditis can cause insufficiency of the aortic valve.

    Dysrhythmia is a deviation in the normal cardiac cycle and can be defined as bradycardia (the heartbeat is too slow), tachycardia (too fast), or arrhythmia (irregular). An *ectopic beat* is defined as a heartbeat that is stimulated by an impulse that originates at a site other than the sinoatrial node. *Paroxysmal tachycardia* is an episode of rapid, closely spaced beats. *Atrial fibrillation* is recognized as a quivering, or waves of incomplete contractions, of the atrium caused by multiple ectopic stimuli. *Ventricular fibrillation,* which occurs during myocardial infarction, is uncontrolled quivering of the ventricles, leading to an absence of contractions (asystole). A *heart block* is improper—or in some cases, no—impulse conduction from the atria to the ventricles. The heart may skip beats or, in the case of a complete heart block, the ventricles may begin to contract on their own, albeit very slowly. Heart blocks are defined as first degree (impulses are delayed but are eventually conducted normally), second degree (impulses are completely obstructed, but only intermittently), or third degree (impulse blockage is complete).

The Respiratory System

▶ OBJECTIVES

SECTION II

Define all highlighted terms.

Characterize the causative agents, and describe the signs and symptoms, of upper respiratory infection and acute bronchitis.

Describe the patterns of spread, causative agents, signs and symptoms of the categories of pneumonia.

Describe the signs and symptoms of respiratory syncytial virus infection.

Characterize the causative agent and signs and symptoms of primary and secondary tuberculosis.

SECTION III

Define all highlighted terms.

Describe the causes and signs and symptoms of chronic pulmonary obstructive disease, chronic bronchitis, and bronchiectasis.

Characterize the disease emphysema, and describe the signs and symptoms of the disorder; define and describe the conditions of "blue bloater" and "pink puffer."

Describe the causes and signs and symptoms of seasonal allergic rhinitis and acute and chronic hypersensitivity pneumonitis.

Characterize the disease asthma, and describe the signs and symptoms of the disorder. Define and describe the condition of status asthmaticus.

SECTION IV

Define all highlighted terms.

Characterize the difference between the ventilation disturbances of suffocation and drowning.

Describe the causes and signs and symptoms of adult respiratory distress syndrome.

Describe the causes and signs and symptoms of respiratory failure, and characterize the two forms of the condition.

Characterize the clinical condition of atelectasis, and describe its causes and signs and symptoms.

Define the condition of pneumoconiosis, and characterize the causes and signs and symptoms of the three types of pneumoconioses.

SECTION V

Define all highlighted terms.

Describe the causes and signs and symptoms of pulmonary hypertension and of pulmonary edema.

Characterize the condition of pulmonary embolism, and describe its causes and signs and symptoms.

Characterize the forms and describe the signs and symptoms of neoplastic conditions affecting the respiratory system: laryngeal carcinoma, primary lung cancer, bronchogenic carcinoma, and secondary lung cancer.

SECTION VI

Define all highlighted terms.

Characterize the conditions and describe the signs and symptoms of pneumothorax, hydrothorax, pleural effusion, empyema, and hemothorax.

Describe the cause and signs and symptoms of the disease cystic fibrosis.

Describe the abnormalities seen in the condition of newborn respiratory distress syndrome.

SECTION ▶ 11-1

I. ANATOMY AND PHYSIOLOGY IN REVIEW

The primary function of the lungs is to be the site of transfer of oxygen from the atmosphere to the blood, and the transfer of carbon dioxide from the blood to the atmosphere. The function of the lungs, then, is **respiration.** Respiration is the combined processes of **ventilation** and **gas exchange.** Ventilation is the movement of air in and out of the lungs, from and to the atmosphere. Ventilation is composed of **inhalation** (moving air in) and **exhalation** (moving air out). Gas exchange occurs across the capillaries in the lungs, where oxygen in the air sacs drifts into the capillary blood, and where carbon dioxide in the capillary blood drifts out into the air sacs. Hemoglobin inside the red blood cells releases the carbon dioxide it picked up in the tissues, and picks up oxygen for transport to the tissues. So the process of respiration is inhalation–gas exchange–exhalation. During this process, other metabolites and certain toxins can also be eliminated with the carbon dioxide. The respiratory system and the process of respiration are shown in Figure 11–1.

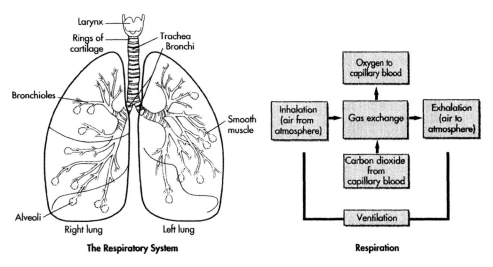

Figure 11–1. The respiratory system and its function.

The functional units of the lungs, where gas exchange takes place, are the air sacs or **alveoli.** Alveoli are very thin-walled terminal structures at the very end of the bronchial tree. A group of alveoli might remind you of a bunch of grapes, with the stems analogous to bronchioles. Alveoli are lined on the inside with epithelial cells called **type I pneumocytes.** Also present are **type II pneumocytes,** which secrete **surfactant.** Surfactant is a vital liquid that decreases the surface tension of lung tissue and prevents the collapse of the air sacs. It is also helpful in lung expansion. Another cell type is the macrophage that acts as a scavenger of foreign material that enters the lungs. In the **interstitial tissue, or septa,** that surrounds the alveoli is the capillary bed that has brought venous blood for oxygenation and will carry away newly created arterial blood.

There are two lungs to carry out respiration. The right lung is divided into three lobes, and the left lung is divided into two lobes. Air moves in and out of the lungs through the **respiratory tree,** also known as the **bronchial tree.** These air passageways very much resemble an upside-down tree. The tree begins with the **larynx,** the entranceway into the **trachea.** The trachea is commonly called the "windpipe." It is the main trunk of the respiratory tree. The trachea splits or forks into two large branches, and the passageway becomes the right and left **bronchi.** The fork is called the **bifurcation.** A bronchus supplies each lung. Bronchi branch off many times, becoming smaller. These smaller airways are called **bronchioles** and they end as alveoli. Smooth muscle runs along the outside of the bronchi and some of the smaller branches. The muscle can constrict or dilate the passageways and control airflow. The trachea and bronchi are lined with **ciliated columnar** epithelial cells. The cilia are tiny, finger-like projections that brush or sweep material from inspired air up and out of the lungs. Inside the bronchi and bronchioles is **mucus,** which acts as a sticky trap for foreign material. The secretion of mucus is increased whenever there is an irritant in the respiratory tree. That irritant may be an infection, or it may be an inhaled substance. Accumulation of mucus is a signal that the lungs need to be cleared, and the **cough reflex** helps expel the irritant.

The rate of ventilation is controlled by the respiratory center in the medulla of the brain. Increased carbon dioxide in the blood stimulates the respiratory center to increase ventilation, or the rate of breathing. This is to blow off and decrease the amount of carbon dioxide while taking on more oxygen. Poor respiration, exercise, and acidosis are all reasons for increased carbon dioxide in the circulation. Another function of the lungs is participating in acid–base balance. You learned in Chapter 3 that the lungs and respiratory center are important compensators in times of acid–base imbalance. Accelerated loss of carbon dioxide in times of acidosis helps raise blood pH.

Ventilation, or the act of breathing, is accomplished primarily through the respiratory muscles, the **diaphragm** and **intercostal muscles.** The diaphragm is the muscular sheet that is under the lungs and separates the thorax (chest) from the abdomen. When the diaphragm contracts, it pulls the lungs down, and they expand. This is helped by the enlargement of the rib cage by the intercostal muscles. This expansion and enlargement decreases the pressure in the lungs to *less than* that of the atmosphere, and so air rushes into the lungs. This is inhalation, or inspiration. Exhalation, or expiration, is a passive process in a healthy person. When the diaphragm relaxes, it pushes the lungs back up. The intercostals relax and collapse the chest cavity. This pushes air back out. In between inspiration and expiration, gas exchange takes place. The movement of the gas molecules is dictated by differences in pressure, or a **pressure gradient.** Molecules move from an area of higher pressure into an area of lower pressure. Carbon dioxide is higher in the blood than it is in the alveoli. Therefore, the carbon dioxide molecules leave the capillaries for the alveoli. Oxygen is higher in the alveoli than in the capillaries. Therefore, it moves from the alveoli into the capillaries. The blood supply for ventilation is provided by the **pulmonary artery** coming from the right ventricle, which carries deoxygenated blood. Oxygenated blood exits the lungs through the **pulmonary vein,** which empties into the left atrium. In between are venules, capillaries, and arterioles.

11-6

The lungs are covered with a thin, double-layered membrane, the **pleura.** The space between the two layers is the **pleural space,** or the **pleural cavity.** This is a potential space, because normally the two layers are collapsed on each other. The pleural cavity contains a small amount of serous fluid that lubricates the surfaces and prevents painful friction during lung movement. The pressure in the pleural cavity is *less than* the pressure in the lungs. In comparison, pleural cavity pressure is negative and the lungs are positive. This creates a partial vacuum that allows the lungs to remain expanded and prevents their collapse.

▶ GENERAL FACTS ABOUT RESPIRATORY DISEASE

11-7

The heart and lungs are so intertwined that they are often called the cardiopulmonary system. Disorder or imbalance in one system adversely affects the other system. You learned in Chapter 10 that cardiac disorders affect the lungs, creating hypertension in the pulmonary circulation or the production of pulmonary edema. Diseases of the lungs also affect the heart. One example given in Chapter 10 was cor pulmonale, where the right ventricle hypertrophied and possibly failed due to severe lung disease. One condition that can cause cor pulmonale is significant pulmonary embolism (see Frame 11-77).

11-8

The respiratory system is open ended and in direct contact with the environment. Because of this, it is very susceptible to disease. Inhalation brings not only oxygen-rich air, but potential pathogens or other harmful substances into the lungs. The following are some categories of lung disease:

1. Upper respiratory infection (URI). The upper respiratory tract consists of the nose, pharynx (throat), larynx (voicebox), and trachea (windpipe). Inhaled viruses cause the common cold that affects these structures, as well as the respiratory disease influenza.
2. Lower respiratory infection (LRI). The lower respiratory tract is the bronchi, bronchioles, and alveoli. Extension of a URI down into the lungs can cause bronchitis or pneumonia. Pneumonia, a very old disease, is still remarkably common. It especially affects immune-suppressed people, including the elderly, chemotherapy patients, and those with AIDS.
3. Allergic disorders. Inhaled allergens can cause hay fever or asthma.
4. Environmental-induced disease. Harmful inhaled substances can cause several of the diseases we will discuss in this chapter. These include pollutants, chemicals, cigarette smoke, and carcinogens. Many of these cases can be prevented, since they are related to occupational exposure and personal habits or behavior.

SECTION ▶ 11. INFECTIOUS DISEASES OF THE RESPIRATORY SYSTEM

▶ UPPER RESPIRATORY INFECTION

11-9

Upper respiratory infection, or **URI,** as it is commonly known, is much more common than infection of the lower respiratory tract. The upper respiratory tract consists of the nose, sinuses, pharynx (throat), larynx (voicebox), and trachea (windpipe). URI is the most common type of infection to plague humans, second perhaps to minor skin infections. URI is best known as the common cold. Colds are caused by viruses, a few of which are influenza A and B, parainfluenza, and rhinovirus ("rhino" means nose). These viruses are present in the air and spread through that route. Affliction tends to be seasonal and occurs most often in fall and winter. URI is usually short lived and self-limiting. People who are predisposed to catching colds include the young, the elderly, and anyone who is immunodeficient or otherwise "run down." In other words, anyone with lowered resistance is susceptible to catching these viruses. It is unfortunate that so many strains of these viruses exist that immunity never develops. For this reason, URI or a cold is an infection that occurs again and again. URI stands for _____(1). It is commonly known as the _____(2). It is caused by _____(3). Because of many strains of viruses, _____(4) never develops.

1. upper respiratory infection
2. common cold
3. viruses
4. immunity

11–10

URI viruses cause acute inflammation of the mucous membrane lining the structures of the upper respiratory tract. Membrane inflammation causes the signs and symptoms of a cold. A case of URI that develops complications can spread to the bronchi, causing acute bronchitis. In children, URI may spread to the middle ear, causing otitis media, which is characterized by an earache. Complications are generally limited to those with poor immune response, such as the populations listed in Frame 11–9. The inflammatory swelling of the mucous membranes of the nose is responsible for the familiar feeling of nasal congestion. The irritation causes the mucous glands to produce a copious amount of a watery secretion. This creates the nuisance of a runny nose. This nasal discharge is medically termed **rhinorrhea.** Sore throat, sneezing, and coughing are further symptoms of viral irritation and inflammation. Malaise, a vague feeling of being unwell, accompanies most colds. In addition to these signs and symptoms, the influenza viruses also cause chills, fever, chest pain, muscle pain, and occasionally gastrointestinal (GI) upset. In the elderly and immune suppressed, influenza virus can progress to pneumonia. The signs and symptoms of URI are caused by _____(1) of the _____(2) along the upper respiratory tract structures. A runny nose is properly termed _____(3). This is due to the secretions of _____(4). Fever and muscle pain often accompany a URI caused by the _____(5) virus.

1. inflammation
2. mucous membranes
3. rhinorrhea
4. mucus
5. influenza

11–11

In severe cases, or in those susceptible populations, a URI may be complicated by a secondary bacterial infection. Remember that a primary infection may so tax the immune system that a secondary invader may gain hold. If bacterial infection develops, the nasal discharge becomes purulent instead of watery. The microorganisms may gain access to the sinuses, causing the pain of sinusitis, or they may spread to the ears. The cough in a bacterial infection often produces a purulent mucus, signaling acute bronchitis. If the bacteria are of the streptococcal variety, strep throat can occur. Invasion of the tonsils causes tonsillitis. (The tonsils are lymph tissue in the throat that filter out bacteria. A high number of bacteria causes their infection.) A complicating factor in URI is the development of a _____(1). The rhinorrhea is then _____(2). Additional conditions that can occur are infection of the sinuses, or _____(3); of the bronchi, or _____(4); and of the tonsils, or _____(5).

1. secondary bacterial infection
2. purulent
3. sinusitis
4. acute bronchitis
5. tonsillitis

11–12

Antibiotics are useless against a cold because viruses are not susceptible to them. However, they are useful in severe cases or in debilitated persons to prevent secondary bacterial invasion. Influenza-caused URI may also be a candidate for antibiotics. If strep throat develops, antibiotics should definitely be administered to prevent rheumatic fever or rheumatic heart disease (Chap. 10). Cases of tonsillitis, sinusitis, and pneumonia are other examples of when antibiotics should be used in URI.

▶ ACUTE BRONCHITIS

11–13

Acute bronchitis is also a common respiratory infection, second to URI. It is sometimes called **tracheobronchitis,** because the affected structures are the upper respiratory tract, including the trachea, and the beginning of the lower tract, which are the bronchi. It is caused by bacteria invading from the upper tract, and inflammation is also the primary symptom-producing reaction. Other irritants such as inhaled dust or gases can cause acute bronchitis. The swelling of the mucous membranes and the production of mucus cause a

1. acute bronchitis
2. tracheobronchitis
3. inflammation
4. cough

productive cough. (A productive cough is one that expels mucus.) Bacterial tracheo-bronchitis often causes fever. Treatment with antibiotics or removal of the irritant usually resolves this condition. Chronic bronchitis is a cause of chronic obstructive pulmonary disease, and will be considered in the next section. Another common upper respiratory infection is _____(1). It is also called _____(2). Again, _____(3) causes the signs and symptoms. The primary sign is a productive _____(4).

► PNEUMONIA

11–14

1. pneumonia
2. pneumonitis
3. *Streptococcus*
4. *Staphylococcus*
5. pneumococcus
6. upper respiratory tract
7. hematogenous

Pneumonia is still a prevalent disease. It is seen most often in the young, elderly, debilitated, immune suppressed, and in those with some other primary illness. Recall from Chapter 4 that it is the typical reason for death in AIDS patients. In infectious pneumonia, 75 percent of the cases are caused by bacteria as opposed to other microorganisms. **Pneumonia** is infectious inflammation of the lungs. It is a historical term for inflammation due specifically to invasion by microorganisms. Nonspecific inflammation of the lungs, not due to infection, is called **pneumonitis.** Pneumonia can develop because of the direct contact the respiratory system has with the environment. The pathogens that most often cause pneumonia are *Streptococcus pneumoniae* and *hemolyticus, Staphylococcus aureus,* and pneumococcus. These organisms reach the lungs through infected secretions from the upper respiratory tract. Hematogenous spread (from the blood) is also a means of developing pneumonia in cases of septic bacteremia. Bacterial pneumonia is a common cause of death in those who are seriously ill with a primary disease. Infectious inflammation of the lungs is _____(1). Noninfectious inflammation is called _____(2). Bacterial pneumonia is most often caused by _____(3), _____(4), and _____(5). These organisms gain access to the lungs following infection of the _____(6). Or they may spread from the blood, which is called _____(7) spread.

11–15

1. alveoli or air sacs
2. fluid or exudate
3. interstitial tissue

Pneumonia can be placed into one of two broad categories. The first is characterized by exudate *within* the air spaces or alveoli. This produces consolidation of the fluid-filled spaces (see Frame 11–16). This type of pneumonia has two patterns of spread. One is called bronchopneumonia (see Frame 11–16), and the other is called lobar pneumonia (see Frame 11–17). The second category, which results in a third pattern of spread, is inflammation of the connective tissue that *surrounds* the alveoli. Within this interstitial tissue lies the blood vessels. This category is interstitial pneumonia (see Frame 11–21), and consolidation (solidification of air spaces) is *not* a feature. Bacteria and viruses are generally the causative agents of the various types of pneumonia. Bronchopneumonia and lobar pneumonia are a category of lung infection in which the _____(1) become filled with _____(2). Interstitial pneumonia is a category in which the infection is confined to the _____(3) outside of the air spaces. The types and patterns of pneumonia are illustrated in Figure 11–2.

11–16

Within the first category of pneumonia is a pattern called **bronchopneumonia.** This is primarily a bacterial infection. *Staphylococcus, Streptococcus,* and pneumococcus all cause this pattern. This is a combination of bronchitis and pneumonia. The infectious inflammation spreads from the bronchi into the alveoli in a spotty or patchy fashion. Infection of the alveoli causes **consolidation.** Consolidation is the filling up of the alveoli with exudate, and the replacement of air. Instead of an empty air sac, the alveoli become solid areas. The function of gas exchange is lost in affected alveoli. These tiny solid areas can be seen on x-ray interspersed throughout normal lung tissue. Bronchopneumonia is the most common form of bacterial pneumonia. It is usually found in the susceptible populations previously mentioned. Another group of predisposed individuals is hospitalized patients. Remember from Chapter

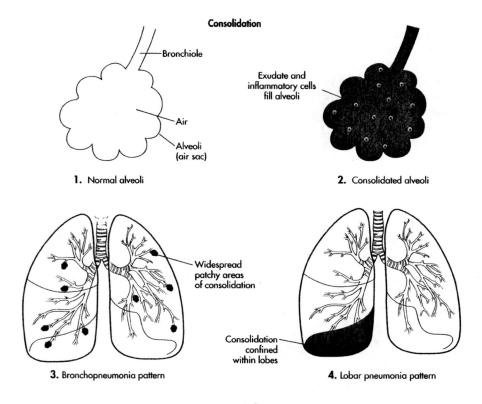

1. Normal alveoli

2. Consolidated alveoli

Bronchiole

Air

Alveoli
(air sac)

Consolidation

Exudate and
inflammatory cells
fill alveoli

Widespread
patchy areas
of consolidation

3. Bronchopneumonia pattern

Consolidation
confined
within lobes

4. Lobar pneumonia pattern

Interstitial

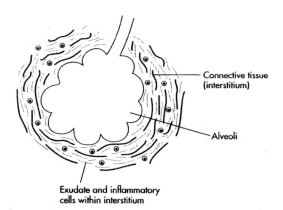

Connective tissue
(interstitium)

Alveoli

Exudate and inflammatory
cells within interstitium

Figure 11–2. Types and patterns of pneumonia.

5 that infection gained through hospital exposure is a nosocomial infection. Nosocomial pneumonia is a major concern for hospitals. The population present is often debilitated by a primary illness, and spread of bacteria through the air is difficult to control. Infectious inflammation of both the bronchi and the lungs is called _____(1). The alveoli fill up with _____(2), which displaces all the _____(3) and turns the air sacs into a _____(4) area. This process is called _____(5). Nosocomial pneumonia is acquired in a _____(6) setting and poses a real threat to debilitated patients.

1. bronchopneumonia
2. exudate
3. air
4. solid
5. consolidation
6. hospital

11–17

1. lobar pneumonia
2. consolidation
3. lobes

Lobar pneumonia is a second pattern of bacterial pneumonia caused specifically by pneumococcus. Pneumococcus is a respiratory tract commensal, which means it is normal flora. Occasionally, pathogenic strains of this bacteria may be spread to others by asymptomatic carriers. Pathogenic strains of pneumococcus usually combine with debilitating factors to produce disease. The microorganisms travel down the respiratory tree into alveoli, causing infectious inflammation. Purulent exudate fills these air sacs, so consolidation is also a feature of lobar pneumonia. This type is so named because it tends to be confined to one or two lobes of the lungs, instead of being spread out as it is in bronchopneumonia. Figure 11–3 is a photograph that compares the patterns of spread in lobar pneumonia and bronchopneumonia. The pneumococci die relatively soon, in about a week, and so complete recovery is generally the rule. This is especially true if the case is treated with the correct antibiotics. The microorganism pneumococcus causes the pattern of infection described as _____(1). Solidification of the alveoli, or _____(2), is also a feature of this type of pneumonia. Areas of infection are confined to particular _____(3) of the lungs.

11–18

Complications related to bacterial pneumonia can sometimes be found in cases that were untreated, in debilitated patients, or in infections with particularly virulent strains of bacteria. If the infection extends outside of the lungs, the pleura will become infected. This is called pleuritis (see Frame 11–90). Pleural effusion will result and it is purulent. A pocket of infection in the lungs may turn into an abscess, whose presence can destroy the surrounding parenchyma (functional tissue) and bronchial walls. Significant lung destruction and resulting fibrosis can lead to chronic lung disease.

11–19

A specific form of bacterial pneumonia is **Legionnaires' disease.** This is a lung infection caused by the bacteria *Legionella pneumophila.* This microorganism grows well in warm moisture, so it may be found growing in air conditioning equipment, humidifiers, or plumbing fixtures. This bacteria may access the lungs by direct inhalation of water droplets from contaminated equipment. Legionnaires' disease can cause massive consolidation and necrosis, so the injury in this type of pneumonia is serious. There is a relatively high mortality

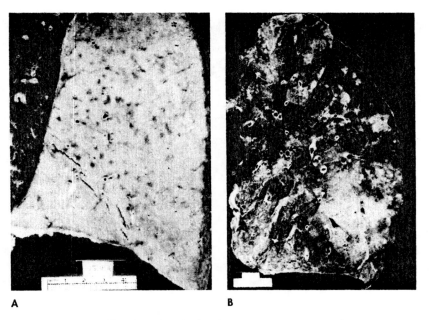

A   B

Figure 11–3. A. Lobar pneumonia. The lobe on the right of the fissure is pale and consolidated. The lobe on the left of the fissure is normal. **B.** Bronchopneumonia. Note the small pale areas of patchy consolidation around bronchioles throughout the lung. *(From Chandrasoma and Taylor,* Concise Pathology, *2nd ed., Appleton & Lange.)*

rate. In the original outbreak in Philadelphia in 1976, at an American Legion conference, 34 of the 200 infected people died. *Legionella pneumophila* is the causative agent of _____(1). This is a _____(2) that can be found growing in the warm _____(3) of some equipment. This pneumonia can cause severe consolidation and _____(4) of the lungs.

1. Legionnaires' disease
2. bacterium
3. moisture
4. necrosis

11–20

There are a variety of signs and symptoms that make up the clinical presentation of bacterial pneumonia. These include fever, chills, difficulty in breathing **(dyspnea),** rapid breathing (tachypnea), and a productive cough that can include bloody sputum **(hemoptysis).** The degree of dyspnea and tachypnea depends on the amount of consolidation present. Remember, consolidation prevents _____(1) exchange. If pleuritis is present, it is painful. Diagnosis of pneumonia is easily accomplished. Auscultation of the chest will reveal the presence of **rales,** or abnormal breath sounds. These abnormal sounds may take the form of roughness, wheezes, crackles, or rattles. A chest x-ray reveals inflammatory infiltrates in consolidated areas. There is leukocytosis on the CBC. [This means the number of _____(2) is increased in order to fight _____(3).] A sputum or mucus specimen is cultured for the pathogen causing the pneumonia. Bacterial pneumonia is effectively treated with correct antibiotics.

1. gas
2. leukocytes or neutrophils
3. infection

11–21

The second category of pneumonia, which produces a third pattern of spread, is **interstitial pneumonia.** This is infectious inflammation of the walls of the alveoli, and of the interstitial tissue in which the alveoli and blood vessels lie. There is little exudate within the air spaces, and a moderate amount can be found in the interstitium. The inflammatory process can interfere with gas exchange between the vessels and alveoli. The infection is usually interspersed or spread evenly throughout all the lobes. Interstitial pneumonia is also known as **primary atypical pneumonia,** because the presenting signs may not be typical of pneumonia. Interstitial pneumonia can be caused by some of the viruses that cause URI, such as influenza A or B, or rhinovirus. Respiratory syncytial virus (see Frame 11–24) will also cause this pattern of infection. More often, interstitial or atypical pneumonia is caused by a bacteria-like organism, *Mycoplasma pneumoniae*. In AIDS patients, *Pneumocystis carinii* is usually the causative agent. Infectious inflammation of the connective tissue and alveoli walls is called _____(1). In contrast to broncho- or lobar pneumonia, there is little _____(2) in the air sacs. Another name for interstitial pneumonia is _____(3). While certain _____(4) can cause interstitial pneumonia, it is more often associated with infection by _____(5). In _____(6) patients, the microorganism _____(7) causes interstitial pneumonia.

1. interstitial pneumonia
2. exudate
3. primary atypical pneumonia
4. viruses
5. *Mycoplasma pneumoniae*
6. AIDS
7. *Pneumocystis carinii*

11–22

As mentioned previously, the clinical picture of interstitial pneumonia may not be typical. The classic signs of pneumonia (fever, cough, respiratory distress) may be absent or mild. Cases which present with classic signs are usually severe. Antibiotic therapy is effective against *M. pneumoniae,* and to prevent secondary bacterial infection in viral cases. There are other diseases of the interstitium that are not infectious in nature, and these will be considered under the topics adult respiratory distress syndrome and pneumoconioses.

11–23

Pneumonia caused by a virus, or viral pneumonia, is an acute disease like bacterial infections. Viral pneumonia often produces an interstitial pattern. Severe cases of upper respiratory infection caused by influenza or respiratory syncytial virus may travel down into the lungs by way of the bronchial tree. Viral pneumonia is contagious, and the transmission is through the airborne route. Viral pathogens are present in the exhaled air and moisture droplets from an infected individual. Viral pneumonia is more common than bacterial pneumonia and is often associated with epidemics. Most cases resolve with proper care, and complications are rare compared to bacterial cases.

11-24

The **respiratory syncytial virus,** or **RSV,** most often affects infants, young children, and the elderly. Infants born prematurely or those with a primary disease, especially respiratory, are susceptible. Children who become infected are usually younger than 3 years of age. RSV pneumonia is generally seasonal, occurring in the winter months. The spread of RSV is by the airborne route from an infected person. An adult with RSV generally presents with mild URI signs. Any adult with a cold must be careful around these susceptible populations, so as not to infect them. The first development that precedes RSV pneumonia is URI or a cold-like state. In babies and children, otitis media (middle ear infection) is often present. The virus then travels down through the bronchial tree. The condition **bronchiolitis** may develop prior to pneumonia, or it may be the only subsequent infection. Bronchiolitis is infectious inflammation of the smaller airways, the bronchioles. It does *not* extend into the alveoli, which defines pneumonia. Bronchiolitis is therefore considered a middle respiratory infection, instead of an upper (nose and throat) or lower (lung) infection. Edema, exudate, and inflammatory debris can partially obstruct some smaller airways. Clinically, RSV bronchiolitis presents with fever, mild dyspnea, a cough, and wheezing due to the partial obstructions. RSV pneumonia causes similar signs, with perhaps worse dyspnea due to interference with gas exchange. Antibiotics are helpful in RSV infection to prevent secondary bacterial pneumonia.

11-25

1. respiratory syncytial virus
2. infants
3. young children
4. elderly
5. upper
6. cold
7. bronchiolitis
8. airways or bronchioles
9. obstruct

RSV stands for _____(1). This is a virus that usually causes more severe disease in _____(2), _____(3), and the _____(4), than it does in adults. Before middle or lower respiratory infection, RSV causes _____(5) respiratory infection, commonly called a _____(6). Middle respiratory tract infection is called _____(7). This is infectious inflammation of the smaller _____(8). The presence of material associated with infection can partially _____(9) the smaller bronchioles.

11-26

With the influenza virus, cases that progress to pneumonia begin as severe upper respiratory infection with debilitation (weakness and lethargy). Usually, most cases of the "flu" are relatively mild. However, from time to time, a particularly virulent strain of the virus emerges. It rapidly spreads through the country in an epidemic that has the potential to kill many of the vulnerable population. Most of the fatal cases are seen in age-related immune incompetency (the very young or old), in the immune suppressed, and in the chronically ill. Influenza pneumonia presents with the typical picture of fever, cough, and dyspnea. Cyanosis may be present depending on the severity of infection. The thickened interstitial tissue can interfere with gas exchange between the capillaries and the alveoli. Prostration (extreme weakness or being "flat out") often accompanies influenza pneumonia. These cases can be easily followed by secondary bacterial infection. This occurs especially during epidemics produced by virulent strains of the virus. The virus kills cells, including the lining of the bronchi, which is an important first line of defense against bacteria. Secondary bacterial invasion is a contributing factor to the high mortality seen in susceptible populations. For this reason, influenza viral pneumonia should be treated with antibiotics as a preventive measure. Flu vaccines are for prevention and are effective only before exposure and infection. Flu vaccines are formulated for specific strains of influenza and are not protective against other strains.

11-27

1. virulent
2. disease
3. vulnerable
4. URI with weakness
5. debilitated or prostrate
6. cyanosis
7. gas

Viral pneumonia caused by the influenza virus develops because particular strains of the virus have become especially _____(1). This means that the microorganism has a powerful ability to cause _____(2). Influenza pneumonia targets _____(3) populations and begins as a severe _____(4). In addition to the usual signs of pneumonia, the patient is without strength, or is extremely _____(5). Bluish discoloration of the skin, or _____(6), indicates infection severe enough as to interfere with _____(7) exchange. An important concern in influenza pneumonia is the development of a secondary _____(8) infection, which raises the number of fatal cases.

The causative agents of fungal pneumonia were presented in Chapter 5 on infectious disease. Primary fungal pneumonia is most often associated with *Histoplasma capsulatum* (**histo-plasmosis**), or with *Coccidioides immitis* (**coccidioidomycosis**). *Histoplasma* is endemic in the Midwest, where this fungus is found in the soil contaminated by bird droppings. *Coccidioides* is found in the soil of the southwest. Fungal pneumonia is a chronic disease and is contracted by inhaling dust contaminated with the organism or its spores. Fungal pneumonia is often asymptomatic in otherwise healthy people. In symptomatic cases, the fungi can cause relatively large single lesions in the lungs, or can be spread out in a diffuse nodular pattern. The reaction to fungal invasion in the lungs is granulomatous inflammation. Healed areas usually contain granulomas that may calcify and easily be seen on an x-ray. The over-all picture of fungal pneumonia, with its chronicity and calcified granulomas, resembles tuberculosis. Acute symptomatic cases present with fever, cough, dyspnea, and some degree of incapacitation. Rarely, in overwhelming infection or in an immune-suppressed individual, either fungus may invade the bloodstream, causing infection in several body systems. The fungus *Histoplasma* causes the disease known as _____(1). *Coccidioides* causes _____(2). These organisms produce _____(3) pneumonia and are contracted by _____(4) contaminated _____(5). Lung tis-sue reacts to fungal invasion with _____(6) inflammation. It is possible, in the right cases, for the fungi to enter the _____(7) and infect other organs.

1. histoplasmosis
2. coccidioidomycosis
3. fungal
4. inhaling
5. dust
6. granulomatous
7. bloodstream

▶ TUBERCULOSIS

Infectious diseases of the respiratory system are reviewed in Table 11–1. Tuberculosis is the last disease we will study. This lung infection caused by *Mycobacterium tuberculosis* was presented in Chapter 5. This once-subdued disease is on the rise again, and can be found in AIDS patients and in immigrants from countries with a high incidence of TB. Tuberculosis is spread via the airborne route, by the coughs or sneezes of an infected individual. In pri-mary tuberculosis, this initial acute infection is often eradicated by the immune response of a healthy adult. The secondary immune response, or hypersensitivity of the immune cells to another exposure, forms the basis of the skin test for TB. Secondary tuberculosis develops if dormant organisms are reactivated from groups called tubercles (a pocket of the organisms surrounded by inflammatory activity). The reactivation and subsequent infection is caused by a decline in immune system function. Once reactivated, the *Mycobacterium* can also spread to other sites, such as the kidneys and bone, through the blood. The lung infection TB is caused by the organism _____(1). It is contracted from an infected individ-ual through the _____(2) route. Most healthy adults overcome a _____(3) infection. A secondary infection may take hold if the organism is _____(4) during a decline in _____(5) protection.

The lesions seen in the lungs during chronic or secondary TB are called **tubercles.** These are clumps of the bacilli that are surrounded by the cells of inflammation and scar tissue. The center of a tubercle will die and become a cheesy **caseous necrosis,** which was described in Chapter 2. The process is called **caseation.** This dead mass soon turns into a liquid, which is coughed up in the sputum. The expulsion of the liquefied tubercle leaves a hole or **cavity** in the lung tissue. This process is repeated until large areas of the lung tissue are destroyed by cavitation. The parenchyma of the lungs can come to resemble Swiss cheese. Erosion around a blood vessel will cause its rupture and the productive cough becomes bloody. The term to describe this (coughing up blood) is _____(1). In addition, secondary bacterial pneumonia is a complication of TB. The characteristic lesions of tuberculosis are called _____(2). The center of these bacteria-filled masses dies and turns into

TABLE 11–1. INFECTIOUS DISEASES OF THE RESPIRATORY SYSTEM

Infection	Cause
Upper respiratory infection (common cold)	Viruses—influenza A & B, parainfluenza, rhinovirus
Acute bronchitis	Bacteria from upper respiratory tract, inhaled irritants
Bronchiolitis	Respiratory syncytial virus (RSV)
Pneumonia	
Bronchopneumonia	Bacteria—*S. pneumoniae, S. hemolyticus, S. aureus,* pneumococcus
Lobar pneumonia	Bacteria—pneumococcus
Legionnaires' disease	Bacteria—*Legionella pneumophila*
Interstitial pneumonia	URI viruses; RSV; bacteria—*Mycoplasma pneumoniae,* protozoa—*Pneumocystis carinii*
Viral pneumonia	URI viruses, RSV, influenza
Fungal pneumonia	Fungi—*Histoplasma capsulatum* (histoplasmosis), *Coccidioides immitis* (coccidioidomycosis)
Tuberculosis	Bacteria—*Mycobacterium tuberculosis*

3. caseous necrosis
4. liquid
5. sputum
6. cavity
7. cavitation

_____(3). This necrotic area later turns into a _____(4), which is coughed up in the _____(5). A hole is left in the lung tissue, which is referred to as a _____(6). Destruction of the lungs is brought about by widespread _____(7).

----- 11–31 -----

An active case of chronic TB presents with fever, a productive and potentially bloody cough, incapacitating weakness, and weight loss. Historically, when TB was more prevalent, this weight loss was responsible for the term "consumption" being used to describe this disease. The infection was consuming, or using up, the patient. Fatal cases are due to large doses of the bacilli, or to poor resistance. Again, most healthy adults overcome acute TB. Treatment for active chronic tuberculosis consists of the long-term administration of the antituberculosis drug isoniazid (INH) combined with rifampin. Surgery may be useful to remove damaged areas of the lungs.

II. REVIEW QUESTIONS

1. b–URI

2. b–excess mucus production by inflamed mucous glands

3. d–bacterial invasion from the upper respiratory tract

1. The common cold is known medically by the abbreviations:
   a. ARDS
   b. URI
   c. COPD
   d. NRDS

2. Rhinorrhea during a common cold is caused by:
   a. excess mucus production by obstructed mucous glands
   b. excess mucus production by inflamed mucous glands
   c. swelling of mucous membrane lining the nasal passages
   d. sneezing to rid the irritant

3. Acute tracheobronchitis is caused by:
   a. long-term inhalation of an irritant
   b. pneumoconiosis
   c. chronic obstructive pulmonary disease
   d. bacterial invasion from the upper respiratory tract

4. Inflammation of the alveoli due to infection is:
   a. pneumonia
   b. pneumonitis
   c. pneumoconiosis
   d. pneumothorax

5. Bronchopneumonia and lobar pneumonia produce exudate in the
   a. _____, while interstitial pneumonia causes inflammation in the
   b. _____.

6. When alveoli become filled with exudate instead of air, this is called:
   a. bronchiectasis
   b. atelectasis
   c. consolidation
   d. rales

7. The infectious inflammation of both the bronchi and lungs is called:
   a. bronchitis
   b. bronchopneumonia
   c. lobar pneumonia
   d. interstitial pneumonia

8. Consolidation is seen in which of the following diseases? (Choose all that are correct.)
   a. bronchopneumonia
   b. interstitial pneumonia
   c. tracheobronchitis
   d. lobar pneumonia

9. Primary atypical pneumonia causes infectious inflammation of the connective tissue among the alveoli. This is also known as:
   a. lobar pneumonia
   b. interstitial pneumonia
   c. Legionnaires' disease
   d. bronchopneumonia

10. A viral pneumonia that most often plagues the very young or old is caused by:
    a. rhinovirus
    b. parainfluenza virus
    c. respiratory syncytial virus
    d. *Legionella pneumophila*

11. A viral pneumonia often associated with epidemics is caused by:
    a. parainfluenza virus
    b. respiratory syncytial virus
    c. rhinovirus
    d. influenza virus

12. Histoplasmosis and coccidioidomycosis are examples of:
    a. fungal pneumonia
    b. viral pneumonia
    c. bacterial pneumonia
    d. pneumonitis

4. a–pneumonia

5. a–alveoli or air sacs
   b–interstitial tissue or septa

6. c–consolidation

7. b–bronchopneumonia

8. a–bronchopneumonia
   d–lobar pneumonia

9. b–interstitial pneumonia

10. c–respiratory syncytial virus

11. d–influenza virus

12. a–fungal pneumonia

13. 1. c–cavitation
    2. b–caseation
    3. d–hemoptysis
    4. a–tubercles

13. Match the terms in the left column that are used in describing tuberculosis, with their definitions in the right column:

a. tubercules   _____ 1. holes left in the lung after coughing up liquefied necroses
b. caseation   _____ 2. tissue death that is cheesy
c. cavitation   _____ 3. coughing up blood
d. hemoptysis   _____ 4. a pocket of TB organisms surrounded by inflammation

SECTION ▶ III. CHRONIC OBSTRUCTIVE PULMONARY DISEASE AND IMMUNE-MEDIATED DISTURBANCE

11–32

1. chronic obstructive pulmonary disease
2. obstruction
3. inflammation
4. destruction
5. bronchioles
6. mucus
7. irritation
8. gas exchange

Chronic obstructive pulmonary disease is common and is known by the acronym **COPD**. COPD is a disorder in which the small airways of the lungs (the smaller bronchi and the bronchioles) are plugged or partially obstructed over a long period of time. This occlusion of the respiratory tree leads to inflammation, degenerative changes, and destruction. This may be permanent depending on the length of duration and the extent of the damage. COPD is a *reaction* to some primary disease state or to a chronic irritant. Therefore, COPD is considered to be a secondary state. The obstruction of the airways is almost always by copious mucus production, with inflammatory material and debris. Most commonly, the mucus production and inflammation is a response to chronic irritation. Occasionally, bacterial infection may also develop, contributing to the obstructive material. No matter what the exact cause or what the obstructive material is, the result common to all states of COPD is ineffective ventilation. Therefore, COPD leads to interference with gas exchange—that is, with the release of CO_2 and the intake of O_2. COPD stands for _____(1). The underlying pathogenesis of COPD is _____(2) of the smaller airways in the lungs. This causes _____(3), degeneration, and possible _____(4), which may be permanent. The obstruction of the smaller bronchi and _____(5) is due to the presence of a great deal of _____(6) and the activities of inflammation. This is usually a response to chronic _____(7). COPD ultimately causes poor ventilation as it interferes with _____(8).

11–33

Of the disease states we are about to discuss, chronic bronchitis and emphysema are the most representative of COPD. Other disorders such as bronchiectasis and asthma are also considered chronic obstructive pulmonary diseases. Chronic bronchitis and emphysema are overwhelmingly caused by cigarette smoking. These two conditions often overlap or coexist together. However, usually one disorder predominates over the other.

▶ CHRONIC BRONCHITIS

11–34

Chronic bronchitis differs from acute bronchitis primarily in cause (infection causing the acute state) and in duration. Chronic bronchitis will develop in reaction to heavy air pollution or to work-related exposure to toxic fumes. About 90 percent of the cases are due to cigarette smoke. The severity of bronchitis seems directly proportional to the number of cigarettes smoked. The symptoms and signs are the same as acute bronchitis, which includes a cough that brings up sputum. As stated, chronic bronchitis is a reaction to long-standing irritation such as smoking, rather than a primary disease. It is defined as the presence of mucus in the airways that causes a productive cough for at least 3 months out of a year for at least 2 years in a row. In response to years of irritation, the mucous membrane lining the bronchi and bronchioles becomes inflamed and swollen. The walls of the airways thicken and the mucous glands undergo hyperplasia. Excessive mucous production combines with swollen membranes and thickened walls to cause partial or complete obstruction of the affected airway. These plugged air tubes become ineffective in ventilation and gas exchange. Clinically, the obstruction causes wheezing as air whistles past the plugs, and shortness of breath indicates ventilation difficulty. Chronic bronchitis may be diagnosed if a productive _____(1) is present for at least _____(2) months during a year, for _____(3) consecutive years. Obstruction of bronchi and bronchioles is due to the presence of _____(4) from hyperplastic glands, _____(5) of the membranes lining the airways, and _____(6) of the walls of the airways. Chronic bronchitis interferes with _____(7).

1. cough
2. three
3. two
4. mucus
5. swelling
6. thickening
7. gas exchange

11-35

In the early stages of chronic bronchitis, the remaining functional lung tissue is enough to maintain an adequate Po_2, or concentration of oxygen in the blood. However, this changes if the situation is not resolved and the airway obstruction spreads. In the later and end stages, hypoxia will develop as well as **hypercapnia** (excessive carbon dioxide in the blood). The swelling and presence of mucus has significantly increased the resistance to air flow through the plugged respiratory tree. The mucus also traps microorganisms that would normally be cleared out, and this makes the sufferer of chronic bronchitis susceptible to frequent respiratory infection. It is not unusual for an individual with chronic bronchitis to experience bronchopneumonia during the winter months. In addition to pneumonia, other complications include bronchiectasis (discussed in the next frame) and emphysema (see Frame 11–38). Early chronic bronchitis has a good chance of resolving if the source of the irritant is stopped. In the majority of cases, this means stop smoking. Later cases progress into emphysema, for which there is no definitive treatment. The later and end stages of chronic bronchitis are hallmarked by insufficient oxygen in the blood or _____(1), and too much carbon dioxide in the blood or _____(2). Individuals with chronic bronchitis suffer from repeated bouts of respiratory _____(3) because _____(4) traps microorganisms. The pathogenesis and complications of chronic bronchitis are illustrated in Figure 11–4.

1. hypoxia
2. hypercapnia
3. infection
4. mucus

▶ BRONCHIECTASIS

11-36

The word root "ectasis" means distention. Therefore, **bronchiectasis** means the dilatation of the bronchi. The bronchioles are also affected **(bronchiolectasis).** This is an enlargement of the internal diameter of the airways that is permanent. The dilation is because of persistent inflammation, swelling, and pressure from mucous plugs. Bronchiectasis is most commonly a sequela of chronic bronchitis. Again, it is a response to a chronic condition, rather than a primary disease. Occasionally, it may follow a viral pneumonia complicated by bacterial infection in children. Other chronic lung diseases, such as TB or cancer, may also cause irreversible airway distention. In bronchiectasis, the walls of parts of the respiratory tree have ballooned outward and become very weak. They eventually necrose and are destroyed. This may take one of two forms: **saccular bronchiectasis,** in which the larger bronchi form round bulges or little sacs; and **cylindrical bronchiectasis,** in which the bronchioles enlarge in tube-like fashion. Since the smooth muscle surrounding the enlarged airways is also destroyed by necrosis, many of the mucous plugs cannot be expelled when coughing. Again, this sets the stage for infection, and small pockets of pus (abscesses) are not unusual. Clinically, the cough that accompanies bronchiectasis often brings up foul material, composed of mucus, pus, and necrotic debris. The patient's breath matches the foulness of the sputum. Figure 11–5 shows the dilated bronchi in bronchiectasis.

11-37

The word "bronchiectasis" describes the condition of smaller airways during COPD, and this condition is _____(1). Bronchiectasis often follows chronic _____(2). The walls of sections of the airways have become weak and _____(3). Larger bronchi balloon out in little bulges called _____(4) bronchiectasis, and bronchioles retain a tube shape during their enlargement, known as _____(5) bronchiectasis. Infection often sets in because

1. distention or dilation
2. bronchitis
3. necrotic
4. saccular
5. cylindrical

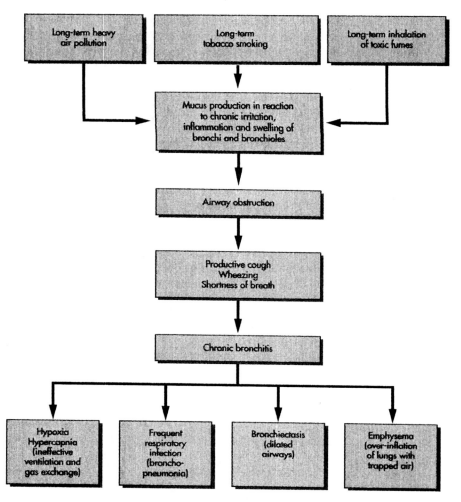

Figure 11–4. The pathogenesis and complications of chronic bronchitis.

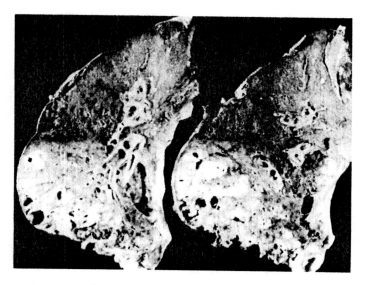

Figure 11–5. Bronchiectasis, showing fibrosis and dilation of bronchi in the lower lobe. Note the dilated bronchi immediately beneath the pleura. *(From Chandrasoma and Taylor,* Concise Pathology, *2nd ed., Appleton & Lange.)*

of the presence of mucous _____(6) that are not expelled when smooth _____(7) is destroyed. Bronchiectasis may be diagnosed upon performance of a **bronchogram,** which is infusion of radiopaque dye into the respiratory tree and x-ray of the lungs. The dilated airways can be seen without great difficulty. The only treatment, if it is to be called that, is to remove the cause of the irritation and hope that the damage is not so advanced that it cannot heal. Antibiotics are necessary to fight secondary infection. Obviously, prevention is best by stopping smoking during early bronchitis. If only one lobe is affected, surgical removal may be indicated.

6. plugs
7. muscle

▶ EMPHYSEMA

11-38

Emphysema is inflation of the lungs by trapped air. The alveoli, or air sacs, at the end of the bronchioles become dilated or enlarged with stagnant air. Emphysema is seen almost exclusively in smokers and is a sequela of chronic bronchitis and bronchiectasis. In addition to being a COPD, it is also considered a ventilation disturbance (see Section IV). In emphysema, air is trapped in diseased alveoli. The oxygen concentration decreases while the concentration of carbon dioxide increases. The exchange of fresh air for this stagnant air is not very effective because the stale air can't be completely exhaled. Pockets of trapped air, which inflate the lungs, are described as the disease _____(1). It follows _____(2) and _____(3) in those who smoke. Stagnant air pockets are high in _____(4), and low in _____(5). This develops because the old air is not completely _____(6).

1. emphysema
2. chronic bronchitis
3. bronchiectasis
4. carbon dioxide
5. oxygen
6. exhaled

11-39

It is believed that cigarette smoke destroys alveoli walls in part by the production of oxygen free radicals, which are molecules that damage cell membranes. The presence of chronic inflammation also causes damage to the walls. Inflammatory cells release proteolytic enzymes, such as protease and elastase, and these enzymes are nonspecific in their destruction. Elastase destroys elastin, an elastic protein in the alveoli walls. The oxygen free radicals also inhibit antiproteolytic chemicals, which are a natural protectant against extensive damage by inflammatory enzymes. With a fair amount of the elastin destroyed, there is less recoil in the alveoli to force out old air. Therefore, when air is inhaled, the alveoli remain enlarged with leftover or trapped air after exhalation. In addition to loss of elastic recoil, the airways are narrowed from long-standing obstruction and destruction. This contributes to loss of efficiency in moving air in and out of the lungs. Eventually, the weakened alveoli rupture and coalesce or blend together. Figure 11–6 compares normal alveoli and ruptured alveoli in emphysema. The fusion of several alveoli into one nonfunctional unit creates a **bulla.** A complication of bulla formation is rupture of the entire large air sac, which introduces air into the pleural space. This disrupts the negative pressure and the vacuum, which allows the lungs to collapse. This is called pneumothorax (see Frame 11–89).

11-40

In emphysema, the walls of the _____(1) are destroyed by oxygen _____(2), and the proteolytic _____(3) that are released during _____(4). Elastase destroys the _____(5) in alveoli walls. This makes them less able to _____(6) when exhaling. After several breaths, the alveoli become enlarged or inflated with _____(7) air. When several alveoli rupture and _____(8), they merge into a large air sac called a _____(9). It is possible that the bulla will also _____(10), leading to a _____(11) lung.

1. alveoli
2. free radicals
3. enzymes
4. inflammation
5. elastin
6. recoil
7. leftover or trapped
8. coalesce
9. bulla
10. rupture
11. collapsed

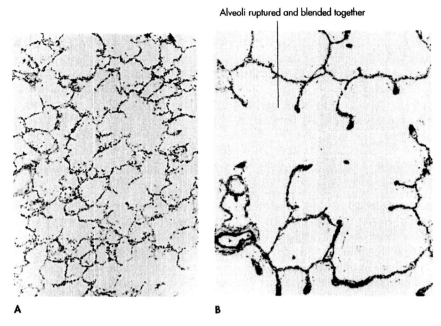

Alveoli ruptured and blended together

A   B

Figure 11–6. A. Normal lung. **B.** Emphysema (taken at the same magnification). Note that the alveoli are larger and fewer in number due to rupture and coalescence. *(From Kent & Hart,* Introduction to Human Disease, *3rd ed., Appleton & Lange.)*

11–41

Early symptoms of emphysema are chronic cough (the presence of chronic bronchitis), shortness of breath, and lack of stamina. Advanced chronic obstructive pulmonary disease presents clinically as one of two forms. A patient who predominantly has chronic bronchitis is described as a **"blue bloater."** This phrase is derived from visible signs in Caucasian patients. Along with persistent episodes of productive cough and dyspnea, a blue bloater develops hypoxia during a prolonged coughing spell. The hypoxia can be severe enough to cause cyanosis (hence the term "blue" in Caucasian patients). Overwork to provide the body with enough oxygen, along with fibrosis around the blood vessels, creates pulmonary hypertension and cor pulmonale. You know that cor pulmonale will lead to right ventricular failure. You also know that a prominent sign of right ventricular failure is the swelling of peripheral edema (hence the term "bloater"). An x-ray of the lungs of a blue bloater shows multiple densities that correspond to the mucus-plugged airways of chronic bronchitis.

11–42

1. dyspnea

A **"pink puffer"** is a COPD patient who predominantly has emphysema. Emphysematous patients have less of a cough with expectoration, and much more difficulty breathing. Difficulty in breathing is called _____(1). This particular type of dyspnea takes the form of tachypnea or rapid, shallow breathing. This type of respiratory movement is responsible for the term "puffer." The destruction of the alveoli has greatly decreased the surface area for gas exchange, and when combined with the inflation of trapped air, this causes the patient to experience feelings of suffocation. Tachypnea produces enough hyperventilation to prevent cyanosis, so Caucasian patients are "pink," not blue. The term pink refers only to the absence of cyanosis. The chest of the emphysematous pink puffer becomes enlarged in what is described as barrel shaped. This is due to a combination of enlargement of the air spaces, loss of elasticity that contracts the lung fields, and working so hard to breathe. Patients with emphysema assume a typical hunched-over posture to breathe. They must use the auxiliary respiratory muscles to move enough air, and hypertrophy of these muscles is a common finding. The x-ray findings in a pink puffer reveal expansion of the lung fields and overinflation. Overinflation is seen as large areas of radiolucency because of the increased air-to-tissue

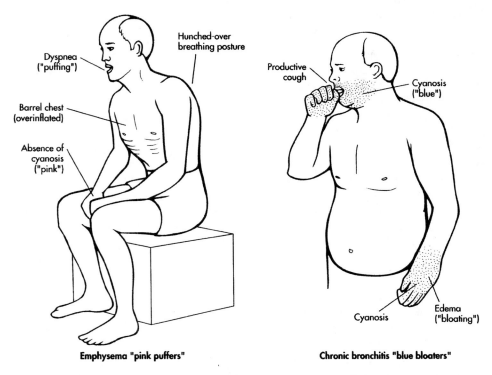

Figure 11–7. Predominant signs in chronic obstructive pulmonary disease. *(Adapted from Damjanov,* Pathology for the Health-Related Professions, *Saunders.)*

ratio. A comparison of the signs of the two major causes of COPD (chronic bronchitis and emphysema) is shown in Figure 11–7.

A COPD patient who presents as a blue bloater predominantly has _____(1). The coloring of the patient is due to _____(2). This develops during episodes of paroxysmal coughing that causes significant _____(3). Pulmonary hypertension and therefore _____(4) follow, and they are because of overwork and _____(5) around the blood vessels. Cor pulmonale leads to right _____(6) failure and the production of peripheral _____(7). This makes the patient look _____(8). A COPD patient who presents as a pink puffer predominantly has _____(9). Cyanosis is avoided because of hyperventilation, which is created by the action of _____(10). This rapid breathing is responsible for the descriptive term _____(11). The chest assumes a _____(12) shape from overinflation, expanded lung fields, and the work of respiration.

1. chronic bronchitis
2. cyanosis
3. hypoxia
4. cor pulmonale
5. fibrosis
6. ventricular
7. edema
8. bloated
9. emphysema
10. tachypnea
11. puffer
12. barrel

11–43

11–44

Before the development of the signs of advanced COPD, a test using an instrument called a **spirometer** may detect chronic obstructive pulmonary disease in its earlier stages. A spirometer measures the movement of air in and out of the lungs and can quantitate the amount. There is no treatment for advanced COPD. Obviously, the source of inflammation and destruction must be stopped to prevent an even earlier death. Supportive measures can be useful to increase the patient's comfort, and these include medications to help clear mucus and physical therapy to increase use of respiratory muscles.

► SEASONAL ALLERGIC RHINITIS

11-45

1. hay fever
2. hypersensitivity
3. allergens

The disorders in the remainder of this section are immune mediated. They develop as a result of the activity of the immune system, both antibody and cell mediated, and incite an inflammatory reaction. The first is extremely well known, **allergic rhinitis.** This is more commonly known as **hay fever.** Hay fever is probably second in frequency only to the common cold. It is not strictly genetic, but certain people tend to be predisposed to allergies. Hay fever seems to be familial, or run in families. It is a type I hypersensitivity reaction (see Chap. 4). The antigens to which antibodies react are called **allergens.** This indicates that the antigen causes allergy, rather than other types of disorders. The most common allergens that produce allergic rhinitis are plant pollens, such as ragweed, grasses, cottonwood, and sagebrush. Other allergens that are ubiquitous (found everywhere) include house dust, animal dander, and molds. Seasonal allergic rhinitis is commonly called _____(1). This is a type I _____(2) reaction to antigens specifically called _____(3).

11-46

Recall from Chapter 4 the various types of antibodies. IgG and IgM work to rid the body of antigens such as bacteria, which can cause infection. IgA is the immunoglobulin found in secretions that form the initial line of defense against foreign invaders. **IgE** is the antibody that is responsible for allergic reactions. IgE attaches itself to **mast cells** found in the mucous membranes lining the nose and surrounding the eyes. When IgE on the mast cells encounters an allergen, it binds or complexes with it. This is the signal for the mast cell to release **histamine.** Remember from Chapter 2 the role of histamine in inflammation. Two important actions that are stimulated by histamine are vasodilation, which increases blood supply to the area, and an increase in vessel permeability, which makes the vessel leaky and allows fluid to accumulate locally. The presence of this edema is responsible for nasal congestion, which is the stuffy feeling that accompanies local swelling. The inflammatory activity also irritates the mucosal cells in the membrane lining. They increase their secretion of mucus, causing a runny nose and watery eyes. The irritation also produces sneezing in an effort to get rid of the offending agent.

11-47

1. IgE
2. mast
3. allergen
4. histamine
5. vasodilation
6. permeability
7. congestion
8. mucus
9. sneezing

The immunoglobulin that mediates allergic rhinitis is _____(1). It is found on _____(2) cells. When this antibody complexes with a (an) _____(3), it stimulates the mast cells to release _____(4). This chemical mediator causes _____(5) and an increase in vessel _____(6). The swelling from local edema causes the feeling of nasal _____(7). Runny nose and watery eyes are because of irritation of the _____(8) glands. The body tries to expel the allergen by _____(9). Treatment for hay fever is symptomatic. Decongestants and antihistamines may provide some relief by interfering with immune and inflammatory activity that causes stuffiness, sneezing, and discharge. Bothersome cases of hay fever may be managed with attempts at **desensitization.** In this process, the offending allergen must be specifically identified by skin testing, or allergy testing. Then, injections of the allergen in tiny amounts are given over a period of time. This is in hope that IgG will be formed against the allergen and destroy it before it is bound by IgE.

► HYPERSENSITIVITY PNEUMONITIS

11-48

Hypersensitivity pneumonitis is an allergic reaction in the alveoli (allergic alveolitis) that is due to inhaling antigens primarily from molds and fungi. These microorganisms grow in plant material like hay and tree bark. They can also be found in bird excrement, dust that contains fungal spores, and animal dander. Some specific types of hypersensitivity pneumonitis are:

1. Farmer's lung, in which the antigens are in moldy hay or grain.
2. Furrier's lung, in which the antigens are in animal skins.
3. Maple bark disease, in which the antigens are in the maple bark.

Hypersensitivity pneumonitis is an allergic reaction that affects the _____(1). The allergens are generally _____(2) or _____(3) that grow in various environments.

1. alveoli
2. molds
3. fungi

.... 11-49 ....

Hypersensitivity pneumonitis can occur in two forms, acute and chronic. In the acute form, the binding of antibody with antigen takes place in the lining of the alveoli. This again stimulates inflammatory activity with its influx of neutrophils and chemical mediators. Complement is also a part of this activity. All of this produces antibody-mediated injury to the lining and walls of the alveoli. Episodes of acute hypersensitivity pneumonitis cause sudden dyspnea that improves when the exposure to the allergen is stopped. Dyspnea is due to the interference in gas exchange when swelling, edema, and other results of inflammation are present in the air sacs. As in all similar conditions, the exchange of gases cannot easily take place through solid material. The acute form of hypersensitivity pneumonitis involves the reactions between _____(1) and allergens. The site of the binding and subsequent reactions is in the lining of the _____(2). This ultimately causes _____(3) to the walls of the air sacs. Dyspnea during periods of exposure is because of interference with _____(4) that develops as a result of inflammation.

1. antibodies
2. alveoli
3. injury
4. gas exchange

.... 11-50 ....

In the chronic form, the injury becomes cell mediated instead of antibody mediated. T lymphocytes are the agents of cell-mediated immune defense. Their activities cause granuloma formation with thickening of the air sacs. Repair or attempts at healing are by fibrosis. Scarring and dilation of the alveoli result in a honeycomb appearance of the lungs. In the chronic form, dyspnea is more pronounced and of longer duration. Hyperventilation occurs in an attempt to compensate for poor gas exchange. Continued exposure to the allergen continues the injury, and the condition will progress to end-stage lung disease and respiratory failure. The only treatment for end-stage lung disease is transplantation. In chronic hypersensitivity pneumonitis, the injury is due to the activity of _____(1) instead of antibodies, so this is called _____(2)-mediated injury. A honeycomb appearance of the lung tissue results from repair attempts in the form of _____(3). The injury and dyspnea in this condition are so severe that over time it progresses to end-stage lung disease and respiratory _____(4).

1. T cells
2. cell
3. fibrosis
4. failure

▶ ASTHMA

.... 11-51 ....

Asthma is labored breathing brought on by spasm of the airways. It occurs in episodes or attacks that can significantly interfere with lifestyle. In addition to being an immune-mediated allergy, it can be considered another chronic obstructive pulmonary disease. This disorder lasts a long time and impairs or obstructs air flow. The allergic form of asthma most commonly occurs in children and young adults. While most cases improve with age, about 50 percent of affected children will have difficulty throughout their lifetime. This allergy also demonstrates a familial tendency to react to certain allergens. The allergens are much like those that cause allergic rhinitis, and some foods are implicated as well. There is a form of asthma not related to allergy that occurs in older adults that we will also discuss. Difficulty in breathing because of spasm in the respiratory tree is _____(1). It is both a (an) _____(2)-mediated _____(3) and a chronic _____(4) pulmonary disease. Allergic asthma is most often seen in _____(5) and young adults.

1. asthma
2. immune
3. allergy
4. obstructive
5. children

.... 11-52 ....

The bronchi and bronchioles of an asthmatic appear to be very sensitive to stimuli. The affected individual is normal in between episodes. Asthma is also a type I hypersensitivity, and the patient frequently has other types of allergies. In asthma, excessive amounts of IgE coat the mucous membrane lining of the airways and also bind to smooth muscle surrounding the bronchioles. When the IgE encounters an allergen and complexes with it, the mast cells release histamine. In addition to its other activities, histamine also stimulates the smooth muscle to contract. The airways become obstructed because of the contraction and squeezing by the muscle. The lumen becomes narrowed, and the resistance to air flow is greatly increased. Dyspnea, or difficult labored breathing, occurs along with wheezing. An asthmatic attack is like trying to breath through a collapsed straw. The wheezing is due to air trying to squeeze through the constricted bronchioles. The dyspnea lasts throughout the muscle spasm. The lumen of the airways is further narrowed by the swelling of mucus membranes, and blocked by mucus production. Moving air in and out becomes very difficult. Most episodes last a moderate amount of time, and asthmatics try to keep medication on hand to shorten the duration. The condition known as **status asthmaticus** is not as common but is much more serious. In this severe episode of constriction, the attack is prolonged and doesn't stop spontaneously. Injections of epinephrine (adrenalin) are necessary. Failure to respond may lead to the need for a **tracheotomy,** in which the trachea is opened with an incision to allow air flow. Respiratory failure and death are not common in asthma, but can be a result of untreated status asthmaticus.

11-53

1. IgE
2. mucous membrane
3. smooth muscle
4. allergen
5. mast cells
6. contract
7. narrows
8. breathing
9. resistance
10. wheezing
11. block
12. status asthmaticus

In asthma, the antibody _____(1) is found on the _____(2) lining of the bronchioles and on the _____(3) surrounding these airways. After it complexes with a (an) _____(4), histamine is released from _____(5). This chemical mediator stimulates the smooth muscle to _____(6). This effectively _____(7) the lumen of the airways, making _____(8) difficult because _____(9) to air flow is increased. The sound an asthmatic makes during an attack is called _____(10). Swelling and mucus further _____(11) the bronchioles. A situation in which the attack goes on and on, with death a possibility, is called _____(12).

11-54

Asthma itself causes no permanent injury to the lungs. As previously mentioned, the severity of attacks decreases with age as the patient "grows out of it," and the prognosis for a normal life is good. Nonallergic asthma seen in older adults is idiopathic. For some reason, the respiratory tree is hypersensitive to stimuli other than allergens. In these cases, psychogenic factors can trigger an attack. These factors include stress, tension, fear, or other emotions felt to an extreme. Irritants that cause bronchitis can also stimulate bronchial constriction, as can respiratory tract infection. Treatment for asthma is largely symptomatic. Bronchodilators such as ephedrine spray are extremely helpful to open the airways during attacks. Some medications are given to prevent degranulation by the mast cells and histamine release. The best management for allergic asthma is to identify the causative allergens through skin testing and to avoid them. Examples of this are to eliminate household dust as much as possible, remove pets from the household, eliminate cigarette smoke and certain foods, and to decrease outside activity during pollen season. Desensitization has been tried in some cases. Nonallergic asthma is managed the same way, that is, to identify the offending agent and remove or avoid it. The causes of chronic obstructive pulmonary disease and immune-mediated disorders are summarized in Table 11–2.

TABLE 11–2. CHRONIC OBSTRUCTIVE PULMONARY DISEASE AND IMMUNE-MEDIATED RESPIRATORY DISEASE

Chronic Obstructive Pulmonary Disease	Immune-Mediated Respiratory Disease
Chronic bronchitis	Seasonal allergic rhinitis
Emphysema	Hypersensitivity pneumonitis
Bronchiectasis	Asthma
Asthma	

III. REVIEW QUESTIONS

1. Blockage of the small airways by mucous plugs over a long period of time is the basic pathogenesis of:
   a. adult respiratory distress syndrome
   b. pneumonia
   c. chronic obstructive pulmonary disease
   d. asthma

2. A productive cough for 3 months out of a year for 2 consecutive years defines:
   a. chronic bronchitis
   b. acute tracheobronchitis
   c. bronchiectasis
   d. emphysema

3. Which of the following are seen in chronic bronchitis? (Choose all that apply.)
   a. increased resistance to airflow through the plugged respiratory tree
   b. frequent infections resulting from trapped mucus and microorganisms
   c. spasm of the smooth muscle around the bronchioles
   d. stale air trapped in alveoli

4. Permanent enlargement of the bronchi is called:
   a. atelectasis
   b. emphysema
   c. bronchitis
   d. bronchiectasis

5. The destruction of elastin in the alveoli, along with other injuries, leaves them less able to recoil and expel stagnant air. This best describes the pathogenesis of:
   a. asthma
   b. emphysema
   c. chronic bronchitis
   d. bronchiectasis

6. A bulla is:
   a. distention of the bronchi in saccular form
   b. an area of abscess
   c. ruptured and coalesced alveoli
   d. a tuberculosis lesion

7. A complication of bulla rupture is:
   a. pneumothorax
   b. hydrothorax
   c. pleural effusion
   d. hemothorax

8. In COPD, a "blue bloater" is associated with the disease a. _____, while a "pink puffer" is associated with the disease b. _____.

9. Seasonal allergic rhinitis is commonly known as:
   a. a cold
   b. the flu
   c. asthma
   d. hay fever

1. c–chronic obstructive pulmonary disease

2. a–chronic bronchitis

3. a–increased resistance to airflow through the plugged respiratory tree; b–frequent infections resulting from trapped mucus and microorganisms

4. d–bronchiectasis

5. b–emphysema

6. c–ruptured and coalesced alveoli

7. a–pneumothorax

8. a–chronic bronchitis; b–emphysema

9. d–hay fever

10. b–the reacting antibody is of the IgG class

11. d–spasm of the smooth muscle surrounding the bronchi, which leaves the bronchi narrowed

12. a–immune mediated

13. b–the release of histamine from mast cells when IgE encounters an allergen

10. Choose the INCORRECT statement about seasonal allergic rhinitis:
   a. the inciting antigens are called allergens
   b. the reacting antibody is of the IgG class
   c. the mast cell releases histamine
   d. symptoms are related to the effects of histamine

11. The basic pathogenesis of asthma is:
   a. destruction of the smooth muscle surrounding the bronchi, which leaves the bronchi permanently dilated
   b. hypersensitivity of the alveoli in response to fungal allergens
   c. intermittent obstruction of the small airways with mucous plugs
   d. spasm of the smooth muscle surrounding the bronchi, which leaves the bronchi narrowed

12. The cause of asthma is:
   a. immune mediated
   b. genetic
   c. idiopathic
   d. a secondary response

13. In asthma, smooth muscle contraction is initiated by:
   a. the release of histamine from neutrophils when IgG encounters an allergen
   b. the release of histamine from mast cells when IgE encounters an allergen
   c. the release of histamine from mast cells when IgG encounters an allergen
   d. the release of elastase from mast cells when IgE encounters an allergen

SECTION ▶ 11-55

IV. DISTURBANCES IN VENTILATION AND INHALATION-BASED DISEASE

Ventilation is made up of all the processes that result in blood being oxygenated and carbon dioxide (CO_2) being eliminated. Adequate ventilation requires all of the following:

1. Movement of oxygen-rich air from the atmosphere, through the entire respiratory tract, down to the level of the alveoli. This is **inhalation** or **inspiration.** Inhalation requires adequate functioning of the respiratory muscles and expansion of the lungs. The expansion of the lungs is permitted largely by differences in pressure gradients in the chest. The pressure is positive inside the lungs (specifically the air sacs), and negative in the pleural space.
2. Movement of oxygen (O_2) molecules from the alveoli through their walls, through the septa (the interstitial tissue between the air sacs), and into the capillaries.
3. Sufficient blood flow through the capillaries so that RBCs and hemoglobin are continuously presented for the exchange of CO_2 for O_2.
4. The release of CO_2 from hemoglobin and the binding of O_2 to hemoglobin.
5. The diffusion of CO_2 in a reverse path just traveled by O_2 (out of the capillaries, through the septa and alveoli walls, into the alveoli).
6. Movement of CO_2 out of the respiratory tract, which is **exhalation** or **expiration.** This requires retraction, or the pulling in of the lungs, the opposite of expansion.

11-56

Any pathology or disease process along this route, or any interference with this process, will cause ventilation disturbance. Therefore, the diseases already discussed—such as COPD, pneumonia, or asthma—cause ventilation disturbance. The classification of the following disorders as ventilation disturbances is arbitrary and meant to facilitate the organization of this chapter. Two additional states that completely disrupt ventilation are drowning and suffocation. **Suffocation** is prevention of inhalation and exhalation by an obstruction in the respiratory tree (usually the upper portion), or by external interference. Examples of internal obstruction are accidentally inhaled foreign bodies, seen usually in children, and inhaled food, seen in adults. External interference can be accidental in the case of children, when they place themselves in a position of running out of air. Or, in cases of adults, it may be deliberate and therefore homicidal. **Drowning** is a form of suffocation in which the respiratory tree is obstructed with fluid. Fluid fills the alveoli instead of O_2 from inspired air. In either suffocation or drowning, the mode of death is systemic anoxia, which most immediately affects the brain. Recovery from partial suffocation or drowning depends on the amount of time the brain was deprived of oxygen, and the degree of permanent brain damage. Suffocation is the stopping of _____(1) and _____(2) by some _____(3) in the _____(4). If suffocation is because of fluid in the alveoli, this is called _____(5). Cause of death in either case is _____(6), and the prognosis for complete recovery depends on the amount of _____(7) injury.

1. inhalation
2. exhalation
3. obstruction
4. respiratory tree
5. drowning
6. systemic anoxia
7. brain

▶ ADULT RESPIRATORY DISTRESS SYNDROME

Adult respiratory distress syndrome, or **ARDS,** is a general term to describe widespread damage to the parenchyma of the lung (in particular the lining of the alveoli), or injury to the interstitial tissue and vessels. ARDS is at the end of the road of many pulmonary disorders that are not resolved. It is another condition that is a secondary reaction rather than a primary disease process. And considering how many pulmonary disorders are themselves secondary states, ARDS can even be called a tertiary reaction. ARDS precedes or comes before respiratory failure. ARDS stands for _____(1). This is a condition that results from other pulmonary _____(2) that have caused widespread _____(3). It represents injury to either the lung _____(4) or to the _____(5) tissue or vessels. ARDS occurs before _____(6).

11-57

1. adult respiratory distress syndrome
2. disorders or diseases
3. damage or injury
4. parenchyma
5. interstitial
6. respiratory failure

ARDS can be due to acute noninfectious interstitial disease. This is injury of a sudden nature that is not caused by infection such as interstitial pneumonia, and that affects the interstitial tissue or septa between the alveoli. Remember, that is where the vessels reside. Some injuries affect the capillaries directly. ARDS also includes a variety of alveolar damage, and in fact has been called diffuse alveolar damage. Here, inflammation of the walls causes thickening and some exudate into the air sacs, although less than in the case of pneumonia. Many injuries can lead to ARDS. The most common reason is shock, and for this reason ARDS used to be called "shock lung." In shock, massive leaking of the contents of blood exude into the interstitial tissue and into the alveoli because of injury to capillary endothelium. Injury to the endothelium can also be due to hypoxia, anoxia, inhalation of a gaseous toxin, chemicals, some drugs, DIC, and inhaled heat from a fire. ARDS, which affects the septa suddenly and not because of infection, is caused by _____(1). ARDS that is due to damage of the air sacs may be called _____(2). A very common reason for ARDS is _____(3), and so this disorder used to be called _____(4) lung. Shock causes injury to the capillary _____(5).

11-58

1. acute noninfectious interstitial disease
2. diffuse alveolar damage
3. shock
4. shock
5. endothelium

Adult respiratory distress syndrome can cause significant impairment in the ability to ventilate (i.e., oxygenate) the blood. It leads to acute respiratory failure. Early signs of respiratory failure occur within 24 hours after the injury. Dyspnea is extreme to the point of gasping for air. Tests for the gaseous content of blood reveal a low P_{O_2} (hypoxemia) and an increased P_{CO_2} (hypercapnia). A chest x-ray shows diffuse consolidation of the lungs with few aerated alveoli. Treatment for ARDS requires placing the patient on a respirator for artificial ventilation. The prognosis in ARDS is guarded. There are many secondary complications such as fatal pneumonia and chronic noninfectious interstitial disease because of extensive fibrosis of the septa. Only about 30 percent of the cases of ARDS survive, and many survivors suffer permanent pulmonary injury. ARDS leads to acute _____(1) because of the

11-59

1. respiratory failure

inability to _____(2) or provide oxygen to the blood. A complication of ARDS in survivors is chronic _____(3) disease because of scarring or fibrosis in the septa.

▶ RESPIRATORY FAILURE

Respiratory failure is lack of oxygen or retention of carbon dioxide because of inadequate functioning of the lungs. This inadequate functioning is, of course, impairment in ventilation. A sufficient amount of oxygen in the blood is measured as the **partial pressure** of oxygen, abbreviated as Po_2. The normal Po_2 is approximately 100 mm Hg. The acceptable limit of carbon dioxide, stated as the partial pressure or Pco_2, is about 40 mm Hg. The values that define respiratory failure are a Po_2 of less than 60 mm Hg (**hypoxemia**) or a Pco_2 of greater than 50 mm Hg (**hypercapnia**). Several of the disorders discussed in this chapter, if severe, can cause respiratory failure. Less than sufficient oxygen in the blood, or too much carbon dioxide, defines _____(1), and this is due to the inability to _____(2) properly. A Po_2 of less than 60 mm Hg is described by the term _____(3). A Pco_2 of greater than 50 mm Hg is described by the term _____(4).

Respiratory failure may take one of two forms. The first is failure of air movement into the lungs, or inadequate inhalation. This is called **alveolar hypoventilation.** This may occur because of:

1. Obstruction in the respiratory tree. Causes include muscular spasm in asthma, inhalation of a foreign body, extreme mucous plugs in chronic bronchitis, and severe exudate in pneumonia.
2. Restriction in movement of the chest wall or in lung expansion. Causes include pleural effusion or pneumothorax (Section VI) and extreme obesity where the movement of the diaphragm is so restricted that breathing occurs in a very shallow manner (Pickwickian syndrome).
3. Nerve or muscle paralysis. Causes include endotoxins in tetanus, poliomyelitis, myasthenia gravis, and muscular dystrophy.
4. Depression of brain function. Causes include drug overdose, hypoxia, and injury to the hypothalamus.

The second form of respiratory failure is either failure of gas exchange because of insufficient diffusion of gases through the tissue or inadequate blood supply to pick up or release gases. This is called a **ventilation–perfusion mismatch.** This means that either enough blood is present for the exchange but there is not enough oxygen, or ventilation is adequate and oxygen is present but there is not enough blood supply to match the gas that is present. A ventilation–perfusion mismatch may occur because of:

1. Destruction of the surface area of the alveoli for gas exchange. Causes include lung diseases such as chronic bronchitis and emphysema.
2. Inadequate circulation in the lungs. Causes include pulmonary embolism.

The result of either type of respiratory failure is generalized hypoxia affecting all body systems, especially the brain. Respiratory acidosis usually develops because of retention of carbon dioxide. Recall from Chapter 3 that high levels of CO_2 will lower the pH of the blood, causing acidosis, which has many ill effects. Unresolved respiratory failure leads to fatal anoxia. The pathogenesis of both types of respiratory failure is depicted in Figure 11–8.

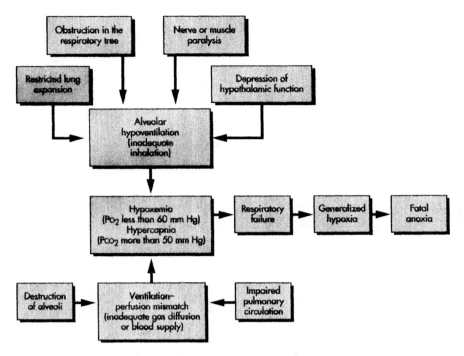

Figure 11–8. The pathogenesis of respiratory failure.

One form of respiratory failure is insufficient air movement into the lungs. This results in _____(1). Alveolar hypoventilation occurs because of some blockage or _____(2) in the _____(3); restriction of movement of the _____(4) wall or _____(5) of the lungs; paralysis of _____(6) or _____(7); or depression of _____(8) function. The other form of failure can occur because of a mismatch between _____(9) and _____(10). Either there is enough _____(11) present but the _____(12) supply is insufficient, or there is enough blood supply but the amount of _____(13) is insufficient. A ventilation–perfusion mismatch may occur if large areas for _____(14) are destroyed by lung disease, or if _____(15) in the lungs is inadequate.

1. alveolar hypoventilation
2. obstruction
3. respiratory tree
4. chest
5. expansion
6. nerves
7. muscles
8. brain
9. ventilation
10. perfusion
11. oxygen
12. blood
13. oxygen
14. gas exchange
15. circulation

▶ ATELECTASIS

Atelectasis simply means collapse of the lungs. This extreme disturbance in ventilation is not a primary disease process, but is secondary to some cause. In many disease states, small localized collapses in the lungs occur with little overall effect on the process of ventilation. However, atelectasis of entire lobes, or of one or both lungs, produces dyspnea that can be severe and lead to death by anoxia. There are two general causes of atelectasis. The *first* is compression of the lungs (pressure applied to them), which comes from the pleural cavity. This can be due to:

1. Air in the pleural space (pneumothorax), which displaces the negative pressure and creates a positive pressure. Positive pressure on the outside of the lungs will collapse them, since negative pressure keeps them expanded. Air may gain entry into the pleural space if in emphysema a bulla ruptures, or if there is traumatic puncture of the lungs.
2. Mechanical pressure by fluid in the pleural space, such as occurs during pleural effusion. The effusion may be a transudate in the case of congestive heart failure, or an exudate in

424   CHAPTER 11 THE RESPIRATORY SYSTEM

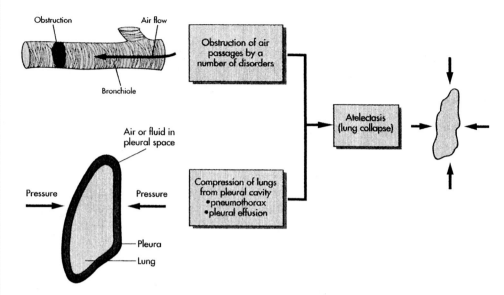

Figure 11–9. Causes of atelectasis.

the case of infection or inflammation. The fluid may also be pus, which defines the condition empyema. These concepts will be presented again in Section VI on pleural diseases.

······· 11–65 ·······

1. collapse
2. compression
3. pleural
4. obstruction
5. air
6. fluid
7. negative
8. expanded
9. mechanical
10. alveoli
11. collapse

The *second* general cause of atelectasis is obstruction of air passages, which prevents inflation of the alveoli. After a while, the air that was present before the obstruction occurred is absorbed, leaving none in the air sacs so they collapse. Any of the previous obstructions we have discussed can cause atelectasis. Whether the collapse is localized or widespread depends on the site of obstruction. The higher up in the respiratory tree that it occurs, the greater the degree of collapse. The causes of atelectasis are summarized in Figure 11–9. Atelectasis means _____(1) of the lungs. It will occur because of _____(2) of the lungs from the _____(3) space, or because of _____(4) somewhere in the respiratory tree. In the case of compression by the pleural cavity, the presence of either _____(5) or _____(6) will cause collapse. The presence of air disrupts the _____(7) pressure in the pleural space, which is normally responsible for keeping the lungs _____(8). Fluid causes _____(9) pressure against the lungs. Obstruction prevents inhalation of further air, so that the _____(10) soon run out of air and _____(11). Widespread atelectasis causes extreme dyspnea to the point of fatality if it is not corrected. If the cause of the collapse is identified quickly and is able to be corrected, the probability of re-expansion and ventilation is good. The causes of disturbances in ventilation that you have studied are reviewed in Table 11–3.

TABLE 11–3. CAUSES OF VENTILATION DISTURBANCE

Pneumonia
COPD—chronic bronchitis, emphysema, bronchiectasis
Asthma
Suffocation
Drowning
Adult respiratory distress syndrome
Respiratory failure
Atelectasis

▶ PNEUMOCONIOSES

The last few examples of pulmonary disorders in this section are inhalation-based diseases. An inhalation-based disease is one in which the injury to the lungs is a primary result of breathing a foreign substance. The substance is generally a chemical that is carried by dust. Large dust particles get filtered out in the nasal passages and do not reach the lungs. The real danger occurs when an irritating substance is found in very fine dust that easily reaches all the way into the alveoli. The substance causes chronic irritation of the interstitial tissue in particular. **Pneumoconioses** are pulmonary disorders that are inhalation based, or are caused by inhaling an irritant. They are a group of *chronic, noninfectious interstitial diseases.* Pneumoconioses are all chronic disorders, because the irritant must be inspired for a long time before there is noticeable damage. Pneumoconiosis can also be described as environmentally induced fibrosis of the lungs, since a major feature is fibrosis of the interstitium. The presence of fibrosis interferes with gas exchange as well as lung expansion, so pneumoconiosis is also a *restrictive* lung disease. Pneumoconioses are pulmonary disorders caused by _____(1) certain irritants that are carried by _____(2) over a _____(3) period of time. The site of injury is the _____(4) tissue. Pneumoconioses is environmentally stimulated _____(5) of the lungs. The presence of scar tissue causes it to be called a _____(6) lung disease as well.

1. inhaling
2. dust
3. long
4. interstitial
5. fibrosis
6. restrictive

The development of a pneumoconiosis is because of long-term occupational exposure, where the harmful substances are carried by dust. In many cases there is a predisposition to develop tuberculosis, because the cells of defense that normally keep this infection in check are occupied with this primary lung disease. The first example of pneumoconiosis is **silicosis.** Silica particles are very reactive in living tissue and incite much inflammation and fibrosis. Silicosis is the most widespread of the pneumoconioses and causes the most damage. Silica is found in many industrial environments, including mining for gold, tin, and coal; metal grinding; sandblasting; stoneworking; and glass cutting.

Inhaled silica found in the bronchi is picked up by phagocytic cells, such as macrophages, and transported across the walls and into the interstitial tissue. As a foreign body, silica stimulates destructive inflammation, and this is followed by significant fibrosis that destroys lung tissue. Immune-mediated damage is also added if the silica combines with body proteins to form an antigen. Removing the source of exposure is not curative, since this condition gets progressively worse. The surface area for gas exchange is permanently destroyed by the activities and repair efforts of inflammation. Clinically, the picture is one of chronic dyspnea. Eventually, the fibrosis around the vessels is so restrictive that the pressure in the vessels rises, and pulmonary hypertension results. As the right side of the heart expends excessive energy to pump blood through the fibrosed septa, right heart failure is not uncommon. This condition (right heart failure as a result of lung disease) is called cor _____(1). In severe cases respiratory failure occurs. There is no specific treatment for silicosis short of a lung transplant. Efforts must be directed towards its prevention by the use of industrial ventilation and filtering masks. Pneumoconioses develop as a result of long-term _____(2) exposure. Substances are inhaled with the _____(3) in the air. The most common and severe pneumoconiosis is _____(4), and the irritant is _____(5). Silica is very _____(6) in tissue, so there is significant inflammation. Injury to lung tissue is the result of destructive _____(7) activity, and of the _____(8) that follows inflammation. Complications of silicosis include increased pressure in the pulmonary vessels, called _____(9), and cor pulmonale, which is _____(10) failure because of lung disease. Pulmonary hypertension and cor pulmonale are because of the restrictive presence of _____(11) in the interstitial tissue.

1. pulmonale
2. occupational
3. dust
4. silicosis
5. silica
6. reactive
7. inflammatory
8. fibrosis
9. pulmonary hypertension
10. right heart
11. fibrosis

11-69

Anthracosis is commonly called coal worker's lung or black lung. Carbon accumulates in the lungs from breathing coal dust. Carbon is an inert material compared to silica and, being less reactive, causes minimal damage. Coal miners are obviously the targeted population for this disorder. Historically, city dwellers were also at risk from breathing soot-laden air, when coal was used as a heat source. Anthracosis is a concern when hard coal is the agent in the environment, since it contains silica. Significant injury in anthracosis occurs from the presence of silica in hard coal. Clinically, most cases are mild and only rarely progress to the severity of silicosis.

11-70

1. neoplasia, cancer, or malignancy

Asbestosis is a well-known pneumoconiosis, since the dangers of asbestos are commonly known. This insoluble particle can be inhaled when working with asbestos rock, or with older building material containing asbestos. Before the danger of asbestos was known, it was widely used in insulation and fireproofing materials. The harmful form of asbestos is not used in materials today. However, *many* older buildings contain asbestos. Asbestosis is a concern when remodeling these buildings, removing old material, or causing their demolition. Undisturbed materials containing asbestos pose less of a threat, since the material is inhaled when dust is created by disturbing the materials. Asbestos particles lead to interstitial fibrosis in much the same way as silica. The results of asbestosis are like silicosis. In addition, asbestos seems to be a carcinogen. A carcinogen is a substance that has been linked to the development of _____(1) (see Chap. 6). Victims of asbestosis have a tendency to develop primary lung cancer, as well as a rare tumor of the pleura associated almost exclusively with asbestosis. The dyspnea seen in asbestosis is caused by fibrosis, as it is in silicosis. Fibrosis causes restriction of respiratory movements and interferes with gas exchange. In asbestosis, in contrast to silicosis, it is rare for the condition to progress to respiratory failure. However, if cancer develops, the demise of the patient is usually related to that.

11-71

1. carbon or coal dust
2. inert
3. silica
4. asbestos
5. old
6. disturbed
7. silicosis
8. fibrosis
9. cancer

In anthracosis, the inhaled substance is _____(1). The carbon in coal is not very reactive, so it is described as _____(2). Significant injury in anthracosis is because of the presence of _____(3) in hard coal. Asbestosis is pneumoconiosis that develops as a result of inhaling _____(4). This material is found in _____(5) building materials. The threat of asbestosis is a concern when these materials are _____(6). The pathogenesis of asbestosis is like _____(7), and the result is interstitial _____(8). Asbestos particles appear to be carcinogenic, so lung and pleural _____(9) may accompany asbestosis.

1. c—widespread lung damage that can result from a variety of diseases or injuries

2. a—shock

IV. REVIEW QUESTIONS

1. Adult respiratory distress syndrome is:
    a. a congenital insufficiency of surfactant that doesn't surface until adulthood
    b. a chronic obstructive pulmonary disease
    c. widespread lung damage that can result from a variety of diseases or injuries
    d. another phrase for respiratory failure

2. The most common cause of ARDS is:
    a. shock
    b. respiratory failure
    c. acute noninfectious interstitial disease
    d. chronic noninfectious interstitial disease

3. A P_{O_2} of less than 60 mm Hg is medically termed a. _____. A P_{CO_2} of greater than 50 mm Hg is medically termed b. _____. These findings indicate the state of respiratory c. _____.

4. In respiratory failure, obstruction of the airways or restriction in lung expansion causes:
   a. acute interstitial disease
   b. alveolar hypoventilation
   c. ARDS
   d. ventilation–perfusion mismatch

5. In respiratory failure, destruction of surface areas for gas exchange or interruption in pulmonary blood supply causes:
   a. chronic interstitial disease
   b. ventilation–perfusion mismatch
   c. alveolar hypoventilation
   d. pulmonary embolism

6. Choose the correct statement about atelectasis:
   a. The term means collapse of the lungs.
   b. It may be caused by compression of the lungs during pleural disease.
   c. It may be caused by obstruction of the airways in which remaining air is absorbed.
   d. All of the above are correct.
   e. None of the above are correct.

7. Long-term inhalation of an irritating chemical in dust, which is often an occupational exposure, is called:
   a. farmer's lung
   b. pneumoconiosis
   c. hypersensitivity pneumonitis
   d. furrier's lung

8. The primary injury associated with pneumoconioses is:
   a. interstitial fibrosis
   b. alveolitis
   c. alveolar fibrosis
   d. primary lung cancer

9. In pneumoconioses, the chemical that causes the most tissue reaction and damage is a. _____. The chemical often associated with the development of cancer is b. _____.

3. a–hypoxemia; b–hypercapnia; c–failure

4. b–alveolar hypoventilation

5. b–ventilation–perfusion mismatch

6. d–All of the above are correct.

7. b–pneumoconiosis

8. a–interstitial fibrosis

9. a–silica; b–asbestos

V. VASCULAR DISORDERS AND NEOPLASIA ◀ SECTION

▶ PULMONARY HYPERTENSION

11–72

We begin our discussion in this section with vascular disorders affecting the lungs. The circulation through the lungs is a low-pressure system compared to the general circulation. Resistance to blood flow is typically minimal. **Pulmonary hypertension** occurs when pressure in this system is increased, which also increases resistance to flow. Pressure and resistance increases when the arteries are narrowed from chronic lung disease, when they are obstructed by many small emboli or a few large ones, or when the respiratory circulation is

1. right
2. lungs
3. resistance
4. pulmonary hypertension
5. narrowing
6. obstruction
7. overload
8. left

overloaded with blood. This overload develops during left-sided heart failure, congestive heart failure, mitral valve stenosis, or in some congenital defects of the heart. Whether the cause of pulmonary hypertension is secondary to lung disease, or to left-sided heart failure, the sequela is cor pulmonale. You know that cor pulmonale is failure of the _____(1) side of the heart as a direct result of pathology in the _____(2). The hypertension, or increased resistance in the circulation of the lungs, creates additional work for the right ventricle as it tries to pump blood through the lungs. If pressure in the pulmonary circulation increases, this increases _____(3) to blood flow. Increased pressure and therefore increased resistance defines _____(4). Pulmonary hypertension can be secondary to the _____(5) of pulmonary arteries, the _____(6) of these arteries by emboli, or by a (an) _____(7) of blood in the lungs. Hypervolemia or excessive blood can occur in the lungs because of pathology in the _____(8) side of the heart.

▶ PULMONARY EDEMA

1. edema
2. pulmonary edema
3. pressure
4. interstitial
5. alveoli
6. air
7. breathe

Pulmonary edema is a relatively common respiratory tract disorder responsible for serious, potentially life-threatening effects. It is the presence of tissue fluid in the septa and alveoli. You know that the presence of fluid in tissues in excess of normal is called _____(1). Edema develops as a result of increased pressure at the venous end of a capillary bed. The pressure squeezes excessive amounts of fluid out of the vessels. Having fluid in the air sacs naturally interferes with breathing. The degree of dyspnea is proportional to the amount of fluid in the lungs. Pulmonary edema severe enough to cause death is very much like drowning. Edema is first present in the interstitial tissue where it has been squeezed from the vessels. At first, the excess fluid is drained away by the lymphatic system. Later, draining efforts are not enough and fluid accumulates in the septa. Then, as fluid flows into the alveoli and fills the air sacs, it displaces the air. Fluid in the septa and air sacs of the lungs is called _____(2). The fluid arrives there because of increased _____(3) in the venules and veins. Edema is present first in the _____(4) tissue (septa) and then flows into the _____(5), where it displaces _____(6). Dyspnea results because it is difficult to _____(7) through fluid.

1. extremities
2. resistance
3. expansion
4. edema
5. lungs

Edema formation in the lungs is different from formation elsewhere in the body. In the extremities, connective tissue is firm and compact. It provides resistance to the fluid escaping from the vessels. It limits the degree of edema, because its own expansion is limited. The resistance works like a compression bandage to limit swelling. The formation of edema is stopped at some point because of limited expansion. In the lungs, the connective tissue is loose and spongy. The absence of tissue resistance, or tissue tension, allows greater amounts of edema to form. Edema forms in the lungs to a greater degree than in the _____(1) because there is much less _____(2) by the connective tissue in the lungs. In the extremities, tissue tension limits the amount of _____(3) that the tissue will undergo. Therefore, this limits the amount of _____(4) formation. There is much less resistance to expansion in the _____(5).

There are several abnormal states that can cause pulmonary edema. The most common causes are left-sided and congestive heart failure. The blood volume in the lungs becomes overloaded because blood backs up behind the failing left ventricle. This overload with blood, or hyperemia, increases the pressure in the pulmonary veins. As you will recall, when this backup of blood develops in the rest of the body, it is called congestion. Pulmonary congestion leads to pulmonary edema, as a result of the congestion. In addition to pulmonary edema (fluid inside the lungs), congestion and increased pressure may cause fluid buildup outside of the lungs, in the pleural space. This is called **hydrothorax.** Hydrothorax can also interfere with breathing or cause dyspnea. The mechanism differs from edema. Instead of displacing the air in alveoli, hydrothorax restricts or limits expansion of the lungs and makes inhalation less effective. The most common causes of pulmonary edema are _____(1) and _____(2). Blood backing up behind the site of failure causes the lungs to become _____(3) with blood. This increases _____(4) in the pulmonary veins. This situation is called pulmonary _____(5), and it leads to _____(6) formation. If fluid accumulates in the pleural space, this is called _____(7). Hydrothorax causes _____(8) by limiting _____(9) of the lungs and therefore limiting the act of _____(10).

1. left-sided heart failure
2. congestive heart failure
3. overloaded
4. pressure
5. congestion
6. edema
7. hydrothorax
8. dyspnea
9. expansion
10. inhalation

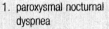

Recall from Chapter 10, on heart disease, that an episode of extreme breathing difficulty, which happens at night while lying down, is called paroxysmal nocturnal dyspnea. This is acute, significant edema formation that is life threatening. This condition has also been called **cardiac asthma,** because the dyspnea resembles a severe asthma attack and is caused by the heart. Other causes of pulmonary edema include:

1. paroxysmal nocturnal dyspnea
2. cardiac asthma

1. Lobar and bronchopneumonia.
2. Electrical shock, which diverts blood to the lungs.
3. Inhalation of some toxic gases, which damages capillary endothelium.
4. Peripheral vasoconstriction, which diverts blood to the lungs.
5. Iatrogenic overload of the general circulation during intravenous therapy. This is most likely to occur in cases of existing congestive heart failure.

Auscultation of the chest in cases of pulmonary edema reveals characteristic rales, in which the abnormal breath sounds are bubbly and moist sounding. Fluid densities can be seen on chest x-ray. Treatment of pulmonary edema must be directed at the inciting cause and should include the use of diuretics to increase water loss from the body. Life-threatening pulmonary edema occurring at night is called _____(1), or sometimes called _____(2) because the cause is heart disease. The pathogenesis of pulmonary edema is reviewed in Figure 11–10.

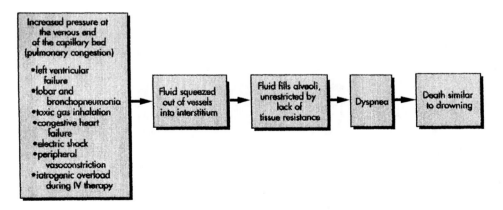

Figure 11–10. The pathogenesis of pulmonary edema.

► PULMONARY EMBOLISM

11–77

1. mass or foreign body
2. circulation
3. thrombus or clot
4. embolism
5. thrombophlebitis

If you will recall, an embolus is a mass or foreign body traveling freely in the circulation. It can be made of several things, such as fat or a clump of bacteria or neoplastic cells. The most common embolus is a thrombus or clot that has broken away from its site of formation. An embolism is a situation in which the traveling mass wedges in a vessel and obstructs blood flow. A **pulmonary embolism** is a mass that has reached the circulation in the lungs and is lodged there. The most common reason for pulmonary embolism is thrombophlebitis. In Chapter 9 you learned that thrombophlebitis is thrombosis or clot formation in the deep veins of the extremities, usually the legs. Breaking off of a piece of this clot gives rise to an embolus, which finds its way to the lungs through the normal path of circulation. Occasionally, a clot may form on the inside wall of the right heart in response to sluggish flow or endocardial injury. This can also give rise to an embolus that travels the short distance to the pulmonary circulation. An embolus is a _____(1) moving freely through the _____(2). The most common embolus is a _____(3). If the embolus gets caught in a vessel and obstructs blood flow, this is called a (an) _____(4). The most common cause of pulmonary embolism is _____(5).

11–78

1. double
2. pathology or disease
3. both

Normally, an embolism can lead to infarction if the affected vessel is completely occluded and blood supply to the local tissue is halted. (Remember that infarction is tissue death or necrosis because of interruption in blood supply.) In the lungs, the blood supply comes from both the aorta (through the bronchial arteries) and from the right heart (through the pulmonary artery). Therefore, because of this double supply, a pulmonary embolism may or may not produce an infarction. However, if there is pathology in both of these vascular systems, an embolism is more likely to cause infarction. An example of this is congestive heart failure, in which supply through the bronchial arteries is compromised. If an embolism then develops in the pulmonary artery, an infarct is likely. This is illustrated in Figure 11–11. Normally, pulmonary embolism is less likely to cause infarction in the lungs, because these organs have a _____(1) blood supply. Infarction has a greater chance of developing if there is _____(2) of _____(3) of these separate supplies.

11–79

The most serious consequence of pulmonary embolism occurs if a large embolus becomes wedged at the fork or bifurcation of the pulmonary artery. This can cause massive infarction of the lungs and death. Any time a blockage occurs in the larger arteries, this produces more tissue death because more tissue is left without circulation. The bifurcation of the pulmonary artery is a branching that leads to many smaller vessels that perfuse many areas of the lungs. A large embolus can also cause acute cor pulmonale when the pressure behind the obstruc-

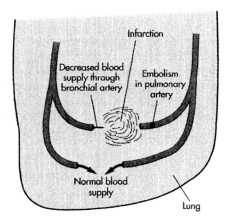

Figure 11–11. Pulmonary embolism and infarction.

tion suddenly rises, which creates tremendous resistance for the right heart. Massive infarction of the lungs can occur if a _____(1) embolus lodges at the _____(2) of the _____(3). Blockage at this site cuts off _____(4) for many areas of the _____(5). The development of cor pulmonale during a large pulmonary embolism is because the _____(6) behind the occlusion rises and causes _____(7) for the right heart.

1. large
2. bifurcation or fork
3. pulmonary artery
4. circulation or blood supply
5. lungs
6. pressure
7. resistance

11-80

The clinical signs of pulmonary embolism vary greatly according to the degree of obstruction. A small embolism may go unnoticed or may cause chest pain. Remember that ischemia causes pain in the affected tissue. An embolism large enough to cause significant infarction produces dyspnea, tachypnea, pain, and hemoptysis. Massive embolism and infarction quickly lead to cyanosis, shock, and death.

▶ LARYNGEAL CANCER

11-81

We will end this section with a discussion of major neoplastic conditions affecting the respiratory system. The first condition is **carcinoma of the larynx,** or **laryngeal cancer.** The larynx is the entryway into the lungs by way of the trachea. It sits at the top of the trachea. The larynx houses the epiglottis, a tissue flap that prevents fluids and food from entering the trachea or windpipe. It also is the site of the vocal cords. For this reason the larynx is sometimes called the "voicebox." Laryngeal cancer is not common in the general population. It is seen largely in heavy smokers, especially those with a long history of heavy alcohol consumption. The type of malignancy is *squamous cell carcinoma,* which can invade any part of the laryngeal structures. Grossly, laryngeal cancer appears as either a large nodule, or nodules, or in ulcer form. This malignancy invades locally and will also metastasize or spread to the lymph nodes of the neck. Untreated laryngeal cancer will metastasize to distant sites. Carcinoma of the larynx causes dyspnea if the cancer is in large nodular form, a form commonly called a tumor. Other clinical manifestations include sore throat, hoarseness, and loss of the voice. Because these signs appear early and are quite noticeable, laryngeal cancer is usually detected early. Therefore, treatment occurs early and the prognosis is relatively good. Treatment consists of surgically excising or removing the tumor or ulcerated area. Radiation can also be effective. The 5-year survival rate of treated laryngeal cancer is about 75 percent.

11-82

Neoplasia of the voice box is usually referred to as _____(1) or _____(2). This malignancy occurs most often in those who _____(3) heavily and combine this habit with heavy _____(4) intake over a long period of time. Laryngeal cancer is of the _____(5) type. It may take the form of a _____(6) or a (an) _____(7). Untreated carcinoma of the larynx will _____(8) locally, or _____(9) to distant organs. Because of prominent signs, this malignancy is usually found _____(10) in the course of the disease.

1. carcinoma of the larynx
2. laryngeal cancer
3. smoke
4. alcohol
5. squamous cell carcinoma
6. nodule
7. ulcer
8. invade
9. metastasize
10. early

▶ PRIMARY LUNG CANCER

11-83

Primary lung cancer is neoplasia that originates in the lungs. It has not spread there from other sites. **Bronchoalveolar carcinoma** is an adenocarcinoma arising not from the respiratory tree, but from the parenchyma of the lungs. In particular, it arises from the alveoli. This primary lung cancer is not caused by smoking, in contrast to our next topic. It is not a common malignancy. If detected early, there is about a 50 percent cure rate after surgical excision. When we think of lung cancer, the form we usually mean is **bronchogenic carcinoma.** Of all cancer that doesn't involve the skin, this form of lung cancer rates among the top three in occurrence, along with breast and colon cancer. It is the most prevalent cause of death from malignancy. Bronchogenic carcinoma is neoplasia of the largest airways in the respira-

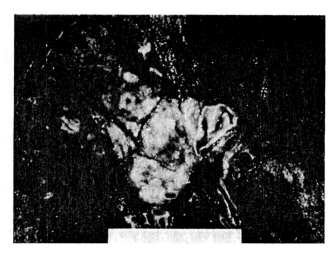

Figure 11–12. Bronchogenic carcinoma. *(From Kent and Hart,* Introduction to Human Disease, *3rd ed., Appleton & Lange.)*

1. primary lung cancer
2. bronchogenic carcinoma
3. largest airways
4. cigarette smoking

tory tree. This tumor is pictured in Figure 11–12. The two leading causes of bronchogenic carcinoma are asbestosis and, more commonly, cigarette smoking. The incidence of lung cancer correlates directly with number of packs smoked per day, along with the number of years the patient has smoked. Cases of lung cancer are seen occasionally in other populations and may be linked with heavy air pollution or industrial fumes. Malignancy that starts or originates in the lungs is called _____(1). The most common form is _____(2), which is cancer of the _____(3) in the respiratory tree. Bronchogenic carcinoma is most often associated with or caused by _____(4).

11–84

1. squamous cell carcinoma
2. adenocarcinoma
3. carcinogens
4. initiation
5. promotion
6. metaplasia
7. squamous cell epithelium
8. adenocarcinoma

There are four histologic types of bronchogenic carcinoma. The two most common are *squamous cell carcinoma* (SCC) and *adenocarcinoma*. The tar component of tobacco smoke contains chemicals (polycyclic hydrocarbons) that are considered carcinogens. Recall from Chapter 6 the concept of carcinogens as either initiators or promoters of cancer, or both. Chemicals in cigarette smoke act as both initiators and promoters of lung cancer. They cause the transformation of normal cells into malignant ones. First, pseudostratified columnar epithelium lining the bronchi undergo metaplasia or a change in form. They become squamous cell epithelium. Metaplasia can be reversible if the cause is removed. Beyond this, the cells become neoplastic. This change to squamous cells is why the SCC form is commonly seen. Adenocarcinoma is associated with neoplastic transformation of the glandular cells. The two most common histologic types of primary lung cancer are _____(1) and _____(2). Chemicals in the tar of tobacco smoke are thought to be _____(3), which can cause both _____(4) and _____(5) of cancer. Pseudostratified columnar epithelium goes through the process of _____(6) and becomes _____(7). Cancer of the glandular cells is called _____(8).

11–85

Of the cases of lung cancer, only about 20 percent have not spread or invaded by the time of diagnosis. In these relatively early cases, about 12 percent may be cured with treatment. In the majority of cases, several manifestations have usually developed by the time of diagnosis. These may include any of the following:

1. A high degree of local invasion with movement of the cancer from the bronchi to the pleural membrane, into the mediastinum, and into the lymph nodes of the chest and neck. About 70 percent of cases have advanced to the invasive state by the time of diagnosis.
2. Invasion of nerves that run through the chest.

3. Obstruction of the airway by the tumor, which causes either local atelectasis after the remaining air is absorbed, or bronchiectasis. Atelectasis means the section of lung has _____(1), and bronchiectasis is permanent _____(2) of the bronchi.

4. Obstruction also causes accumulation of secretions in the airways, and the trapping of microorganisms. This easily leads to pneumonia or abscess formation. Pneumonia may be the cause of death before the malignancy causes death.

5. Distant metastasis through the circulation to the liver, brain, or bones (the most common organs that are invaded).

Travel by the cancerous lung cells to structures in the chest is called local _____(3). The tumor may block or _____(4) the air passages, causing _____(5) or _____(6). It may predispose the patient to developing fatal _____(7).

1. collapsed
2. dilation
3. invasion
4. obstruct
5. atelectasis
6. bronchiectasis
7. pneumonia

11-86

Some of the clinical features of lung cancer are common to any type of malignancy. These are pain, anorexia, weight loss and cachexia, and weakness. Features specific for lung cancer include dyspnea (from bronchial obstruction), chronic cough (from bronchial irritation), frequent lung infections, and hemoptysis. Hemoptysis occurs if the tumor erodes into a blood vessel and causes bleeding. The smoker who has lost a lot of weight and has a bloody cough should be evaluated immediately for lung cancer. Distant spread will produce signs according to the invaded organ. There may be evidence of liver malfunction, neurologic disorder, or pathologic (disease-caused) bone fractures. Another aspect of primary bronchogenic carcinoma is paraneoplastic syndrome. If you remember from Chapter 6, this is the secretion of hormone-like chemicals by the tumor. The chemicals in this instance mimic parathyroid hormone, adrenocorticotropic hormone, and antidiuretic hormone. Disorders may arise from the reaction of the body to these fake hormones. Lung cancer is first suspected from the appearance of a chest x-ray. It can only be confirmed by cytology of the sputum, a bronchial wash, or a biopsy. A biopsy is accomplished with the use of a bronchoscope, a lit tube inserted into the trachea. In the few cases diagnosed as early bronchial cancer, surgical excision offers a fair prognosis if invasion or metastasis has not occurred. In most cases, metastasis has occurred and radiation and chemotherapy are used to extend life. The prognosis is poor, with about a 10 percent 5-year survival rate. Primary lung cancer is considered incurable for the most part.

▶ SECONDARY LUNG CANCER

11-87

Secondary lung cancer is malignancy in the lungs that has metastasized there from some other primary site. It is metastatic neoplasia or a metastasis. The lungs are a very common site for metastasis to occur. If you will remember, this spread of cancer cells is by way of the circulation. Clumps of tumor cells get filtered out in the tiny capillaries of the lungs and grow there. Neoplastic cells in the lymphatic circulation also end up in the lungs. Both carcinomas (cancer of epithelial tissues) and sarcomas (cancer of connective tissues) will spread to the lungs. The most common primary malignancies to move to the lungs are cancers of the breast, colon, liver, stomach, ovaries, cervix, and kidneys. If on an x-ray it can be shown there is only a single tumor, its excision affords a fair prognosis. More likely, there are multiple defined lesions, which are described as a "cannonball" pattern; or the malignancy appears in a diffuse (spread-out) pattern. The presence of widespread cancerous lesions offers no hope in the postponement of death. Cancer of the lungs that has arrived there from some other site is called _____(1). Metastatic lung cancer is _____(2) common/uncommon (circle one). The two major classifications of neoplasia, _____(3) and _____(4), will both spread to the lungs through either the _____(5) or the _____(6) system. Give three examples of organ cancer that will metastasize to the lungs: _____(7), _____(8), and _____(9).

1. secondary lung cancer
2. common
3. carcinomas
4. sarcomas
5. bloodstream or circulation
6. lymphatic
7., 8., and 9. breast, colon, liver, stomach, ovaries, cervix, kidneys (any three of these)

V. REVIEW QUESTIONS

1. d–pulmonary hypertension

2. b–pulmonary edema

3. d–Paroxysmal nocturnal dyspnea is also called cardiac shock.

4. c–clots from the deep leg veins (thrombophlebitis)

5. a–the embolus becomes lodged in the major bifurcation of the pulmonary artery

6. c–laryngeal carcinoma

7. c–either nodules or ulcers

8. a–bronchogenic carcinoma

1. If the arteries in the lungs become narrowed from disease, or if the lungs are overloaded with blood, this may cause:
   a. cor pulmonale
   b. pulmonary edema
   c. pulmonary embolism
   d. pulmonary hypertension

2. Excessive tissue fluid in the interstitial tissue and in the alveoli is:
   a. pulmonary embolism
   b. pulmonary edema
   c. pulmonary hypertension
   d. pulmonary infarction

3. Choose the INCORRECT statement about pulmonary edema:
   a. Edema forms to a greater extent in the lungs because there is less resistance in this spongy tissue.
   b. The most common cause of pulmonary edema is heart failure.
   c. Events preceding edema are hypervolemia, increased pressure, and pulmonary congestion.
   d. Paroxysmal nocturnal dyspnea is also called cardiac shock.

4. The most common cause of pulmonary embolism is:
   a. clots from the wall of the right heart (mural thrombosis)
   b. septic emboli
   c. clots from the deep leg veins (thrombophlebitis)
   d. neoplastic emboli

5. Massive infarction and death may occur during pulmonary embolism if:
   a. the embolus becomes lodged in the major bifurcation of the pulmonary artery
   b. the embolus becomes lodged in a smaller branch of the pulmonary artery
   c. the embolus becomes lodged in any branch of the bronchial artery
   d. any of the above locations will cause massive infarction and death

6. "Throat cancer," seen in heavy smokers who also drink to excess, is properly described as:
   a. mesothelioma
   b. bronchogenic carcinoma
   c. laryngeal carcinoma
   d. bronchoalveolar carcinoma

7. The condition described in Question 6 will appear as:
   a. nodules
   b. ulcers
   c. either nodules or ulcers
   d. none of the above

8. Common primary lung cancer is properly described as:
   a. bronchogenic carcinoma
   b. bronchoalveolar carcinoma
   c. metastatic pulmonary carcinoma
   d. pulmonary carcinoma

9. The most common cause of primary lung cancer is:
   a. asbestosis
   b. smoking
   c. metastases
   d. idiopathic

10. In primary lung cancer, metaplasia of pseudostratified columnar epithelium eventually leads to:
    a. adenocarcinoma
    b. mesothelioma
    c. undifferentiated carcinoma
    d. squamous cell carcinoma

11. In primary lung cancer, bronchiectasis, atelectasis, and pneumonia may result from:
    a. invasion of local structures in the chest
    b. metastasis to other sites
    c. obstruction in the respiratory tree
    d. any of the above

12. Malignancy of the lungs that has spread there from a primary site is called a. _____.

9. b–smoking

10. d–squamous cell carcinoma

11. c–obstruction in the respiratory tree

12. a–secondary lung cancer

VI. OTHER DISORDERS OF THE RESPIRATORY SYSTEM ◄ SECTION

► DISEASES OF THE PLEURA

11-88

The pleural membrane is made of two layers. The layer that covers the outside of the lungs is the visceral pleura, and the layer that lines the inside of the thorax or chest is the parietal pleura. The area between these two layers is the pleural space or cavity. Normally, this is a potential space, meaning that the area is collapsed between the two layers. It contains only a small amount of serous fluid to lubricate the movements of respiration. But it has the potential to become an actual cavity if it fills with fluid or air. This forms the basis for several pleural diseases, which are illustrated in Figure 11–13. The pressure in the pleural cav-

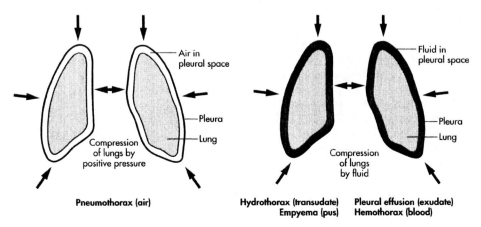

Figure 11–13. Disease of the pleura.

ity is negative, or less than the pressure inside of the lungs. It is this pressure difference that helps keep the lungs expanded.

If air should enter the pleural cavity, this space now has a positive pressure. This pushes on the lungs from all sides, causing them to collapse. The term for collapsed lung is _____(1). This condition is called **pneumothorax,** which literally means air in the chest cavity. The cause of pneumothorax can be external or internal. External causes introduce air from the atmosphere, and these include stab wounds, gunshot wounds, or fractured ribs that protrude outward. Internal causes release air from inside the lungs, and these include the rupture of bullae in emphysema and fractured ribs that puncture the lungs. Atelectasis caused by pneumothorax can be quite severe, depending on the amount of air in the pleural cavity. Clinically, this causes severe dyspnea and even cyanosis. Severe pneumothorax is a life-threatening state and must be treated on a emergency basis. In a procedure called **pleurocentesis,** extreme dyspnea is relieved by removing the air through aspiration. A catheter is placed into the pleural cavity and the air is drawn out. This allows the lungs to reinflate. If the original cause of the pneumothorax can be successfully treated, usually with surgical repair, the prognosis is good for permanent reinflation and function. Air in the pleural space is called _____(2). The presence of pneumothorax causes the lungs to _____(3). The air may be introduced from the _____(4) by penetrating trauma, or it may come from inside the _____(5) in certain diseases. Atelectasis produces the clinical sign of _____(6), which if severe enough leads to visible deficiency in oxygen or _____(7).

Before we discuss the next pleural disorder, we need to review the difference between a transudate and an exudate. A transudate is tissue fluid outside of the vessels that does not contain very much protein or any cells. It occurs in conditions that are *not* due to inflammation. An exudate is tissue fluid loaded with both protein and cells, and it *is* associated with inflammation. The presence of tissue fluid in the pleural space is called either **hydrothorax** or **pleural effusion.** In hydrothorax (water in the chest), the fluid is a transudate. It is most often caused by congestive heart failure, which you will recall results in generalized edema. In pleural effusion, the fluid is an exudate. It is most often associated with inflammation of the pleura. This inflammation is called **pleuritis** or **pleurisy.** If you will remember, inflammation creates an effusion that is an exudate. Pleuritis is often an infectious state and it has spread there from a lung infection. Examples are the spread of bacterial pneumonia (in which the exudate can be purulent), and viral pneumonia (in which the exudate is more serous). Tuberculosis is another lung infection that can move into the pleura and create pleural effusion. Pleurisy also occurs as a result of tumors of the lungs, or with a penetrating injury. These last examples cause inflammation that is not based on infection, but exudate is still produced. Transudate fluid in the chest cavity is called _____(1). Exudate fluid in the chest cavity is called _____(2). The difference between these two fluids is whether or not they are associated with the process of _____(3). Hydrothorax is not associated with _____(4), but _____(5) is a result of inflammation. Inflammation of the pleura is called _____(6) or _____(7). Often, it is an extension of _____(8) from the lungs.

The presence of a significant amount of fluid will cause the same results as pneumothorax, that is, collapse of the lungs. If you will remember from Frame 11–64, as we discussed atelectasis, pleural disorders were cited as a major cause. A complication of pleuritis that produces a purulent exudate is the formation of **adhesions,** thick bands of scar tissue that run from one free surface to another. The adhesions form as a result of the high amount of fibrin in the exudate. Their presence can limit lung expansion or movement, so this is a restrictive state. Clinically, pleuritis or pleurisy is seen as extremely painful inspirations because of all the nerves that are affected. Taking a breath creates stabbing pain. Fluid in the pleural space is easily seen on x-ray and a portion can be sampled to determine the cause. First, the fluid must be characterized as transudate or exudate by testing protein levels and looking for inflammatory cells. If it is a pleural effusion, it can further be characterized by bacteriologic tests for causative microorganisms, or with cytology to look for neoplastic cells. Since pleurisy, pleural effusion, and hydrothorax are all secondary conditions, treatment must be directed at the primary cause. A significant amount of hydrothorax or pleural effusion will cause _____(1) of the lungs, known medically as _____(2). A complication of purulent effusion during pleurisy is the formation of bands of scar tissue called _____(3). These fibrotic strands can restrict or _____(4) the amount of movement by the lungs.

1. collapse
2. atelectasis
3. adhesions
4. limit

11-92

If the exudate in the pleural cavity is purulent, or composed of pus, this is specifically called **empyema.** This is not very common and requires a massive bacterial infection of the lungs with purulent exudate. The cause of empyema is primarily a ruptured lung abscess. An abscess may form in lung tissue in any of the following circumstances:

1. empyema
2. rupture
3. abscess

1. Aspiration or drawing infected material into the lungs. This is a concern during oral surgery to treat infectious states such as an abscessed tooth or tonsillitis.
2. Bronchopneumonia, especially those cases caused by *Staphylococcus.*
3. Obstructive bronchiectasis, which traps microorganisms.
4. Septic pulmonary embolism in which the embolus is a clump of bacteria.
5. The spread of infection from other internal organ abscesses, for example, from the liver.

As a compressive state, severe empyema can cause atelectasis and dyspnea. Pus in the pleural cavity is called _____(1). It most often develops following _____(2) of a (an) _____(3) in the lungs.

11-93

Hemothorax is blood in the pleural cavity. The cause may be trauma to pulmonary vessels (a penetrating wound or rib fracture), or erosion into them by a tumor. Either case causes bleeding into the pleural space. Severe hemothorax causes atelectasis and dyspnea. Removal of the blood is called **thoracocentesis.** Withdrawal of the blood allows reexpansion of the lungs. The cause of the bleeding must be found and surgically corrected. Tumors of the pleura are either primary or secondary. Primary pleural neoplasia is rare and the tumor is called a **mesothelioma.** It can be a sequela of asbestosis (see Frame 11–70). **Secondary pleural neoplasia** is more common, and results from invasion of primary lung cancer, or from metastasis of cancer elsewhere in the body. Breast and ovarian cancer seem especially prone to move to the pleura. The pleural effusion may be aspirated and examined for neoplastic cells to confirm the diagnosis. Metastatic pleural cancer holds the same poor prognosis as metastatic lung cancer. Blood in the chest cavity is called _____(1). Severe bleeding can cause _____(2) and _____(3), so it must be stopped. Tumors of the pleura may be primary as in the case of a _____(4), which is associated with _____(5). Or they may have _____(6) there from another site.

1. hemothorax
2. atelectasis
3. dyspnea
4. mesothelioma
5. asbestosis
6. metastasized

► CYSTIC FIBROSIS

11-94

Cystic fibrosis is a genetic disease of the exocrine glands seen in young children. The parents are heterozygous carriers, each having one recessive gene for the disease. The affected offspring will be homozygous for the recessive cystic fibrosis gene and will manifest the disease. Cystic fibrosis causes the exocrine glands of the body to produce abnormal secretions. The various glands that are affected include the mucus glands, sweat glands, and glands of the pancreas that produce the digestive enzymes. The primary abnormality of the secretions from these glands are that they are very thick or viscous. Therefore, they have a tendency to block or plug the exocrine ducts. In the respiratory system, the trachea and bronchi become obstructed with thick mucus. The child is susceptible to many respiratory infections as a result. Bacteria are trapped by the viscous mucus and multiply rapidly. The blocked airways cause bronchiectasis and also atelectasis, once remaining air is absorbed. Even though cystic fibrosis affects several parts of the body, including the digestive system, death is generally from respiratory causes. Pneumonia may be the cause, or areas of lung collapse and dyspnea can lead to eventual respiratory failure.

---

1. genetic
2. young children
3. secretions
4. exocrine glands
5. viscous
6. block or obstruct
7. bronchi
8. respiratory infection
9. pneumonia
10. respiratory failure

The cause of cystic fibrosis is _____(1) or hereditary. The affected population is _____(2). The disease produces abnormality in the _____(3) from _____(4). The abnormality is a very thick or _____(5) secretion. This tends to _____(6) various ducts. In the lungs, the trachea and _____(7) become obstructed. Victims of cystic fibrosis have many bouts with _____(8). The cause of death is generally infection of the lungs or _____(9), or ultimately, _____(10). The pancreas is the digestive organ that is targeted in cystic fibrosis, and changes the disease causes there are responsible for its name. The ducts that release digestive enzymes become blocked by thick secretions. This means the enzymes are not present in the intestines to digest food. Maldigestion and malabsorption result. The pancreatic glands swell with mucus and become cystic (meaning little sacs), and fibrosis occurs around the cystic glands. The sweat glands are also abnormal. The sweat they produce is excessive and very high in salt. Excessive body water loss through the sweat makes the child susceptible to heat exhaustion. The diagnostic test for cystic fibrosis is called the sweat test, which measures the amount of sodium chloride in the perspiration. Advances in the treatment of cystic fibrosis have prolonged life from childhood into early adulthood. This includes antibiotics to decrease the incidence of respiratory infection, respiratory therapy to decrease mucous congestion, and digestive enzyme supplements given with meals.

▶ NEWBORN RESPIRATORY DISTRESS SYNDROME

---

1. newborn respiratory distress syndrome
2. hyaline membrane disease
3. surfactant
4. expand
5. atelectasis
6. hyaline membrane
7. gas exchange
8. premature
9. maturation

Newborn respiratory distress syndrome (NRDS) is also known as **hyaline membrane disease,** and it is a very important cause of neonatal death. ("Neo" means new and "natal" refers to birth.) Normally, at birth, the presence of a secretion called **surfactant** reduces the surface tension in the lungs. This allows the alveoli to inflate and the lungs to expand. Surfactant is produced by the pneumocytes relatively late in gestation. The lack of this vital chemical, or insufficient amounts of it, means that the lungs will remain in their collapsed or atelectatic fetal state, even after birth. While they are collapsed, a false membrane made of proteins (including fibrin) is formed. This protein sheet lines the bronchioles and the walls of the air sacs. This membrane is called a hyaline membrane, and it is formed in response to injury, which in this case is widespread atelectasis. Figure 11–14 is an excellent photograph of hyaline membrane formation. The presence of this protein in the alveoli severely impairs gas exchange. Newborn respiratory distress syndrome is usually seen in premature babies and is a result of lack of time for maturation. In other words, the baby was born before the lungs were ready or able to function. In premature neonates, there are several body systems that are not mature enough to function effectively. A significant cause of death in newborns is _____(1), also called _____(2). This condition results from a lack of the chemical _____(3). This chemical allows the alveoli and lungs to _____(4). In NRDS, they remain collapsed or in a state of _____(5). In response to this injury, a sheet of protein is formed, and this is called the _____(6). It lines the air passages and greatly interferes with _____(7). The population affected with this condition is _____(8) neonates. It can be summed up as a lack of _____(9) of the lungs.

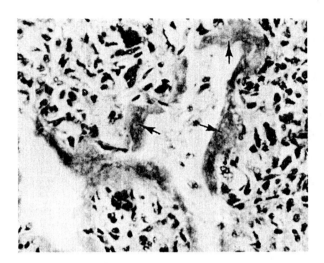

Figure 11–14. Microscopic view of hyaline membranes *(arrows)* in pulmonary alveoli during newborn respiratory distress syndrome. *(From Kent and Hart,* Introduction to Human Disease, *3rd ed., Appleton & Lange.)*

11–97

Premature neonates with NRDS who are undiagnosed and untreated will die within 48 hours. Recognition of this syndrome early, and proper treatment, changes the prognosis. The baby must be attached to an artificial ventilator, which will breathe for the baby and allow sufficient time for the lungs to mature. The overall survival rate is about 50 percent, depending on the age of the neonate. There may be some permanent lung damage. NRDS is easy to recognize. First, a premature birth is a red flag. Then, within an hour, extreme dyspnea develops, which is very labored and rapid breathing with grunting sounds. Cyanosis is recognizable within 6 hours. In some pregnancies, it may be desirable to terminate the pregnancy prior to the natural birth time. For this reason, it is critical to be able to predict the survival probability of the baby outside of the mother. Maturation of the lungs is assessed with a test called the lecithin/sphingomyelin ratio, more commonly known as the L/S ratio. Both of these lipids are present in amniotic fluid. The amount of sphingomyelin remains constant, even to birth. However, the amount of lecithin increases as maturity nears. A rise in lecithin, in comparison to sphingomyelin, corresponds to surfactant activity and lung development. If the ratio is greater than 2 (twice as much lecithin), there is adequate surfactant for the baby to survive. A ratio of less than 1.5 means that NRDS is likely outside of the uterus. Therefore, the L/S ratio is helpful to determine if elective premature delivery is safe for the baby.

VI. REVIEW QUESTIONS

1. Please match the pleural diseases in the left column with their descriptions in the right column:

   a. empyema
   b. hydrothorax
   c. pneumothorax
   d. hemothorax
   e. pleural effusion

   _____ 1. blood in the pleural cavity
   _____ 2. pus in the pleural cavity
   _____ 3. transudate in the pleural cavity
   _____ 4. exudate in the pleural cavity
   _____ 5. air in the pleural cavity

2. All of the disorders in Question 1 may cause:
   a. atelectasis
   b. bronchiectasis
   c. adhesions
   d. pleurisy

1. 1. d–hemothorax;
   2. a–empyema; 3. b–hydrothorax; 4. e–pleural effusion;
   5. c–pneumothorax

2. a–atelectasis

3. b–pleural effusion

4. d–purulent pleuritis

5. 1. c–pneumothorax;
   2. e–hemothorax;
   3. a–hydrothorax;
   4. d–empyema; 5. b–pleural
   effusion

6. a–mucus glands; b–thick or
   viscous

7. b–respiratory tree blockage,
   leading to pneumonia caused
   by trapped microorganisms

8. c–It is a genetic defect in
   which the gene that produces
   surfactant is missing.

3. Pleurisy or pleuritis is most often associated with:
   a. pneumothorax
   b. pleural effusion
   c. hydrothorax
   d. empyema

4. Adhesions may be a complication of:
   a. hemothorax
   b. empyema
   c. hydrothorax
   d. purulent pleuritis

5. Please match the pleural diseases in the left column with their causes in the right column:
   a. hydrothorax   _____ 1. penetrating chest trauma or ruptured bullae
   b. pleural effusion   _____ 2. vessel trauma
   c. pneumothorax   _____ 3. congestive heart failure
   d. empyema   _____ 4. ruptured lung abscess
   e. hemothorax   _____ 5. inflammation of the pleura

6. Cystic fibrosis is a genetic disease in which the secretions from a. _____ are
   very b. _____.

7. Cause of death in cystic fibrosis is usually due to:
   a. pancreatic duct blockage, maldigestion, and malabsorption to the point of starvation
   b. respiratory tree blockage, leading to pneumonia caused by trapped microorganisms
   c. dehydration and heat exhaustion caused by excess sweat and salt loss
   d. death is due to any of these causes

8. Choose the INCORRECT statement regarding newborn respiratory distress syndrome:
   a. It is a major cause of death in premature babies.
   b. It represents a lack of maturity of the lungs.
   c. It is a genetic defect in which the gene that produces surfactant is missing.
   d. Lack of surfactant prevents expansion of the lungs.

CHAPTER ► SUMMARY

► **SECTION II**

Perhaps the most common human affliction is *upper respiratory infection* (URI), customarily referred to as the "common cold." URI is caused by viruses (e.g., influenza A and B, parainfluenza, rhinovirus) that spread through the air from person to person. Immunity to URI fails to develop because many strains of the viruses exist. Complications of URI, which may include otitis media (middle ear infection) and secondary bacterial infection, are generally limited to individuals with poor immune response to the causative virus. *Acute bronchitis,* also known as *tracheobronchitis,* is caused by bacterial infection, inflammation, or inhaled dust or gases. The primary sign of tracheobronchitis, which affects both the upper and lower respiratory tracts, is a productive (mucus-expelling) cough.

Pneumonia is infectious inflammation of the lungs caused by the invasion of microorganisms (usually bacteria). The microorganisms reach the lungs following infection of the upper respiratory tract. *Bronchopneumonia* occurs as the result of the infection spreading from the bronchi into the alveoli, causing the alveoli to fill with exudate; this process is termed "consolidation." It is the most common type of pneumonia. *Lobar pneumonia* is caused specifically by the pneumococcus bacterium and also results in alveolar consolidation. In contrast to the diffuse patchy spread of bronchopneumonia, lobar pneumonia is generally confined to one or two lobes of the lungs. *Legionnaires' disease,* caused by the bacterium *Legionella pneumophila,* infects the lungs via inhalation of water droplets from contaminated fixtures (air conditioners, humidifiers, plumbing, etc.). This form of pneumonia can cause consolidation and necrosis of the alveoli; therefore, there is a relatively high mortality rate associated with Legionnaire's disease. *Interstitial pneumonia,* or primary atypical pneumonia, is characterized by infectious inflammation of the walls of the alveoli and the surrounding interstitial tissue. Little exudate is seen in this type of pneumonia, which can be caused by certain bacteria or viruses.

The *respiratory syncytial virus* (RSV), which most often infects infants, young children, and the elderly, is transmitted from an infected person by the airborne route. The disease presents as a mild URI in adults; in babies and infants otitis media is often present. Bronchiolitis and pneumonia may develop. Infection with a particularly virulent strain of the *influenza virus* can progress to pneumonia, which can be fatal to individuals who are immune incompetent or chronically ill. Secondary bacterial infection, which occurs especially during epidemics of influenza pneumonia, is often a contributing factor to the high mortality rate seen in "flu" outbreaks. *Primary fungal pneumonia* is classified, depending on the causative fungus, as histoplasmosis or coccidioidomycosis. Fungal pneumonia is contracted by inhaling dust contaminated with the fungus or its spores, and the condition can cause lesions in the lungs. Calcified granulomas in the lungs are often seen in fungal pneumonia.

Tuberculosis is an infection of the lungs caused by *Mycobacterium tuberculosis.* An initial acute infection (primary tuberculosis) is often cleared by the individual's immune system. Secondary tuberculosis results if mycobacteria are reactivated from tubercles (clumps of the dormant bacteria surrounded by inflammatory cells and scar tissue) in the lungs. As the disease progresses, the core of the tubercles becomes a caseous necrosis, which liquefies and is expectorated. Repetition of this process results in large areas of lung tissue destruction by cavitation.

► SECTION III

In *chronic obstructive pulmonary disease* (COPD), the bronchi and bronchioles are plugged or partially obstructed over a long period of time. Since the condition is a reaction to a primary disease or a chronic irritant, COPD is considered a secondary state. Whatever the cause of the airway obstruction, ineffective ventilation is the result of COPD. *Chronic bronchitis,* which differs from acute bronchitis in cause and duration, develops as the result of air pollution or exposure to toxic fumes. The vast majority of cases are due to smoking. Signs and symptoms are identical to those of acute bronchitis. Hypoxia and hypercapnia develop in the later stages of the disease. Sufferers of chronic bronchitis may also experience bronchospneumonia, bronchiectasis, and/or emphysema.

In *bronchiectasis,* the walls of the respiratory tree have become distended and weakened, leading to eventual necrosis. In *saccular* bronchiectasis, larger bronchi form round bulges, while in *cylindrical* bronchiectasis, the bronchioles enlarge in tube-like fashion. In both cases, infection results when mucus plugs cannot be expelled by coughing.

The disease *emphysema,* a condition seen almost exclusively in smokers, occurs when the alveoli become dilated with stagnant air. Oxygen concentration decreases and carbon dioxide concentration increases in the diseased lungs. Damage to the alveoli occurs by oxygen free radicals (found in cigarette smoke) inducing chronic alveolar inflammation, leading to tissue destruction via the release of proteolytic enzymes. Weakened alveoli may rupture or fuse, forming nonfunctional bullae. An individual with early symptoms of emphysema may present as a "blue bloater" (due to cyanosis and edemic swelling) or a "pink puffer" (due to tachypnea and characterized by an absence of cyanosis).

Seasonal allergic rhinitis is a general term to describe certain immune-related disorders. *Allergic rhinitis* ("hay fever"), classified as a type I hypersensitivity reaction, involves immune reactivity against specific antigens such as plant pollens, house dust, animal dander, and molds. Allergic rhinitis is mediated by immunoglobulin E (IgE), an antibody that induces mast cells to release histamine, which in turn causes inflammation. *Hypersensitivity pneumonitis,* which can be either acute (antibody mediated) or chronic (cell mediated), is an allergic reaction in the alveoli due to antigen inhalation. Farmer's lung, furrier's lung, and maple bark disease are examples of this form of allergic reaction.

Asthma is characterized by dyspnea precipitated by spasm of the airways. This condition is also classified as type I hypersensitivity. Excessive IgE in the airways, upon antigen encounter, causes contraction of the smooth muscles of the airways in response to histamine from mast cells. The lumen becomes narrowed, causing resistance to air flow. In the condition of *status asthmaticus,* the attack is prolonged and does not stop spontaneously; injections of epinephrine and/or a tracheotomy may be necessary.

▶ SECTION IV

The processes that result in blood being oxygenated and carbon dioxide being eliminated are collectively called *ventilation.* COPD, pneumonia, and asthma cause ventilation disturbance. *Suffocation* (the prevention of inhalation and exhalation by respiratory obstruction) and *drowning* (suffocation in which the respiratory tree is filled with fluid) are also classified as ventilation disturbances. *Adult respiratory distress syndrome* (ARDS), considered a secondary rather than a primary reaction, is a general term to describe widespread damage to the parenchyma of the lungs. The condition can be due to acute noninfectious interstitial disease or to shock. ARDS leads to acute respiratory failure due to the inability to oxygenate the blood.

Respiratory failure is characterized as a lack of oxygen (hypoxemia) or retention of carbon dioxide (hypercapnia) because of inadequate lung functioning. The condition may be due to failure of air movement into the lungs or inadequate inhalation (alveolar hypoventilation), or to insufficient diffusion of gases through the tissue (ventilation–perfusion mismatch). The result of respiratory failure is generalized hypoxia affecting all body systems. Atelectasis, or collapse of the lungs, is a secondary condition resulting from compression of the lungs by pneumothorax (air in pleural space) or pleural effusion (fluid in pleural space), or from obstruction of the air passages. If the condition affects entire lobes of the lungs, dyspnea and death by anoxia can result.

Other forms of pulmonary disorders are inhalation based. *Pneumoconioses,* a group of chronic disorders, occur from long-term inhalation of an irritant carried by dust. *Silicosis,* the most widespread and most damaging of this group of disorders, results from inhaled silica transported across the bronchial walls into the interstitial tissues. *Anthracosis* (coal miner's lung, black lung) results from carbon accumulation in the lungs. *Asbestosis* is the result of the inhalation of asbestos, a chemical formerly used for fireproofing in buildings.

▶ SECTION V

Pulmonary hypertension occurs when resistance to blood flow in the lungs is increased. The condition can result from chronic lung disease, from emboli, or when respiratory circulation is overloaded with blood due to heart malfunction. *Pulmonary edema,* a potentially life-threatening disorder, is the presence of tissue fluid in the septa and alveoli. The condition develops as the result of increased pressure at the venous end of a capillary bed. In the most severe cases, death is like drowning. Left-side and congestive heart failure and pulmonary congestion can lead to pulmonary edema, and can lead to hydrothorax (fluid accumulation in the pleural space outside the lungs). Other causes of pulmonary edema are lobar and bronchopneumonia, electrical shock, toxic gas inhalation, peripheral vasoconstriction, and iatrogenic overload of the general circulation during intravenous therapy.

A *pulmonary embolism* is a blood-borne mass that has reached the lungs and become lodged. The most common reason for pulmonary embolism is thrombophlebitis. Infarction can result from a pulmonary embolism, the most serious case being if the embolus becomes wedged at a bifurcation of the pulmonary artery.

Several neoplastic conditions affecting the respiratory system can occur. *Laryngeal cancer* (carcinoma of the larynx), a relatively uncommon form of cancer that occurs most frequently in heavy smokers, is a squamous cell carcinoma. The malignancy can metastasize to the cervical lymph nodes and, left untreated, can spread to distant sites in the body. *Primary lung cancer* is neoplasia that originates (i.e., has not spread there from other sites) in the lungs. *Bronchoalveolar carcinoma* is an adenocarcinoma arising from the alveoli. *Bronchogenic carcinoma,* of which four distinct histologic types are recognized, is neoplasia of the largest airways in the respiratory tree. The leading causes of this form of lung cancer are cigarette smoking and asbestosis. Only about 20% of primary lung cancers have not metastasized or invaded at the time of diagnosis. *Secondary lung cancer* is malignancy in the lungs that has metastasized there from another primary site, most commonly from the breast, colon, liver, stomach, ovaries, cervix, and kidneys.

▶ SECTION VI

Pneumothorax occurs when air enters the pleural cavity, causing the lungs to collapse. The condition can be caused by trauma to the pleural cavity (wounds, fractured ribs) or from the rupture of bullae in emphysema. *Hydrothorax* (literally, "water in the chest"), is the condition of transudate fluid in the pleural space, most often caused by congestive heart failure. In *pleural effusion,* a condition associated with inflammation of the pleura, the pleural spaces contain exudate fluid. This is referred to as pleuritis or pleurisy, and it may be caused by bacterial pneumonia or tuberculosis. Because of the high amount of fibrin in the exudate, thick bands of scar tissue (adhesions) may form, which may limit lung expansion. If the exudate in the pleural cavity is purulent because of a ruptured lung abscess, the condition is called *empyema. Hemothorax* ("blood in the chest") can be caused by trauma or a tumor. Bleeding into the pleural space causes atelectasis and dyspnea; withdrawal of the blood (thoracocentesis) allows for reexpansion of the lungs. Primary and secondary pleural neoplasias are often the cause of hemothorax.

Cystic fibrosis is a genetic disease of the exocrine glands seen in young children. In the disease, the secretions of the mucus, sweat, and pancreatic glands produce abnormally viscous secretions, thereby blocking the exocrine ducts. The trachea and bronchi become obstructed, resulting in a high susceptibility to respiratory infections. Additionally, the affected child suffers from maldigestion and malabsorption, heat exhaustion, and fibrosis of the cystic glands. In the *newborn respiratory distress syndrome* (NRDS), or hyaline membrane disease, lack of a secretion called surfactant reduces the surface tension of the lungs. The result is that the lungs remain in their atelectic (collapsed) fetal state, leading to the production of a false membrane in the bronchioles and walls of the air sacs. The net result of this condition is a severe impairment of gas exchange.

CHAPTER 12

The Gastrointestinal System

▶ OBJECTIVES

SECTION II

Define all highlighted terms.

Describe the causes and signs and symptoms of stomatitis.

Describe the causative agents and signs and symptoms of tonsillitis, strep throat, scarlet fever, and "thrush."

Characterize the causes and signs and symptoms of dental caries, periapical abscess, gingivitis, periodontitis, and molar impaction.

Describe the condition of oral neoplasia.

Define and characterize the causes and signs and symptoms of sialoadenitis.

Describe how neoplasia affects the salivary glands.

SECTION III

Define all highlighted terms.

Describe the causes and signs and symptoms of esophagitis, and cite the most common type of esophagitis.

List the potential complications of chronic esophagitis.

Characterize the condition of a hiatal hernia, and list the suspected causes of the condition.

Describe the relationship between hiatal hernia and reflux esophagitis.

Describe the condition of esophageal cancer.

Describe the cause and signs and symptoms of esophageal varices and achalasia.

Describe the various forms of gastritis (acute, acute hemorrhagic, chronic), and characterize the causes and signs and symptoms of each.

Describe the forms of ulcer (peptic, gastric, duodenal), and characterize the causes and signs and symptoms of each.

Relate the presence of *Helicobacter pylori* to gastritis and gastric ulcer.

List and explain the complications of chronic peptic ulcer.

Describe the condition and patterns of gastric neoplasia.

SECTION IV

Define all highlighted terms.

Describe the three mechanisms of diarrhea, and characterize the causes and signs and symptoms of each.

Describe the forms of enteritis, and characterize the causes and signs and symptoms of each.

Describe the conditions of inflammatory bowel disease and ischemic bowel disease. Characterize the causes and signs and symptoms of both.

List the potential complications of ischemic bowel disease.

Define and describe the condition of ileus, and characterize the causes and signs and symptoms of mechanical and paralytic ileus.

Describe the causes and signs and symptoms of the conditions of malabsorption, maldigestion, and malnutrition.

Describe the most common neoplasia of the small intestines.

Describe the condition of appendicitis, and characterize the causes and signs and symptoms.

SECTION V

Define all highlighted terms.

Describe the causes and signs and symptoms of idiopathic ulcerative colitis and pseudomembranous colitis.

Describe the association between ulcerative colitis and neoplasia.

Describe the conditions of diverticulosis and diverticulitis.

Characterize the condition of neoplasia of the colon, and describe the causes and signs and symptoms.

Describe the forms of peritonitis, and characterize the causes and signs and symptoms of each form.

State the clinical significance of peritoneal adhesions.

Describe the different forms of ascites.

SECTION VI

Define all highlighted terms.

Describe the conditions of irritable bowel syndrome and hemorrhoids, and characterize the causes and signs and symptoms of both.

SECTION ▶ I. ANATOMY AND PHYSIOLOGY IN REVIEW
12-1

The **gastrointestinal system** is often called the **digestive tract** or the **alimentary tract.** Its main functions are **digestion** of food, **absorption** of nutrients, and **excretion** of wastes. The GI system, as we will abbreviate it here, is another body system in direct contact with the environment. It is essentially an open system from the mouth to the anus. All of the main GI organs are hollow or tubular in structure. They all have the same four layers (mucosa, submucosa, muscularis, and serosa), with some differences in the types of epithelium of the mucosa. In the abdominal cavity the outer covering of the organs, the serosa, becomes the **peritoneum.** Like the pleura of the thoracic cavity, the peritoneum is composed of the visceral layer on the organs and the parietal layer which lines the abdomen. The main organs of the GI system are the **mouth; pharynx; esophagus; stomach; small intestine** (the **duodenum, jejunum,** and **ileum); large intestine** (the **colon); rectum;** and **anus.** The accessory organs that are vital in digestion and processing of nutrients are the **pancreas, liver,** and **gallbladder.** Diseases of these accessory organs are presented in the next chapter. The digestive tract is shown in Figure 12–1.

12-2

In the abdomen is a connective tissue sheath, the **mesentery,** that suspends and anchors the many loops of the bowels so that they do not become entangled. Within the mesentery are the vessels, lymphatics, and nerves that supply the digestive organs. The blood supply to the intestines is through the **mesenteric arteries,** and the venous return is handled by the **portal system,** which continues to the liver. Nutrients are absorbed into the capillary beds in the walls of the intestines, and this blood, which is now venous, goes to the liver for the processing of nutrients. The lymphatic system of the intestines has a major role in nutrient absorption. It consists of blind-ended ducts in the walls of the intestines, which are called **lacteals.** The lacteals eventually empty into the thoracic duct, which empties into the circulation in the heart.

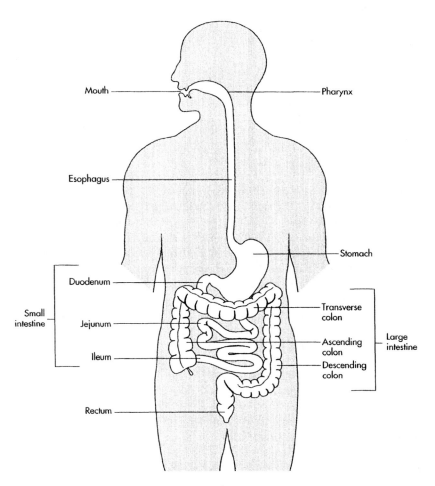

Figure 12–1. The main organs of the digestive tract.

As mentioned in Frame 12–1, the function of the alimentary tract is the digestion and absorption of nutrients in food. Many separate and complex activities work together to prepare the nutrients for absorption. Each section of the GI tract has its own individual function, and each section helps prepare the nutrients for assimilation (use) by the body. These sections and their specific functions are:

1. The mouth, which serves as a receptacle for **ingestion,** or the taking in of food into the body.
2. The teeth, jaw bones, and muscles that provide for **mastication** or chewing of the ingested food. This is the first step in the breakdown of food, and it is a mechanical action that results in smaller pieces that must be digested. Chemical breakdown begins here as well as when saliva from the **salivary glands** mixes with the food. Saliva contains the enzyme **amylase,** which starts the breakdown of carbohydrates.
3. The pharynx and esophagus provide a path for swallowing or **deglutition.** Swallowing is voluntary at first, and then once in the esophagus it is involuntary. At this point, and *throughout the rest of the digestive tract,* **peristalsis** moves the food though the organs. Peristalsis is waves of smooth muscle contractions that push or propel material through the system. The muscle movement also mixes the food with digestive juices.
4. The salivary glands, stomach, and the duodenum of the small intestine are responsible for **digestion.** This is the chemical breakdown of nutrients in food into compounds that can be absorbed through the walls of the intestines. The chemicals largely responsible are var-

ious **enzymes,** which are biochemical catalysts. Once food enters the stomach and is mixed with digestive juices, it is in a liquid form known as **chyme.** In the stomach, hydrochloric acid and the enzyme pepsin begin digestion (the walls of the stomach are protected from the acid by mucus). In the duodenum, many more chemicals are added to the chyme. These include enzymes from the pancreas such as amylase for starch digestion, lipase for fat digestion, and trypsin for protein digestion. **Bile** from the liver and gallbladder is added to the chyme in the duodenum for fat absorption. Bile will emulsify fat, that is, cause it to mix with water. The tiny globules of fat mixed with water are called **micelles.** Disaccharidase is also added for starch digestion and dipeptidase for protein digestion from the duodenum.

12-4

5. The jejunum and ileum of the small intestine serve as sites for **absorption** or the bringing of digested nutrients across their walls and into the lymph and blood supply. The different nutrients (carbohydrates, fats, and proteins) are absorbed in different sections of the intestines. Water and electrolytes are absorbed in the large intestine. The small intestine are very effective at what they do because of the arrangement of the mucosa. The mucosa is in the form of **villi,** which are numerous finger-like projections that cover the entire mucosal surface. The purpose of this configuration is to provide much more surface area for absorption than would otherwise be possible within the abdomen. Each villi contains a capillary bed (with arterial and venous ends) and a lacteal. These vessels stand ready to receive the absorbed nutrients and transport them to the liver and other sites.
6. The large intestine (colon) is responsible for water absorption and, together with the rectum, is responsible for **excretion.** This is the ridding of solid waste. Once water is absorbed from the liquid chyme, it becomes solid. This waste is undigested food and metabolic by-products of metabolism from the liver. The waste is moved along and stored in the rectum.
7. The anus passes the solid waste from the rectum out of the body during **defecation.** The solid waste is known as **feces** or **stool.**

12-5

The various secretions of the GI tract include enzymes, as mentioned. Enzymes split complex compounds such as starch into simple ones such as sugar, so they can be absorbed. The release or secretion of the enzymes is carefully controlled by a variety of hormones also secreted by the digestive tract. The hormones serve as a chemical signal that the enzymes are needed for action. In addition to hormonal control, digestion and absorption are governed by the autonomic nervous system.

SECTION ▶ ## II. DISEASES OF THE MOUTH AND SALIVARY GLANDS

▶ INFECTIOUS DISEASES OF THE MOUTH

12-6

A variety of oral disorders are inflammatory in nature. The medical term for inflammation in the mouth is **stomatitis.** A very common inflammation due to infection is a viral disorder, **herpes simplex type I.** This herpesvirus (a close relation to the genital herpes simplex type II) causes **vesicles** or blisters on the lips. This especially occurs at the junction of the membrane of the lip and the skin. Herpes oral vesicles are commonly known as "cold sores." This condition recurs again and again throughout the life of the affected individual. After the initial infection, which is transmitted orally, the virus retreats into nearby nerve ganglia and remains in a latent state. Outbreaks of the infection are reactivated by several factors including stress and sunlight. Reactivation of the latent virus by a fever has earned it the common name of "fever blisters." When the herpesvirus moves from the nerve back to the surface, it reproduces in such numbers it causes the classical blister. This blister soon erodes or breaks open into a painful ulcer. The lesions can become quite extensive in the immune suppressed. In the normal individual, they heal spontaneously in a week or two. The topical application of an antiviral drug such as acyclovir decreases the severity of outbreak and length of duration. However, as with genital herpes, there is no permanent cure.

Aphthous stomatitis, or **aphthous ulcers,** are commonly known as "canker sores." These are also recurrent lesions, and are shallow, painful ulcers on the tongue and the insides of the lips and cheeks. The cause of these erosions is unknown. An agent has never been identified. This common malady may be stress related. Canker sores also heal on their own. Lesions around the lips that are blisters are caused by the virus _____(1). Another term for blister is _____(2). They break open and become _____(3). These lesions are commonly called _____(4). In between outbreaks, the virus is in a _____(5) state, residing in _____(6). Ulcers inside the mouth, whose cause is unknown, are medically known as _____(7) or _____(8). The common descriptive phrase is _____(9). The general term for inflammation of the oral cavity is _____(10).

1. herpes simplex stomatitis type I
2. vesicle
3. ulcers
4. cold sores
5. latent
6. nerve ganglia
7. aphthous stomatitis
8. aphthous ulcers
9. canker sores
10. stomatitis

The tonsils are two groups of lymphoid tissue located on either side of the base of the throat. They function like lymph nodes and filter foreign matter, especially bacteria, from the juices in the mouth. If the bacterial count in the mouth should become very high, it is likely the increased numbers that are filtered out in the tonsils will lead to their infection. This defines **tonsillitis.** If you will remember from Chapter 5, dose or numbers of bacteria present is one determining factor in the development of an infection. A common bacteria that can build to infectious numbers in the mouth is streptococci. Acute tonsillitis causes swelling of this tissue, pain in the back of the throat, and **dysphagia** or difficulty in swallowing. Pus may accumulate in the tonsils. Tonsils contain deep crypts that can harbor bacteria after an acute infection. This pocket of smoldering infection can easily lead to chronic infection, which manifests as episodes of a very sore throat. The treatment for repeated episodes of tonsillitis used to be surgical removal. Today, effective antibiotics for a sufficient amount of time may be able to eradicate the infection and avoid the need for surgery. Infection of the tonsils is called _____(1). This develops because of high _____(2) of bacteria in the mouth. The microorganism most associated with tonsillitis is _____(3). Chronic tonsillitis may develop because of pockets of _____(4) that remain hidden deep in the tissue.

1. tonsillitis
2. numbers
3. streptococci
4. bacteria

A common infection mentioned previously in this text, and one that often coincides with tonsillitis, is **strep throat.** This is infection of the tonsils and the pharynx or throat by *Streptococcus pyogenes.* Fever and malaise accompany a sore throat. In addition to swollen tonsils, the wall of the pharynx becomes covered with a film of white infectious exudate. The lymph nodes of the neck may become enlarged and tender. **Scarlet fever** during strep throat is a condition in which the particular strain of streptococci produces a toxin that causes a red rash on the skin of the face or neck. A suspected case of strep throat should be cultured for the causative agent because other infections can cause a sore throat with exudate production. These include some viral infections, diphtheria (uncommon now), and oral gonorrhea. Strep throat should be treated with an effective antibiotic for a sufficient amount of time to avoid the complications of rheumatic fever, glomerulonephritis of the kidneys, and rheumatic heart disease. Strep throat is caused by the microorganism _____(1). A film of _____(2) develops that covers the wall of the _____(3). A reaction to a toxin from the bacteria causes a red _____(4) on the skin, and this is known as _____(5).

1. *Streptococcus pyogenes*
2. exudate
3. throat or pharynx
4. rash
5. scarlet fever

Candida albicans is the causative agent of a fungal infection of the mouth called **candida albicans stomatitis** or **oral candidiasis.** This infection is also called **thrush.** *Candida* is part of the normal flora of the mouth. It is held in check by other organisms and the immune system. If uncontrolled by the immune system, it causes opportunistic infection (see Chap. 5). Thrush is seen in the immune suppressed, and especially in AIDS patients. The presence of this infection is a red flag to alert the clinician to investigate the presence of AIDS. White

1. fungal
2. *Candida albicans*
3. immune suppressed
4. opportunistic

plaques cover the mucosa inside the mouth and may slough, leaving raw ulcers. In AIDS patients, and other severely debilitated patients, thrush has the potential to become systemic. Thrush is a _____(1) infection of the mouth caused by _____(2). It develops in those who are very _____(3). This type of infection is called a (an) _____(4) infection.

▶ DISEASES OF THE TEETH AND GUMS

12-11

A very common malady of the teeth is **dental caries.** This is infectious inflammation of the layers of a tooth, with varying degrees of destruction. Dental caries are commonly known as cavities. Cavities produce holes in the layers of a tooth as a result of destruction during infection by bacteria. Cavities are much more prevalent in childhood, but they may develop in adulthood if dental hygiene is poor. Saliva is somewhat protective because it contains the bacterial defense enzyme, lysozyme. However, as we discuss the pathogenesis of dental caries, you will see that this defense is inadequate in the face of poor hygiene. A tooth is composed of several layers. The enamel is the outer covering that is visible. It is a very hard structure in order to withstand mastication. The strength of the enamel is due to calcification. However, it is not unusual for the enamel to develop tiny cracks or fissures. In this case, any infection present can burrow its way to the next underlying layer, the dentin. The dentin is also calcified and therefore hardened. It makes up most of the mass of the tooth. This main structure contains channels that communicate with the pulp, the inner layer of the tooth. The pulp is soft connective tissue containing vessels and nerves. At its base is the root of the tooth with small openings through which nerves and vessels enter. Infection that has reached the dentin can access the pulp and the root of the tooth through the channels.

12-12

1. dental caries
2. destruction
3. cavities
4. dentin
5. enamel
6. pulp
7. nerves
8. root

Bacterial infection of the layers of a tooth is called _____(1). It produces holes in the layers because of various degrees of _____(2). Dental caries are commonly called _____(3). An infection may reach the second layer of the tooth, the _____(4), if there are tiny cracks in the outer layer, the _____(5). From there, the infection may travel to the soft inner layer, the _____(6). This layer contains the vessels and _____(7). The point of entry of vessels and nerves is called the _____(8) of the tooth. Infection may also reach here.

12-13

1. plaque
2. organic acids
3. dentin
4. infection

When food debris is caught and remains around the teeth, bacteria ferment the carbohydrates and produce organic acids. Colonies of active bacteria, decaying food particles, and products of bacterial fermentation produce a thick film called **plaque.** The formation and presence of plaque on the teeth is the first step in the creation of dental caries. The organic acids in the plaque begin to decalcify and erode the tooth enamel. As a small area of the enamel gradually erodes, this allows bacteria and acids to enter the tooth and continue to destroy underlying layers. Once in the dentin, the acids cause greater destruction than in the enamel. A larger cavity is created compared to the small hole in the enamel. Once through the dentin, bacteria enter the soft tissue or pulp and cause a true infectious inflammation. Inflammation of the pulp causes the familiar tooth pain of dental caries. The infection may travel deeper into the root and surrounding tissue. This deep decay often produces a **tooth abscess,** or **periapical abscess,** around the nerve that enters the pulp. This pus-containing sac around the root leads to greater and persistent pain. The associated lymph nodes in the neck may become swollen and painful, and a fever may be present. The abscess may extend even deeper in the bone of the jaw, infecting the bony structure. A film around the teeth that is made of bacteria, food remains, and fermentation products is called _____(1). The products of fermentation that erode tooth enamel are _____(2). The next structure to be entered and worn away is the _____(3). Once bacteria and acids reach the pulp, a true _____(4) exists. If the infection descends into the root area and produces pus there, it is called a _____(5) or a _____(6). It is possible for the infection to extend into the _____(7) of the jaw.

12–14

Treatment for dental caries consists of removing the diseased portion of the tooth and replacing the eroded structures with an inert metal, in a procedure commonly known as a filling. An abscess requires antibiotics and usually surgical draining. A root canal (removing the infected pulp and sealing the canals) may be necessary, depending on the extent of infection. Tooth extraction is generally the last resort. Obviously, prevention of cavities, or their early detection and treatment, is best. Preventative measures include fluoridated water, proper dental hygiene, a diet restricted in simple sugars, and professional cleaning and check-ups.

12–15

Another consequence of plaque is **gingivitis,** or infectious inflammation of the gums surrounding the teeth. Inadequate brushing and flossing allows plaque to build up around the base of the teeth. As bacteria colonize the soft tissue of the gums, they become red, slightly swollen, and fragile. A hallmark sign of gingivitis is gums that bleed easily, for example, when brushing. Gingivitis precedes periodontal disease (described in the next frame), which is deep destruction of the gums. In gingivitis, a space or pocket develops around the base of the teeth that allows plaque to descend under the gum line. Over time, the plaque becomes calcified, and this hardened product is **tartar.** Another term for tartar is **dental calculus.** The presence of tartar further inflames the gums. Gingivitis should be treated as soon as it is apparent to prevent deeper infection of the periodontal tissue. Teeth should be cleaned professionally by a dental hygienist to remove plaque and tartar before it causes further damage. Antibiotics may be indicated to clear up any remaining infection. Inflammation of the gums caused by infection is called _____(1). It is first produced by the presence of _____(2) around the teeth and gums. Infected gums appear _____(3) and swollen, and _____(4) easily. After plaque has reached below the gum line, it calcifies into _____(5) or _____(6). The significance of gingivitis is that, untreated, it leads to _____(7) disease.

1. gingivitis
2. plaque
3. red
4. bleed
5. tartar
6. dental calculus
7. periodontal

12–16

Periodontitis, or **periodontal disease,** is infectious inflammation of the periodontal membrane, which is the deep extension of the gingiva down into the tooth socket (its resting place in the jaw bone). This is a continuation of the events of gingivitis on a deeper level. Deep pockets become laden with bacteria. The combination of bacteria, plaque, and tartar produces an inflammation that loosens the ligaments that hold the teeth in place. These ligaments are the fibers of the periodontal membrane, which are destroyed by the infection. The tooth may die if the blood supply is impeded by infection at the root canal. If pus exudes from the gums, this condition is called **pyorrhea.** Periodontal disease causes the teeth to become very loose, and movements such as chewing further destroy the anchoring membranes. Along with dental caries, periodontal disease is a common cause of tooth loss. The presence of continuous infection causes **halitosis,** or foul breath. Deep infection of the bone leads to resorption, or bone loss. Prevention is the most effective treatment for periodontal disease. Infection of the deep gingiva around the tooth socket is called _____(1) or _____(2). This deep gingiva is specifically called the _____(3). The _____(4) or fibers that hold the _____(5) in place are destroyed by deep _____(6). The exudation of pus from the gums is called _____(7). A common result of periodontitis is _____(8). The events of tooth infection by bacteria, causing dental caries and periodontal disease, are illustrated in Figure 12–2.

1. periodontitis
2. periodontal disease
3. periodontal membrane
4. ligaments
5. tooth
6. infection
7. pyorrhea
8. tooth loss

12–17

The third molars at the back of the mouth are commonly called the wisdom teeth. These erupt (emerge from under the gums) relatively late in life, at around 17 to 21 years of age. Wisdom teeth do not appear in all people. In those who have their third molars, **molar impaction** is not unusual. Often there is not enough room for these teeth to erupt because of their angle of emersion, or because of adjacent teeth. Lack of room causes them to butt against teeth already present, causing an impaction (obstruction in emerging). Interference in

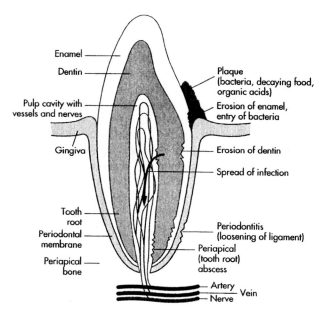

Figure 12–2. Formation of dental caries and periodontitis.

1. emergence
2. third
3. wisdom
4. teeth

their eruption causes continued pain that is relieved only by extraction of the wisdom teeth. Molar impaction is prevention of _____(1) of the _____(2) molars, commonly known as _____(3) teeth. Emergence is blocked by the angle or by other _____(4).

▶ ORAL NEOPLASIA

12-18

1. epithelial
2. squamous cell carcinoma
3. lower lip
4. best

Oral neoplasia, or cancer of the mouth, is the squamous cell carcinoma type. If you will remember from Chapter 5, neoplasia is classified according to the cells of origin. Carcinoma is cancer derived from _____(1) cells or tissue. Since the mouth is lined with epithelium, the cancer there is carcinoma, instead of a sarcoma. The development of oral neoplasia is associated with tobacco use, including pipe smoking, and with chronic alcohol consumption. All structures of the mouth are susceptible to cancer; however, the most common site for carcinoma is the lower lip. In many cases, a chronic sore or crack in the lip that doesn't heal seems to precede the cancer. The prognosis for lip carcinoma is good, since it metastasizes late and it is very responsive to treatment (surgical excision or radiation). Carcinoma of the tongue has a less favorable outcome. It will spread more rapidly and may have already done so by the time it is detected. Carcinoma of the pharynx has the worst prognosis because it is highly malignant. Usually, the first sign of pharyngeal cancer is enlargement of the regional lymph nodes, which means it has already moved there. Oral neoplasia is the _____(2) type. The most common site of cancer of the mouth is the _____(3). This cancer has the _____(4) prognosis in regards to spread and treatment.

12-19

There are several ways in which oral neoplasia may manifest. The mucosal surface may show **leukoplakia** (white plaques) or **erythroplasia** (red plaques). In these raised flat areas is the start of malignancy. If the tissue is examined histologically, various stages of metaplasia can be identified. The lesion is classified as precancerous. Cancer may also be present as ulcers (erosions) or nodules (bumps). When oral neoplasia metastasizes, the local lymph nodes in the neck are the first sites of spread. Therefore, enlargement of these structures is an important early clue of the nature of the cancer.

▶ DISEASE OF THE SALIVARY GLANDS

12–20

The two most important disorders of the salivary glands are inflammation and neoplasia. Inflammation of the salivary glands is called **sialoadenitis.** The inflammation causes a painful swelling accompanied by a disturbance in function. Either too much saliva is produced, or not enough. The most common cause of sialoadenitis is a viral infection, generally known as the mumps. This infectious inflammation is also known as **parotitis** because the mumps virus targets the largest gland, the parotid gland. Mumps is seen more often in children than in adults. This is an acute condition that heals spontaneously. The phrase that means that a disorder resolves on its own is "self-limiting." Bacterial infections of the salivary glands can cause obstruction of the ducts, leading to a very dry mouth from lack of saliva and even greater swelling. Bacterial infections are often chronic. If pus is present, the condition is called **suppurative sialoadenitis.** Another cause of gland inflammation is autoimmune destruction where immune cells, especially lymphocytes, infiltrate the glands and hamper their function. Inflammation of the salivary glands is called _____(1). The most common cause is infection by a (an) _____(2), commonly known as the _____(3). Sialoadenitis caused specifically by the mumps virus is also known as _____(4), because it affects the _____(5) gland. A bacterial infection that produces pus is called _____(6).

1. sialoadenitis
2. virus
3. mumps
4. parotitis
5. parotid
6. suppurative sialoadenitis

12–21

The salivary glands are also candidates for the development of cancer. The parotid gland is affected most often, and cancer is another reason for gland enlargement. While some cases are malignant, most are benign and very slow growers. As a space-occupying lesion, even a benign tumor can cause problems. Several nerves course through salivary gland tissue. A large tumor can press on the facial nerve and cause paralysis of the facial muscles. It is very fortunate most salivary gland neoplasia is benign because it does not respond well to removal. Since it is intertwined among nerves, complete removal is impossible, and recurrence of the tumor is common. In contrast to malignant oral cancer, neoplasia of the salivary glands is usually _____(1). Difficulties arising from these tumors are because of their presence as a _____(2) lesion. Diseases of the mouth and salivary glands are summarized in Table 12–1.

1. benign
2. space-occupying

TABLE 12–1. DISEASES OF THE MOUTH AND SALIVARY GLANDS

Disease	Causative Agent or Contributing Factors
Herpes simplex type I stomatitis	Herpes simplex type I virus
Aphthous stomatitis (canker sores)	Idiopathic, possibly stress induced
Tonsillitis	Streptococci or other bacteria
Streptococcal pharyngitis (strep throat, scarlet fever)	*Streptococcus pyogenes*
Thrush (candida albicans stomatitis, oral candidiasis)	*Candida albicans*
Dental caries (cavities), periapical abscess (tooth abscess)	Inadequate oral hygiene, which allows bacterial infection of tooth layers
Gingivitis	Continuation of the events of dental caries or a result of plaque
Periodontitis (periodontal disease)	Continuation of the events of gingivitis at deepest levels
Oral squamous cell carcinoma	Tobacco use, heavy alcohol consumption
Sialoadenitis, parotitis (mumps)	Mumps virus, chronic bacterial infection, autoimmune destruction
Sialoadenoma	Idiopathic

II. REVIEW QUESTIONS

1. d–stomatitis

2. b–bacteria in the mouth, especially streptococci, increase to infectious numbers

3. c–*Streptococcus pyogenes* of the scarlet fever strain

4. a–dental caries

5. c–plaque

6. b–infection during caries formation reaches the area where the nerves enter the pulp

7. d–gingivitis

1. The medical term for inflammation in the mouth is:
   a. gingivitis
   b. laryngitis
   c. parotitis
   d. stomatitis

2. In general, tonsillitis develops when:
   a. infection from a tooth abscess spreads to the tonsils
   b. bacteria in the mouth, especially streptococci, increase to infectious numbers
   c. virulent pathogens are ingested
   d. one is exposed to an individual with infectious tonsillitis

3. Tonsillitis, a white exudate covering the throat, and a red rash on the face or neck, are most consistent with:
   a. oral candidiasis or thrush
   b. *Staphylococcus aureus* of the scarlet fever strain
   c. *Streptococcus pyogenes* of the scarlet fever strain
   d. herpes simplex type I
   e. aphthous stomatitis

4. Penetration and destruction of tooth enamel and dentin, followed by infection of the pulp, describes the pathogenesis of:
   a. dental caries
   b. dental calculus
   c. periapical abscess
   d. periodontal disease

5. Decalcification and erosion of tooth enamel is accomplished by organic acids found in a thick film called:
   a. tartar
   b. dental calculus
   c. plaque
   d. pyorrhea

6. A periapical or tooth abscess is created when:
   a. bacteria reach infectious numbers during caries formation
   b. infection during caries formation reaches the area where the nerves enter the pulp
   c. infection during tonsillitis drains into a tooth root
   d. periodontal disease reaches the deep pocket of the tooth socket

7. Plaque under the gum line, which calcifies and produces inflammation of the gums, describes:
   a. pyorrhea
   b. periodontitis
   c. halitosis
   d. gingivitis

8. Periodontitis is a consequence of unresolved:
   a. periapical abscess
   b. inflammation of the periodontal ligaments
   c. gingivitis
   d. molar impaction

9. In periodontal disease, tooth loss is the result of:
   a. destruction of the fibers or ligaments of the periodontal membrane by infectious inflammation
   b. deep infection in the root canal
   c. tartar formation
   d. destruction of the pulp by infectious inflammation

10. The most common malignancy of the mouth is:
    a. adenocarcinoma of the lip
    b. squamous cell carcinoma of the lip
    c. adenocarcinoma of the tongue
    d. squamous cell carcinoma of the pharynx

11. Parotitis is:
    a. sialoadenitis caused by the mumps virus
    b. suppurative sialoadenitis caused by bacteria
    c. inflammation of the small salivary glands caused by the presence of benign neoplasia
    d. inflammation of the salivary glands as a consequence of tonsillitis

8. c–gingivitis

9. a–destruction of the fibers or ligaments of the periodontal membrane by infectious inflammation

10. b–squamous cell carcinoma of the lip

11. a–sialoadenitis caused by the mumps virus

III. DISEASES OF THE ESOPHAGUS AND STOMACH ◄ SECTION

► INFLAMMATORY AND OBSTRUCTIVE DISORDERS OF THE ESOPHAGUS

.... 12-22 ......

Inflammation of the esophagus is called **esophagitis.** There are several causes. One is infection by a fungus such as *Candida albicans,* or by a virus such as herpesvirus. Infectious esophagitis is not common and is seen in immune-suppressed patients. Chemical esophagitis will develop after swallowing a caustic chemical. A caustic compound is one that is irritating or harmful to living tissue. Chemical esophagitis is generally associated with accidents in children. The most common esophageal inflammation by far is **reflux esophagitis.** This is inflammation of the lower end of the esophagus because of the backflow or reflux of acid from the stomach. At the lower end of the esophagus is a sphincter, called the lower esophageal sphincter, or LES. A sphincter is a ring of smooth muscle in a hollow or tubular organ. Its function is to constrict (close) or dilate (open) that area of the organ to direct or control the flow of fluid. The LES functions to close the distal end of the esophagus after a bolus of food has passed by and entered the stomach. Therefore, the LES usually prevents stomach acid from washing back into the esophagus. Reflux esophagitis develops due to LES incompetency. The sphincter fails to close adequately, allowing acid to enter and irritate and inflame the tissue. Painful ulcers may develop. There is no mucus present in the esophagus to protect the lining, as there is in the stomach. Esophagitis is _____(1) of the _____(2). The most common reason for this inflammation is the condition called _____(3). The inflammation affects the _____(4) end, where the lower esophageal _____(5) is located. Reflux esophagitis may develop because of _____(6) of this sphincter, which

1. inflammation
2. esophagus
3. reflux esophagitis
4. lower or distal
5. sphincter
6. incompetency

means it does not _____(7) adequately. Failure to close as it should allows _____(8) to enter the esophagus and eat away at the tissue.

The presence of a hiatal hernia (described in the next frame) may causes LES incompetency. In fact, hiatal hernia is a common cause of reflux esophagitis. Other causes that decrease the tone of the muscle of the sphincter are smoking and caffeine. The amount of inflammation is responsible for the signs and symptoms of esophagitis. Mild discomfort, commonly known as heartburn, presents itself as a burning sensation in the chest. Esophagitis that has progressed to ulcers causes more severe pain. The effects of reflux esophagitis are often felt after eating, when the stomach has been activated and produces more acid. The constant inflammation causes changes in the epithelial lining that may be precancerous. Chronic ulceration can lead to scarring of the area. If you will remember from Chapter 2, fibrotic tissue contracts as part of the healing process. If a scarred area of a hollow organ contracts, it can produce **stenosis,** which is a narrowing or stricture of the organ at that site. Therefore, stenosis can interfere with the passage of food. Mild to moderate cases of reflux esophagitis are managed with antacids to decrease the acidity of the gastric contents, a bland diet, and the avoidance of alcohol. A common reason for reflux esophagitis is a hiatal _____(1). The discomfort is directly related to the amount of _____(2) present. Chronic ulcers, when healing, lead to formation of _____(3) when the scar tissue _____(4). Stenosis can interfere with the passing of _____(5) through the esophagus.

There is a hole in the diaphragm through which the esophagus passes before joining the stomach. This hole is called the **hiatus.** A **hernia** is the bulging of tissue or organ parts through some hole or opening. A **hiatal hernia** is the sliding of the upper part of the stomach (the cardia) through the hiatus or diaphragmatic hole. The cardia then ends up sitting with the lower part of the esophagus in the chest, as seen in Figure 12-3. The cause of hiatal hernia is unclear, but it is fairly common. Obesity predisposes to the condition, and worsens it if it is already present. Some cases are asymptomatic but many cause incompetency of the LES. This is because the presence of the stomach bunched up against it interferes with efficient muscle contraction and closure. Therefore, reflux esophagitis may accompany hiatal hernia, with heartburn or indigestion after eating. The most common management for most cases is to avoid irritating diets (spicy foods and alcohol) and to take antacids. Weight loss decreases the incidence and severity of the episodes. Very troublesome cases can be surgically corrected by suturing or tacking the cardia in place. If the upper part of the stomach pushes through the diaphragmatic hole, this is called a _____(1). The most common symptoms associated with hiatal hernia are because it can cause the condition _____(2). This is because the protruding stomach interferes with the function of the _____(3).

▶ NEOPLASTIC AND OTHER DISORDERS OF THE ESOPHAGUS

Cancer of the esophagus presents as squamous cell carcinoma and is highly malignant. Usually, by the time it is diagnosed it has spread to lymph nodes and the mediastinum. The type of cancer is carcinoma because the esophagus is lined with _____(1) tissue. In this country, neoplasia of the esophagus is not common compared with neoplasia of the rest of the GI tract. However, the incidence of this cancer around the world varies, with many more cases appearing in China and South Africa. This suggests it is related to the presence of some carcinogen in the environment. In this country, esophageal cancer is linked to smoking and heavy alcohol use. The carcinoma may grow as a focal (local) mass or tumor that protrudes into the lumen with potential obstruction. Or it may be present as a diffuse (spread out) thickening of the walls, which decreases the size of the lumen. Clinically, the patient experiences painful dysphagia, which is difficulty _____(2), due to the narrowed lumen. The obstruction may be severe enough to prevent the passage of solid food,

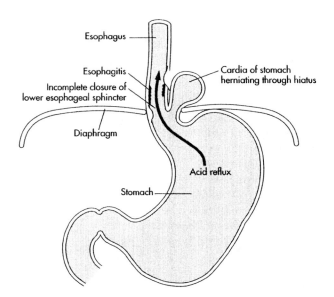

Figure 12–3. Hiatal hernia and reflux esophagitis.

which then regurgitates back into the throat. The patient loses weight because of the difficulty in obtaining adequate nutrition. Death from cancer of the esophagus is particularly unpleasant, since the obstruction progresses to the point that even liquids, including saliva, cannot be swallowed. Because metastasis before detection is common, the prognosis is poor. Fewer than 5 percent of patients live 2 more years. Surgery to remove the cancer leaves only some of the esophagus, which must be anastomosed (connected) to the stomach or replaced with a section of the colon.

Neoplasia of the esophagus is of the _____(1) type. It is characterized as being highly _____(2). It may develop as a local mass or _____(3), or become a diffuse _____(4). Either case _____(5) the lumen of the esophagus. The patient with esophageal cancer presents with difficulty swallowing or _____(6). This obstruction prevents the passage of _____(7) and, in late stages, even the passage of _____(8).

12-26

1. squamous cell carcinoma
2. malignant
3. tumor
4. thickening
5. narrows or decreases
6. dysphagia
7. food
8. liquids

12-27

Esophageal varices are varicose veins of the esophagus. You learned in Chapter 9 that varicose veins are veins that are dilated and filled with pooled blood. The cause of esophageal varices is a backup of blood, which increases the pressure and dilates the veins. The backup is due to interference in drainage of the portal vein in the liver. This interference causes obstruction of drainage of veins behind the liver in the circuit of blood flow. The portal vein most often is obstructed because of cirrhosis of the liver (see Chap. 13). This is massive scarring or fibrosis of the liver in response to chronic inflammation (such as chronic active hepatitis), or in response to other damage (such as chronic alcoholism). Fibrotic tissue contracts so massive scarring shrinks the entire liver and compresses blood flow. This creates portal hypertension. (Portal refers to liver.) Portal hypertension leads to congestion or stagnation of blood in veins behind the liver in the circuit of blood flow. The extreme danger of esophageal varices is potential rupture of the veins because of the high pressure. This can result in massive hemorrhage that can be fatal. As the blood pours into the esophagus and stomach, vomiting of blood is seen clinically. Vomiting blood is called **hematemesis.** Varicose veins of the esophagus are called _____(1). Increased pressure in the liver is created because of massive scarring or _____(2) of that organ. Fibrotic tissue shrinks or _____(3). This compresses or obstructs _____(4).

1. esophageal varices
2. fibrosis
3. contracts
4. blood flow

5. veins
6. esophagus
7. rupture
8. hemorrhage
9. hematemesis

As a result, congestion builds in _____(5) behind the liver in the path of blood flow. This causes veins in the _____(6) to dilate and become filled with blood. Because of the high pressure, it is possible that those veins will _____(7), and result in massive _____(8). Clinically, this bleeding will produce vomiting of blood or _____(9).

12-28

1. achalasia
2. passage
3. dysphagia

Achalasia is sporadic tension of the lower esophageal sphincter. This is the opposite of LES incompetency seen in reflux esophagitis. Instead of being too relaxed, in achalasia the smooth muscle of the sphincter enters a spasm and is unable to relax. This blocks the passage of food and causes dysphagia. The patient experiences the sensation of food sticking in the lower chest region. The cause of achalasia is idiopathic; however, degeneration of the nerve cells around the sphincter has been demonstrated histologically. If the lower esophageal sphincter becomes spastic, the tension creates the condition _____(1). The tightening interferes with the _____(2) of food, and this inability to swallow effectively is called _____(3).

▶ INFLAMMATORY DISORDERS OF THE STOMACH

12-29

1. inflammation
2. mucosa
3. erosions
4. ulcers
5. irritants
6. chemical
7. alcohol
8. aspirin

Gastritis is inflammation of the stomach lining, which is the mucosa. We will discuss **acute gastritis** first. This is inflammation that leads to shallow erosions of the superficial epithelium, or to deeper ulcers of the mucosa. One cause of acute gastritis is a deficiency of the blood supply to the stomach. The damage suffered by the mucosal cells because of ischemia makes them more vulnerable to stomach acid. The acid then can cause irritation and inflammation. Interruption in circulation can occur during shock, or when increased levels of circulating steroids are present during stress. A second, more common cause of acute gastritis is the ingestion of irritants that cause a chemically induced inflammation. Alcohol is a potent irritant, and it also increases acid production. Several drugs, including aspirin and other anti-inflammatory agents, can irritate the stomach lining. Stomach upset is a common side effect of aspirin ingestion. Excessive coffee and spicy foods may cause irritation. Cases of staphylococcal food poisoning are usually accompanied by a toxin that causes some damage. Other types of infection can cause gastroenteritis, infectious inflammation of the stomach and intestines (see Frame 12–43). Gastritis is _____(1) of the lining or _____(2) of the stomach. The inflammation may cause shallow _____(3) or deeper _____(4) of the mucosa. A common cause of acute gastritis is the ingestion of _____(5) that cause a _____(6) inflammation. Common gastric irritants include the beverage _____(7), and the drug _____(8).

12-30

Clinically, acute gastritis presents as a range of symptoms from mild discomfort to stabbing pain. Nausea may be present. Deeper ulcers can cause some bleeding, and more severe cases may have vomiting of bloody gastric juice. These cases are usually a result of excessive alcohol intake. The name applied to this condition is **acute hemorrhagic gastritis.** Most cases of acute gastritis are mild and resolve after a short while if the irritant is removed.

12-31

Chronic gastritis presents a different picture and has different causes. Along with inflammation there is atrophy or wasting away of the mucosa. For this reason it is also known as **chronic atrophic gastritis.** One theory about its cause is that it is autoimmune in nature. There may be immune-mediated damage in which autoantibodies destroy the gastric mucosal cells, causing atrophy of the lining. This same condition will lead to pernicious anemia, as we discussed in Chapter 9. Destruction of gastric cells leads to lack of intrinsic factor secreted by the cells. Intrinsic factor is required for the absorption of the B vitamins necessary for red blood cell maturation. Genetic predisposition may be a cause of chronic gastritis. Also, infection with **Helicobacter pylori** may be a contributing factor. *H. pylori* is present in the stomach of about 20 percent of the population. It is a small bacterium that lives in the mucosa. Its presence and colonization of the stomach lining creates a chronic low-grade inflammation that seems to worsen with age. (The presence of *H. pylori* does not always cause chronic gastritis, because many cases are asymptomatic.) The significance of chronic *Helicobacter* gastritis is its possible role in the development of stomach ulcers or of stomach cancer. Chronic inflammation in any tissue causes some metaplasia (change in form) in the responding cells. Metaplasia has the potential to become precancerous since neoplastic cells are the epitome of a change in form.

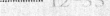

The difference between acute and chronic gastritis is that in chronic gastritis _____(1) occurs along with inflammation. Another name for this state is _____(2). It may be caused by _____(3)-mediated damage in which _____(4) destroy mucosal cells and lead to _____(5) of the lining. In this case chronic atrophic gastritis is related to _____(6) anemia. The bacteria _____(7) is also suspected in chronic gastritis. It colonizes the stomach lining and may cause a low-grade _____(8) in response to its presence. It has been considered that *H. pylori* infection may predispose to the development of stomach _____(9) or _____(10). Clinically, chronic gastritis causes **dyspepsia,** or indigestion, because of a deficiency of pepsin and hydrochloric acid. Atrophy of the mucosa causes a loss of the enzyme and acid-secreting cells.

1. atrophy
2. chronic atrophic gastritis
3. immune
4. autoantibodies
5. atrophy
6. pernicious
7. *Helicobacter pylori*
8. chronic inflammation
9. ulcers
10. cancer

On a deeper level, inflammation and erosion of the mucosa can lead to the development of a **peptic ulcer.** "Peptic" refers to stomach and small intestines. An ulcer is a lesion that begins as inflammation and turns into an area of necrosis. When the dead tissue sloughs off, a hole is left. A **gastric ulcer** (of the stomach specifically) may be created when mucosa that doesn't secrete acid comes into contact with the acidic gastric juice. Gastric juice also contains pepsin, a proteolytic enzyme that will digest surfaces. These vulnerable sites include the lesser curvature of the stomach and the lower esophagus. The upper duodenum is a very common site of ulcer formation. In this case it is called a **duodenal ulcer.** Acid and pepsin eat away and erode the surface mucosa, then penetrate the deeper layers of the muscle. An ulcer appears as a well-defined deep hole surrounded by inflammation. This is well shown in Figure 12–4. Vascular granulation tissue lines this crater and fibrosis lies underneath. Erosion often involves surrounding blood vessels, so bleeding is a common feature of peptic ulcer. A peptic ulcer is _____(1) and _____(2) of the mucosa on a deeper level than in gastritis. An ulcer looks like a well-defined _____(3) after a layer of _____(4) tissue has sloughed off. Ulcers of the stomach are

1. inflammation
2. erosion
3. hole
4. necrotic

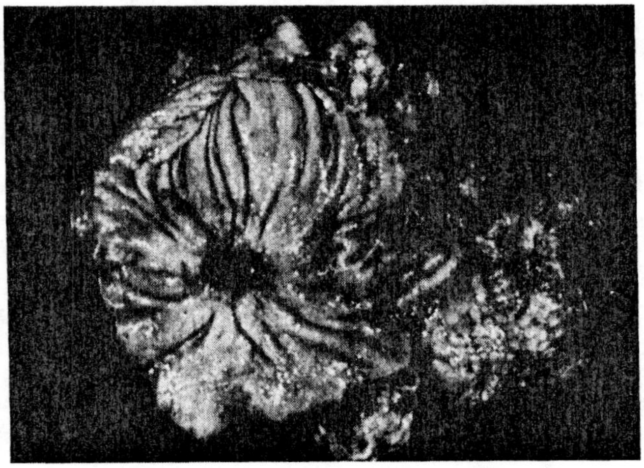

Figure 12–4. Chronic peptic ulcer. A large punched-out ulcer below the level of the mucosa. *(From Chandrasoma and Taylor,* Concise Pathology, *2nd ed., Appleton & Lange.)*

5. gastric ulcers
6. duodenal ulcers
7. acid
8. acid
9. proteolytic enzymes or pepsin
10. bleeding

called _____(5), while ulcers of the first part of the small intestine are called _____(6). Peptic ulcers develop when mucosa that doesn't secrete _____(7) is bathed with gastric juice containing _____(8) and _____(9). A common occurrence of peptic ulcer is _____(10) because of erosion of blood vessels.

12-34

The exact cause of peptic ulcers is unknown. The underlying pathogenesis seems to be a combination of damage to the mucosa along with exposure to stomach acid and enzymes. Mucosa that does not secrete acid is normally protected from digestion by acidic stomach juice. The lining epithelial cells form a barrier with their tight junctions that prevent acid from entering further. This barrier can be damaged by the same chemical irritants that cause gastritis. A break in the integrity of the barrier allows acid to penetrate the submucosa. Laxity or excessive relaxation of the pyloric sphincter at the stomach's exit can allow reflux of irritating alkaline contents from the duodenum into the stomach. Or, in the reverse case, it could allow stomach acid to enter the duodenum. Stress plays a role in development, because the steroid hormones increase the activity of the vagus nerve that stimulates acid secretion. Considering how many people use alcohol to relieve stress (which irritates and further acidifies the stomach), it is no wonder peptic ulcers are as prevalent as they are. Infection with *Helicobacter pylori* has been implicated as a cause of peptic ulcer. Cases in which this bacteria is present heal well after antibiotic treatment to eliminate *H. pylori*. Suspected cases of *H. pylori* can be confirmed by a positive culture of stomach contents or by seeing the organism in a biopsy specimen. Genetic predisposition is another suspected factor in ulcer development.

12-35

1. damage
2. mucosa
3. acid
4. enzymes
5. barrier
6. junctions
7. epithelial
8. submucosa

The fundamental cause of peptic ulcers appears to be a combination of _____(1) of the _____(2), which is then exposed to _____(3) and _____(4). Protection of the underlying tissue is usually accomplished by the _____(5) that is created by the tight _____(6) of the _____(7) cells. A break in the barrier allows acid and enzymes to enter the _____(8). Peptic ulcers present with a range of symptoms depending on the severity of injury. These include nausea, vomiting, and weight loss. Pain is very common and is due to the action of acid on raw surfaces and muscle spasms. Pain with a duodenal ulcer usually occurs later after a meal when stomach contents begin to be released into the first part of the small intestine. The effect of eating on the pain of peptic ulcers often depends on the location of the ulcer. These effects range from relief of pain to no change or to worsening of the pain.

12-36

1. hemorrhage
2. iron deficiency
3. black, tarry
4. digested

The complications of peptic ulcers can be quite serious, depending on the severity of the ulcer. The first is *hemorrhage*. Erosion into vessels causes bleeding. Small amounts of blood loss over a long period of time, or chronic bleeding, leads to iron deficiency anemia. Clinically, gastric hemorrhage is seen as **melena.** This is stool with a black, tarry appearance. This appearance is because the stool contains digested blood that has traveled the digestive tract. Melena is the most common manifestation of hemorrhage. A situation with greater consequences is **hematemesis.** This is vomiting blood. It occurs with large hemorrhages into the stomach that cause vomiting. Significant or massive hematemesis can cause shock or even death. Hematemesis most often develops as a result of the next complication of a gastric ulcer, which is *penetration*. In penetration, the ulcer erodes completely through the stomach wall and into the pancreas, which lies next to the stomach. Erosion of the larger vessels of the pancreas produce hematemesis. Damage from the ulcer also causes pancreatitis, inflammation of that gland (see Chap. 13). Pancreatitis is a painful condition with its own set of potentially serious consequences. Erosion into blood vessels by an ulcer causes the complication _____(1). Small volumes of blood loss over time lead to _____(2) anemia. Clinically, the stool has a _____(3) appearance. This is because of the presence of _____(4) blood. This condition is described as _____(5). If there is a large hemorrhage into the stomach, this causes _____(6) of blood. This state is described as _____(7). This often accompanies another complication known as _____(8). Here, the ulcer has eaten its way through the _____(9) and into the _____(10).

5. melena
6. vomiting
7. hematemesis
8. penetration
9. stomach wall
10. pancreas

12-37

1. cicatrization
2. stenosis

Cicatrization is another complication, which is excessive contraction of scar tissue to the point of deformity. If this occurs with a healing ulcer, it could cause stenosis or narrowing of a region of the stomach. Cicatrization of a hollow structure can be compared to drawing purse strings tightly. This most often develops around the pylorus, and so it is called **pyloric stenosis.** Contraction of the tissue where stomach contents are supposed to exit amounts to a blockage. In response to this obstruction, continual vomiting may occur. Sustained loss of stomach fluid can lead to dehydration and metabolic alkalosis from acid or hydrogen ion loss. A complication of duodenal ulcer is *perforation.* This is like penetration, except instead of breaking into an adjacent structure like the pancreas, the ulcer punches out a hole in the intestinal wall. This allows spillage of gastric contents into the abdomen. This causes intense inflammation of the abdominal cavity, or peritonitis (see Frame 12–83). Stomach acid and digestive enzymes wreak havoc on the peritoneal cavity. Peritonitis is an extremely painful condition that must be treated as an emergency because it has life-threatening consequences. Please refer to Figure 12–5 for an overview of peptic ulcers and their complications. If during healing, the scar tissue contracts too much, this is called _____(1). In a hollow organ, cicatrization produces narrowing or _____(2). This acts as an obstruction and produces

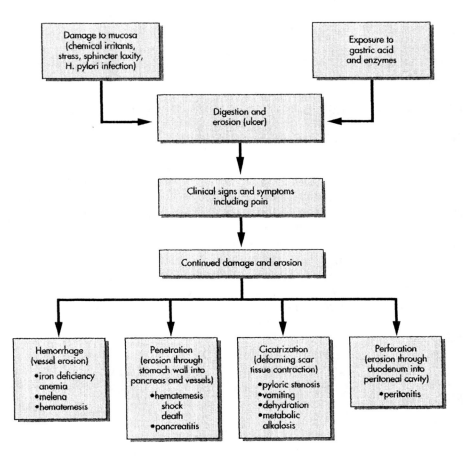

Figure 12–5. The pathogenesis and complications of peptic ulcers.

3. vomiting
4. dehydration
5. metabolic alkalosis
6. duodenal
7. intestinal
8. gastric contents
9. inflammation
10. peritonitis

ongoing _____(3). This can result in _____(4) and _____(5) from fluid and acid loss. A perforation is when a (an) _____(6) ulcer erodes through the _____(7) wall and creates an opening into the peritoneal cavity. Through this opening, _____(8) leak out. This causes widespread _____(9) of the abdominal cavity, which is called _____(10).

12-38

There are two approaches to treating peptic ulcers, medical and surgical. Most cases can be improved to the point of healing with a medical approach. The goal of medical therapy is to decrease the acidity of stomach contents so the damaged tissue may recover. Drugs used to accomplish this are antacids, antihistamines, and anticholinergics (histamine and acetylcholine both stimulate acid secretion). Managing stress and a bland diet are very helpful. Irritants such as alcohol must be avoided. Cases with *H. pylori* infection should be treated with antibiotics. In some cases, vagotomy (cutting the vagus nerve) may be helpful, since this nerve stimulates acid secretion. Severe cases usually require surgical intervention. A partial gastrectomy is a procedure in which part of the stomach is removed. In particular, acid-secreting sections are excised to remove the source of further damage. Loss of a portion of the stomach leads to some degree of malabsorption and weight loss. Surgery may be required to repair the damage of the complications of peptic ulcers such as massive bleeding, perforation, and peritonitis.

▶ GASTRIC NEOPLASIA

12-39

1. carcinoma

Since the stomach is an epithelial-lined organ, the classification of cancer of this organ would be _____(1). In particular, it is an adenocarcinoma because it affects the glandular epithelial cells. Stomach cancer is less common than colon cancer. Its incidence in this country has decreased over the years. This is believed to be due to improved food processing and sanitation. The cause of gastric neoplasia has not been proven, but diet is suspected to play a role. Specifically, the presence of nitrosamines may be linked to the development of cancer. Nitrosamines are generated when bacteria in food convert nitrates to nitrites. The presence of bacteria and nitrites are higher in food that has not been properly processed.

12-40

1. mucosa
2. metastasize
3. lumen
4. focal
5. fungating
6. polypoid
7. diffuse
8. thick
9. stiff

Adenocarcinoma of the stomach arises from the gastric mucosa. It may spread through the walls of the stomach and metastasize to regional lymph nodes, the liver, other abdominal organs, and the lungs. There are several patterns of stomach cancer. One is the formation of a cauliflower-like mass that bulges out into the lumen of the stomach. Since a mass is localized, this pattern is *focal*. The mass may vary slightly in appearance, earning it the descriptions *fungating* (like a mushroom), or *polypoid* (like a polyp). Another manifestation may be an irregularly shaped ulcer in the mucosa. This is the *ulcerative* form. A third pattern is *diffuse,* where the cancer is within the wall of the stomach causing it to thicken and stiffen. Significant thickening also decreases the space inside the gastric lumen. Stomach cancer develops in the gastric _____(1). It may spread or _____(2) to other sites. The formation of a mass that projects into the _____(3) of the stomach is a _____(4) pattern. It may look like a mushroom and be called _____(5), or like a polyp and be called _____(6). If the neoplasia is inside the stomach wall, this pattern is called _____(7). This causes the wall to become _____(8) and _____(9).

TABLE 12–2. DISEASES OF THE ESOPHAGUS AND STOMACH

Disease	Causes or Contributing Factors
Reflux esophagitis (heartburn, ulcers)	Inadequate closure of the lower esophageal sphincter with backflow of stomach acid due to lifestyle or hiatal hernia
Hiatal hernia	Idiopathic, predisposed to by obesity
Esophageal squamous cell carcinoma	Possibly environmental carcinogen, lifestyle (tobacco, heavy alcohol use)
Esophageal varices (varicose esophageal veins)	Portal vein congestion and hypertension in liver cirrhosis
Achalasia	Spasm of lower esophageal sphincter
Acute gastritis	Ischemia, ingestion of irritants (alcohol, spicy food, aspirin)
Chronic atrophic gastritis	Possibly autoimmune destruction of mucosal cells, infection with *Helicobacter pylori*
Peptic ulcer (gastric or duodenal)	Mucosal injury, gastric acid and enzymes, chemical irritants, stress, infection with *H. pylori*
Gastric adenocarcinoma	Idiopathic, diet

12–41

The signs and symptoms of stomach cancer are those common to cancer (pain, anorexia, weight loss, and anemia). Additional signs of stomach cancer are stomach distress or dyspepsia, the presence of an abdominal mass or enlarged stomach, vomiting caused by obstruction, and hematemesis. The prognosis for gastric neoplasia is poor because it tends to be detected late and it has usually metastasized by then. Before finishing this section, you may review the diseases of the esophagus and stomach by referring to Table 12–2.

III. REVIEW QUESTIONS

1. Reflux esophagitis is produced by:
   a. achalasia (spasticity) of the lower esophageal sphincter
   b. overproduction of stomach acid
   c. rupture of esophageal varices
   d. lower esophageal sphincter incompetency (failure to close)

2. A complication of chronic severe reflux esophagitis is:
   a. stenosis
   b. hiatal hernia
   c. achalasia
   d. esophageal varices

3. Sliding of the upper part of the stomach through the diaphragmatic hole describes:
   a. pyloric stenosis
   b. hiatal hernia
   c. dyspepsia
   d. umbilical hernia

4. Hiatal hernia often causes:
   a. esophageal varices
   b. esophageal achalasia
   c. reflux esophagitis
   d. gastritis

1. d–lower esophageal sphincter incompetency (failure to close)

2. a–stenosis

3. b–hiatal hernia

4. c–reflux esophagitis

5. a–varicose; b–pressure;
   c–liver; d–hemorrhage

6. a–acute gastritis

7. c–low-fiber diet

8. b–peptic ulcer

9. d–an ulcer

10. c–Damaged mucosa
    exposes submucosa to ero-
    sion by acid and enzymes.

11. 1. c–hemorrhage;
    2. a–penetration;
    3. b–cicatrization;
    4. d–perforation

5. Esophageal varices are a. _____veins of the esophagus, so dilated because of increased b. _____in the venous circulation usually due to c. _____ disease. Rupture causes massive d. _____.

thrombosed	stenosis	varicose
kidney	pressure	heart
volume	liver	hemorrhage
shock		

6. Excessive ingestion of irritants such as alcohol and aspirin can cause:
   a. acute gastritis
   b. reflux esophagitis
   c. chronic atrophic gastritis
   d. gastric ulcer

7. Which of the following is NOT suspected as a cause of chronic atrophic gastritis?
   a. autoantibody damage of gastric mucosal cells
   b. genetic predisposition
   c. low-fiber diet
   d. *Helicobacter pylori* infection

8. The lower esophagus, lesser curvature of the stomach, and upper duodenum are the most common sites for development of:
   a. carcinoma
   b. peptic ulcer
   c. gastroenteritis
   d. *Helicobacter pylori* infection

9. A sharply outlined deep hole in gastric mucosa, surrounded by inflammation and containing granulation tissue and fibrosis, describes:
   a. a vesicle
   b. a canker sore
   c. a diverticulum
   d. an ulcer

10. Which of the following BEST describes the pathogenesis of peptic ulcer?
    a. Autoantibodies stimulate gastric mucosal cells to greatly increase acid production.
    b. Overactivity of the vagus nerve increases acid production.
    c. Damaged mucosa exposes submucosa to erosion by acid and enzymes.
    d. Genetic predisposition combines with *H. pylori* infection to produce chronic inflammation.

11. Match the complications of peptic ulcer in the left column with the correct description in the right column:
    a. penetration   1. _____ seen as melena or hematemesis depending on the site
    b. cicatrization   and severity
    c. hemorrhage   2. _____ erosion into the pancreas which may cause hematemesis
    d. perforation   or pancreatitis
                        3. _____ creates pyloric stenosis and obstruction
                        4. _____ causes peritonitis when intestinal contents are released
                              into the abdomen

12. Cancer of the stomach, or gastric neoplasia, may appear in all of these forms EXCEPT:
    a. ulcerative
    b. diffuse
    c. fungating
    d. polypoid
    e. it appears in none of these forms
    f. it may appear in any of these forms

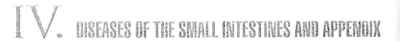

IV. DISEASES OF THE SMALL INTESTINES AND APPENDIX ◀ SECTION

▶ INFECTIOUS AND INFLAMMATORY DISORDERS OF THE SMALL INTESTINES

12–42

While vomiting is the hallmark of stomach distress, diarrhea is associated with intestinal disorders. **Diarrhea** is stool that is too loose, generally created by the presence of too much water or other fluid in the intestinal lumen. Of the mechanisms of diarrhea, there are three types that we will refer to. They are:

1. **Osmotic diarrhea.** The presence of excess solutes in the intestines (material not absorbed) draws water or solvent into the lumen. This follows the principle of osmosis discussed in Chapter 3. As too much water is retained in the lumen, this leads to a loose stool. Osmosis is the principle behind stool softeners. The material draws water into the intestines. Malabsorption leads to osmotic diarrhea. Malabsorption may or may not be caused by damage to the intestinal mucosa, through which material is absorbed.
2. **Inflammatory mucosal diarrhea.** In severe inflammation, large amounts of exudate fluid are produced and released into the lumen. Blood and mucus may contribute to the liquid contents, which makes for a loose stool.
3. **Secretory diarrhea.** During several bacterial infections (*E. coli,* cholera, *Shigella*), toxins are released by the microorganisms that stimulate cyclic AMP production by the mucosal cells. Cyclic AMP is an enzyme that regulates passage of solute and solvent across cell membranes. Increased production of this enzyme leads to a great outpouring or secretion of sodium and water into the small intestines. In this manner, an electrolyte imbalance may be created with sodium loss.

Diarrhea is defined as too much _____(1) in the _____(2). Osmotic diarrhea is created when unabsorbed _____(3) in the intestines draw _____(4) into the lumen. The state of _____(5) can cause osmotic diarrhea. In cases of great inflammation, _____(6) may leak into the lumen, along with _____(7) and _____(8). This is called _____(9). Some bacterial infection produces a chemical or _____(10), which causes _____(11) diarrhea. This is because the toxin increases production of _____(12), which allows the passage of a great amount of _____(13) and _____(14) into the intestinal lumen.

12–43

The term that means inflammation of the intestines is **enteritis** ("entero" referring to intestines). While chemical irritation is often responsible for gastritis [inflammation of the _____(1)], infectious states usually cause enteritis. Infectious enteritis often occurs in combination with infectious inflammation of the stomach (**gastroenteritis**) or with infectious inflammation of the colon (**enterocolitis**). Infections of the gastrointestinal tract are acquired from a contaminated environment. They are generally spread by the fecal–oral route, such as through contaminated food or water, or hand-to-mouth practices. Some infections are caused by highly virulent organisms that are not destroyed by stomach acid. [Viru-

2. disease

lent refers to an organism's ability to cause _____(2).] Other types of infection are caused by less virulent or weaker organisms. In these cases, either the organisms were ingested in very large numbers, or else they had a chance to grow and multiply before ingestion. This is the case with staphylococcal and *Salmonella* food poisonings. Leaving food unrefrigerated for a period of time or improper cooking can allow numbers to increase. Recall that dose is a factor in development of infection (see Chap. 5). Bacteria that cause enteritis (or gastroenteritis or enterocolitis) lead to diarrhea through two mechanisms. One is the release of a toxin that causes secretory diarrhea. There is no invasion and injury to the mucosa. Examples of this are cholera, *E. coli* infection, and staphylococcal food poisoning. Another mechanism is invasion of the mucosa in which the bacteria colonize and damage the intestinal walls. Inflammation and exudation is the result. This may be seen with *Campylobacter, Shigella,* and *Salmonella.* Some bacteria can act in both manners.

12–44

1. inflammation
2. intestines
3. infection
4. gastroenteritis
5. enterocolitis
6. environment
7. virulent
8. numbers
9. toxin
10. secretory
11. invasion
12. exudate
13. inflammatory mucosal

Enteritis is _____(1) of the _____(2). It is most often caused by _____(3) by microorganisms. Simultaneous inflammation of the stomach is called _____(4), while simultaneous inflammation of the colon is _____(5). GI infections develop from contact with the contaminated _____(6). They may develop in two ways: first is the ingestion of a powerful or _____(7) organism, and second is the ingestion of greater _____(8) of weaker organisms. Infectious diarrhea may develop in response to a _____(9) from the organisms. In this case it is a _____(10) type of diarrhea. Or there may be damaging _____(11) of the mucosa, with inflammation and _____(12) production. This is a _____(13) type of diarrhea.

12–45

1. *E. coli*
2. pathogenic
3. enterohemorrhagic
4. enterotoxigenic
5. enteroinvasive
6. cholera
7. toxin
8. dehydration
9. electrolyte imbalance
10. hypovolemic shock

Some microorganisms that cause infectious enteritis (or stomach and colon infection) are described in this frame and the next. These were presented in Chapter 5 on infectious disease, and you are referred back to that chapter for more detail on their mechanisms.

Most strains of *Escherichia coli* are harmless normal flora of the intestines. However, a few pathogenic strains do exist. They can be divided into four types:

1. Enteropathic *E. coli.* This strain causes severe diarrhea in infants.
2. Enterohemorrhagic *E. coli.* This strain causes a hemorrhagic or bleeding infection of the colon (colitis).
3. Enterotoxigenic *E. coli.* This strain causes a secretory diarrhea. It is commonly known as "traveler's diarrhea." People who are new to a particular environment, especially one in which sanitation practices are questionable, have not developed as much immunity as the residents. The clinical effects of traveler's diarrhea range from inconvenience to incapacitation.
4. Enteroinvasive *E. coli.* This strain invades the intestinal mucosa.

Cholera is caused by the pathogen *Vibrio cholerae.* Its mechanism is secretory diarrhea because of its toxin. There is no tissue invasion. Cholera produces intense vomiting and voluminous diarrhea (described as rice-water stool). Untreated cases quickly lead to life-threatening dehydration, electrolyte imbalance, and hypovolemic shock. About one third of untreated cases are fatal within a few days.

_____(1) is usually a harmless normal flora, but _____(2) strains do exist. Colonic bleeding is caused by _____(3) *E. coli,* secretory diarrhea is caused by _____(4) *E. coli,* and mucosal invasion is caused by _____(5) *E. coli. Vibrio* causes the serious disease _____(6). Secretory diarrhea is produced in response to a _____(7). Severe fluid loss can lead to _____(8), _____(9), and _____(10).

12-46

Staphylococcal food poisoning is another type of infectious enteritis. *S. aureus* growing in food causes vomiting and diarrhea because of its toxin. Therefore, the mechanism of diarrhea would be _____(1). The onset of illness is shortly after eating (1 to 4 hours) because it affects the stomach and upper small intestine. Food poisoning should be suspected when several people become ill after eating the same thing.

Salmonella food poisoning is also called *salmonellosis*. Many species of *Salmonella* cause enteritis. The mechanism may be either toxin-induced secretory diarrhea, or damage from invasion of the mucosa. In this case, blood and mucus may be present in the diarrhea. It also causes vomiting. Its onset is later, about 1 to 2 days, because it affects the lower intestine and the effects of invasion must accumulate. It should be suspected in delayed group illness with a history of food dishes in common.

Campylobacter is a bacteria that produces diarrhea because of invasion and colonization. This is also called *campylobacteriosis*. It affects the intestines and colon so it would be called infectious _____(2).

Shigella can produce abdominal pain and a very watery diarrhea. This is also called *shigellosis* or *bacterial dysentery*. It has both a secretory and invasive component. Intestinal wall inflammation often produces ulcers. A state of **dysentery** may develop. This is more severe than diarrhea. The stool is very watery but also contains significant amounts of blood and mucus. It may also contain bits of sloughed tissue from the intestinal walls. Bacterial dysentery often affects the colon, and colitis causes **tenesmus,** or straining when passing stool. Untreated cases can last a long time, leading to dehydration and weight loss. Shigellosis is often associated with epidemics.

1. secretory
2. enterocolitis

12-47

In differentiating between causes of food poisoning, timing is helpful. In staphylococcal cases, the timing is _____(1) after ingestion. With salmonellosis it is _____(2). In addition to toxin production like *Staphylococcus, Salmonella* also _____(3) the mucosa. One bacteria that causes infectious enterocolitis is _____(4). Dysentery may be a feature of infection with _____(5), often called _____(6) or _____(7). Erosions or _____(8) may be present in intestinal walls. Dysentery is differentiated from diarrhea by the presence of large amounts of _____(9), _____(10), and pieces of _____(11) tissue. Colitis during bacterial dysentery can cause straining at stool, called _____(12).

1. shortly
2. delayed or later
3. invades
4. *Campylobacter*
5. *Shigella*
6. shigellosis
7. bacterial dysentery
8. ulcers
9. blood
10. mucus
11. sloughed
12. tenesmus

12-48

Enteritis caused by viruses is much more common than bacterial enteritis. There are many viruses that may cause GI upset, but the most common are *rotavirus* (affecting infants and children), and *Norwalk agent* (affecting adults). Viruses invade the mucosa of the upper small intestine, where they grow inside the cells and damage them. Viral gastroenteritis is commonly called "intestinal flu." For 2 or 3 days, there is vomiting, diarrhea, fever, and abdominal cramping. Viral gastroenteritis is self-limiting and resolves without complications in a short while. Instead of the environment serving as the source of infection, as it is with bacterial enteritis, viral infections are transmitted from infected individuals. It tends to be seasonal and occur in epidemics in the winter months. The medical phrase for intestinal flu is _____(1). It is much _____(2) common than _____(3) enteritis. The virus most often affecting babies and children is _____(4), while _____(5) afflicts adults. The source of viral gastroenteritis is _____(6).

1. viral enteritis
2. more
3. bacterial
4. rotavirus
5. Norwalk agent
6. infected individuals

The last type of microorganism to be considered is the protozoa. The most common in this country to affect the small intestines is *Giardia lamblia*. Enteritis caused by *Giardia* is called *giardiasis*. This one-celled organism may be found in water contaminated by animal feces, having been passed from the animal's intestines. Municipal water treatment plants are sufficiently effective in removing this microorganism from the drinking water. Danger of giardiasis exists when drinking or accidentally ingesting raw, untreated water such as from lakes or streams. *Giardia* does not invade the mucosa but it does heavily colonize the surface. Its presence interferes with absorption of material from the intestinal lumen. When malabsorption exists, the type of diarrhea that can develop is _____(1) diarrhea. The most common protozoal enteritis in this country is _____(2), caused by _____(3). It is contracted by ingesting _____(4) contaminated by animal _____(5). It grows profusely on the surface of the _____(6), interfering with _____(7) and therefore causing diarrhea. Table 12–3 reviews the causes of infectious disease of the gastrointestinal tract.

Our next topic is **inflammatory bowel disease (IBD).** There are two separate diseases that fall under this heading. The first affects sections of the small intestines. It is called **regional enteritis** and it is also known as **Crohn's disease.** The second disorder affects the colon and is called ulcerative colitis. Ulcerative colitis will be discussed in Section V on colon diseases. Inflammatory bowel disease is a chronic condition characterized by repeated episodes of inflammation of the small and large bowel. It is difficult to separate regional enteritis from ulcerative colitis. They share the same underlying pathogenesis and have many features in common. These features include the population affected (generally Caucasians), a familial tendency, changes in the mucosa, and complications. However, they are traditionally considered by most sources to be two separate diseases. Regional enteritis is _____(1) of parts of the _____(2). Another name for this disease is _____(3). The same disorder, when it affects the colon, is called _____(4). Both of these diseases fall under the heading of _____(5).

The cause of regional enteritis is idiopathic. Genetic predisposition and autoimmune damage have been considered as possible causes or inciting factors. Stress or intense emotional distress may play a role in recurring episodes. Inflammatory bowel disease is chronic inflammation that most often affects the terminal ileum (the end of the last section of the small intestines), the appendix, and the colon. It is interesting to note that about 30 percent of IBD cases have inflammation of structures outside the intestines, in the skin, joints, liver, and eyes. In the intestines, this inflammation produces ulcers in the mucosa and extends through the

TABLE 12–3. MICROORGANISMS ASSOCIATED WITH INFECTIOUS GASTROENTERITIS, ENTERITIS, OR ENTEROCOLITIS

Microorganism	Features of Infection
Escherichia coli	
Enteropathic	Severe diarrhea in infants
Enterohemorrhagic	Bleeding of the colon
Enterotoxigenic	Traveler's diarrhea in new unsanitary environment
Enteroinvasive	Invasion of intestinal mucosa
Vibrio cholerae	Cholera—severe secretory diarrhea due to toxin
Staphylococcus aureus	Food poisoning due to toxin with acute onset
Salmonella	Salmonellosis or food poisoning due to either toxin or mucosal invasion with later onset
Campylobacter	Campylobacteriosis with mucosal invasion
Shigella	Shigellosis or bacterial dysentery with invasion of mucosa, ulcers, blood, and mucus
Rotavirus	Viral gastroenteritis ("intestinal flu") with mucosal cell invasion
Norwalk agent	
Giardia lamblia	Giardiasis due to ingestion of water contaminated by animal feces

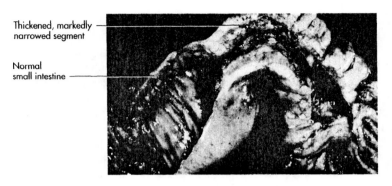

Thickened, markedly narrowed segment

Normal small intestine

Figure 12–6. Crohn's disease, showing significant narrowing and thickening of a segment of small intestine. (*From Chandrasoma and Taylor,* Concise Pathology, *2nd ed., Appleton & Lange.*)

1. ileum
2. appendix
3. colon
4. inflammation
5. intestines
6. ulcers
7. thickening
8. decreases or narrows
9. stiff
10. scar tissue
11. motility
12. peristalsis

wall. This thickens the wall. Granuloma formation is common and fibrosis is also a feature. The thickening of the walls causes the lumen to become narrowed in sections. This can be seen in Figure 12–6. The scarring stiffens the affected sections, causing them to lose flexibility. The appearance of the mucosa is described as "cobblestone" because affected areas are dispersed among normal areas. Figure 12–7 is an excellent example of this configuration. As the inflammation reaches the outside of the intestines, it involves the serosa. Fibrosis on the external surface leads to the formation of adhesions, or bands of scar tissue. These bands run among the loops of intestines and gather or hold them. This interferes with motility and peristalsis. Significant adhesion formation causes chronic obstruction, which is a complication of regional enteritis. The structures affected in inflammatory bowel disease are the end of the _____(1), the _____(2), and the _____(3). Some cases of IBD have _____(4) in structures outside of the _____(5). The lesions seen in regional enteritis are _____(6) of the mucosa, and _____(7) of the walls. The thickening _____(8) the lumen of involved sections. Fibrosis makes the walls _____(9). A complication of chronic regional enteritis is adhesions, the formation of bands of _____(10). Adhesions can cause parts of the intestines to stick together, thereby interfering with _____(11) and _____(12).

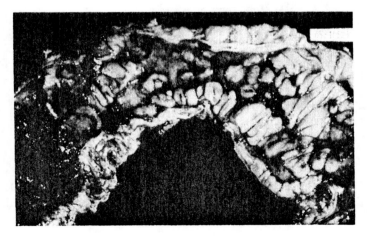

Figure 12–7. Crohn's disease, showing the typical cobblestone appearance of the mucosa. (*From Chandrasoma and Taylor,* Concise Pathology, *2nd ed., Appleton & Lange.*)

Regional enteritis may be hard to diagnose for a long period because the signs are vague. The signs are diarrhea, cramps, melena, and weight loss. The damage to the intestines by chronic inflammation leads to some degree of malabsorption, and therefore to malnutrition. Electrolyte imbalance and nutritional deficiency are common effects. Later in the course of the disease, constipation may become a feature. The narrowed lumen combined with adhesion formation interferes with the ability to move material along the digestive tract. Signs of inflammation outside the GI tract correspond to the affected structure, such as dermatitis (skin) and arthritis (joints). Regional enteritis is definitively diagnosed through endoscopy and biopsy. Endoscopy is the use of a flexible hollow tube with a light and viewing device at the end. This allows internal lesions to be seen. Because it is hollow, it is possible to pass pincers through it to take a tissue sample for biopsy. Treatment for regional enteritis is aimed at controlling the severity of episodes and relieving the signs. This is done with anti-inflammatory medications, which include corticosteroids and azulfidine. In severe cases, where hemorrhage or perforation is a threat, surgery is required. The diseased sections are removed or resected. However, it is not unusual for regional enteritis to develop later in the remaining normal sections.

▶ ISCHEMIC BOWEL DISEASE

1. blood supply
2. oxygen
3. damage
4. atherosclerosis
5. clot or thrombus
6. hypotension
7. heart failure

Infarction of the intestines (death due to absence of blood supply and oxygen) occurs as a dramatic result of obstruction or complete occlusion of arteries. Ischemia (damage due to decreased blood supply and oxygen) is a more subtle injury. Ischemia may be widespread or patchy depending on the cause. Conditions that interfere with the blood supply to the intestines include:

1. *Atherosclerosis* of arteries supplying the intestines (see Chap. 9). As you know, atherosclerosis is a common condition and a chronic one.
2. *Partial thrombosis* of the veins draining the intestines (see Chap. 9).
3. *Systemic hypotension* or shock. This may worsen any pre-existing condition such as atherosclerosis.
4. *Congestive heart failure,* which produces systemic hypoperfusion and episodes of hypotension.

Ischemia of the intestines is insufficient _____(1) and therefore insufficient _____(2), which causes _____(3) to the tissue. Narrowing of the arteries by fat plaques, or _____(4) is one cause of ischemia. In thrombosis, a vein is blocked by the presence of a _____(5) which interferes with blood supply. Shock produces systemic _____(6), and periodic hypotension is also a feature of congestive _____(7).

1. severity

The effects of intestinal ischemia depend on the severity of interruption in blood supply. Mild cases cause edema, slight hemorrhage, and some necrosis of the mucosa. The damage does not affect the entire wall of the intestine. Healing is without complications and with minimal fibrosis. With a moderate amount of damage there is more scarring after healing. This may lead to cicatrization and stenosis or stricture. The effect of intestinal stenosis (whatever the cause) is shown in Figure 12–8. Greater amounts of fibrosis are also seen in chronic conditions like atherosclerosis. A severe episode of ischemia causes greater hemorrhage, ulceration, and complete loss of areas of the mucosa. It is often complicated with infection by normal intestinal flora (the coliforms), which are now able to penetrate deep into the intestinal wall. If the cause of severe ischemia is not removed, it may proceed to infarction. This may occur if a partially blocked vessel becomes completely blocked. The necrosis extends through the full thickness of the wall. The area becomes gangrenous and is very likely to rupture. Rupture is associated with a high death rate. In intestinal ischemia, the amount of tissue damage depends on the _____(1) of

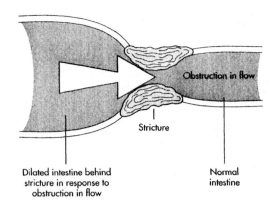

Figure 12–8. Intestinal stenosis or stricture.

interruption in _____(2). In mild cases the effects do not involve the entire _____(3) and there is minimal scarring or _____(4). With greater damage there is more _____(5) once it has healed. This may lead to the complication of _____(6), which is _____(7) or stenosis. A worst case of ischemia is often complicated by _____(8) with coliforms. This is because loss of more mucosa allows the bacteria to _____(9) into the wall. Severe ischemia that is not relieved may lead to tissue death or _____(10). A section of affected intestinal wall undergoes _____(11) completely through. Gangrene and _____(12) are likely.

2. blood supply
3. wall
4. fibrosis
5. scarring
6. cicatrization
7. stricture
8. infection
9. penetrate
10. infarction
11. necrosis
12. rupture

12-55

Clinically, the signs of ischemic bowel disease depend on the duration and extent of injury. The abdomen may become rigid because of pain (intestinal angina). Remember that ischemic tissue is painful. This presentation is called an "acute abdomen," which will be discussed in the last section. Diarrhea is present with a variable amount of blood. Chronic ischemia will lead to weight loss because of malabsorption. (Any time the intestinal walls are diseased, this interferes to some degree with their function of absorbing nutrients.) Infarction and rupture cause septic peritonitis (see Frame 12–84). The patient goes into shock and will die unless this is repaired during emergency surgery.

► INTESTINAL OBSTRUCTION

12-56

A term from the Greek that means obstruction of the intestines is **ileus**. This is any type of blockage that prevents material from moving forward. An obstruction may be a physical impediment, in which case it is a **mechanical ileus.** Or it may be a lack of normal intestinal peristalsis or movement, in which case it is a **nonmechanical** or **paralytic ileus.** During obstruction, pressure from mounting chyme or fecal material increases behind the site and the section also dilates. The pressure may kill the tissue of the walls (pressure necrosis) or cut off blood supply (infarction). In mechanical ileus especially, the pressure and necrosis may build to the point of gangrene and rupture. In a rupture, chyme and digestive enzymes or fecal material spills into the abdominal cavity. Millions of intestinal bacteria also enter the abdominal cavity. The presence of enzymes or bacteria causes widespread chemical inflammation, or infectious inflammation, respectively. This condition is peritonitis (see Frame 12–83). Intestinal rupture and peritonitis are fatal if not treated aggressively on an emergency basis. Ileus means _____(1) of the _____(2). Material in the bowels is not allowed to _____(3) forward. A physical blockage is called _____(4). Lack of intestinal motility is called _____(5). The

1. obstruction
2. intestine
3. move
4. mechanical ileus
5. nonmechanical or paralytic ileus

6. pressure
7. pressure necrosis
8. infarction
9. rupture
10. abdominal cavity
11. inflammation
12. peritonitis

_____(6) behind the site of obstruction rises. The pressure may cause _____(7) or _____(8). The danger is if the pressure rises to the point of _____(9). In this case, intestinal contents are released into the _____(10), causing widespread _____(11). This condition is called _____(12).

12–57

1. caught
2. hole
3. blood vessel
4. blood
5. strangulated hernia
6. infarction
7. rupture
8. twist
9. suspended
10. kinked or twisted
11. infarction

The causes of mechanical or obstructive ileus are described in this frame and the next.

1. A **mass** or space-occupying lesion such as a tumor or gallstones.
2. A **hernia** in which a section of the intestine gets caught in or bulges through a hole in the abdominal wall. The affected section becomes kinked, and material is prevented from moving through. The vessels are squeezed at the site where the intestines are caught. If the blood supply is cut off, then the section is strangled. This is called a **strangulated hernia.** The danger of a strangulated hernia is infarction and rupture. The most common hernias are:
   A. an inguinal hernia, where a loop of intestine slides through the inguinal canal and into the scrotum or under the skin;
   B. an umbilical hernia, where the intestine may protrude through the wall around the umbilicus or naval; and
   C. a hiatal hernia, where the intestine projects up through the hole in the diaphragm.
3. **Volvulus,** which is twisting of a section of small intestine ("twisted bowel"). The bowels are suspended by hanging connective tissue called the mesentery. Therefore the intestines are not anchored and are relatively free floating. In a volvulus, the bowels have rotated around in the mesentery. The vessels have also become twisted and therefore kinked. This leads quickly to infarction. A volvulus must be straightened out during emergency surgery.

An intestinal hernia is when a loop of bowel gets _____(1) in a _____(2) in the abdominal wall. In addition to the intestine being compressed at the site, the _____(3) may also be squeezed. This may cut off _____(4) supply. If this occurs, the condition is described as a _____(5). The complications of a strangulated hernia are _____(6) and _____(7). A volvulus is a _____(8) in a section of intestine. This may occur because the intestines are _____(9) in mesentery and are able to move freely. The vessels may also become _____(10), which again interferes with blood supply and may lead to _____(11).

12–58

1. band
2. scar tissue

4. **Adhesions,** as mentioned earlier, are bands or strings of scar tissue in the abdominal cavity. They run from one free surface to another, causing the affected structures to be stuck together. When adhesions join loops of bowel together, it interferes with peristalsis and movement of material. Adhesions form after an inflammatory reaction in the abdomen. The inflammation is often the fibrinous type (see Chap. 2), so fibrin is present in a great amount and it organizes into stringy threads. Adhesions may follow a bout of peritonitis, surgery after which fibrosis develops around the manipulated tissue, or after perforation of a peptic ulcer.
5. **Intussusception,** during which a section of intestine pushes forward into itself like a collapsing telescope. It is similar to pulling a sleeve partially inside out. The medical term for this is **invagination.** The junction of the invagination obstructs movement of material and may compromise blood supply. The presence of a tumor, increased intestinal motility, and acute enteritis predispose to an intussusception.
6. **Stenosis,** or narrowing, is the last example of causes of mechanical ileus. Cicatrization is the most common reason for stenosis.

An adhesion is a _____(1) of _____(2) that forms between two structures, connecting them together. Adhesions between intestinal loops decrease

_____(3). These fibrous cords form after _____(4) in the abdominal cavity. Intussusception is the _____(5) of one section of the intestine inside another. For greater understanding, it is compared to a _____(6) telescope. Cicatrization, or excessive _____(7) of scar tissue, can cause obstruction by creating _____(8). Figure 12–9 illustrates the causes and complications of mechanical ileus.

3. peristalsis
4. inflammation
5. invagination
6. collapsing
7. contraction
8. stenosis

12–59

The causes of paralytic ileus include:

1. Severe pain, during which sphincters in the intestines enter a spasm and fail to relax to let material pass.
2. Peritonitis, during which a significant accumulation of pus from infection surrounds the intestine and prevents contraction of smooth muscle. Appendicitis and perforated ulcer are two conditions that may lead to infectious peritonitis.
3. Severe enteritis, where the inflammation interferes with neuromuscular transmission.

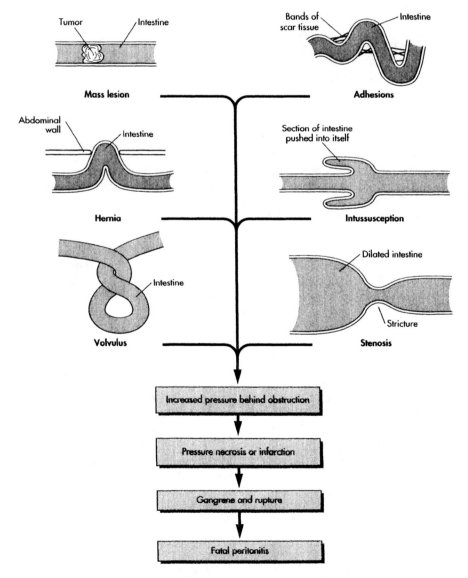

Figure 12–9. Causes of obstructive ileus and complications.

1. nonmechanical or
   paralytic ileus
2. obstruction
3. motility

4. Nerve damage during spinal cord trauma, which leaves sections of the intestines denervated (without nerve transmission).

Severe pain, infection, inflammation, and nerve interruption may cause _____(1). This means there is no physical _____(2), but there is lack of intestinal _____(3).

12–60

Complete mechanical obstructions are acute and present as emergencies. The pain is severe and the abdomen is rigid and distended with fluid and gas. Vomiting may be profuse and produce a foul, greenish material. The strain of vomiting increases the risk of rupture. Constipation is complete since nothing, not even gas, can be passed. Emergency surgery is required for mechanical ileus. The physical abnormalities must be corrected (a herniated loop pulled out, a volvulus untwisted, adhesions broken down). Areas of necrotic or gangrenous sections must be removed. The ends of the remaining sections are joined together in a procedure called **anastomosis.**

► MALABSORPTION

12–61

1. absorption
2. nutrients
3. function
4. disease
5. surgical
6. GI tract
7. short bowel

The primary function of the small intestines is to absorb nutrients from food. The prefix "mal" means bad. Therefore, **malabsorption** means bad or inadequate absorption of nutrients, and represents a failure in function. Any primary disease that damages intestinal structure or alters the absorptive surface may cause enough interference with function that malabsorption results. Malabsorption has already been mentioned as a complication of a primary disease, such as infectious enteritis or regional enteritis. Since this failure is the result of a primary disease, it can be called **secondary malabsorption.** (In Frame 12–65 we will discuss an example of primary malabsorption.) In addition to injury from disease, secondary malabsorption can be created after surgical removal of parts of the GI tract. Examples include surgery for peptic ulcer, trauma, Crohn's disease, and obstructive infarction. Surgery that removes enough of the GI tract to produce secondary malabsorption leads to **short bowel syndrome.** Short bowel syndrome is defined as a loss of a significant amount of functional intestine because of *either* disease or surgical removal. There is literally a decrease in the length of functional bowel and a proportional loss of absorptive area. Depending on the amount of loss, short bowel syndrome can cause malnutrition (see Frame 12–64), since nutrients, vitamins, and minerals are poorly absorbed. Malabsorption is poor _____(1) of _____(2), and this represents a failure in _____(3) of the GI tract. Secondary malabsorption may result after damage from a primary _____(4). It may also be created after _____(5) removal of parts of the _____(6). Loss of so much of the GI tract that it creates secondary malabsorption is called _____(7) syndrome.

12–62

1. digestion
2. absorbed
3. malabsorption
4. enzymes

Another related concept is **maldigestion.** This is failure to adequately digest or break down food so that it can be absorbed. Naturally, it follows that if food cannot be first digested properly, then it will not be able to be absorbed. Therefore, maldigestion leads to malabsorption. Maldigestion may exist because of several causes. Atrophy of the stomach, or atrophic gastritis, fails to produce hydrochloric acid and proteolytic enzymes. Lack of digestive enzymes from the pancreas is a major cause of maldigestion. When the pancreas does not release sufficient quantities of enzymes, this is called pancreatic insufficiency (see Chap. 13). One cause of this is continual damage that eventually destroys the exocrine portion of the pancreas. This damage is seen in chronic pancreatitis (see Chap. 13). Other causes of maldigestion include cystic fibrosis (which you will recall severely affects the pancreas), and obstructed bile flow from the liver or gallbladder (see Chap. 13). Maldigestion is insufficient _____(1) of food so that nutrients are not available in necessary form to be _____(2). Therefore, maldigestion will lead to _____(3). The most significant cause of maldigestion is lack of enough digestive _____(4) from the _____(5). Disease of the pancreas may so impair its output of enzymes that the condition is described as _____(6).

5. pancreas
6. pancreatic insufficiency

12-63

Clinically, malabsorption appears as weight loss in adults and stunted growth in children. Because fat is not absorbed, but instead is passed with the stool, the stool is pale and greasy. Unabsorbed fat in stool is **steatorrhea.** The stool is very malodorous, or has a great stench, because of bacteria metabolizing the fat. There is an excess of stool volume because of all the material that is passed instead of being absorbed. For this reason, the stool is sometimes described as "bulky." Additional signs of malabsorption are because of malnutrition, which is described in the next frame.

12-64

It makes sense that both maldigestion and malabsorption eventually lead to poor nutrition. The term for this would be _____(1). **Malnutrition** is defined as a deficiency of required nutrients, which include proteins, lipids, fat-soluble vitamins (A, D, E, and K), and minerals. The clinical signs of malnutrition are many. Some of them are:

1. malnutrition

1. Anemia from protein deficiency. Related to this is edema caused by hypoalbuminemia.
2. Amenorrhea or lack of menstruation.
3. Bleeding tendencies from lack of vitamin K.
4. Bone weakness and hypocalcemia from lack of vitamin D.
5. Lethargy or weakness.
6. Hair loss.
7. Delayed healing.
8. Muscle wasting.
9. Electrolyte imbalance.

12-65

Primary malabsorption is caused by an intrinsic defect in intestinal function. It is not the result of damage from some previous disease or surgical loss of bowel. Of the primary malabsorption disorders, **celiac disease** is the most common. It is also known as **celiac sprue,** and **gluten hypersensitivity enteropathy.** This last name is the most descriptive, for it is indeed a disease of the intestines caused by hypersensitivity to gluten. Gluten is a plant-based protein found most notably in wheat products. You know from Chapter 4 that hypersensitivity is an immune reaction commonly known as an allergic reaction. This allergy to gluten is most likely due to genetics, although the exact mechanism of inheritance has not been established. Since the immune reaction to this foreign substance is an allergy, the antigen (gluten) would be called an _____(1). The presence of gluten in the diet incites the production of antibodies and their attack of this allergen. Since gluten is absorbed in the intestines, this is the site of attack and therefore the site of damage. The mucosa becomes chronically inflamed. This leads to degeneration of the villi, and they become shortened and flattened. Atrophy would be another word to describe this loss of epithelial tissue and the loss of function. These projections also become thickened by infiltration with immune cells. Obviously, absorption though such abnormal epithelial structures becomes seriously impaired.

1. allergen

12-66

Failure in absorption *not* related to pre-existing disease or surgical removal of bowel is called _____(1). The most well-known example is _____(2) disease, also called celiac _____(3) and _____(4). The etiology is thought to be _____(5) in nature. The underlying pathogenesis is a _____(6) or _____(7) reaction. The allergen is _____(8), a protein found in _____(9). The immune-mediated damage occurs in intestinal walls, where it causes the villi to become _____(10) and _____(11). Another word to describe the changes is _____(12). These epithelial "fingers" also become thickened with infiltration by _____(13). Clinically, celiac disease is first expressed in childhood after eating wheat-based cereals. Diarrhea and cramps are the predominant signs and symptoms.

1. primary malabsorption
2. celiac
3. sprue
4. gluten hypersensitivity enteropathy
5. immune mediated
6. hypersensitivity
7. allergic
8. gluten
9. wheat
10. short
11. flat
12. atrophy
13. immune cells

TABLE 12–4. CLASSIFICATION AND FEATURES OF MALABSORPTION

Classification	Cause
Primary malabsorption	Defective intestinal absorption Celiac disease (celiac sprue, gluten hypersensitivity)
Secondary malabsorption	Short bowel syndrome Primary intestinal disease (enteritis), which interferes with absorption Surgical removal of parts of GI tract Maldigestion (atrophic gastritis, pancreatic insufficiency, cystic fibrosis, cholestasis)

Features
Weight loss in adults, stunted growth in children
Steatorrhea
Malnutrition

These discomforts disappear if gluten grains are removed from the diet. Gluten hypersensitivity enteropathy is definitively diagnosed through biopsy, which shows the typical changes in the villi. The treatment is a gluten-free diet, which allows the mucosa to regenerate back to normal. Table 12–4 reviews the classification, causes, and features of malabsorption.

▶ INTESTINAL NEOPLASIA

12–67

1. carcinoid
2. glandular mucosa
3. neuroendocrine
4. liver
5. carcinoid

Cancer of the small intestines is uncommon compared to cancer of the large intestines (colorectal cancer, Frame 12–77). Of the few small bowel neoplasia, carcinomas are rare. Lymphoma of the gastrointestinal lymphoid tissue does occur, and it is similar to the lymph node lymphoma discussed in Chapter 9. The most common malignancy is a **carcinoid,** which arises from the glandular cells in the mucosa. This is considered a "neuroendocrine tumor" and is often present as multiple nodules. Carcinoid is a low-malignancy cancer, meaning it grows very slowly. However, it will metastasize to the lymph nodes and liver. Once it has reached the liver, **carcinoid syndrome** is likely to occur. This is somewhat like the paraneoplastic syndrome described in Chapter 6, where a tumor secretes compounds with hormone-like activity. Since carcinoid is of neuroendocrine origin, the tumor does secrete hormone-like chemicals once it has reached the liver. These secretory products enter the bloodstream and cause constriction of bronchi and wheezing, watery diarrhea, abdominal pain, and even fibrosis of the right heart valves. The most common malignant neoplasia of the small intestines is a _____(1). Its origin is from _____(2). It is therefore classified as a _____(3) tumor. It exhibits the typical secretory behavior of a neuroendocrine tumor once it has reached the _____(4). Clinically, the signs are described as _____(5) syndrome.

▶ APPENDICITIS

12–68

Appendicitis is acute inflammation of the appendix caused by obstruction and infection. The appendix is a hollow cul-de-sac near the ileocecal junction (where the small intestine meets the cecum of the large intestine). It has no apparent function. It does, however, have a tendency to trap fecal material in its blind end, which predisposes to obstruction. The cause of acute inflammation of the appendix may be related to a diet containing high amounts of red meat and low amounts of fiber. It usually affects young adults. Often, the inflammation is related to the presence of a **fecalith,** which is a hard mass of feces that blocks the appendix ("lith" refers to stone). This blockage is also described as an impaction, and it may lead to infection by intestinal bacteria. During acute appendicitis, the appendix becomes red and swollen, with ulcers in its mucosa. Figure 12–10 compares a normal appendix with an inflamed one that contains a fecalith. The predominating organism isolated from an infected appendix is generally *E. coli*. The peritoneum surrounding the appendix also becomes inflamed. The complications of acute appendicitis are of serious concern. The entire sac may become a large abscess, causing localized peritonitis. The infection may spread to the liver. A common complication of an untreated case is perforation. If the appendix becomes necrotic and gangrenous, it will rupture. This allows fecal material, bacteria, and pus into the abdominal cavity. The widespread peritonitis that results is generally fatal if not treated in time. This treatment includes aggressive antibiotic therapy and surgical lavage (flushing) of the abdomen.

12-69

Appendicitis is _____(1) of the _____(2). It most likely develops because of _____(3) and _____(4) of this appendage. The obstruction is with _____(5) material, which when it is hardened, is called a _____(6). The infection is most often caused by the bacteria _____(7). A common complication of acute appendicitis is _____(8). This is rupture of the necrotic and _____(9) appendix. This allows fecal and infectious material into the abdomen, causing widespread _____(10), which is potentially fatal. Clinically, the pain of acute appendicitis causes the abdomen to be rigid, and this is another suspicion on the list when managing a case with the acute abdomen presentation. The right lower quadrant of the abdomen is very tender on palpation during later stages. Fever, nausea, and vomiting accompany the classic presentation. Leukocytosis (increased numbers of neutrophils and bands on a CBC) is present and indicates an inflammatory condition. If perforation occurs, the relief from swelling often causes the pain to subside. Therefore, rupture should be suspected in these cases. The treatment is surgical removal of the appendix (appendectomy) to prevent complications.

1. inflammation
2. appendix
3. obstruction
4. infection
5. fecal
6. fecalith
7. *E. coli*
8. perforation
9. gangrenous
10. peritonitis

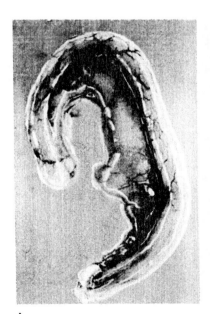
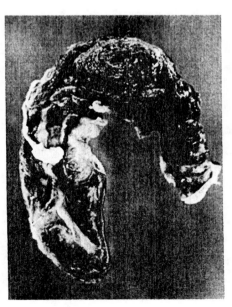

A   **B**

Figure 12–10. A. A normal appendix. **B.** Appendicitis. The appendix is swollen and inflamed with a fecalith present in the lumen *(arrow). (From Kent and Hart,* Introduction to Human Disease, *3rd ed., Appleton & Lange.)*

Because the danger of perforation and peritonitis is so grave, the general policy is to perform an appendectomy if appendicitis is suspected, rather than proven.

IV. REVIEW QUESTIONS

1. e–None of these descriptions are correct.

2. b–infectious states caused by ingested bacteria

3. a–invasion of the walls, causing inflammatory mucosal diarrhea; d–stimulation of cyclic AMP, causing secretory diarrhea

4. a–blood; b–mucus; c–tissue

5. c–viral gastroenteritis

6. a–1. osmotic

7. c–inflammatory bowel disease

1. Of the following descriptions of the mechanisms of diarrhea, which is correct?
   a. Inflammatory mucosal diarrhea is the presence of unabsorbed solutes, which draws water in the lumen.
   b. Secretory diarrhea is an outflux of exudate with blood and mucus.
   c. Osmotic diarrhea is stimulation of cyclic AMP with copious loss of sodium and water.
   d. All of these descriptions are correct.
   e. None of these descriptions are correct.

2. Enteritis, gastroenteritis, and enterocolitis are:
   a. inflammatory states caused by ingested irritants
   b. infectious states caused by ingested bacteria
   c. inflammatory states caused by poor diet and genetic predisposition
   d. infectious states caused by exposure to infected individuals

3. During bacterial infection of the small intestines, the two mechanisms that produce diarrhea are (choose two):
   a. invasion of the walls, causing inflammatory mucosal diarrhea
   b. invasion of the walls, causing secretory diarrhea
   c. stimulation of cyclic AMP, causing osmotic diarrhea
   d. stimulation of cyclic AMP, causing secretory diarrhea

4. Bacterial dysentery causes severe watery diarrhea containing a._____, b. _____, and sloughed dead c. _____.

5. The most common type of infectious gastroenteritis is:
   a. bacterial gastroenteritis
   b. giardiasis
   c. viral gastroenteritis
   d. dysentery

6. *Giardia lamblia* (giardiasis) causes a. _____ diarrhea because of its heavy colonization and interference in absorption.
   1. osmotic   2. secretory   3. inflammatory mucosal   4. dysentery

7. Regional enteritis is classified as:
   a. ischemic bowel disease
   b. infectious enteritis
   c. inflammatory bowel disease
   d. obstructive bowel disease

8. Features of regional enteritis include (choose all that apply):
   a. paralytic ileus
   b. extraintestinal inflammation
   c. mucosal ulcers
   d. volvulus
   e. thickening of the walls
   f. granuloma formation
   g. diverticula
   h. adhesion formation
   i. ischemic necrosis

9. Thrombosis, atherosclerosis, and systemic hypotension may produce:
   a. ischemic bowel disease
   b. inflammatory bowel disease
   c. mechanical ileus
   d. paralytic ileus

10. Which of the following is NOT a potential complication of ischemic bowel disease?
    a. cicatrization and stenosis
    b. infection
    c. infarction and rupture
    d. intussusception

11. Ileus is the medical term for:
    a. infectious enteritis
    b. intestinal obstruction
    c. inflammatory bowel disease
    d. ischemic bowel disease
    e. malabsorption

12. Which of the following is NOT a potential complication of intestinal obstruction?
    a. cicatrization
    b. pressure necrosis
    c. infarction
    d. rupture
    e. peritonitis

13. Please match the causes of mechanical ileus in the left column with the correct description in the right column:
    a. intussusception
    b. strangulated hernia
    c. volvulus
    d. adhesions
    e. stenosis

    1. _____ loop of bowel caught in a hole in the abdominal wall with blood supply cut off
    2. _____ threads of fibrotic tissue joining bowel loops together
    3. _____ contraction of fibrosis causing narrowing of the lumen
    4. _____ invagination of one section of bowel into another
    5. _____ rotation or twisting of bowels

14. Short bowel syndrome is:
    a. a congenital defect in which parts of the small intestine are missing
    b. a result of celiac sprue in which the villi become shortened
    c. loss of a significant amount of functional bowel as a result of disease or surgery
    d. hyperactivity in peristalsis so that absorption time is shortened

8. b–extraintestinal inflammation; c–mucosal ulcers; e–thickening of the walls; f–granuloma formation; h–adhesion formation

9. a–ischemic bowel disease

10. d–intussusception

11. b–intestinal obstruction

12. a–cicatrization

13. 1. b–strangulated hernia;
    2. d–adhesions;
    3. e–stenosis;
    4. a–intussusception;
    5. c–volvulus

14. c–loss of a significant amount of functional bowel as a result of disease or surgery

15. d–secondary malabsorption

16. a–malabsorption;
    b–maldigestion

17. a–steatorrhea; b–malab-
    sorption

18. c–celiac sprue

19. a–carcinoid

20. d–The coliform most often
    isolated from an infected
    appendix is *Clostridium diffi-
    cile.*

15. Short bowel syndrome causes:
    a. primary malabsorption
    b. Crohn's disease
    c. celiac disease
    d. secondary malabsorption

16. List two general failures in intestinal function that lead to malnutrition:
    a. _____ b. _____

17. Pale, greasy, bulky stool is medically described by the term a. _____, and
    is a clinical sign of b. _____.
    melena   malnutrition   steatorrhea
    hematemesis   malabsorption   carcinoid

18. Allergy or hypersensitivity to the wheat protein gluten is seen in the disease:
    a. Crohn's disease
    b. ulcerative colitis
    c. celiac sprue
    d. short bowel syndrome

19. Cancer of the small intestines most often takes the form of:
    a. carcinoid
    b. adenocarcinoma
    c. lymphoma
    d. squamous cell carcinoma

20. Choose the INCORRECT statement about acute appendicitis:
    a. The underlying pathogenesis is impaction by hardened feces and infection.
    b. A low-fiber diet contributes to the incidence of inflamed appendix.
    c. Rupture and peritonitis are life-threatening complications of acute appendicitis.
    d. The coliform most often isolated from an infected appendix is *Clostridium difficile.*

SECTION ▶ ## V. DISEASES OF THE LARGE INTESTINES AND ABDOMINAL CAVITY

▶ INFLAMMATORY DISORDERS OF THE LARGE INTESTINES

12–70

Idiopathic ulcerative colitis was introduced in Section IV as one of two disorders of the
intestines that are classified as chronic inflammatory bowel disease. Ulcerative colitis is
chronic inflammation of the colon and rectum, and of the appendix in some cases. Its cause
is unknown, as is the cause of regional enteritis. The same factors are suspected, and include
stress or emotional upset as well as autoimmune and genetic factors. There are several differences in pathology between regional enteritis and ulcerative colitis. In ulcerative colitis,
there is a diffuse (spread-out) inflammation of the colonic mucosa instead of the patchy
appearance seen in regional enteritis. Following inflammation, ulcers later develop. Areas of
the mucosa atrophy and inflammatory polyps may develop, as seen in Figure 12–11. The
fragile, damaged lining bleeds easily. Infection by intestinal bacteria is common. The ulcers
spread throughout the colon. Only the lining is affected. The entire wall does not become
inflamed as it does in regional enteritis. Granuloma and adhesion formation are also absent.
Instead of thickening, the wall of the colon becomes thinned and dilation may occur. A
dilated, enlarged colon is described as **megacolon.** One feature the two diseases have in

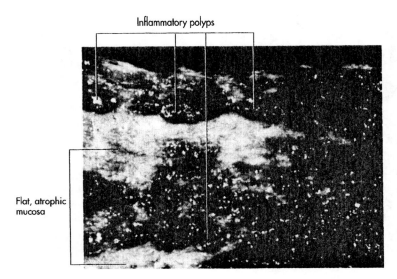

Inflammatory polyps

Flat, atrophic mucosa

Figure 12–11. Chronic ulcerative colitis, with flat areas of atrophied mucosa and inflammatory polyps. *(From Chandrasoma and Taylor,* Concise Pathology, *2nd ed., Appleton & Lange.)*

common is inflammation of other body structures outside of the intestines. Idiopathic ulcerative colitis is classified as chronic _____(1). The differences in the course of disease between regional enteritis and ulcerative colitis are that in ulcerative colitis the pattern is _____(2) instead of patchy; the wall of the colon is _____(3) instead of thick because _____(4) does not affect the entire wall; and there are no _____(5) or _____(6) formations. After inflammation, erosions or _____(7) develop through much of the colon. It is common for _____(8) of other parts of the body to coexist with ulcerative colitis, as it does in regional enteritis.

1. inflammatory bowel disease
2. diffuse
3. thin
4. inflammation
5. granuloma
6. adhesion
7. ulcers
8. inflammation

12–71

A very important complication of ulcerative colitis, not seen with regional enteritis, is increased risk of cancer. In prolonged cases, where the inflammation has been present for years, the eventual dysplasia of the epithelial tissue becomes pre-neoplastic. The concept of continual injury followed by abnormal regeneration has been previously presented as a possible precursor of cancer. About 30 percent of the cases develop adenocarcinoma of the colon. Clinically, idiopathic ulcerative colitis presents as intermittent episodes of weight loss, colicky cramps, diarrhea with pus and mucus, and rectal bleeding. Chronic blood loss leads to iron deficiency anemia. Medical management of these long-standing cases includes stress reduction, avoidance of irritating foods, and corticosteriods to decrease inflammation. In prolonged cases, a cure is desirable and achieved by surgical removal of the colon. This eliminates the significant risk of cancer. The procedure is called a colostomy or ileostomy. A permanent opening is created in the abdominal wall and the end of the remaining bowel (the ileum) is attached to the opening. Feces are passed through the abdominal opening and into a collecting bag (a colostomy bag). The inconvenience that this creates in one's lifestyle must be weighed against the troublesome episodes of the disease and risk of cancer. Chronic inflammation or chronic injury to epithelial tissue may lead to dysplastic regeneration, which may be pre-_____(1). This is probably the basis for the increased incidence of _____(2) among ulcerative colitis victims.

1. neoplastic or cancerous
2. colon cancer

Pseudomembranous colitis is inflammation of the colon caused by the intestinal bacteria *Clostridium difficile.* The bacteria are normally found in small numbers in the colon. It has the ability to secrete a necrotizing (tissue-killing) toxin. Pseudomembranous colitis, while possibly due to other causes, is most commonly a complication of oral antibiotic therapy. The prolonged use or overuse of broad-spectrum antibiotics kills much of the protective normal flora in the colon. Without their presence, *C. difficile* multiplies into great numbers. This overgrowth is accompanied by the release of toxin. The toxin causes necrosis of the mucosa. A **pseudomembrane** (false membrane) is formed and it is made of fibrin, inflammatory cells, mucus, and dead tissue. This exudate is sticky and adheres to the mucosa. The pseudomembrane can cover a large area. Other microorganisms such as *Staphylococcus* and *Shigella* have also shown the ability to produce necrotizing toxins. The clinical presentation of pseudomembranous colitis is acute severe diarrhea with blood. Sloughing of the false membrane and tissue loss are responsible for the bleeding. This condition must be recognized early and treated aggressively, since the toxins can cause death. The treatment, ironically, is antibiotics. However, the antibiotic is not broad spectrum but is specific for *C. difficile.*

1. enterocolitis

Bacterial infections of the colon were first introduced in Section IV. Bacterial infection of the intestines is enteritis. Bacterial infection of the intestines *and* colon is _____(1). The mechanisms were presented earlier. Toxins from bacteria stimulate cyclic AMP, which produces a secretory diarrhea of the small intestines. Or microorganisms invade and colonize the colon walls, causing direct injury and diarrhea. Organisms that specifically infect the colon include *E. coli, Campylobacter, Salmonella,* and *Shigella.* Infection of the colon often produces **tenesmus,** which is spastic straining brought on by irritation of nerves that control evacuation of bowels, or bowel movements. **Dysentery** is infectious inflammation of the colon that causes a severe, watery diarrhea and abdominal pain. Bacterial invasion and tissue damage cause blood, mucus, pus, and necrotic tissue to be present in the diarrhea of dysentery.

▶ DIVERTICULA

1. diverticula
2. mucosa
3. muscle fibers
4. diverticulosis
5. age
6. diet
7. fiber
8. constipation

Diverticula (the singular form is **diverticulum**) are small pouches that form in the intestinal wall and protrude outward, not into the lumen. The mucosal lining pushes through the muscle fibers of the wall, creating indentations. These numerous tiny sacs are about pea sized. Diverticula of the sigmoid colon are the most clinically significant. The presence of many diverticula defines the condition **diverticulosis.** The cause of diverticulosis seems to be related to age and diet. The number of diverticula increases with age as tissue weakens, and diverticulosis is common among the elderly. A diet that is low in fiber, or lacks enough roughage, creates constipation, which favors the development of diverticula. In constipation the stool is too hard and is difficult to move. This causes straining to evacuate the bowels. The pressure herniates the mucosa and submucosa, so that they bulge through the muscular layer at points of relative weakness in the walls (where vessels enter). Tiny outpouches in the walls of the intestines are called _____(1). They are caused by the _____(2) pushing or bulging through the _____(3) of the walls. A significant number of diverticula is called _____(4). Their development appears to be related to old _____(5) and a _____(6) low in _____(7). Straining to pass hard stool, or _____(8), favors the formation of diverticulosis.

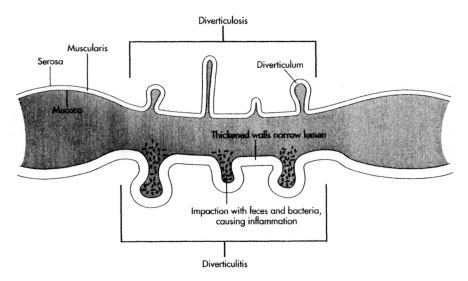

Figure 12–12. Diverticulosis and diverticulitis.

12–75

Diverticulosis is relatively asymptomatic and not a great problem unless complications develop. The most common complication is **diverticulitis,** which is infectious inflammation of the tiny sacs. It should be easy to imagine how these depressions in the colon walls become impacted with feces over time. Bacteria become trapped inside, causing infection and inflammation, and add to the obstruction. As in appendicitis, bacteria trapped in the sacs are able to multiply into numbers capable of causing infection. The walls in the area become thickened by the inflammation, narrowing the lumen and further interfering with the passage of stool. Another less common but more serious complication is rupture or perforation of the infected diverticula. This may lead to abdominal abscess formation, adhesions, and peritonitis. The most common complication of diverticulosis is _____(1). This is inflammation caused by _____(2). The infection develops after _____(3) and _____(4) obstruct the diverticula. The passage of stool may be hindered when the walls become _____(5) in reaction to the inflammation. Diverticulosis and diverticulitis are illustrated in Figure 12–12.

1. diverticulitis
2. infection
3. feces
4. bacteria
5. thickened

12–76

While diverticulosis causes few if no signs, diverticulitis produces abdominal pain and tenesmus. The stool often contains blood. Severe diverticulitis clinically resembles carcinoma of the colon. Diverticula are easily seen during barium enema and x-ray studies. Medical management of diverticulitis includes administration of antibiotics. A change to a fiber-rich diet should decrease the incidence of further episodes. Severe cases prone to recurrent infection may require surgical excision of the colon.

▶ NEOPLASIA OF THE COLON

12–77

The majority of malignant neoplasia of the colon is of the adenocarcinoma type. Malignant neoplasia is much more common in the large intestine or colon than it is in the small intestines. Colon cancer is the third most common malignancy in this country behind lung and breast cancer. Even though this is a cancer that is relatively easily diagnosed (in part because of its location), it is still a leading cause of death. This may be due to the avoidance of regular checkups. Management of colon cancer is aimed at regular screening (checking for blood in the stools) and early diagnosis. The most common form of colonic adenocarcinoma is focal tumor formation (versus diffuse thickening). The tumor protrudes into the lumen. Many cases involve the sigmoid colon and the rectum, and protruding rectal tumors can be palpated during a routine physical exam.

The etiology of colon cancer is most likely due to the influence of carcinogenic factors such as genetics and diet. Some people have a strong hereditary predisposition for colon cancer, and this may be due to the possession of oncogenes or a deficiency in tumor suppressor genes. Those people whose relatives have had colon cancer are at higher risk than the general population and should be screened regularly. The diet most associated with adenocarcinoma of the large intestines contains high amounts of red meat (especially when grilled over charcoal, which increases carcinogens), high amounts of fat, and low amounts of fiber. Chronic inflammatory conditions, most notably idiopathic ulcerative colitis, also seem to predispose to cancer development. Malignant neoplasia of the _____(1) intestines is much more common than it is in the _____(2) intestines. Malignancy of the large intestines is of the _____(3) type. It is not hard to detect, but it still a leading cause of _____(4). The most common form is a protruding _____(5), which can be _____(6) during a rectal examination. Three carcinogenic factors associated with colon cancer are _____(7) predisposition, poor _____(8), and chronic _____(9).

Neoplasia of the colon may be benign or malignant. The growth begins as a **polyp,** which is a round mass of tissue that projects into the lumen. A **pedunculated polyp** is attached to the mucosa by a stalk. This is shown in Figure 12-13. The polyp is produced by overgrowth of epithelial tissue or mucosa on the tips of villi. Some remain benign, and others are transformed into malignancy by carcinogenic factors. The incidence of polyp formation increases with age. A benign polyp is an adenoma, while a malignant one is an adenocarcinoma tumor.

In colorectal adenocarcinoma, at least half are located around the rectosigmoid area, where the colon ends and the rectum begins. Most tumors begin as premalignant neoplastic polyps. Other forms include plaques and ulcerations. Often, there is infiltration of the colon wall around its entire diameter, which narrows the lumen. This is a circumferential stenosis, which can be seen in Figure 12-14. This can be felt rectally and is described as a "napkin-ring" stricture. Although the growth of colorectal cancer is relatively slow, advanced cases metastasize to local lymph nodes and then to the liver, where death is inevitable. Neoplasia of the colon usually begins as growths known as _____(1). A polyp sitting on a stalk is called a _____(2). The most common site for colorectal cancer is around the _____(3) area. Infiltration of the wall _____(4) the lumen, and the stricture that can be palpated is compared to a _____(5). Death in colon cancer is because of _____(6) to the _____(7).

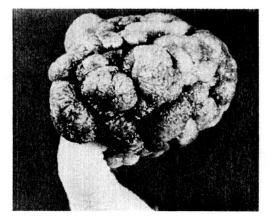

Figure 12-13. A pedunculated polyp of the colon. *(From Chandrasoma and Taylor,* Concise Pathology, *2nd ed., Appleton & Lange.)*

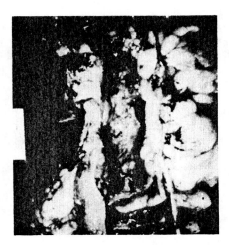

Figure 12–14. Carcinoma of the colon, showing the circumferential stenosing type of growth. *(From Chandrasoma and Taylor, Concise Pathology, 2nd ed., Appleton & Lange.)*

12–81

Clinically, there are no signs of early colorectal adenocarcinoma. It can, however, be detected by routine health checks that screen for the presence of occult blood in the stool. Occult means hidden, so the blood is not grossly visible. A positive occult blood test is followed by an endoscopic exam and biopsy of abnormal areas. Cases advanced enough to produce signs exhibit typical findings of cancer including pain and weight loss. Signs particular to colon cancer include visible blood in the stool. The surfaces of tumors are scraped during stool passage, and the ulcerated surfaces bleed. The presence of the tumors as space occupying-lesions interferes with the passage of stool, creating constipation. The stool produced is often ribbon-like. Iron deficiency anemia because of chronic bleeding is a common finding. Colon cancer can be cured if it is detected soon enough and the colon is surgically removed before metastasis. The location of most of the tumors makes removal easier. The prognosis for colorectal adenocarcinoma is good if it is found before metastasis. If it has already spread to the liver, the prognosis is grave.

► DISORDERS OF THE ABDOMINAL CAVITY

12–82

The abdominal cavity is properly termed the **peritoneal cavity.** Like the thorax or chest, this is a compartment that houses the vital organs. Like the chest, it is also lined with a double-layered serous membrane called the **peritoneum.** The visceral layer covers the abdominal organs, and the parietal layer lines the cavity. The peritoneum is very absorptive, that is, it easily absorbs many materials that may gather in the abdominal cavity. Examples of materials that can be absorbed include blood and medications. Transfusions in neonates, or the administration of some drugs, may be accomplished with an intraperitoneal (IP) infusion, which is injection directly into the abdominal cavity. Unfortunately, the peritoneum also absorbs toxins or infectious materials just as well. The substances absorbed by the peritoneum enter the general circulation.

1. inflammation
2. peritoneum or abdominal cavity
3. irritants
4. infection
5. localized
6. generalized

Peritonitis is inflammation of the peritoneal cavity due to chemical irritants or infection by bacteria. It may be localized (confined to one area) or generalized (widespread). Inflammation because of chemical irritation, not infection, is called **sterile peritonitis.** Causes of sterile peritonitis include:

1. A ruptured gallbladder or common bile duct, which releases bile into the abdominal cavity. Bile contains inflammatory bile acids.
2. Acute pancreatitis, in which digestive enzymes are spilled into the abdominal cavity from areas of injury in the pancreas.
3. Surgical material, such as talc powder on gloves, which enters the abdomen.

Sterile peritonitis generally produces a localized inflammation at the site of contact between the irritant and the peritoneum. Peritonitis is _____(1) of the _____(2). It may be caused by chemical _____(3) or by _____(4) by bacteria. If the inflammation is contained in one area, this is _____(5) peritonitis. If it covers a wide area, this is _____(6) peritonitis.

Infectious or **septic peritonitis** develops when bacteria from the intestines gain entry into the abdominal cavity. Entry is gained through the rupture of a diseased abdominal organ or penetrating trauma. Of these coliforms, *E. coli* is the most predominant of the infectious agents. Depending on the ruptured organ, fecal material may also be spilled into the abdomen. Whether infectious peritonitis is localized or becomes generalized depends on the size of the rupture and the amount of infectious material introduced into the cavity. A small perforation or hole in an inflamed organ usually produces localized infectious peritonitis. Causes include perforation associated with acute appendicitis, peptic ulcer, regional enteritis, and diverticulitis. The exudate that always accompanies infectious peritonitis contains sticky fibrin, which organizes to wall off or confine the infection to the initial area of spill. Adhesions (see Frame 12–87) often develop.

1. bacteria
2. rupture
3. organ
4. size
5. amount
6. localized
7. fibrin
8. generalized

In generalized infectious peritonitis, there is perforation of a diseased section of the digestive tract on a greater scale, with the release of more bacteria and fecal material. The disease states listed in Frame 12–84 can cause generalized infection if the rupture is significant. In addition, a common cause of generalized peritonitis is rupture of a sizeable portion of intestine when a section becomes necrotic or gangrenous. Disease states of the intestines that lead to necrosis and large ruptures include strangulated hernia, intussusception, volvulus, complete intraluminal obstruction, and penetrating intestinal trauma. In ulcerative colitis, the dilated colon (megacolon) is also susceptible to rupture (toxic megacolon). Infectious peritonitis is the result of intestinal _____(1) entering the abdomen. Coliforms and fecal material gain entry into the abdomen through a hole or _____(2) in a diseased _____(3). Infectious peritonitis may be localized or generalized depending on the _____(4) of a rupture or the _____(5) of foreign material that is spilled. In small perforations, the peritonitis is usually _____(6) or held in check. This holding is accomplished by _____(7), which closes off the area. A large perforation or great amount of foreign material in the abdomen causes _____(8) peritonitis.

In generalized infectious peritonitis, the walling-off response is insufficient. The infection cannot be contained and spreads throughout the peritoneal cavity. The toxins from the organisms, and other harmful substances in the exudate, are absorbed into the general circulation. This produces toxemia and septic shock that is easily fatal. The formation of adhesions can cause intestinal obstruction, which is a further complication. Clinically, infectious peritonitis presents as severe abdominal pain and rigidity (extreme tension) of the abdominal muscles. This is described as "guarding" the abdomen and is a presentation of the acute abdomen. Systemic signs and symptoms associated with infection and shock are also present and include fever, leukocytosis, hypotension, and collapse. Generalized infectious peritonitis is treated as an emergency. Potent antibiotics must be administered intravenously. Surgical management must include repair of the inciting perforation and peritoneal lavage. This is suctioning out as much exudate as possible, followed by flooding the abdominal cavity with sterile saline to literally wash out the infection and stop the absorption of harmful substances. Shock is treated with fluids to maintain blood pressure, corticosteroids, and correction of acid–base imbalance. Even today, the prognosis for generalized infectious peritonitis is guarded. The pathogenesis of septic shock in generalized infectious peritonitis is the _____(1) of toxins from bacteria that enter the _____(2). Figure 12–15 outlines the pathogenesis of the three types of peritonitis that you have just studied.

1. absorption
2. general circulation

12–87

After inflammation of the abdominal cavity (sterile or infectious), the fibrin in the exudate matures or organizes into tough, fibrous scar tissue. This dense connective tissue takes the form of stringy bands, instead of acting as a patch for a tissue defect. These bands are called **peritoneal adhesions.** Any inflammatory condition within the abdomen, including surgical activity, can cause adhesion formation. Therefore, the same diseases that were cited as causing peritonitis can also lead to adhesion formation. Adhesions link parts of the gastrointestinal tract and other organs together. Tough threads run from one free surface to another, tying the structures together. The most clinically significant result is intestinal obstruction. In these cases, surgery is required to break down the adhesion. An adhesion is a stringy _____(1) of _____(2) that forms after inflammation. Its origin is _____(3), which is found in exudate. Adhesions tie parts of the _____(4) tract together. This may lead to intestinal _____(5).

1. band
2. scar tissue
3. fibrin
4. gastrointestinal
5. obstruction

12–88

Ascites is the presence of excess fluid in the abdominal cavity. The abdomen becomes distended or swollen. There are three kinds of fluid that may accumulate. The fluid may be a transudate (low in protein and lacking inflammatory cells), which closely resembles tissue fluid. Its accumulation is usually the result of increased pressure in an organ that squeezes fluid into the abdomen. In cirrhosis of the liver, or portal hypertension (see Chap. 13), fluid leaks from the liver. In nephrotic syndrome (see Chap. 14), fluid is lost from the kidneys. In congestive heart failure (see Chap. 10), pressure backs up into the liver and fluid then leaks from this organ. During generalized peritonitis, the fluid is an exudate (high in protein and containing inflammatory cells). Exudate that is bloody is often associated with carcinoma that has metastasized to the peritoneum. The least frequent type of fluid is chyle, which is milky fluid containing fat. It may build up when the thoracic duct or intestinal lymph vessels are obstructed. Ascites is too much _____(1) in the _____(2). A serous fluid low in protein is a _____(3), and it may accumulate when _____(4) in certain organs is _____(5). This causes fluid to be _____(6) into the abdomen. Inflammatory fluid high in protein and cells is a (an) _____(7), and it is associated with generalized _____(8). Blood in ascites may be caused by the presence of _____(9).

1. fluid
2. abdominal cavity
3. transudate
4. pressure
5. increased
6. squeezed
7. exudate
8. peritonitis
9. carcinoma

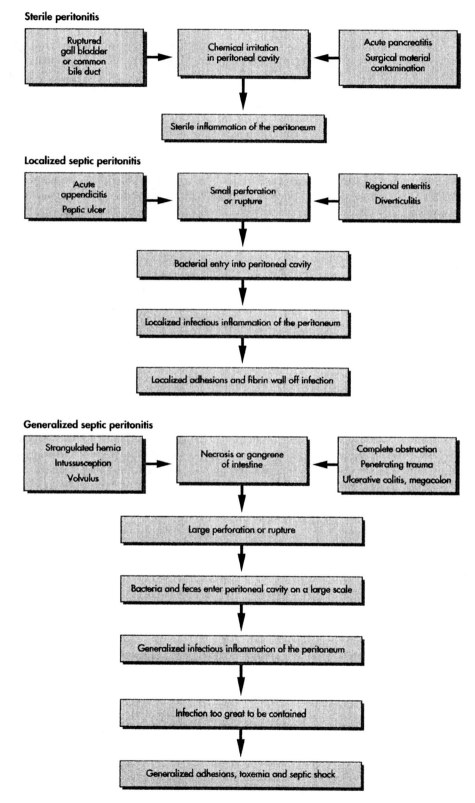

Figure 12–15. The pathogenesis of peritonitis.

V. REVIEW QUESTIONS

1. Idiopathic ulcerative colitis is classified as:
   a. ileus
   b. ischemic bowel disease
   c. neoplastic bowel disease
   d. inflammatory bowel disease
   e. secondary malabsorption

2. Features of idiopathic ulcerative colitis that SEPARATE it from regional enteritis are (choose all that apply):
   a. extraintestinal inflammation
   b. inflammation and thickening of the walls
   c. diffuse inflammation
   d. thinning of the walls and dilation
   e. ulceration of the mucosa
   f. absence of granuloma formation
   g. infection
   h. absence of adhesion formation

3. A complication of ulcerative colitis not seen with regional enteritis is:
   a. increased risk of adenocarcinoma of the colon
   b. gangrene and rupture
   c. obstruction
   d. diverticulum formation

4. Which of the following statements about pseudomembranous colitis is INCORRECT?
   a. It is infectious inflammation of the colon usually caused by *Clostridium difficile*.
   b. It develops when an immune-suppressed individual becomes vulnerable to opportunistic infection.
   c. A toxin from the bacteria causes necrosis and sloughing of the mucosa.
   d. A false membrane composed of inflammatory exudate adheres to the walls.

5. Diverticulosis is:
   a. the presence of a single large protrusion of the colon mucosa out through the muscle of the wall
   b. a congenital deformity where the sigmoid colon ends as a blind sac or diverticulum
   c. infectious inflammation of diverticula
   d. the presence of many small protrusions of the colon mucosa out through the muscle of the wall

6. Diverticula formation is favored by the presence of which of the following factors? (Choose all that are correct.)
   a. advanced age
   b. high-fiber diet
   c. chronic diarrhea
   d. low-fiber diet
   e. chronic inflammation
   f. chronic constipation

1. d–inflammatory bowel disease

2. c–diffuse inflammation; d–thinning of the walls and dilation; f–absence of granuloma formation; h–absence of adhesion formation

3. a–increased risk of adenocarcinoma of the colon

4. b–It develops when an immune-suppressed individual becomes vulnerable to opportunistic infection.

5. d–the presence of many small protrusions of the colon mucosa out through the muscle of the wall

6. a–advanced age; d–low-fiber diet; f–chronic constipation

7. b–fecal impaction and trapped bacteria in diverticulosis

8. c–colon and rectum

9. a–a polyp

10. c–around the rectosigmoid junction

11. b–inflammation of the abdominal cavity caused by bacterial infection spread over a wide area

12. a–generalized infectious peritonitis

13. d–absorption of toxins and other infectious material through the peritoneum and into the bloodstream

14. a–3. adhesions

7. Diverticulitis develops as a result of:
   a. an extension of infectious bacterial enterocolitis
   b. fecal impaction and trapped bacteria in diverticulosis
   c. an extension of ulcerative colitis
   d. constipation or hard stool

8. The most common gastrointestinal neoplasia affects the:
   a. stomach
   b. small intestines
   c. colon and rectum
   d. esophagus

9. In colorectal cancer, a focal precancerous growth that protrudes into the lumen is described as:
   a. a polyp
   b. a napkin-ring stricture
   c. hyperplastic villi
   d. an adenocarcinoma

10. Most cases of large bowel adenocarcinoma are located:
    a. in the end or distal portion of the rectum
    b. in the transverse colon
    c. around the rectosigmoid junction
    d. in the sigmoid colon

11. Generalized septic peritonitis is:
    a. inflammation of the abdominal cavity caused by chemical irritation in a confined area
    b. inflammation of the abdominal cavity caused by bacterial infection spread over a wide area
    c. inflammation of the abdominal cavity caused by chemical irritation spread over a wide area
    d. inflammation of the abdominal cavity caused by bacterial infection in a confined area

12. Intestinal obstruction followed by necrosis and rupture usually causes:
    a. generalized infectious peritonitis
    b. generalized sterile peritonitis
    c. localized infectious peritonitis
    d. localized sterile peritonitis

13. In generalized infectious peritonitis, septic shock develops because of:
    a. severe systemic hypotension when venous circulation pools in abdominal vessels
    b. thrombosis of abdominal vessels by bacterial emboli
    c. entry of bacteria into the bloodstream through diseased intestinal walls
    d. absorption of toxins and other infectious material through the peritoneum and into the bloodstream

14. Inflammation within the abdominal cavity may end with the creation of
    a. _____ from fibrin in the exudate.
    1. ascites   2. cicatrization   3. adhesions   4. abscesses

15. The most significant complication of peritoneal adhesions is:
    a. rigidity in the abdominal wall
    b. intestinal obstruction
    c. peritonitis
    d. septic shock

16. The accumulation of excess fluid in the abdominal cavity is called _____.

15. b—intestinal obstruction

16. ascites

VI. OTHER DISORDERS OF THE GASTROINTESTINAL SYSTEM ◀ SECTION

▶ CONGENITAL MALFORMATIONS AND OTHER BIRTH DEFECTS

12-89

The information about birth defects that affect the digestive tract is presented for your awareness and for the sake of completion. These are malformations that occur in the developing embryo. Most require surgical repair in babies to prevent death. The most common defects are:

1. **Cleft lip** and **cleft palate.** A failure of fusion (joining) between the nasal and maxillary processes (the upper roof of the mouth) creates a fissure or common area between the mouth and nasal cavity.
2. **Esophageal atresia.** This in an incomplete tube formation where the distal portion or end of the esophagus is missing. Actually, it is connected to the trachea, creating a tracheo-esophageal fistula, and the upper portion of the esophagus is a blind sac.
3. **Pyloric stenosis.** The distal section or outlet end of the stomach is greatly narrowed because the muscle has thickened or hypertrophied. This is the most common of the congenital abnormalities, second to Meckel's diverticulum. The stricture prevents the stomach from emptying. The result is projectile vomiting in an affected newborn after feeding.
4. **Congenital diaphragmatic hernia.** A large hole in the diaphragm allows a significant portion of the intestines to push into the chest and interfere with breathing.
5. **Hirschsprung's disease.** This is an abnormality of the nerve cells that control bowel movements. Lack of proper innervation leads to inability to evacuate feces. Stool builds up, causing great distention of the colon (megacolon). Hirschsprung's disease causes chronic constipation and abdominal distention.
6. **Meckel's diverticulum.** This is a large tubular sac or outpouch of the ileum. Meckel's diverticulum is asymptomatic except when the diverticulum becomes impacted with chyme and bacteria. Then the obstructive inflammation resembles appendicitis.
7. **Anal atresia.** In this condition, the end of the rectum is missing. The blind tube does not connect to the anus. A fistula, or abnormal opening from the rectum into the bladder or vagina, is common.

▶ MISCELLANEOUS DISORDERS OF THE GASTROINTESTINAL SYSTEM

12-90

A very troublesome condition is **irritable bowel syndrome,** also known as **spastic colon.** As the name implies, this is overactivity of the large bowel. There are no physical lesions that accompany this disorder, as there are in the organic diseases we have already studied. Inflammation, ulcers, or masses are absent. Instead, irritable bowel syndrome is a disturbance in function of peristalsis or movement. The exact cause is unknown but it is strongly suspected to be related to stress or emotional upset. Therefore, instead of being an organic disease, it may be classified as psychosomatic. It is well known that the autonomic nervous system can adversely

1. overactivity
2. lesions
3. function
4. stress
5. emotional upset

affect the digestive tract. Clinically, spastic colon resembles other intestinal upsets. There are episodes of diarrhea, gas accumulation, and cramping. While there is no specific treatment, increasing fiber in the diet helps to regulate motility. Episodes of disturbance are made worse by certain irritating foods (spicy foods, alcohol, and caffeine, for example), and so these substances should be avoided. In irritable bowel syndrome there is _____(1) of the large bowel. This is not because of physical _____(2) that are seen in organic diseases, but due to disturbance in _____(3). This disturbance is believed to be brought on by _____(4) or _____(5).

12–91

1. hemorrhoids
2. varicose
3. piles
4. pressure
5. inflamed
6. swollen

Hemorrhoids are varicose veins of the rectum and anus, so they are dilated veins filled with stagnant blood. Hemorrhoids, also called "piles," may develop internally in the rectum, or externally around the anus. The likelihood of developing hemorrhoids seems to be related to a genetic or familial predisposition, the existence of varicose veins in the legs, and a low-fiber diet. The actual cause of piles is probably increased pressure in the rectal or anal region that interferes with venous drainage and causes dilation. Constipation, frequent straining to pass stool, and pregnancy are some conditions that increase pressure in this area. Hemorrhoids become inflamed easily and that accounts for the pain associated with swelling. Ulceration of the veins may occur and bleeding is common. Most cases are successfully managed medically, rather than requiring surgery, as was done in the past. Increasing fiber in the diet, stool softeners, and creams to relieve swelling and pain are the general approach to treatment. Dilated or engorged veins of the rectum and anus are medically termed _____(1). They are actually _____(2) veins. A common term for hemorrhoids is _____(3). Hemorrhoids may develop when there is increased _____(4) present in the region. Hemorrhoids are painful if they become _____(5) and _____(6).

VI. REVIEW QUESTIONS

1. f–none of the above

2. b–increased pressure around the rectum or anus

1. In irritable bowel syndrome, the pathologic lesions that are found are (choose all that are correct):
   a. ulcers of the mucosa
   b. inflammation of the walls
   c. obstructing masses
   d. stenosis
   e. diverticula
   f. none of the above

2. The cause of hemorrhoids is most likely:
   a. low-fiber diet
   b. increased pressure around the rectum and anus
   c. genetics
   d. vasculitis of the rectum and anus

CHAPTER ▶ SUMMARY

▶ **SECTION II**

A common cause of the condition *stomatitis* (literally, inflammation of the mouth) is infection by the virus herpes simplex type I. Infection causes *vesicles* ("cold sores") on the lips, which may recur for the lifetime of the individual. Factors that contribute to vesicle recurrence include stress, sunlight, and fever. *Aphthous stomatitis* ("canker sores") is the condition of recurrent lesions inside the mouth, the cause of which is unknown. As with herpes-induced vesicles, canker sores heal spontaneously.

Pus accumulation in the tonsils leads to swelling, pain, and dysphagia (difficulty in swallowing); this condition is called *tonsillitis.* "Strep throat" is infection of the tonsils and pharynx, specifically with the bacterium *Streptococcus pyogenes,* leading to fever, malaise, and a sore throat. Infection by a particular strain of *Streptococcus* may lead to scarlet fever, so named because of the appearance of a red rash on the face. *Oral candidiasis* ("thrush") is caused by *Candida albicans,* a fungus that is part of the normal flora of the mouth. The condition is seen most often in the immune suppressed and in AIDS patients.

Dental caries (cavities) are characterized by infectious inflammation, with varying degrees of destruction, of the layers of a tooth. Cavities result from the production of organic acids by bacterial colonies in the areas around the teeth, leading to decalcification and erosion of the tooth enamel. If bacteria invade the root of the tooth, a *periapical abscess* may occur. *Gingivitis* (infectious inflammation of the gums) is the result of plaque (composed of bacteria, decaying food, and organic acids) on the gum tissue. Gingivitis often precedes more severe periodontal disease, such as tartar accumulation underneath the gum line. Accumulation of bacteria, plaque, and tartar within the periodontal tissue leads to *periodontitis,* a condition that can lead to loosening and/or loss of the teeth. Individuals with periodontitis may have *pyorrhea* (pus exuding from the gums) and *halitosis* (foul breath).

Oral neoplasia (cancer of the mouth) is of the squamous cell carcinoma type. This condition, the most common site of which is the lower lip, can result from smoking and from chronic alcohol consumption. Carcinoma of the tongue and of the pharynx can also occur. Oral neoplasia may manifest as white plaques (leukoplakia) or red plaques (erythroplasia).

Inflammation of the salivary glands *(sialoadenitis),* is most commonly caused by a viral infection ("mumps"). Other causes include bacterial infection, autoimmune damage to the salivary glands, or neoplasia. If pus is present in a salivary gland, the condition is called suppurative sialoadenitis. Swelling and disturbances of saliva production and secretion can occur in sialoadenitis or, in the case of cancer of the salivary glands, paralysis of the facial muscles.

▶ SECTION III

Inflammation of the esophagus *(esophagitis),* a relatively rare condition, can be caused by fungal or viral infection, or by swallowing a caustic chemical. *Reflux esophagitis,* due to the backflow of stomach acid, is the most common form of esophageal inflammation. This condition can lead to esophageal stenosis, thereby inhibiting the passage of food into the stomach. A *hiatal hernia* occurs when the upper part of the stomach slides through the hiatus, the opening in the diaphragm through which the esophagus passes. A hiatal hernia interferes with closure of the lower esophageal sphincter and can lead to reflux esophagitis.

Cancer of the esophagus, which presents as a squamous cell carcinoma, is highly malignant. Since the incidence of this type of cancer varies worldwide, it may be due to an environmental carcinogen. *Esophageal varices* are varicose veins of the esophagus. This condition results from an interference in drainage of the portal vein (most often due to cirrhosis of the liver), causing a backup of blood and an increase in pressure and dilation of the esophageal veins. This situation can in turn lead to rupture of the veins. A characteristic sign of ruptured esophageal veins is *hematemesis* (vomiting blood).

Achalasia is sporadic tension of the lower esophageal sphincter (LES), a condition that results in dysphagia. *Acute gastritis* is inflammation of the stomach lining that leads to erosions of the epithelium or to ulcers of the mucosa. The condition can be caused by a deficient blood supply to the stomach, as may be seen in shock or by the presence of steroids in the circulation. Many other factors (irritant chemicals, alcohol, aspirin, caffeine, bacteria) can lead to acute gastritis. In the condition of *chronic gastritis,* inflammation and atrophy of the mucosa are seen, leading to dyspepsia and pernicious anemia. Autoimmune destruction, bacterial infection, or genetic predisposition have all been implicated as the cause of chronic gastritis.

A *peptic ulcer* results from inflammation and eventual necrosis of the mucosal cells of the stomach and small intestine. Ulcers develop due to the action of acid and digestive enzymes on the mucosa. "Gastric" and "duodenal" define ulcers localized in the stomach and duodenum, respectively. The cause of peptic ulcers is unclear, but chemical irritants, relaxation of the pyloric sphincter, stress, alcohol, genetic predisposition, or bacteria may contribute to their formation. Complications include hemorrhage (manifested by melena and hematemesis), cicatrization (which could lead to pyloric stenosis), dehydration, perforation (resulting in a spillage of stomach contents into the abdomen), and peritonitis.

Adenocarcinoma of the stomach, which arises from the gastric mucosa, may metastasize to the regional lymph nodes, the liver and other abdominal organs, and the lungs. Several patterns of stomach cancer are seen: focal (localized in the stomach), ulcerative (irregularly shaped ulcer in the mucosa), and diffuse (within the stomach wall).

▶ SECTION IV

Diarrhea (loose, watery stool), can be of three types: osmotic (due to excess water being drawn into the intestinal lumen), inflammatory mucosal (due to severe inflammation), and secretory (due to bacterial infection). *Enteritis* (inflammation of the intestines) can occur in combination with infectious inflammation of the stomach *(gastroenteritis)* or colon *(enterocolitis).* Such infections can generally be traced to a contaminated environment. Examples of microbes that can cause enteritis are *Staphylococcus, Salmonella, Vibrio cholerae, Campylobacter, Shigella* (which can lead to dysentery, colitis, and tenesmus), and several strains of *Escherichia coli.* Certain viruses (e.g., rotavirus, Norwalk agent) can cause enteritis, as can certain protozoa (e.g., *Giardia lamblia*).

Crohn's disease, also called regional enteritis, is a form of *inflammatory bowel disease* (IBD). The condition is characterized by repeated episodes of inflammation of the small and large intestines. In approximately one third of the cases, inflammation occurs in other tissues (e.g., skin, joints, liver, eyes). *Ischemic bowel disease* is caused by inadequate blood supply to the intestines, due to atherosclerosis, partial thrombosis of the intestinal veins, systemic hypotension (shock), or congestive heart failure. Effects of intestinal ischemia range from edema and slight hemorrhage to necrosis of large areas of the intestinal mucosa.

Intestinal obstruction *(ileus)* may occur from a physical blockage of the intestine *(mechanical ileus)* or from the absence of intestinal peristalsis *(paralytic ileus).* Mechanical ileus can be caused by a tumor, gallstones, a hernia, a volvulus, adhesions, intussusception, or intestinal stenosis. Pain and peritonitis are examples of causes of paralytic ileus. The significance of intestinal obstruction is potential rupture and fatal peritonitis.

Malabsorption, or inadequate absorption of nutrients from the intestinal lumen, may result as a complication of a primary disease (e.g., infectious or regional enteritis) or following surgery in the GI tract. *Short bowel syndrome* occurs due to a loss of functional intestine from disease or surgery. *Maldigestion,* or malabsorption of food due to inadequate digestion, may be due to atrophic gastritis, lack of pancreatic digestive enzymes, cystic fibrosis, or obstructed bile flow. Primary malabsorption is caused by a defect in intestinal function. Celiac disease (gluten hypersensitivity enteropathy) is the most common form of primary malabsorption.

Intestinal neoplasia is most commonly of the carcinoid type, in which a malignancy arises from glandular cells in the mucosa. This form of tumor can metastasize to the lymph nodes and liver, resulting in carcinoid syndrome (a condition in which a tumor secretes hormone-like compounds). Acute inflammation of the appendix *(appendicitis)* is caused by obstruction and infection. The condition may result from a *fecalith* (impaction by hardened feces). A common complication of appendicitis is perforation, which can cause lethal peritonitis.

▶ SECTION V

Idiopathic ulcerative colitis is chronic inflammation of the colon and rectum. Its precise cause is unknown, but stress, autoimmunity, and genetic predisposition are suspected. In contrast to regional enteritis, diffuse inflammation of the colonic mucosa is suspected in ulcerative colitis. The condition can lead to an enlarged colon (megacolon), and a complication is increased risk of cancer. The disease *pseudomembranous colitis* is necrosis of the colon mucosa caused by a toxin released by the intestinal bacteria *Clostridium difficile.* Other bacteria that specifically infect the colon include *E. coli, Campylobacter, Salmonella,* and *Shigella. Tenesmus* (spastic straining during bowel movements) and dysentery are often the result of infection of the colon. In *diverticulitis,* small pouches that protude outward from the lumen of the large intestine (diverticula) become infected with bacteria, leading to interference with stool passage and possibly perforation of the infected diverticula.

Neoplasia of the colon is most frequently of the adenocarcinoma type, and may be benign or malignant. Neoplasia usually begin as a premalignant polyp. At least half of the colorectal adenocarcinomas arise in the rectosigmoidal area. Advanced cases of colorectal cancer may metastasize to the lymph nodes and liver.

Peritonitis is inflammation of the peritoneal (abdominal) cavity. The condition may be classified as sterile peritonitis (due to bile acids, digestive enzymes, or surgical materials) or infectious (septic) peritonitis (bacterial infection due to perforation of an infected organ). Conditions that can lead to infectious peritonitis include acute appendicitis, peptic ulcer, regional enteritis, diverticulitis, or disease states of the intestines (e.g., strangulated hernia, intussusception, volvulus). Adhesion formation, toxemia, and septic shock are complications of infectious peritonitis. *Ascites* is the presence of excess fluid in the abdominal cavity. The accumulated fluid may be characterized as transudate, exudate, or chyle.

▶ SECTION VI

Irritable bowel syndrome (spastic colon) is a disturbance in function of peristalsis of the colon. The condition is thought to be psychosomatic in origin. *Hemorrhoids* ("piles") are varicose veins of the rectum and anus. The likely cause of hemorrhoids is increased blood pressure in the rectal and/or anal region that interferes with venous drainage and causes dilation.

CHAPTER 13

The Liver, Gallbladder, and Pancreas

▶ OBJECTIVES

SECTION II

Define all highlighted terms.

Explain the relationship between the signs of liver failure and the effects on normal function.

Relate the types of jaundice to specific disease processes, and explain why or how jaundice develops for each category.

State the serum chemical responsible for causing jaundice.

Describe the complications of obstructive jaundice.

Recognize the clinical descriptions of ascites and edema, and state the mechanisms responsible for producing ascites and edema.

List causes of hemorrhage in liver disease.

Describe the signs of hepatic encephalopathy, the toxin responsible for it, and three events that precipitate encephalopathy.

Explain how portal hypertension and portal–systemic shunting develop.

Outline the relationship between hypertension, shunting, and clinical signs.

Explain the cause for hematemesis in liver disease and why it occurs.

Outline the features and prognosis for zonal necrosis, focal necrosis, bridging necrosis, and massive necrosis.

Explain why there is such a difference in prognosis for the various patterns of necrosis.

SECTION III

Define all highlighted terms.

Outline the features of transmission and various stages of disease for hepatitis A, B, C, D, and E.

List the complications of chronic active hepatitis.

Explain the concept of a carrier.

State the cause of hepatic lipidosis and explain the mechanism of injury to liver cells.

Describe cirrhosis.

Cite factors that contribute to the signs of cirrhosis.

Relate the presence of cirrhosis to signs of liver failure.

State the most common form of hepatic neoplasia.

List two disease conditions that can predispose to primary liver cancer.

SECTION IV

Define all highlighted terms.
Describe the pathogenesis or development of cholecystitis.
State the most common cause of cholecystitis.
List the complications of cholecystitis.
Understand the relationship between cholelithiasis, cholestasis, cholecystitis, and cholangitis.
Describe the formation of gallstones.
Relate the development of gallbladder carcinoma to pre-existing conditions.

SECTION V

Define all highlighted terms.
Explain the mechanism of injury in acute pancreatitis and give the most probable causes of pancreatitis.
State the signs of acute pancreatitis.
Describe changes in digestion that accompany pancreatitis.
Discuss the development and results of acute hemorrhagic pancreatitis.
Relate chronic pancreatitis to pancreatic insufficiency and steatorrhea.
Understand the basic abnormality in cystic fibrosis and the glands that are affected.
State the most common location of a tumor in pancreatic adenocarcinoma and an early sign caused by this location.

SECTION ▶

13-1

I. ANATOMY AND PHYSIOLOGY IN REVIEW

The liver, gallbladder, and pancreas are called the accessory organs of the digestive system because of their contribution to digestive and metabolic processes. The liver is considered to be the largest and perhaps the most complex of the visceral or internal organs. It is impossible to assign more importance to one vital organ than another. Failure of the heart, brain, or kidneys results in death. However, the liver is the real workhorse of the body because of the diversity or variation of normal function. Most of the functions can be divided into four categories, which often overlap each other:

1. Metabolism of nutrients.
2. Synthesis of various products.
3. Detoxification of several compounds.
4. Secretion of products and excretion of waste.

13-2

Hepatocytes are the functioning cells of the liver. The nutrients that are metabolized are carbohydrates, proteins, and fats. Storage of excess nutrients, including minerals and vitamins, occurs in the liver. Carbohydrates absorbed from the intestines undergo several changes as the liver maintains the blood glucose levels at normal. The maintenance of normal blood sugar is essential for all body functions, including the brain. Should the glucose or sugar level drop below a certain point, this is defined as **hypoglycemia,** which, if severe, causes coma. This situation is prevented by the liver's manipulation of **glycogen,** which is the storage form of glucose. Carbohydrate metabolism is complex and will not be reviewed here.

13-3

The metabolism of proteins occurs in the form of building and breaking down. Dietary protein provides the basic amino acids that the liver uses to produce or synthesize important plasma proteins that play a part in several body functions. Almost all plasma or blood proteins are made by the liver, except for the antibodies. Nutrients beyond the body's immediate needs are converted to fat and stored. One specific type of fat, cholesterol, is produced by the liver as an important part of bile. The absorption of ingested fats results in either immediate use by the liver or in conversion to **lipoproteins.** Lipoproteins are the transport form of fats as they are carried in the bloodstream to their storage place, **adipose** tissue.

13-4

The liver creates or synthesizes many proteins of the body, including metabolic enzymes and albumin. **Albumin** is responsible for **osmotic pressure,** as you learned in Chapter 2. Osmotic pressure attracts and holds fluid in the vessels. Therefore, decreased albumin levels can result in excessive fluid loss into the tissues, which is **edema.** Other proteins made by the liver are the clotting factors **fibrinogen** and **prothrombin,** which prevent hemorrhage. Vitamin K is necessary for the synthesis of these factors. **Bile acids,** or **bile,** are another product of the liver. Dietary fats and fat-soluble vitamins cannot be absorbed from the intestines without the presence of bile. Before the lipid enzymes can digest fat, it must be **emulsified** by bile. That is, fat molecules are surrounded and dissolved by the bile, making them water soluble.

13-5

The liver can detoxify many compounds. A toxin is a substance that is poisonous or chemically harmful to the body. Detoxification is the process of turning these substances into soluble compounds that can be excreted by the body. An **endogenous** toxin is produced by the body, such as bilirubin and ammonia. An **exogenous** toxin is usually ingested, though some chemicals may be absorbed through the skin. Examples of ingested toxins are drugs, alcohol, and chemicals. The blood supply of the liver helps to ensure that ingested substances are acted upon by the liver *before* they reach the rest of the body. This is an important protective "clearinghouse" function of the liver. **Kupffer's cells** are phagocytic cells among the hepatocytes that assist in this protective function by removing (ingesting) bacteria and other foreign particles that have entered the system.

13-6

Solubility is the key to ridding the body of compounds. Insoluble means that the compound will not dissolve during urine or stool formation, and therefore cannot be passed out of the body. Many compounds are insoluble as they reach the liver. **Conjugation** is the process of turning them into soluble compounds by joining them with other substances that *are* soluble. In this way the entire compound can be excreted. **Bilirubin** is a substance that must be conjugated. Bilirubin is the end result of hemoglobin breakdown. Unconjugated bilirubin is neurotoxic in newborn babies, and buildup can cause brain damage. In older individuals, buildup produces jaundice, which we will study shortly. Certain steroid hormones must also be conjugated and excreted so that they do not have a prolonged effect on the body. **Ammonia** comes from protein metabolism, and it is also produced by intestinal bacteria and can be absorbed. Ammonia is very toxic to the central nervous system and must be excreted. The liver metabolizes it to **urea,** which is a compound the kidneys can easily excrete.

13-7

Secretion is the act of synthesizing or making a product and then releasing it. **Excretion** is the elimination of waste. The liver does both. As products that are formed and released, proteins and bile acids are secreted. Bilirubin has been labeled as a waste product and is excreted into the bile, before the bile is secreted into the intestine. Urea as a waste product is excreted, along with detoxified hormones, drugs, and chemicals. These substances enter the bloodstream where they are filtered out by the kidneys.

13-8

The liver is unique because it has a dual or double supply of blood. This feature makes infarcts in the liver much more rare than at other sites of the body. The **hepatic artery** accounts for about 25 percent of the total blood flow through the liver. The primary purpose is to provide oxygen to the hepatocytes. The **portal vein** supplies the other 75 percent and is rich with all of the nutrients just absorbed from the gastrointestinal tract, where this vein originates. It also contains any ingested drugs, alcohol, or chemicals. Figure 13–1 represents blood supply to the liver or hepatic circulation. Because of this portal circulation, the contents of the blood may be acted upon by the liver as it performs its various functions before the blood reaches the heart and is pumped to the rest of the body. The structural framework of the liver cells contributes to the efficiency of the flow through the liver. They are arranged in **cords** or columns (rows), with **sinusoids** or spaces between these rows. This allows for exposure to the blood on all sides of the cells and therefore maximum clearing efficiency by the cells. The sinusoids are also lined with the phagocytic Kupffer's cells, which remove particles as they flow by. Each individual unit of arrangement is called a **lobule.** Figure 13–2 will help you to understand this structure.

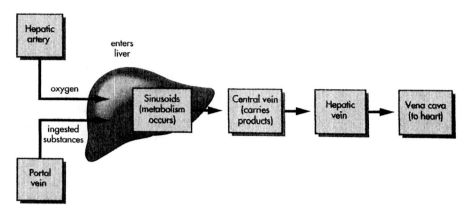

Figure 13–1. Hepatic circulation.

The gallbladder is a small, muscular sac that buds off of the common bile duct. It is located under the liver on the right side of the upper abdomen. Its primary functions are to concentrate bile by removing water and to store bile until it is needed in the duodenum for fat digestion. The pathway of bile passage is called the **biliary tree.** It is like a tree in that the beginning of this system is tiny and numerous, like the upper limbs of a tree. It ends in a large singular passage, like a trunk. The smallest ducts are intrahepatic, which means they are

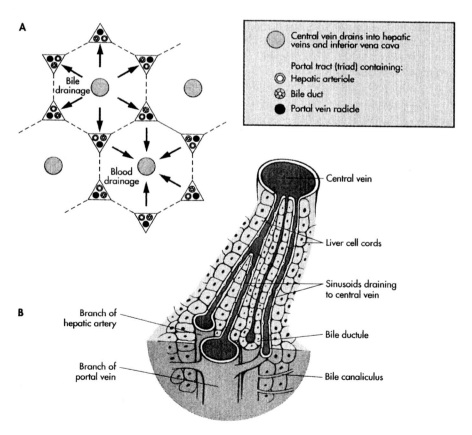

Figure 13–2. Structural framework of a liver lobule. **A.** Top view of lobules in relation to each other. **B.** Cross-sectional view of a liver lobule. *(Adapted from Chandrasoma and Taylor,* Concise Pathology, *2nd ed., Appleton & Lange.)*

found in the liver. They are called **canaliculi.** From the canaliculi the bile leaves the liver through the hepatic ducts and enters the gallbladder by way of the cystic duct. The presence of fatty food in the duodenum causes a hormone to stimulate the gallbladder to contract and release bile. The bile passes back out the cystic duct and exits the biliary tree through the common bile duct. Figure 13–13 in Section IV shows the relationship between the liver, gallbladder, duodenum, and pancreas.

13–10

The pancreas is a long, narrow glandular organ located behind the stomach in a horizontal position. It is arbitrarily divided into the head, body, and tail. The head of the pancreas is closely aligned with the duodenum, and this is important in how some pancreatic diseases manifest themselves. The pancreas is an organ of secretions that are divided into two categories. The **endocrine** portion consists of the glands of "internal" secretions. These are the **islands of Langerhans,** which are patches of **alpha** and **beta** cells in the parenchyma. As endocrine glands, these groups of cells release their products directly in the circulation without the use of ducts. The two products are the hormones **insulin** and **glucagon.** Insulin lowers blood glucose by assisting glucose across cell membranes into cells. Glucagon raises blood glucose by inhibiting insulin and increasing glycogenolysis. The diseases associated with glucose metabolism were discussed in Chapter 8. The **exocrine** portion consists of glands of "external" secretions. These secretions are enzymes of digestion and make their way into the intestines through ducts. These digestive enzymes pass out of the pancreas through the pancreatic duct, which empties into the duodenum. The enzymes are **amylase, trypsin** and its derivatives, and **lipase.** Amylase breaks down carbohydrates, trypsin digests proteins, and lipase acts on fats or lipids.

II. GENERAL CONCEPTS OF LIVER DISEASE ◀ SECTION

▶ LIVER FAILURE

13–11

The diseases presented in Section III can cause **hepatocellular failure** if the condition is severe enough to overcome the powers of regeneration. In this case the liver cells would be replaced with nonfunctioning _____(1) tissue or fibrosis. Signs of liver failure are directly related to the loss of normal functions. The predominant plasma protein that the liver manufactures is _____(2). This protein is responsible for maintaining _____(3) pressure. As the failing liver is unable to perform its work, this creates lower than normal amounts of albumin in the blood, or **hypoalbuminemia.** This causes an upset in normal fluid distribution because of loss of osmotic pressure. As fluid is lost into the tissues this is seen as swelling in the extremities, called _____(4). More importantly, cellular metabolic functions are upset as a result of the fluid imbalance. Transport failure occurs because albumin and many other plasma proteins are responsible for taking substances to various parts of the body where they are needed. As levels of clotting factors fall, bleeding tendencies may develop. In liver failure one important disturbance in metabolic function is the decrease in synthesis of plasma _____(5). These proteins include albumin and clotting _____(6), which prevent bleeding.

1. scar
2. albumin
3. osmotic
4. edema
5. proteins
6. factors

13–12

The liver fails in its detoxification duties. As bilirubin is unable to be conjugated, the insoluble unconjugated form builds up, causing jaundice. Jaundice will be discussed shortly. Any drugs in the system will not be metabolized properly and can build to toxic levels, even if the dose was normal. This is a critical consideration when giving medication to a person with liver failure. As steroid hormones remain active beyond their normal range, there can be several undesirable effects. Perhaps one of the most dramatic results is seen when the liver is not able to convert the neurotoxin ammonia to soluble urea for excre-

1. liver or hepatocellular
2. bilirubin
3. drugs
4. hormones
5. ammonia
6. detoxification

····· 13–13 ·····

1. disease
2. ammonia
3. poison
4. hepatic encephalopathy
5. protein
6. ammonia

tion. This causes a condition called hepatic encephalopathy, which is presented in the next frame. Four substances that can build to harmful levels during _____(1) failure are _____(2), _____(3), _____(4), and _____(5). The inability to turn these substances into harmless compounds is a failure in the process of _____(6).

Hepatic encephalopathy is a dramatic result of failure in ammonia detoxification. First, let us examine the literal meaning of the phrase. **Hepatic** always refers to liver. You know the suffix **"pathy"** means _____(1). **"Encephalo"** refers to brain. Therefore, hepatic encephalopathy means a disorder of the brain caused by the liver. This is a mental disorder caused by a toxic buildup. It is seen as a deterioration or breakdown in mental processes. There is loss of memory, confusion, and personality change. The neurotoxin that causes this is _____(2). By neurotoxin, we mean it acts as a (an) _____(3) to the nervous system. As the condition worsens, the patient progresses into a stupor (not very responsive) and then into a coma (not responsive at all). Seizures are common. Death is the end result. The effects are also seen as **ataxia,** which is incoordination of movements and trembling. Hepatic encephalopathy can be brought on by a heavy protein meal, absorption of intestinal bacteria ammonia, or bleeding in the GI system. Bleeding of dilated esophageal veins is not uncommon in liver disease. The mechanism during bleeding is that the large amount of protein in the blood is digested as if it were dietary. Protein breakdown produces ammonia. The severe and possibly fatal mental effects during liver failure are called _____(4). This can be caused or made worse by a heavy load of _____(5) absorbed from the intestines. A toxic breakdown product of protein is _____(6). Whenever a disease is approaching the end of its course and can only result in death, it is described as **end stage.** Therefore, liver failure could also be called end-stage liver disease.

····· 13–14 ·····

1. pressure
2. portal vein
3. entrance
4. liver
5. resistance
6. back pressure
7. path of less resistance or detour

Portal hypertension can be a feature of liver failure. To define portal hypertension, we need only look at the word meanings. "Portal" refers to an entrance, and in this case means the entrance of blood vessels into an organ. Commonly, it is understood to mean the entrance of the portal vein from the intestines into the liver. Hypertension is increased pressure in blood vessels. This is the same as saying increased blood pressure. So we can say portal hypertension means increased _____(1) in the _____(2) at the site of _____(3) into the _____(4). The cause is an obstruction to blood flow through the organ. You have already learned about the garden hose analogy of what happens because of obstruction to flow. If the flow meets with _____(5), the pressure increases behind the obstruction, or there is increased back pressure. Also, the fluid will tend to take a path of less resistance, which can be thought of as a detour. A more specific cause of portal hypertension is chronic liver disease that has left a great deal of scar tissue or fibrosis in the organ. This is called **cirrhosis,** which will be presented shortly. Figure 13–3 illustrates portal hypertension and the changes in circulation that we will consider next. Two effects of increased resistance to flow are increased _____(6) and the fluid taking a _____(7).

····· 13–15 ·····

One of the effects of portal hypertension is the development of **portal–systemic anastomoses.** An anastomosis is all of the secondary blood vessel connections (or possible routes for a detour). Some sources call this an increase in **collateral circulation.** This is a series of other routes for the blood to reach the vena cava. As the obstructed flow takes these secondary routes, the vessels dilate (enlarge) and become engorged (overfilled) with blood. Dilated, engorged vessels are called **varicose.** One set of these vessels runs along the esophagus. When they become varicose, this is called **esophageal varices.** Unfortunately, these collateral veins are not designed to handle the extra load without some problem occurring, usually in the form of hemorrhage. Esophageal varices tend to rupture and bleed. This is probably due to the relative trauma of continued swallowing or can happen if the patient develops esophagitis. A patient with ruptured esophageal varices will vomit the blood from

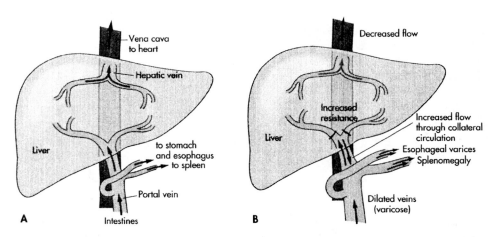

Figure 13–3. Portal hypertension and circulatory changes (shunting). **A.** Normal circulation to and through the liver. **B.** Obstruction to blood flow.

their stomach. The term for vomiting blood is **hematemesis.** A varicose vein is described as _____(1) and _____(2). A varicose vein can develop if there is an increase in _____(3) circulation. This increased secondary circulation is also called a portal–systemic _____(4). The most likely problem from the overdistention of the veins is _____(5), and this is usually seen in esophageal _____(6). Bleeding esophageal varices will present as vomiting blood or _____(7).

1. dilated
2. engorged
3. collateral
4. anastomosis
5. hemorrhage
6. varices
7. hematemesis

13–16

In addition to vessels becoming enlarged, the backflow of blood naturally ends up in the organs that the vessels are draining. One of these organs is the spleen. The spleen is a "solid" organ compared to the hollow stomach and intestines. The spleen also becomes distended with the extra blood and becomes enlarged. **Splenomegaly** describes this enlarged organ ("megaly" means large). The enlarged organ can be **palpated,** or felt, by the hands of the physician or seen on an x-ray. _____(1) means enlarged spleen, and in the case of portal hypertension is due to excessive _____(2) in the organ.

1. splenomegaly
2. blood

13–17

The change in the majority of normal blood flow to other pathways is called a **portal–systemic shunt.** A shunt means to turn to a side pathway. The obstruction shunts the blood (diverts it) through the anastomosis channels (see Fig. 13–3). Its significance is that much of the blood supply bypasses the hepatocytes. Therefore, the cells cannot process the substances in the blood. The detoxification function is bypassed, allowing harmful substances to reach the general circulation. One example is ammonia produced by bacteria in the intestines. You already know the nervous system effects of this compound, which causes a mental disorder known as hepatic _____(1). Bacteria or their endotoxins can also reach the general circulation, causing septicemia or endotoxic shock. Because of portal _____(2) tension, blood flow through the liver meets with increased _____(3). This causes the flow to be turned away to other channels, which is described as a portal–systemic _____(4). The harmful result of a shunt is the detour around the hepatocytes, not allowing them to perform the important function of _____(5). The relationship between the concepts you have just learned is that, because of hypertension due to obstruction, the blood shunts through the anastomoses. The anastomoses are the pathways for the shunt, or diverted flow.

1. encephalopathy
2. hyper
3. resistance
4. shunt
5. detoxification

13–18

1. ascites

One sign of portal hypertension is **ascites.** Ascites is plasma or fluid (not blood) in the abdominal cavity that has oozed out of the liver because of the increased pressure within the organ itself. The liver is normally spongy and holds a lot of blood. Increased pressure comes from the scar tissue of chronic disease contracting inward. Like squeezing a sponge, it forces fluid from the organ into the abdomen. This contributes to the fluid imbalance seen in liver failure. Fluid from the liver in the abdomen is called _____(1). Ascites is seen as a distended or enlarged abdomen. Pressure contributes to the production of ascites, as does hypoalbuminemia.

► JAUNDICE

13–19

1. icterus
2. yellow or orange
3. skin, sclera, and other tissues
4. bilirubin
5. jaundice
6. sign

Jaundice is not a disease, it is a sign of disease and does not always mean liver disease. **Jaundice** describes a yellowish or orange-tinged appearance of skin and other tissues, including the sclera or whites of the eyes. The etiology of jaundice is the excessive amounts of bilirubin in the circulation, which has built up and been deposited in the tissues, therefore staining the tissues. (Bilirubin has a yellow-orange color and is a bile pigment.) Another term sometimes used to describe the yellow staining is **icterus.** Jaundice, or (another term) _____(1), is a _____(2) discoloration of the _____(3) caused by buildup of _____(4) in the circulation. Icterus or _____(5) is not a disease but is a _____(6) of disease. Bilirubin is the end compound produced from hemoglobin breakdown after red blood cells have reached the end of their life span. In its natural state, bilirubin is insoluble and cannot be eliminated very well from the body. The liver extracts unconjugated bilirubin from the blood passing through the sinusoids. The liver then conjugates (joins) the bilirubin to soluble glucuronic acid, and the entire soluble complex is excreted into the bile. Bile will reach the intestines, and after its role in fat absorption, becomes part of the stool and is passed from the body.

13–20

There are three categories of pathologic (disease-associated) jaundice, and they are named according to the cause. It may or may not be due to liver disease. The names of the categories are related to where the disturbance is in the flow of processes in the body. The flow is always forward, as in the case of circulation. If the disturbance is occurring *before* the flow reaches an organ, the condition might be labeled as **pre-.** Conversely, problems developing *after* the organ has performed its function may be labeled as **post-.** This is represented in Figure 13–4.

13–21

1. before
2. bilirubin

In **pre-hepatic** or **hemolytic jaundice,** there is upset in the processes _____(1) (when?) the flow reaches the liver. The second term is specific for the cause, hemolysis of RBCs. Since the bile pigment _____(2) (hemolytic) is the breakdown product of RBCs and hemoglobin, it makes sense that excessive hemolysis leads to excessive levels of bilirubin. The causes for the increased hemolysis were presented in Chapter 9 on hemolytic anemias. So this is jaundice *not* due to liver disease, but due to another pathology that precedes (comes before) the liver. The mechanism for jaundice is that the liver is sim-

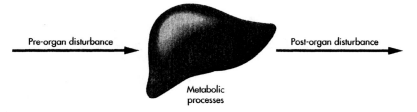

Figure 13–4. Categories of functional disturbance in the body.

ply unable to keep up with the extra bilirubin. It conjugates as much as possible but levels of unconjugated bilirubin build up in the circulation and ultimately stain the body tissues. In hemolytic jaundice levels of both forms of bilirubin are increased (conjugated and unconjugated). However, there is a greater increase in the unconjugated form because of the backup of all the extra bilirubin. Remember, unconjugated bilirubin is insoluble and is not easily _____(3) from the body. Jaundice due to increased destruction of RBCs is called _____(4) or _____(5) jaundice. The liver is not _____(6) but is not able to conjugate the extra _____(7) load.

In cases of actual disease of the liver, there is also an increase in unconjugated bilirubin because the hepatocytes are damaged and not able to function properly. This is called **hepatic jaundice.** Processing bilirubin for excretion into the bile is one of the _____(1) functions of the liver. In contrast to pre-hepatic jaundice, levels of conjugated bilirubin are decreased. Table 13–1 compares the forms of bilirubin in the three types of jaundice. Hepatic jaundice is also called **hepatocellular jaundice,** since the primary cause is insufficiency in liver function. Another term for hepatic jaundice is _____(2), because the disease is in the _____(3) itself.

13–22

In **post-hepatic** or **obstructive jaundice,** the liver functions normally, but once the bile components, including bilirubin, are secreted into the various ducts, the bile is blocked. The blockage can be a tumor or more commonly a gallstone. Since the normal pathway for the bile leads to the intestine, an obstruction causes the bile to seek another path. In particular, it backs up through the passageways from which it came. The bilirubin has been conjugated normally, and it is this form that spills over into the circulation and becomes elevated. Conjugated bilirubin is _____(1) soluble/insoluble (choose one), and therefore as it passes through the kidneys it can be _____(2) as waste. Bilirubin in the urine causes the urine to be dark. Bilirubin in the urine is a good indication of this type of jaundice. Obstructive jaundice is also called _____(3) because the upset is _____(4) (where?) the liver in terms of flow of normal processes. Bile cannot enter the intestine because of a _____(5), and therefore bilirubin _____(6) into the blood. Conjugated bilirubin is excreted by the kidneys, so bilirubin will be found in the _____(7) and it will look _____(8). Look at Table 13–1 again to compare the types of jaundice and forms of bilirubin elevations. **Cholestasis** is a term that describes the results of the obstruction. Stasis means stopping and chole- refers to bile. Therefore, cholestasis means the flow of bile is _____(9).

13–23

Another sign that is seen in obstructive jaundice is clay-colored (pale) or **acholic** stools. Acholic means lacking the presence of bile. The prefix "a" or "an" means "without" or "absence," and "chol" refers to bile. Bile ultimately gives the stool its characteristic brown color. If bile doesn't reach the intestine in normal amounts, the stool will not be brown. Acholic stool is _____(1) in appearance and lacks its normal _____(2) color. Acholic stool is a good indication of _____(3) jaundice.

13–24

TABLE 13–1. LEVELS OF THE FORMS OF BILIRUBIN IN JAUNDICE

Category of Jaundice	Unconjugated Bilirubin (Indirect)	Conjugated Bilirubin (Direct)	Stool Color	Urine Bilirubin
Hemolytic (Pre-hepatic)	Very increased ↑↑	Increased ↑	Normal	Absent
Hepatic	Increased ↑	Decreased ↓	Normal	Absent
Obstructive (Post-hepatic)	Normal →	Increased ↑	*Pale	*Present

*Features present only in obstructive form.

13-25

1. fats
2. bleeding
3. complication
4. infection
5. malabsorption
6. bleed
7. liver

In post-hepatic jaundice there are problems that arise from the obstruction itself. These secondary effects are often called **complications.** The first complication is the likelihood of infection in the biliary tree or liver because of cholestasis. Any bacteria that have gained access from the intestines have a chance to colonize the area because of the lack of bile movement. **Malabsorption** is very likely since bile is not reaching the intestine. You know that bile is necessary for the absorption of _____(1). Therefore, in the absence of bile, fat as well as fat-soluble vitamins are not absorbed. One fat-soluble vitamin that is required to synthesize the clotting factor prothrombin is vitamin K. Deficiency of vitamin K and therefore prothrombin would lead to _____(2) tendencies. Finally, direct damage to the hepatocytes can occur if the condition persists. The mechanism for this injury is pressure necrosis as the backup of bile increases pressure within the liver. Chemical irritation caused by the stasis almost certainly contributes to this secondary liver disease. Look at Table 13–2 to understand these consequences. A problem that is a result of a preceding condition is called a secondary effect. This can also be labeled a _____(3). Cholestasis can result in four complications: bacterial _____(4); _____(5) of fats and some vitamins; a tendency to _____(6); and secondary _____(7) disease.

▶ HEPATIC TOXICITY AND NECROSIS

13-26

There are many agents that can act as **hepatotoxins,** that is, have a damaging effect on the liver by chemical action. Toxic may be thought of as poisonous. These agents include various environmental chemicals, poisons, medications, and even viruses. The injury is either caused directly by the agent or as a reaction because of hypersensitivity. The amount of injury can range from mild cellular swelling to necrosis and accompanying inflammation.

13-27

1. hepatotoxin

Medication or **drug-induced** toxicity generally is mild but can cause considerable damage in a susceptible individual. During the detoxification process of drugs in the liver, intermediary compounds that are formed can be toxic. An example of this is the common pain reliever acetaminophen. One group of people who are susceptible to toxic damage are those with a pre-existing liver disease. As normal function is impaired, even normal doses of common drugs can cause injury if they are not processed for elimination. Drugs are an example of an agent that can act as a _____(1) and injure the liver through their chemical nature. The commonly used gas anesthetic halothane is infamous for causing severe massive necrosis of the liver in a very small percentage of patients. This is the most serious example of drug-induced hepatotoxicity. The pattern of necrosis that is produced is called the **acute hepatitic pattern.** (We will be discussing patterns of necrosis in the following frames.)

TABLE 13–2. COMPLICATIONS OF OBSTRUCTIVE JAUNDICE

Infection
  Intestinal bacteria
    Liver abscess
Malabsorption
  Lack of bile in intestine
    Fats
    Vitamin K
      Bleeding tendencies
Liver cell damage
  Cholestasis
    Pressure
      Chemical irritation and injury

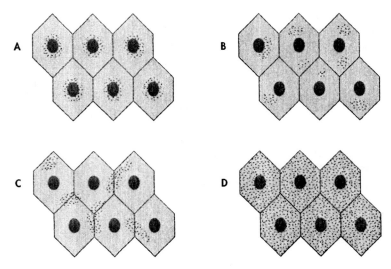

Figure 13–5. Patterns of liver necrosis as seen in lobules. **A.** Zonal distribution. **B.** Focal distribution. **C.** Bridging necrosis. **D.** Massive necrosis.

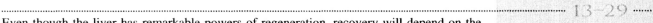

13–28

1. zonal distribution
2. focal distribution
3. bridging hepatic necrosis
4. viruses
5. Massive necrosis
6. viruses
7. poisons

Necrosis of the liver usually appears in specific patterns. The arrangement of hepatocytes is identical in every part of the liver. The liver is divided into several lobes, and these are further divided into lobules. Each lobule is the same in cellular layout and blood supply (refer back to Fig. 13–2). When toxic injury is severe enough to cause necrosis, it may affect each lobule in the same physical pattern. In this case the necrosis is described as a **zonal distribution,** meaning the same area is affected in each lobule. **Focal distribution** is a spotty or random pattern, so that the site of necrosis varies with each lobule. **Bridging hepatic necrosis** is more extensive and reaches outside of the lobules to other areas (hence, bridging). This type of widespread necrosis is often seen with the viruses of hepatitis. **Massive necrosis** involves huge areas and is characteristic of acute fulminant hepatitis caused by viruses or can be due to poisonous reactions. If each necrotic area in a lobule is the same as other lobules, the pattern is described as a _____(1). If the pattern is not the same but is scattered, this is a _____(2). Necrosis spreading beyond the confines of a lobule is called _____(3) and may be caused by _____(4). _____(5) is the most severe extent and may also be caused by _____(6) or some _____(7). These patterns are illustrated in Figure 13–5.

13–29

1. zonal
2. focal
3. structural framework

Even though the liver has remarkable powers of regeneration, recovery will depend on the amount and severity of injury. Obviously, there will be some point at which the severity overcomes the ability to regenerate. After both zonal and focal necrosis, the prognosis is good for complete regeneration. The damage is not as severe as the other types and *most importantly, the structural framework is not destroyed.* This means the newly formed cells are placed as

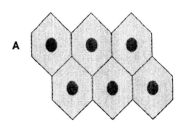

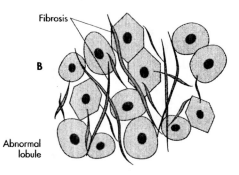

Figure 13–6. Comparison of regeneration with nodule formation. **A.** Normal regeneration by following the guidance of the intact foundation. **B.** Nodule formation when there is no guiding foundation.

they should be and will not cause problems just by their physical location. The best prognosis for regeneration comes after the damage of _____(1) or _____(2) necrosis, where the injury is not severe. The most important part that is left intact is the _____(3), which acts as a guide for the placement of new cells.

····· 13–30 ···

In bridging hepatic necrosis the prognosis is fair because recovery is possible if the cause of injury can be removed in time. Often, in this type of necrosis, areas of the structural framework are also destroyed. The regeneration takes place in the form of **nodules** or large groups of randomly placed cells. This leads to the production of **macronodular cirrhosis,** or a bumpy scarred liver. Figure 13–6 compares structured regeneration and nodule formation. In cases of massive necrosis, while recovery is still possible, acute liver failure is more likely,

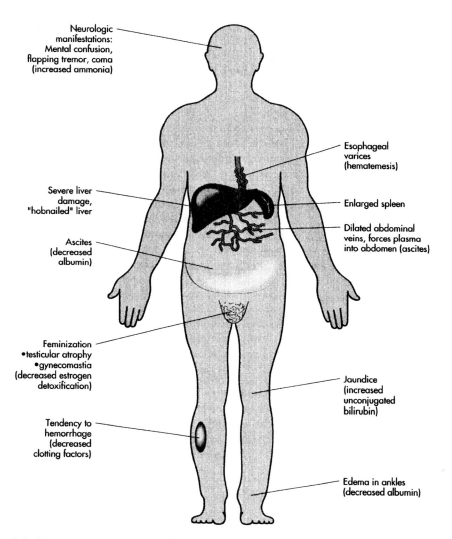

Figure 13–7. Clinical presentation in liver failure and portal hypertension. *(Adapted from Mulvihill,* Human Diseases: A Systemic Approach, *4th ed., Appleton & Lange.)*

and so the prognosis is poor. Any regeneration that takes place is again in the form of nodules, which leads to cirrhosis. The severity often leads to shunting of blood supply and further disorder. The prognosis is worse for bridging and massive necrosis because of the formation of _____(1), which are groups of randomly placed _____(2). Placement is random because of the destruction of the guiding _____(3) framework. This causes the condition _____(4), which has its own consequences. Acute liver failure is usually seen with _____(5) necrosis. The clinical presentation and other effects of liver failure that you have learned in this section are represented in Figure 13–7.

1. nodules
2. cells
3. structural
4. macronodular cirrhosis
5. massive

II. REVIEW QUESTIONS

1. The world "hepatic" pertains to the _____.

2. Choose the correct statement:
   a. Hypoalbuminemia means greater than normal amounts of albumin in the blood.
   b. The signs of liver failure are directly related to loss of normal function.
   c. Hypoglycemia causes an upset in normal fluid distribution.
   d. Liver failure leads to increased production of plasma proteins.

3. Liver failure may cause:
   a. toxic buildup of drugs given in normal doses
   b. mental disturbances
   c. hypoalbuminemia and a deficiency in clotting proteins
   d. only one of the above
   e. all of the above

4. Please complete this sentence:
   A central nervous system disruption that can be seen in liver failure is called
   a. _____ _____. This is caused by buildup of the neurotoxin
   b. _____. These effects can be made worse when there is a heavy load of
   c. _____ absorbed from the intestines.

5. Please answer the following questions as true or false:
   a. _____ Portal hypertension causes decreased resistance to blood flow through the liver, so this causes the flow to increase through the sinusoids.
   b. _____ One effect on veins because of portal hypertension is that they become varicose.
   c. _____ Gastric varices are a serious effect of portal hypertension and have a tendency to rupture and bleed.
   d. _____ An enlarged spleen, or splenomegaly, is a common occurrence in portal hypertension.

6. When the circulation bypasses much of the liver, and the hepatocytes do not have the opportunity to detoxify harmful substances, this describes:
   a. esophageal varices
   b. ascites
   c. portal–systemic shunt
   d. portal–systemic anastomoses

7. Define ascites: _____.

1. liver

2. b–The signs of liver failure are directly related to the loss of function.

3. e–all of the above

4. a–hepatic encephalopathy; b–ammonia; c–protein

5. a–false; b–true; c–false; d–true

6. c–portal–systemic shunt

7. fluid in the abdomen coming from the liver

8. 1. c–pre-hepatic
   2. a–post-hepatic
   3. b–hepatic

9. b–obstructive

10. bile or bilirubin pigment

11. a–malabsorption; b–bleeding; c–infection; d–secondary liver disease

12. a–true; b–true; c–false; d–true

13. 1. d–massive necrosis
    2. b–focal distribution
    3. a–zonal distribution
    4. c–bridging necrosis

14. a–bridging; b–massive

8. Please match these three types of jaundice with their cause:
   a. post-hepatic   1. _____ RBC hemolysis
   b. hepatic   2. _____ obstruction in bile flow
   c. pre-hepatic   3. _____ diseased liver

9. One type of jaundice will cause visible signs in the urine and stool. This type is:
   a. physiologic
   b. obstructive
   c. hemolytic
   d. hepatic

10. Acholic stool means that the stool is lacking _____.

11. List four complications of obstructive jaundice:
    a.
    b.
    c.
    d.

12. Please answer the following questions as true or false:
    a. _____ Pre-existing liver disease makes one more susceptible to drug-induced toxicity.
    b. _____ Necrosis of the liver often appears in recognized patterns.
    c. _____ The most serious hepatic necrosis is zonal distribution.
    d. _____ The prognosis following liver necrosis depends on the amount of structural framework that remains intact.

13. Please match these patterns of liver necrosis with their physical description:
    a. zonal distribution   1. _____ the largest areas of necrosis
    b. focal distribution   2. _____ a random pattern
    c. bridging necrosis   3. _____ the same area in all lobules
    d. massive necrosis   4. _____ extending to other areas

14. Macronodular cirrhosis is a likely result of a. _____ necrosis or b. _____ necrosis.

SECTION ▶ III. DISEASES OF THE LIVER

▶ VIRAL HEPATITIS

13–31

1. inflammatory

By literal definition, viral hepatis would be inflammation of the liver caused by a virus. While this is true to some degree, swelling and necrosis of the hepatocytes are the true direct injury. The classic stages of the inflammatory response are replaced with hepatocellular necrosis, but remember, necrosis in living tissue produces a (an) _____(1) response. In the United States there are about five viruses that cause hepatitis. We will study these viruses by dividing them into categories of transmission. Hepatitis is a disease of rather long course and recovery. Differences between the types of hepatitis exist in the incubation period, severity of signs, and prognosis. Table 13–3 compares the features of the hepatitis viruses.

TABLE 13–3. FEATURES OF HEPATIC VIRUSES

	HAV	HBV	HCV	HDV	HEV
Fecal–oral transmission	+	–	–	–	+
Body fluid transmission	–	+	+	+	–
Epidemic outbreaks	+	–	–	–	+
Chronic stage	–	+	++	+	–
Carrier state	–	++	+	+	–
Cirrhosis	–	+	++	+	–
Carcinoma	–	+	+	+	–

Enteric Hepatitis

You have learned that the term "enteric" pertains to the _____(1) system. Hepatic viruses in this group are shed and acquired mainly through the gastrointestinal route. This route is often called the **fecal–oral mode of transmission.** The virus is shed in the stool or feces and to some degree in the urine. Food or water sources may become contaminated with even a tiny amount of the infected excrement and be ingested, thus infecting the exposed person. This type of hepatitis is usually associated with institutions such as schools, restaurants, or nursing facilities. Any situation where an infected food handler may pass on the virus to relatively large groups of people can result in an epidemic of enteric viral hepatitis. Since poor sanitation perpetuates this disease, the best way to prevent it is through good personal hygiene and sanitary regulations. The simple act of hand washing is a good first line of defense. The mode of transmission of _____(2) source hepatitis is often called the _____(3) route, which describes the spread of the virus.

13–32

1. gastrointestinal
2. enteric
3. fecal–oral

Hepatitis A (HAV) is the most common of the enteric transmitted viruses. It is sometimes known as **infectious hepatitis.** It has the shortest incubation period, about 2 to 6 weeks. The signs experienced by the patient may be confused with having the flu. HAV produces mild illness compared to blood-borne viruses. There is anorexia, lethargy, low-grade fever, and nausea. Jaundice is possible but not usually seen. The liver may be tender and enlarged. Write the term for enlarged liver: _____(1). The prognosis for HAV is good for complete recovery. Antibodies in the blood mean lifelong immunity. There is no development into a chronic condition and there is no carrier state. The initials that refer to hepatitis A are _____(2), and the disease is also known as _____(3). The signs can look like the _____(4). The prognosis is _____(5) because HAV does not result in a _____(6) condition or a _____(7) state. **Hepatitis E** is also enteric or fecal–oral in mode of transmission and was specifically identified only recently. Prior to identification, it was part of a group known as non-A, non-B hepatitis. It is rare compared to HAV. It is also associated with epidemic outbreaks. All other characteristics are very like HAV and will not be discussed.

13–33

1. hepatomegaly
2. HAV
3. infectious hepatitis
4. flu
5. good
6. chronic
7. carrier

Blood-Borne Hepatitis

Blood-borne transmission is probably more accurately called **parenteral,** because there are other avenues of access for these viruses besides through the blood. However, blood exchange plays a major role in transmission. Remember that parenteral means entry into the body *not* through the _____(1). Some examples of the parenteral transmission of these viruses include blood transfusion, sharing of needles among drug users, needle sticks occurring to health care workers, transplacentally or perinatally, and unprotected sex. In short, any exchange of or exposure to body fluids may lead to infection. The main route

13–34

1. alimentary canal or GI system

2. body fluids

13-35

1. intensity
2. ill
3. jaundiced

13-36

1. massive
2. function
3. failure

13-37

1. chronic active hepatitis
2. recovery
3. hepatocytes
4. cirrhosis
5. liver cancer

13-38

1. carrier
2. shed

13-39

of transmission of viruses that cause hepatitis through parenteral means is through the exchange of _____(2).

Hepatitis B, or HBV, was previously known as **serum hepatitis,** which describes its mode of transmission. HBV no longer has that distinction since at least one other virus has been named that is transmitted through the blood. HBV has a long incubation period, ranging from 2 to 6 months. The signs of hepatitis B are somewhat like HAV, in that there is gastrointestinal disturbance such as anorexia, nausea, and weight loss. However, the intensity is worse in the case of HBV. Patients are much more ill with bouts of vomiting, diarrhea, and severe fatigue. Jaundice is usually a feature. Two major differences between the signs of HAV and HBV are that in HBV the _____(1) is worse so the patient is much more _____(2), and the patient looks visibly _____(3).

Another difference is cases of HBV is the possible lack of complete recovery and sudden turns for the worse. **Acute fulminating hepatitis** is a fatal course this disease may take in a few cases. Understanding the word "fulminating" will help you to picture the events and outcome. Fulminating describes an explosive, runaway process ranging out of control. The literal definition is "to occur suddenly with great intensity." The Latin means "to flare up." This particular manifestation of HBV causes necrosis in large areas of the liver, which you now know is called _____(1) necrosis. Widespread areas of death mean the hepatocytes are not available to perform their normal _____(2). The liver's loss of ability to function is called liver _____(3). Most cases of acute fulminating hepatitis proceed to death in about a week.

Lack of complete recovery from acute HBV can be seen in several ways. First, is the production of cirrhosis, which is a permanent condition you will learn about shortly. Hepatocellular carcinoma or liver cancer can be another result. These have been linked to a preceding condition called **chronic hepatitis.** In this instance the immune system was not able to kill all of the virus, and the virus retreats into the hepatocytes and stays in the liver. Persistence of the virus as shown by blood tests for longer than 6 months after the first illness defines chronic hepatitis. There are two types: **chronic persistent hepatitis,** which is mild with little permanent damage; and **chronic active hepatitis,** or **CAH,** which has complications. Two life-threatening complications of CAH are the development of cirrhosis and primary liver cancer, both attributed to the slow, steady destruction of the liver over time. "CAH" stands for _____(1), and is due to lack of complete _____(2) from the acute stage. Antibodies are not able to eradicate all of the virus and it goes into hiding in the _____(3). Two complications resulting from CAH can be _____(4) and _____(5).

Another pathway of the course of HBV is to produce a **carrier** state in someone who has been exposed. A carrier is a person infected with an agent, who is not experiencing any visible signs of illness but may be shedding the agent. Obviously, this is a serious matter, since protective measures are not going to be taken unless a person knows he or she is a carrier. The most frequent means of identifying healthy carriers is through routine blood screening tests when these individuals donate blood. If an individual appears to be healthy but actually harbors an infectious agent and is able to pass it to others, that person is called a _____(1). A carrier is able to _____(2) a virus without seeming to be sick.

Hepatitis C, or HCV, produces illness in the patient that is similar to severity to HBV. The clinical signs are usually indistinguishable from HBV. The mode of transmission appears to be limited to direct blood exposure, as in a transfusion. Transfusion-associated hepatitis was expected to decrease after the discovery of the specific HBV antigen and the development of a test for it. However, this was not the case. Because of ongoing hepatitis from transfusions that was *not* due to HBV, scientists called this probable group of agents **non-A, non-B hepatitis.** Recently, one agent was isolated from this group. This was hepatitis C, and it was shown to be the cause of the majority of transfusion-transmitted infections. The incidence has now decreased, since blood banks have a way to screen donors for the virus. HCV has an incubation period of 2 weeks to 6 months. Two liver viruses that are very alike in signs and severity are _____(1) and _____(2). The primary route of transmission of HCV or _____(3) is through exposure to _____(4). Before the identification of and testing for HCV, it was known as part of a group of viruses called _____(5). It is now known that _____(6) was a major cause of transfusion-transmitted infection. Compared to HBV, the prognosis is worse for HCV because the development of chronic active hepatitis is of much higher incidence. More cases of cirrhosis have been documented. However, the chances of a carrier state are much smaller.

1. HBV
2. HCV
3. hepatitis C
4. blood
5. non-A, non-B hepatitis
6. HCV

13–40

Hepatitis D, or the **delta** virus, is a defective virus that can only live and replicate in the presence of HBV. Therefore, it is not found as disease by itself. The significance is that if it is present along with HBV, the chances of acute fulminant hepatitis, chronic active hepatitis, and cirrhosis are greater. This is because of the increased injury to the liver cells and strain on the immune system.

▶ HEPATIC LIPIDOSIS

13–41

The term "lipid" means fat. **Hepatic lipidosis** is fatty liver. In this condition, fat, particularly triglyceride, becomes deposited or builds up inside the hepatocytes. This is shown in Figure 13–8. As the cell becomes filled with fat, this infiltration causes the cell to degenerate. Therefore, degeneration is the mechanism of injury here. As the tiny organelles in the cytoplasm are crowded and squeezed by the abnormal presence of fat, they are unable to function normally or may stop altogether. During an autopsy a fatty liver appears enlarged, greasy, and yellow. A fatty liver is referred to as _____(1). Crowding and pressure by fat on the _____(2) in the cell cytoplasm interferes with their normal _____(3). The mechanism of injury is _____(4). Remember that the liver plays a major role in the metabolism of nutrients. Fat normally makes its way through the cells as it is prepared for storage or as it is being changed to a usable energy source.

1. hepatic lipidosis
2. organelles
3. function
4. degeneration

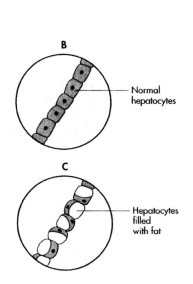

Figure 13–8. Hepatic lipidosis. **A.** Lobule with cords of hepatocytes **B.** Cord of normal hepatocytes. **C.** Hepatocytes infiltrated and compressed by fat.

13-42

1. alcoholism
2. diet
3. vitamins
4. calories
5. food or calories

Poor dietary habits can produce hepatic lipidosis. An imbalanced diet may lack important vitamins required for the cells to metabolize fat properly. Overeating or excessive calories in the form of ethanol is usually the cause. Ethanol is drinking alcohol. In addition to the "empty calories," alcohol inhibits glycogen synthesis and cell metabolism. Alcoholics experience chronic fatty liver due to their constant heavy intake over a long period of time. Alcoholism is a leading cause of fatty liver. Continued damage to the cells by the fat infiltration leads to necrosis, and as it continues, usually leads to cirrhosis. More will be said shortly about alcohol and cirrhosis. On the other hand, complete lack of food intake or starvation can contribute to hepatic lipidosis. As body stores of fat are released from adipose tissue, it all converges on the liver for processing and can overwhelm the cells and remain there. A major cause of hepatic lipidosis is _____(1). This is one of several factors in a poor _____(2) that can cause fatty liver. An imbalanced diet may lack certain _____(3) necessary for proper metabolism. Too many _____(4) or not enough _____(5) can upset normal fat processing by the liver.

► CIRRHOSIS

13-43

1. fibrosis
2. scarring
3. damage or necrosis

Cirrhosis is an end-stage liver disease, because once it develops to any great extent the prognosis is grave. It is debatable whether to actually call cirrhosis a disease. Literally, it is fibrosis or scarring of the liver in response to injury or necrosis over a long period of time. It is a morphologic response to chronic destruction, which means there are changes in the physical structure of the lobules as a result of continual damage. Large areas of structural framework have been destroyed. Recall that hepatocytes regenerate in a prolific manner after injury. Also remember that the framework upon which the new cells will be laid is vital. This is because efficient function depends on how the cells are laid out in order to allow maximum blood flow through the sinusoids and exposure of the cells to the blood. Regeneration without a guiding foundation leads to the formation of **nodules** or groups of new cells existing in a very disorganized fashion. Loss of the guiding framework is a critical factor that causes the problems that go with cirrhosis. Grossly, these nodules make the liver look bumpy, as you can see in Figure 13–9. The disorganization is a tremendous interference in function. Cirrhosis literally means _____(1) or _____(2) of the liver because of a long duration of _____(3). The

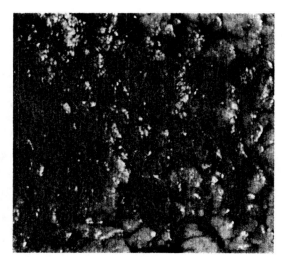

Figure 13–9. Cirrhosis of the liver (cut surface) showing diffuse nodularity. *(From Chandrasoma and Taylor, Concise Pathology, 2nd ed., Appleton & Lange.)*

_____(4) eventually is destroyed so that new cells are produced haphazardly in groups called _____(5). These nodules, which visibly look like _____(6), are part of a great disorganization that prevents the liver from performing its normal _____(7).

13–44

4. framework
5. nodules
6. bumps
7. function

Another factor that causes serious hindrance to function is the presence of the scar tissue. Some of the fibrous tissue serves as replacement of hepatocytes that undergo necrosis. Once these cells are gone forever there is no mechanism to replace their part in liver function. You know that scar tissue performs none of the _____(1) of the original tissue. Also recall that an area of fibrosis will shrink as it matures in a process called _____(2). A diseased liver is often enlarged before cirrhosis. The maturing scar tissue of cirrhosis causes the entire organ to shrink and become smaller than normal. This contraction causes obstruction to blood flow and portal hypertension. Cirrhosis is a (an) _____(3)-stage liver disease that results in the liver becoming _____(4) than normal. This shrinking causes circulatory obstruction and _____(5).

1. function
2. contraction
3. end
4. smaller
5. portal hypertension

13–45

Chronic active hepatitis can lead to cirrhosis. Severe toxic injury from a poison can produce enough necrosis and scarring to result in the condition. Malnutrition that leads to severe and long-standing lipidosis is another mechanism for the development of cirrhosis. A few cases are classified as idiopathic, which means the cause is _____(1). The most common cause of cirrhosis is chronic alcoholism. Alcohol is thought to be a direct toxin to hepatocytes. In addition, there appear to be secondary contributions through malnutrition and lipidosis. For this reason cirrhosis due to alcohol is often called **fatty nutritional cirrhosis** to show this relationship. You already know that chronic lipidosis can cause _____(2) or fibrosis of the liver. The fatty change in the liver can be seen in Figure 13–10.

1. unknown
2. cirrhosis

13–46

Unfortunately, cirrhosis is asymptomatic (shows no signs) until it reaches the point where it is irreversible. It will continue to progress to complete liver failure. As in many disease processes, the signs of cirrhosis are often interrelated. As the first imbalance causes the second imbalance, it in turn makes the first problem worse in a downward spiral. The first group of signs is caused by contraction of the scar tissue. Refer back to Frame 13–44 and list two results of the contraction: _____(1) and _____(2). Now look back to Frames 13–15 through 13–18 and list four effects of portal hypertension: _____(3), _____(4), _____(5), and _____(6). A serious consequence of esophageal varices is _____(7). Hemorrhage that follows rupture can lead to shock and further necrosis of the liver due to ischemia. Hepatic encephalopathy is the result of blood bypassing its normal route through the liver, and we call this detour a _____(8). The toxic compound causing encephalopathy is _____(9) that has been absorbed from the intestines. Another consequence of the constriction is obstructive jaundice, because the bile canaliculi are closed down. Absence of bile prevents proper absorption of _____(10) and fat-soluble vitamins such as vitamin K. Vitamin K is required for the liver to produce proteins that are _____(11).

1. obstruction to blood flow
2. portal hypertension
3. esophageal varices
4. hepatic encephalopathy
5. splenomegaly
6. ascites
7. bleeding
8. shunt
9. ammonia
10. fat
11. clotting factors

13–47

In addition to shunting, altered blood flow deprives liver cells of their own supply. This hastens the onset of liver failure, as injured cells then suffer additional injury from ischemia. Ascites is made worse by the lack of albumin production, and edema is also seen. Lack of clotting factors can result in gastrointestinal bleeding and hematemesis. In addition to possible shock, the protein overload from the digested blood can precipitate or worsen hepatic encephalopathy. Death often results following coma. Patients who survive with cirrhosis are at higher risk for developing liver cancer. These effects of cirrhosis are actually the events of liver failure, as was shown in Figure 13–7.

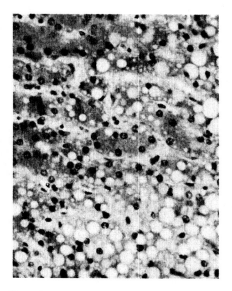

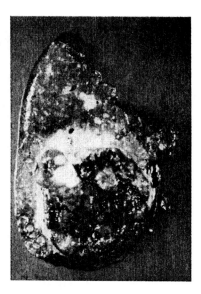

Figure 13–10. Macrovaculor fatty change of the liver in alcoholism. The large fat globules in the cytoplasm appear as empty spaces that have displaced the nucleus to the side. *(From Chandrasoma and Taylor,* Concise Pathology, *2nd ed., Appleton & Lange.)*

Figure 13–11. Hepatocellular carcinoma, showing a large solitary nodule that is grossly encapsulated except in one area. *(From Chandrasoma and Taylor,* Concise Pathology, *2nd ed., Appleton & Lange.)*

▶ NEOPLASIA

13–48

1. cancer or neoplasia
2. liver or hepatocytes
3. spread to another site where the cancer then grows

Hepatocellular carcinoma is the last liver disease we will consider. As the name implies, hepatocellular carcinoma means _____(1) of the _____(2). An example may be seen in Figure 13–11. Neoplasia or cancer of the liver can be divided into two categories, primary and secondary. Secondary cancer is due to metastasis of neoplasia from the primary or original site to the liver. Referring back to Chapter 6 on neoplasia, write the definition of metastasis: _____(3). Secondary liver cancer is by far more common than primary cancer. An example of secondary or metastatic cancer is shown in Figure 13–12. The most common sites of primary cancer are the breast, stomach, colon, pan-

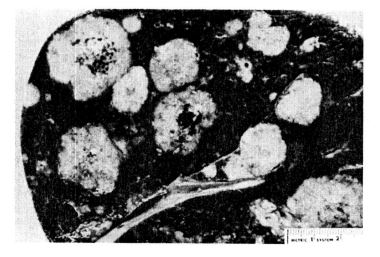

Figure 13–12. Liver metastases in a patient who presented with jaundice and an undiagnosed carcinoma of the colon. *(From Kent and Hart,* Introduction to Human Disease, *3rd ed., Appleton & Lange.)*

creas, and lung. Lymphomas can also spread to the liver, as can malignant melanoma which is skin cancer. The vast blood supply and clearinghouse function of the liver make this organ especially susceptible to metastasis through a hematogenous route. By hematogenous we mean the cancer spreads by way of the _____(4). Primary hepatocellular carcinoma may be called a **hepatoma** to indicate that the cancer is arising from the hepatocytes. **Cholangiocarcinoma** (about 20 percent of the cases) means that the cancer originates from the intra-hepatic bile ducts. Secondary liver cancer occurs _____(5) often than primary cancer. The liver is susceptible because of its _____(6) supply. Primary neoplasia may be a _____(7) or a _____(8) depending on where the cancer cells are growing.

4. blood supply or circulation
5. more
6. blood
7. hepatoma
8. cholangiocarcinoma

One cause of primary hepatocellular carcinoma is suspected to be cirrhosis. The mechanism for this is perhaps related to chronic excessive stimulation of the hepatocytes to regenerate. This continual nodular regrowth may set the stage for uncontrolled growth of de-differentiated hepatocytes. You have learned that neoplasia literally means abnormal _____(1). Another factor in the development of a neoplasm is chronic active hepatitis that is seen with HBV. Finally are the cases of idiopathic neoplasia in a normal liver. Three possible causes of primary hepatocellular carcinoma are _____(2), _____(3), and _____(4).

13-49

1. new growth
2. cirrhosis
3. chronic hepatitis
4. idiopathic

The signs of liver cancer depend on the location of the tumor or tumors. For example a tumor pressing on the portal vein would cause portal hypertension and the accompanying signs. The ascites in this case is also bloody, which is an important diagnostic clue. (Remember, erosion of blood vessels and bleeding is a feature of cancerous growth—Chap. 6.) Bile duct obstruction would produce jaundice. Weight loss and abdominal pain are common. The development of liver failure with its signs is part of end-stage disease as the functioning parenchyma is replaced with cancer cells.

13-50

III. REVIEW QUESTIONS

1. One manner of transmission of hepatitis viruses is by the eneric route which is also known as:
   a. fecal–oral
   b. blood borne
   c. parenteral
   d. hematogenous

1. a–fecal–oral

2. Please match these hepatitis viruses with their associated characteristics. Going down the column on the right, match the letter of the characteristic with **every** correct virus on the left:
   1. HAV _____   a. enteric transmission
   2. HBV _____   b. blood borne transmission
   3. HCV _____   c. carrier state
   4. HDV _____   d. chronic state
   5. HEV _____   e. epidemics
                     f. dependent on HBV
                     g. mild illness
                     h. more severe illness

2. 1. e, a, g
   2. b, c, d, h
   3. b, c (possible), d, h
   4. f, h
   5. a, e, g

3. Acute fulminating hepatitis is associated with:
   a. HCV and bridging necrosis
   b. HAV and massive necrosis
   c. HCV and zonal necrosis
   d. HBV and massive necrosis

3. d–HBV and massive necrosis

4. a–cirrhosis; b–carcinoma

5. A healthy appearing person who is infective, which means able to shed disease-causing organisms

6. a–HCV; b–transfusions

7. a–fatty liver; b–pressure on the organelles interferes with function

8. c–nutritional factors

9. d–massive fibrosis

10. c–disorganized regeneration and scar tissue contraction

11. a–portal hypertension; c–liver failure

12. a–hepatocellular carcinoma; b–secondary

13. a–true

4. Of the following conditions, choose the two that can be the result after chronic active hepatitis:

   lipidosis   portal hypertension   jaundice
   cirrhosis   liver failure   carcinoma

   a. _____
   b. _____

5. Define the word "carrier." _____

6. The hepatitis virus that used to be called non-A, non-B is a. _____ and the primary mode of transmission was through blood b. _____.

7. Hepatic lipidosis means a. _____. What happens to the hepatocytes in this condition? b. _____

8. The etiology of hepatic lipidosis is primarily due to:
   a. viral infection
   b. liver cancer
   c. nutritional factors
   d. all of the above

9. Cirrhosis is:
   a. a viral infection
   b. a neoplasm
   c. fat deposits
   d. massive fibrosis

10. Two mechanisms of disease production in cirrhosis are:
    a. fat deposits and toxic injury
    b. toxic injury and scar tissue contraction
    c. disorganized regeneration and scar tissue contraction
    d. disorganized regeneration and fat deposits

11. Two major classifications of the signs of cirrhosis are due to: (choose two)
    a. portal hypertension
    b. liver cancer
    c. liver failure
    d. jaundice

12. The medical terminology for liver cancer is a. _____. The type of cancer that is most common is b. _____ primary / secondary (choose one).

13. True or false: Chronic liver disease can be a precursor of primary hepatocellular carcinoma a. _____.

IV. DISEASES OF THE GALLBLADDER

Diseases of the gallbladder often affect the other accessory organs of digestion. Figure 13–13 shows the relationship between the liver, gallbladder, duodenum, and pancreas. Diseases of this small simple organ are few. There are two major gallbladder disorders, inflammation and obstruction. Infection and neoplasia do occur, and are considered to be results of inflammation and obstruction. Inflammation and obstruction are very closely related in that one may lead to the other and both usually occur together. In fact, some authors say that the

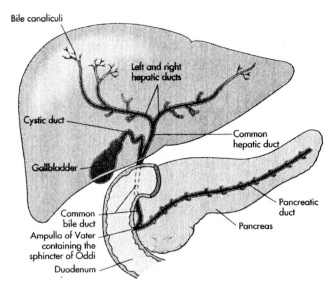

Figure 13–13. Anatomy of the biliary system and accessory organs of digestion. *(Adapted from Chandrasoma,* Concise Pathology, *2nd ed., Appleton & Lange.)*

terms describing these diseases (cholecystitis and cholelithiasis) are synonymous and can be used interchangeably. The two major disorders of the gallbladder are _____(1) and _____(2) and they are closely _____(3) to each other.

1. obstruction
2. inflammation
3. related

▶ ACUTE CHOLECYSTITIS

13–52

Try to determine the meaning of this word. Frame 13–24 associates the word part "chol" with _____(1). You know that the suffix "itis" means _____(2). Cyst refers to a saclike structure, in this case the gallbladder. Write here what you think cholecystitis is describing: _____(3). If you said this word means "inflammation of the bile-containing gallbladder," you are correct. Edema and swelling accompany the inflammation. The primary cause is obstruction somewhere in the passageway that prevents bile from exiting. The obstruction may be a tumor, abscess, or other "space-occupying lesion." The most common blockage is due to stones (gallstones). Since the bile is static (is not moving), it becomes more concentrated, and this causes a severe irritation due to chemical injury to the tissues. Therefore, this chemical irritation develops because of cholestasis. The blockage may be in the neck of the gallbladder or in the cystic or common bile duct. The primary cause of cholecystitis is a (an) _____(4), and this is most commonly due to _____(5). The cause of inflammation is chemical _____(6) from the concentrated bile. The stopping of bile, which allows it to become concentrated, is called _____(7).

1. bile
2. inflammation
3. (Continue reading this frame)
4. obstruction
5. stones
6. injury
7. cholestasis

13–53

The signs of acute cholecystitis are brought about after eating a heavy meal, especially a meal high in fat. Pain is experienced in the upper right quadrant of the abdomen, and the patient is fevered, nauseous, and vomiting. The enlarged organ may be palpated during a physical exam.

13–54

The complications of cholecystitis can be life threatening. The swelling compromises blood supply and can be severe enough to produce an infarction and gangrene of the gallbladder. Remember that an infarction is an area of _____(1) caused by loss of _____(2). A swollen, impacted gallbladder can rupture, causing possible fatal peritonitis due to rapid shock. Backflow into the ducts of the liver results in stasis there that leads to necrosis of the cells surrounding the ducts and cirrhosis if the

1. necrosis
2. blood supply

condition persists. This is called **biliary cirrhosis.** As the bile becomes more concentrated, this predisposes to more stone formation, which exacerbates (worsens) the condition. Several life-threatening complications of cholecystitis are _____(3), _____(4), _____(5), _____(6), and _____(7).

▶ CHOLELITHIASIS

The word element "lith(o)" means stone, so **cholelithiasis** is stone formation of bile origin. This is commonly referred to as gallstones. Another term is **biliary calculi.** Calculi means a hard formation, as in a stone. The relationship between cholelithiasis and normal bile flow is shown in Figure 13–14. Gallstones are present in many forms. They can be large or small, singular or multiple. They may fill the gallbladder, as seen in Figure 13–15. Many tiny stones are called "gravel," and as these filter out of the gallbladder they can obstruct the cystic duct. Imagine sand pouring down through an hourglass but the constricted area of the glass being too small to let the sand pass. The signs of an acute obstruction will be discussed shortly. If there is no obstruction the presence of gallstones causes a low-grade inflammation known as chronic cholecystitis. The common name for cholelithiasis is _____(1). Another medical term that can be used in place of cholelithiasis is _____(2). Gallstones cause signs of disease if they result in a (an) _____(3).

Bile is mainly cholesterol, bile salts, bilirubin, and water. The bile salts help to keep the cholesterol *in solution,* or *dissolved* in the bile. Some theories of stone formation say that abnormal bile production by the liver, where there are not enough bile salts, is responsible. There appears to be a genetic predisposition, since some ethnic populations have a higher incidence of this condition. Whatever the reason, cholelithiasis is *precipitation (falling out of solution)* of the cholesterol, bilirubin, and calcium normally dissolved in bile. Obesity plays a role in cholelithiasis, and this may be due to higher cholesterol levels. Also, women have a higher incidence. Gallstones occur when cholesterol, bilirubin, and calcium are no longer _____(1) in solution. Four explanations for stone formation are _____(2), _____(3), _____(4), and _____(5).

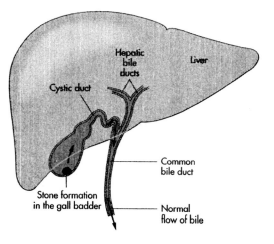

Figure 13–14. Cholelithiasis (gallstone formation) and the normal flow of bile.

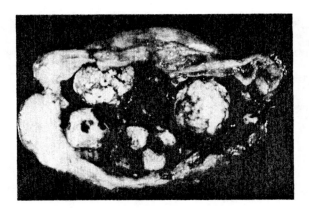

Figure 13–15. Gallbladder filled with multiple mixed gallstones. The wall shows diffuse thickening due to fibrosis. *(From Chandrasoma and Taylor,* Concise Pathology, *2nd ed., Appleton & Lange.)*

13–57

Cholelithiasis is often asymptomatic, depending on the size and shape of the stones. However, when obstruction occurs there is extreme pain and the other signs that go along with an inflamed gallbladder. (Remember, these two conditions are related.) As a complication of sudden obstruction, cholecystitis is the result. The irritating cholestasis may be in the gallbladder or reach into the liver. As you learned earlier, the blockage of bile causes a type of jaundice known as _____(1) jaundice or _____(2) jaundice. Therefore, cholelithiasis and cholestasis are mechanisms of obstructive jaundice. Examine Figure 13–16 to understand these complications. Another complication of obstruction may be **cholangitis.** Cholangitis is infection of the gallbladder and portions of the biliary tree. Look back at Frame 13–25. _____(3) can cause infection because bacteria have a chance to colonize in one place. This is an ascending infection as organisms from the intestines gain access to the compromised area. These organisms can reach the liver and produce an abscess. Look at Figure 13–17 to see the relationship between cholelithiasis, cholestasis, cholecystitis, and cholangitis.

1. obstructive
2. post-hepatic
3. Cholestasis or stasis

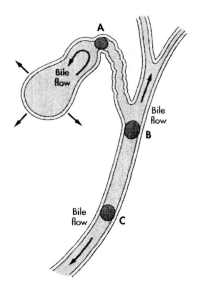

Figure 13–16. Complications of gallstone obstruction. **A.** Obstruction in the cystic duct causes acute cholecystitis with pain, possible rupture, and peritonitis. **B.** Obstruction in bile flow produces biliary cirrhosis and obstructive jaundice due to cholestasis. **C.** Obstruction of the common bile duct produces obstructive jaundice due to cholestasis, cholangitis, and pancreatitis.

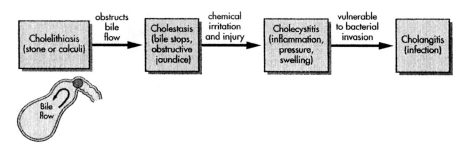

Figure 13–17. Pathogenesis of biliary tract disease.

▶ CARCINOMA OF THE GALLBLADDER

13-58

1. metastasized

Malignant cancer does occur in the gallbladder but it is rare. It is thought to be a consequence of chronic untreated cholelithiasis and cholecystitis. Therefore, it can be said that gallstones may predispose to neoplasia. The prognosis may be poor because by the time it is detected, often the cancer has spread or _____(1) to the liver.

IV. REVIEW QUESTIONS

1. a–cholecystitis; b–cholelithiasis; c–inflammation; d–stones

2. c–a stone or stones

3. b–complications

4. a–true; b–true; c–true; d–true

1. The two major diseases of the gallbladder are a. _____ and b. _____. One term means c. _____ of the gallbladder and the other term means d. _____ in the gallbladder or its ducts.

2. The most common cause of cholecystitis is:
   a. a tumor
   b. an abscess
   c. a stone or stones
   d. any space-occupying lesion

3. Infarction and rupture are _____ of cholecystitis.
   a. causes
   b. complications
   c. predisposing factors
   d. the etiology

4. Please mark as true or false:
   a. _____ Gallstones form when cholesterol, bilirubin, and calcium fall out of solution.
   b. _____ Biliary calculi is another term for cholelithiasis.
   c. _____ Cholecystitis is usually secondary to cholelithiasis.
   d. _____ Inflammation and obstruction can predispose the gallbladder to infection and cancer.

V. DISEASES OF THE PANCREAS ◀ SECTION

As we reviewed in Section I, the pancreas is responsible for glucose metabolism by insulin and glucagon, and for nutrient digestion by several enzymes made by the pancreas. It is important to realize that these enzymes are in an inactive state while they are in the pancreas. It is actually their precursor substances that are released. They are activated or converted to the working form outside of the pancreas, in the intestines where they are supposed to act. A major disease of the pancreas (pancreatitis) involves a disorder in this mechanism. The enzymes begin to act while still in the pancreas, creating destruction of the organ. A long-term consequence of chronic destruction or severe acute injury is malabsorption due to inability of this organ to perform its role in the digestive process.

▶ ACUTE PANCREATITIS

As the name implies, acute pancreatitis is _____(1) of the _____(2). Acute pancreatitis is one of several conditions that make up the clinical presentation of an **acute abdomen.** An acute abdomen is the presentation of a patient in moderate to severe pain that indicates the possibility of an emergency. Other causes of an acute abdomen are acute appendicitis, a perforated ulcer, and acute cholecystitis. This inflammation of the pancreas can range from mild to severe. The digestive enzymes become activated and begin the digestive process while still in the pancreas. This is called **autolysis** or **autodigestion,** because the enzymes digest or "eat" the tissue within this organ. In other words, the organ begins to digest itself ("auto"). Another term would be **enzymatic necrosis,** because the enzymes kill or destroy the cells in the process of digestion. The reaction by the organ is acute inflammation and edema. The amount of destruction dictates the severity of signs in the patient. The most severe presentation can lead to fatality if **acute hemorrhagic pancreatitis** has developed (Fig. 13–18). In this instance, the digestion has eroded into the blood vessels and internal bleeding results. Hemorrhage of a large amount can easily produce shock and death. Acute pancreatitis presents as an emergency that must be differentiated from other conditions in a clinical presentation known as a (an) _____(3). The mechanism for destruction is the activation of _____(4) that are located _____(5) the pancreas. Three terms that describe the injury are _____(6), _____(7),

1. inflammation
2. pancreas
3. acute abdomen
4. enzymes
5. in
6. autolysis
7. autodigestion

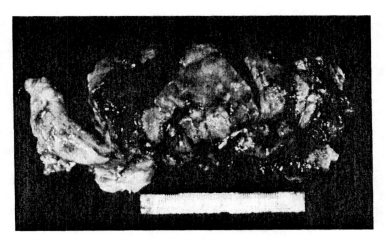

Figure 13–18. Acute hemorrhagic pancreatitis. *(From Mulvihill,* Human Disease: A Systemic Approach, *4th ed., Appleton & Lange.)*

8. enzymatic necrosis
9. acute hemorrhagic pancreatitis
10. blood vessels
11. bleeding or hemmorhage

and _____(8). A fatal consequence may be seen in the development of _____(9), because the enzymes have eaten their way into the _____(10). The cause of death is internal _____(11).

13-61

The signs of pancreatitis are pain (mild to severe) in the upper abdomen that is felt through to the back. Because of the pain the abdomen is rigid and the patient is described as "guarding" the abdomen. Guarding means the patient resists palpation. (Pain, rigidity, and guarding are seen in the acute abdomen in general.) Nausea and vomiting accompany the pain. The stimulation of a meal can bring on an attack. Acute hemorrhagic pancreatitis may present as shock. Blood pressure is decreased, heart rate is increased, extremities are cold, and there may be loss of consciousness.

13-62

1. alcohol
2. meal
3. cholelithiasis
4. pancreatic duct
5. idiopathic

The cause of pancreatitis is not well understood. There are several theories and it is safe to say many cases are idiopathic. Some relationships have been indicated by studies of these cases. Excessive alcohol intake is a contributing factor. Alcohol is a strong stimulus of pancreatic secretions. A heavy, fat-laden meal combined with high amounts of alcohol have been implicated in acute hemorrhagic pancreatitis. Chronic cholelithiasis or the presence of gallstones is thought to cause inflammation and swelling of the pancreatic duct, therefore preventing the release of the enzymes after they have been stimulated by a meal. A stone may actually obstruct the duct. Any duct obstruction, such as a tumor, combined with the stimulus to secrete can lead to pancreatitis. Blunt trauma to the abdomen can fracture the organ and allow the release of enzymes. The mumps virus can cause a mild, self-limiting case as this virus affects salivary and related glands. A lifestyle factor in the development of pancreatitis is the excessive intake of _____(1), especially when combined with a heavy _____(2). A chronic gallbladder disease known as _____(3) may obstruct the _____(4). Some cases are baffling in their cause and are classified as _____(5).

13-63

If a large area of the organ is destroyed, or widespread atrophy takes place, the sequel to this disease is severely impaired digestion. Maldigestion leads to malabsorption ("bad" digestion and "bad" absorption). Nutrients must be digested before they are absorbed. Malabsorption causes malnutrition and interference in normal body function.

► CHRONIC PANCREATITIS

13-64

1. chronic pancreatitis
2. malabsorption
3. diabetes
4. pancreatic insufficiency
5. steatorrhea

Continued bouts of acute pancreatitits, or continual low-grade inflammation, lead to the chronic condition. The patient experiences either the acute signs or mild ongoing discomfort. The organ injury and destruction is a slow progression like cirrhosis of the liver. This is most often associated with chronic alcoholism. As the exocrine and endocrine glands are destroyed, permanent malabsorption and diabetes are the consequences. Some sources classify this problem as an organ failure, since the pancreas loses its ability to perform normal function. A term for this loss is **pancreatic insufficiency.** There are additional enzymes in the digestive tract that can provide absorption of carbohydrates and proteins, although this absorption is less than optimal. However, fats have no secondary means of absorption, so pancreatic insufficiency generally shows itself as large amounts of fat in the stool. This is called **steatorrhea.** Grossly, the stool is greasy and foul smelling. Laboratory tests point to the diagnosis of pancreatic insufficiency through the demonstration of steatorrhea. Failure of the pancreas is a result of the disease known as _____(1). Loss of function as glands are destroyed lead to _____(2) and _____(3). The loss of function is called _____(4). The diagnosis of insufficiency is made in part by the demonstration of _____(5). Figure 13–19 illustrates some causes of chronic pancreatitis.

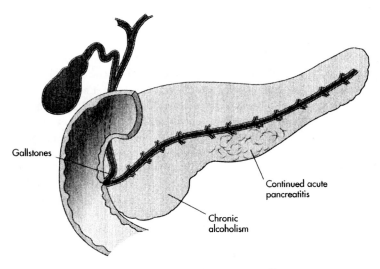

Figure 13–19. Causes of chronic pancreatitis.

► CYSTIC FIBROSIS

Cystic fibrosis is a genetic or hereditary disease affecting children. Many exocrine glands of the body are abnormal, especially those producing mucus, digestive enzymes, and sweat. This condition is also known as **fibrocystic disease.** In the pancreas, abnormally thick mucus blocks or obstructs the exocrine ducts, causing them to dilate or become cystic. Fibrosis surrounds the cystic pockets. This obstruction prevents release of enzymes and pancreatitis may occur. Maldigestion, malabsorption, and malnutrition are seen in these children. Chapter 11 on respiratory disease described the most life-threatening effects of cystic fibrosis, which also stem from thick mucus and blocked air passages. Respiratory failure is the usual cause of death. A genetic disease of children that is fibrocystic disease is more commonly known as _____(1). The abnormality is in exocrine _____(2) throughout the body. The disease develops because thick _____(3) blocks or _____(4) ducts or air passages. Children with this disease appear _____(5). Some results of gland obstruction in several parts of the body are reviewed in Figure 13–20.

1. cystic fibrosis
2. glands
3. mucus
4. obstructs
5. malnourished

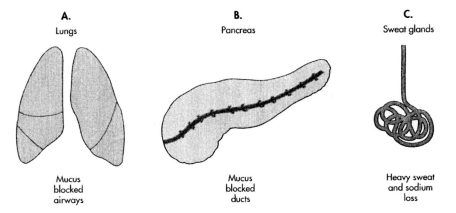

A. Lungs   **B.** Pancreas   **C.** Sweat glands

Mucus blocked airways   Mucus blocked ducts   Heavy sweat and sodium loss

Figure 13–20. Results of obstruction of exocrine ducts by very thick secretions in cystic fibrosis. **A.** Mucus-blocked airways (bronchial obstruction), recurring respiratory infection (trapped bacteria causes pneumonia), and difficulty breathing (bronchiectasis and lung collapse). **B.** Mucus-blocked pancreatic ducts (pancreatitis), maldigestion, malabsorption, and malnutrition. **C.** Heavy sweating with high salt concentration in sweat (sodium loss), and electrolyte imbalance (low sodium or hyponatremia).

▶ NEOPLASIA

Cancer of the pancreas in general is called an **adenocarcinoma.** "Adeno" refers to gland, and the pancreas can be thought of as a giant gland. There is an increase in the occurrence of this type of cancer that is thought to be due to lifestyle. Cigarettes contribute to the development, as well as diet high in fat and meat. The continual stimulation of the organ leads to hyperplasia, which you know can be a precursor to neoplasia. There also seems to be a link with diabetes. The prognosis depends on the location of the tumor because some locations cause little or no signs until the cancer is advanced. Metastasis easily occurs to the liver, stomach, and duodenum. Neoplasia of the pancreas is called _____(1) because the pancreas is largely made of _____(2). The occurrence of this type of cancer is _____(3) and could be related to _____(4).

Suspicion of pancreatic adenocarcinoma begins with the signs. If the tumor is located in the head of the pancreas, which is most common, this causes the earliest sign. The space-occupying lesion presses on the duodenum and common bile duct, obstructing this structure. Obstructive jaundice is the result and is an important sign (Fig. 13–21). Tumors in the body or tail have no early specific signs. Therefore, their prognosis is worse because they are not discovered until later. Generalized signs are present in all cases and are impaired digestion, weight loss, and pain. In pancreatic adenocarcinoma, the prognosis depends on the _____(1) of the tumor because this determines if early specific _____(2) develop. Obstructive _____(3) is a sign when the tumor is in the _____(4) of the pancreas. This is due to the blockage of the _____(5). The most common location of the tumor is in the _____(6) of the pancreas.

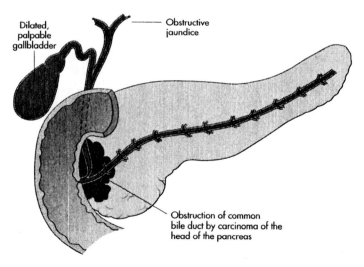

Figure 13–21. Adenocarcinoma of the head of the pancreas, causing biliary obstruction.

V. REVIEW QUESTIONS

1. The basic mechanism of injury in acute pancreatitis is:
   a. enzymatic necrosis
   b. autolysis
   c. autodigestion
   d. all of the above
   e. none of the above

2. Acute pancreatitis and several other painful conditions make up the clinical presentation known as:
   a. encephalopathy
   b. gastrointestinal distress
   c. shock
   d. acute abdomen

3. The most life-threatening form of inflammation of the pancreas is:
   a. acute hemorrhagic pancreatitis
   b. acute pancreatitis
   c. chronic pancreatitis
   d. pancreatic insufficiency

4. Please mark as true or false:
   a. _____ A patient presenting with an acute abdomen who goes into shock should be suspected as having chronic pancreatitis.
   b. _____ The exact cause of pancreatitis is not well understood.
   c. _____ Malnutrition leads to malabsorption and this causes maldigestion.
   d. _____ Repeated episodes of acute pancreatitis can lead to chronic pancreatitis.

5. Chronic pancreatitis results in:
   a. steatorrhea
   b. pancreatic insufficiency
   c. malabsorption and diabetes
   d. all of the above
   e. none of the above

6. The abnormality in cystic fibrosis is in:
   a. many endocrine glands
   b. many exocrine glands
   c. pancreatic ducts only
   d. respiratory air passages only

7. The most common location of a pancreatic adenocarcinoma tumor causes:
   a. weight loss
   b. pain
   c. obstructive jaundice
   d. impaired digestion

1. d–all of the above
2. d–acute abdomen
3. a–acute hemorrhagic pancreatitis
4. a–false; b–true; c–false; d–true
5. d–all of the above
6. b–many exocrine glands
7. c–obstructive jaundice

CHAPTER SUMMARY ▶

▶ SECTION II

The signs of liver disease are directly related to interference in normal functions. Hypoalbuminemia and hemorrhage result from decreased synthesis of albumin and clotting factors. Jaundice is a combination of interference in detoxification and excretion. Hepatic encephalopathy develops when portal hypertension causes shunting and blood ammonia bypasses detoxification. Hypoalbuminemia causes a decrease in osmotic pressure, which allows fluid to escape into the tissues as edema. In addition to increased ammonia levels, impaired detoxification can allow medications to build to dangerous levels. Hepatic encephalopathy is the name of the mental effects that are produced by toxic levels of the compound ammonia. Neurotoxin is the term applied to this compound that affects the brain. Amounts of ammonia are related to amounts of protein ingestion or bleeding in the GI tract. A portal–systemic shunt is a detour of blood away from normal routes through the liver to connecting pathways called *anastomoses*. As blood distends the secondary vessels they become swollen or varicose. Varicose veins along the esophagus are called esophageal varices. They have a tendency to bleed. Hemorrhage of esophageal varices can trigger an episode of encephalopathy. The shunt itself contributes to encephalopathy and other deficiencies in detoxification, since much of the blood volume does not flow through the sinusoids. A portal–systemic shunt develops when inelastic scar tissue acts as an obstruction and produces portal hypertension. The increased pressure creates an increase in resistance to flow, which causes the shunt. The scar tissue follows chronic liver disease and is referred to as cirrhosis. Splenomegaly and ascites are signs of a portal–systemic shunt.

Jaundice is an easily recognized sign that may mean liver disease. It is divided into three categories: pre-hepatic or hemolytic, hepatic, and post-hepatic or obstructive. Deposits of bilirubin in body tissues cause the yellowish stain of the skin, sclera, and mucus membranes. Pre-hepatic jaundice is due to excessive hemolysis of RBCs, which leaves more bilirubin than normal to be processed. Hepatic jaundice is due to injured or diseased hepatocytes that are unable to conjugate bilirubin in normal amounts. Post-hepatic jaundice is from obstruction in the flow of bile after it is formed and released from hepatocytes. The most common obstruction is cholelithiasis, and this causes cholestasis. Bilirubin spills over into the urine, making it darker. Decreased bile in the intestines leads to acholic stool, which is another sign of obstructive jaundice. Post-hepatic jaundice differs from the other types of jaundice because of complications such as malabsorption of fats and some vitamins. Malabsorption results from lack of bile in the intestines. Liver toxins (hepatotoxins) can cause necrosis of hepatocytes in particular arrangements and in varying amounts. Patterns of necrosis are named after these locations and amounts. The prognosis depends on the pattern, with zonal and focal distributions having better outcomes than bridging and massive necrosis. While regeneration of the liver is excellent, destruction of the structural framework leads to randomly placed groups of cells called nodules, which create macronodular cirrhosis with its complications.

▶ SECTION III

The viruses that cause hepatitis are contracted through either the fecal–oral route (enteric hepatitis) or through exchange of blood or body fluids (blood-borne hepatitis). The enteric borne viruses are hepatitis A and E. They are associated with poor hygiene, unclean or crowded conditions, and outbreaks (epidemics). Viruses that are blood borne, such as hepatitis B and C, can also be described as parenteral in transmission. Illness caused by HBV is worse than with HAV or HEV. Sequela to active hepatitis due to HBV include the possibility of fatal acute fulminant hepatitis, chronic hepatitis, and a carrier state. Chronic active hepatitis or CAH can produce cirrhosis or neoplasia. A carrier is an infected person who shows no signs of illness but is infectious, that is, able to infect others with the virus. Hepatitis C used to be grouped in with other hepatitis viruses called non-A, non-B until its relatively recent isolation. The clinical course can usually not be differentiated from HBV. HCV was a major cause of transfusion–transmitted hepatitis. HCV has a higher incidence of the development of chronic active hepatitis.

Hepatic lipidosis is infiltration of the liver by fat or lipid. The infiltration causes the cells to degenerate and lose function. The biggest contributor to fatty liver is improper diet, especially in the form of excessive calories from alcohol abuse. Starvation can also cause lipidosis. Cirrhosis is extensive scarring of the liver as a result of chronic injury. While CAH may result in cirrhosis, alcoholism predominates as the cause along with contributing factors such as malnutrition and lipidosis. The random regeneration of cells produces bumpy nodules whose disorganization decreases the ability to function. The fibrosis, which replaces working cells, contributes further to the permanent loss of overall function. As the scarred areas contract and pull inward, portal hypertension results from this obstruction to circulation. The increased resistance causes the flow to seek paths of lesser resistance and therefore bypasses normal routes through the sinusoids. This portal–systemic shunting causes ascites, esophageal varices, hepatic encephalopathy, and splenomegaly. Additional effects include bleeding of the varices and bile obstruction that decreases absorption of vitamin K necessary to make clotting proteins. The cirrhotic liver ultimately fails completely. Carcinoma of the liver is usually from the spread of cancer from other sites, or is secondary. Primary hepatocellular carcinoma can be either a hepatoma (arising from liver cells) or cholangiocarcinoma (arising from bile duct cells). Cirrhosis and chronic hepatitis due to HBV are considered risk factors in the development of primary liver cancer.

▶ SECTION IV

Disease of the gallbladder are mainly obstruction and inflammation, with infection and cancer also occurring. Cholecystitis is inflammation that generally is from an obstruction. Gallstones are the most common obstruction encountered. Cholestasis results from the obstruction and causes chemical irritation and therefore inflammation. Gangrene and rupture are important complications of the swollen inflamed condition. Cholelithiasis is the presence of a stone or stones of varying size and number. The stones form when compounds such as cholesterol, bilirubin, and calcium turn solid in the bile, instead of remaining dissolved. Cholelithiasis causes obstruction, cholestasis, and cholecystitis. Cholangitis, or an ascending infection by intestinal bacteria, can become a part of this picture. Untreated chronic cholelithiasis can predispose to carcinoma of the gallbladder.

▶ SECTION V

Acute pancreatitis results when digestive enzymes become activated inside the organ, or if release of the activated enzymes are blocked in the pancreatic duct. The mechanism of injury is digestion and therefore destruction of the pancreatic tissue. If the autolysis or enzymatic necrosis erodes blood vessels, this can cause fatal shock from the bleeding. This is acute hemorrhagic pancreatitis. Inflammation of this digestive organ is often idiopathic but a relationship with excessive alcohol and fatty diet is suspected. Maldigestion and malabsorption are related to the degree of organ destruction. Alcoholism can cause chronic pancreatitis, which often is a low-grade progression towards organ impairment. This impairment can be called pancreatic insufficiency due to loss of digestive function. Pancreatic insufficiency is suspected if steatorrhea, or excessive fat in the stool, can be demonstrated. Cystic fibrosis is a genetic abnormality of several exocrine glands in the body. Thick mucus production blocks ducts causing glands to swell or become cystic and fibrotic. Pancreatitis may result from the obstruction and malnutrition is one of several problems in affected children. Abnormality in the lungs is the most life-threatening result of this disease. Adenocarcinoma, or cancer of the pancreas, is another lifestyle-related neoplasm that has been linked to smoking and improper diet. Location of the cancerous growth determines the signs in the patient, which influence the timing of the diagnosis and prognosis. Tumors in the head of the pancreas are most common and produce the earliest signs, such as obstructive jaundice.

CHAPTER 14

The Urinary System

▶ OBJECTIVES

SECTION II

Define all highlighted terms.

Describe the condition of polycystic kidney disease, and characterize the causes and signs and symptoms of the disease.

SECTION III

Define all highlighted terms.

Characterize and describe the causes and signs and symptoms of the glomerular diseases glomerulonephritis, glomerulopathy, glomerulosclerosis, nephritic syndrome, and nephrotic syndrome.

Distinguish between the diseases acute and chronic glomerulonephritis. Describe the types of both, and characterize the causes and signs and symptoms of each type.

Describe the conditions of pyelonephritis, pyelitis, and pyonephrosis, and characterize the causes and signs and symptoms of each.

Describe the condition of cystitis, and characterize the causes and signs and symptoms of the disease.

SECTION IV

Define all highlighted terms.

Describe the causes and signs and symptoms of the metabolic disorders diabetic nephropathy, glomerulosclerosis, and papillary necrosis.

Characterize the causes and signs and symptoms of the forms of urolithiasis.

Describe the causes and signs and symptoms of the circulatory-associated disorders acute tubular necrosis and renal cortical necrosis.

Describe the effects of atherosclerosis and hypertension on renal function.

Describe and characterize the causes, signs and symptoms, and differences of acute and chronic renal failure.

SECTION V

Define all highlighted terms.

Compare and contrast the urinary-associated neoplasias renal carcinoma and bladder carcinoma. Describe the possible causes and signs and symptoms of both.

532

I. ANATOMY AND PHYSIOLOGY IN REVIEW

The urinary system is made up of two **kidneys,** two **ureters,** the urinary **bladder,** and the **urethra,** as shown in Figure 14–1. Within the kidneys are the areas of the cortex, medulla, and renal pelvis. The kidneys form urine. The ureters connect the kidneys to the bladder and conduct urine from the kidneys to the bladder. The bladder stores urine until it is eliminated from the body in the process of **urination, or micturition.** The urine exits the bladder through the urethra, which opens outside of the body.

The function of the urinary system is to form and eliminate **urine.** Urine contains waste products that must be eliminated or else their presence is toxic to the body. **Blood urea nitrogen, or BUN,** is a significant toxin that is responsible for **uremia, or uremic poisoning.** BUN is an end product of protein breakdown. Potassium, as you know from Chapter 3, must not be allowed to accumulate in the circulation since hyperkalemia can cause bradycardia and cardiac arrest. Sodium, water, hydrogen ions, and creatinine are other substances whose concentrations are regulated by the kidneys. The water content of urine is part of the regulatory mechanism that maintains normal hydration. ADH (antidiuretic hormone) from the pituitary gland is a vital hormone in governing the amount of water that is resorbed back into the blood from the pre-urine filtrate. Resorption of fluid from the filtrate produces a concentrated urine. Less than 10 percent of the blood volume that is filtered by the kidneys is excreted from the body. Aldosterone from the adrenal glands is necessary to govern sodium and potassium exchange and, therefore, the balance of these electrolytes.

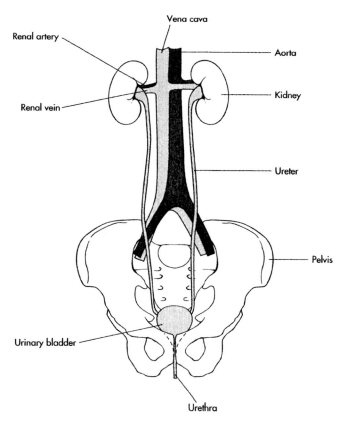

Figure 14–1. The urinary system.

The functional unit of the kidney is the **nephron,** as shown in Figure 14–2A. There are over a million nephrons in each kidney. This structure is responsible for forming urine from the blood that filters through it. The blood supply of the kidneys, which furnishes the blood to be filtered, is by way of the renal arteries that branch off the aorta. The structures of a nephron are the **glomerulus,** several sections of **tubules,** and the **collecting ducts.** The glomerulus is surrounded by the **Bowman's capsule.** The glomeruli and convoluted sections of the tubules are located in the cortex of the kidneys. Henle's loop and collecting ducts are located in the medulla.

Figures 14–2B and C show the components of a glomerulus in detail. The glomerulus is a specialized bed of capillaries that selectively filter substances from the blood flowing through it. Fluids and solutes from the blood enter the lumen of the nephron and become the **primary filtrate.** The primary filtrate in healthy kidneys never contains protein or red blood cells because these substances are too large to pass through the selectively permeable basement membrane of this capillary bed. The primary filtrate will become urine after passing

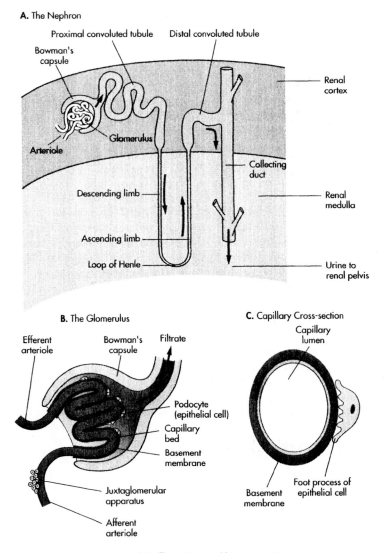

A. The Nephron

Proximal convoluted tubule

Distal convoluted tubule

Bowman's capsule

Renal cortex

Glomerulus

Arteriole

Collecting duct

Descending limb

Renal medulla

Ascending limb

Loop of Henle

Urine to renal pelvis

B. The Glomerulus

Efferent arteriole

Bowman's capsule

Filtrate

Podocyte (epithelial cell)

Capillary bed

Basement membrane

Juxtaglomerular apparatus

Afferent arteriole

C. Capillary Cross-section

Capillary lumen

Foot process of epithelial cell

Basement membrane

Figure 14–2. The nephron and its components.

thorough the rest of the nephron and being modified. The tubules that make up the remainder of the nephron consist of the **proximal convoluted tubule, Henle's loop** (made up of a descending limb, nephron loop, and ascending limb), and the **distal convoluted tubule.** Most of the fluid content of the filtrate is resorbed back into the circulation, and specific substances such as electrolytes, ions, and minerals are added to the filtrate. There are capillary networks that surround the tubules. A constant exchange of substances between the capillaries and tubules takes place as the filtrate passes through. **Resorption** is drawing substances back into the blood from the filtrate, while **secretion** is adding substances to the filtrate from the blood. Glucose is resorbed, drugs are secreted, and potassium is exchanged for sodium. Hydrogen ions are either secreted or resorbed, depending on the pH of the blood. This function is part of the acid–base balance mechanisms that were discussed in Chapter 3. When the blood is too acidic, more hydrogen ions are secreted (eliminated) to raise the pH. When the blood is too alkaline, more hydrogen ions are resorbed (retained) to lower the pH. The end product of all the activity of the nephron, urine, enters the collecting ducts. The collecting ducts of all the nephrons empty into the renal pelvis, which is a collecting space. From there, the urine enters the ureters, which conduct urine to the bladder for storage until it is eliminated.

In addition to the vital function of filtering waste and excreting it, the kidneys also have a secretory function. The kidneys secrete **renin,** which is a hormone important in the homeostatic function of maintaining or raising blood pressure (see Chap. 3). There is a group of cells called the **juxtaglomerular apparatus** in the walls of the arterioles that supply the glomeruli. The juxtaglomerular apparatus secretes renin, which is converted to **angiotensin.** Angiotensin causes vasoconstriction that raises blood pressure. The kidneys also secrete the growth factor **erythropoietin,** which stimulates the production of red blood cells in the bone marrow (see Chap. 9). That is why chronic kidney disease can cause anemia. Insufficient erythropoietin leads to insufficient erythropoiesis.

▶ GENERAL CONSIDERATIONS IN URINARY SYSTEM DISEASE

Before we begin the study of disease of the urinary system, there are a few important points to consider. The excretory function of the kidney obviously depends on the health and normal function of these organs. However, factors outside of the kidneys will affect their function. The formation of urine requires a certain blood pressure to filter the blood through the glomerulus. As you know, blood pressure is affected by hydration, blood volume, cardiac output, regulatory hormones, and blood vessels (specifically arteries). Also, formation of urine then requires its elimination. Blockages of ureters, the bladder, or urethra ultimately interfere with this excretory function. Therefore, in addition to **renal** causes of failure (disease of the kidneys themselves), there are also categories of **prerenal** and **postrenal** failure. Prerenal causes are most often due to insufficient blood pressure, such as during shock or cardiac insufficiency. Postrenal causes are generally obstruction in the elimination tracts, such as bladder stones or urethral stenosis.

Hypertension, atherosclerosis, and diabetes are other events outside of the kidneys that significantly affect their function. Hypertension and atherosclerosis cause narrowing of renal arteries and subsequent renal ischemia. This ischemia especially damages the delicate glomeruli, causing hardening **(glomerulosclerosis).** The vascular damage during the microangiopathy of diabetes causes similar injury to the glomeruli **(diabetic glomerulosclerosis).** The tubules of the nephrons are very sensitive to oxygen deprivation. Their complex function demands oxygen. During shock or heart failure, hypoxia or anoxia quickly leads to **tubular necrosis.** Therefore, systemic hypoperfusion and ischemia can significantly hinder kidney function.

Disease of the urinary system will cause either localized or systemic symptoms. Localized symptoms include flank pain associated with infection of the kidneys, or painful urination during bladder infection. Spastic pain, or urinary colic, is associated with stones of the ureters. Abnormal kidney function will produce several changes in the composition of urine. The volume of urine may be abnormal, such as excessive **(polyuria)**, decreased **(oliguria)**, or absent **(anuria)**. The urine can contain abnormal elements such as protein **(proteinuria)**, glucose **(glucosuria)**, blood **(hematuria)**, or pus **(pyuria)**. Infection of the kidneys or bladder may produce systemic symptoms consistent with infection, such as fever, chills, and malaise. Renal failure produces **uremia**, or **uremic poisoning.** This is an apt description because the body literally becomes poisoned by the harmful waste that is retained. An end stage of chronic uremia is depression of the central nervous system, which can lead to coma and death.

II. DEVELOPMENTAL DEFECTS ◀ SECTION

▶ POLYCYSTIC KIDNEY DISEASE

Developmental defects of the urinary tract are quite common. However, many of these do not cause enough interference in function that they produce signs. Many structutral anomalies or abnormalities of the urinary tract are found during routine examinations. The only disorder we will consider with any detail affects the kidneys. This is **polycystic kidney disease**, or **PKD.** PKD is the most significant developmental defect of the urinary system. It is a genetic disease with an autosomal dominant inheritance pattern. The underlying pathogenesis is an idiopathic obstruction of some tubules in both kidneys. The collecting ducts do not open into the renal pelvis as they should. Because of the obstruction, fluid builds up. Two consequences are the formation of many cysts of varying size and great enlargement of both kidneys. The presence and pressure of the cysts gradually compresses the normal tissue, which can be seen in Figure 14–3, and this interferes with

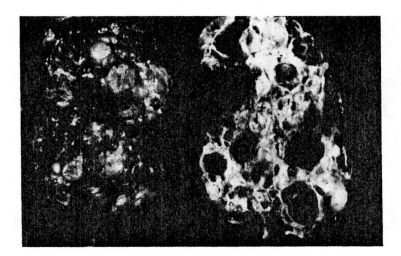

Figure 14–3. Polycystic kidney disease in an adult. Note the destruction of renal parenchyma due to the presence of multiple cysts. *(From Chandrasoma and Taylor,* Concise Pathology, *2nd ed., Appleton & Lange.)*

1. polycystic kidney disease
2. genetic or inherited
3. obstruction
4. renal pelvis
5. fluid
6. cysts
7. enlarged
8. function
9. failure

14-10

function. This interference is generally not suspected until adulthood. The affected individual generally develops chronic renal failure and hypertension by young to mid-adulthood. To prevent death from uremia, a kidney transplant is the only viable treatment option. The most important developmental defect of the urinary system affects the kidneys, and this is _____(1). The cause of PKD is _____(2). In this disorder, there is _____(3) of tubules within the kidneys and failure of the collecting ducts to empty into the _____(4). As a result, _____(5), accumulates and causes the formation of fluid pockets, or _____(6). Both kidneys also become very _____(7). The pressure of the cysts eventually interferes with _____(8), and the affected individual develops chronic renal _____(9).

Other developmental defects of the kidneys of which you should be aware include:

1. Renal agenesis. This is the presence of only one kidney because the second organ did not form (agenesis is "without creation"). Unilateral, or one-sided, renal agenesis is usually not problematic, but bilateral agenesis, or absence of both kidneys, is obviously incompatible with life.
2. Horseshoe kidney. Instead of two separate kidneys, the two organs have fused into one curved kidney at the midline.
3. Cystic renal dysplasia. This is abnormal enlargement of only one of the kidneys.
4. Dysplastic (multicystic) kidney. Here, there is malformation of the nephrons, and cysts form. This is usually seen in cases of malformation of other parts of the urinary tract. Any symptoms that may be present depend of the amount of parenchyma that is abnormal.

II. REVIEW QUESTIONS

1. c–a genetic or inherited disease

2. b–obstruction of tubules and collecting ducts so that urine backs up and causes cyst formation with swelling of the kidneys

3. c–gradual interference with function due to pressure, with uremia and chronic renal failure in adulthood

1. The cause of polycystic kidney disease is:
   a. idiopathic
   b. a spontaneous anomaly
   c. a genetic or inherited disease
   d. a birth defect caused by a teratogen

2. The pathogenesis of polycystic kidney disease is based on:
   a. the formation of cysts in the kidneys while in utero
   b. obstruction of tubules and collecting ducts so that urine backs up and causes cyst formation with swelling of the kidneys
   c. obstruction of the renal pelvis by cysts so that urine backs up and causes swelling of the kidneys
   d. obstruction of the tubules by fibrosis following in utero infection, so that prefiltrate backs up and causes cyst formation with swelling of the kidneys

3. The result of polycystic kidney disease is:
   a. acute renal failure in infancy due to uremia
   b. death from uremia in early childhood
   c. gradual interference with function due to pressure, with uremia and chronic renal failure in adulthood
   d. acute necrosis of the renal parenchyma due to pressure, with uremia and acute renal failure by adolescence

III. INFLAMMATORY AND INFECTIOUS DISEASES ◄ SECTION

► GLOMERULAR DISEASES

14–11

There are several classifications of glomerular diseases, depending on their cause and other features. Table 14–1 in Section IV summarizes them for you. The first classification is anti-body-mediated, or immunologic, disease. The injury to the glomerulus that is produced in these cases is called **glomerulonephritis.** Antibodies in the blood appear to be attracted to the specialized capillaries of the glomeruli. The basement membrane of these capillaries filter such large amounts of blood that their exposure to injurious agents is significant. In systemic autoimmune disease, antibodies and antibody–antigen complexes are frequently deposited in the basement membrane of the glomerular capillaries. These are either type II (cytotoxic) or type III (immune complex) hypersensitivity mechanisms. An allergic reaction might also describe these events. The immune deposits in the glomeruli cause inflammation (hence the name glomerulonephritis). There are some immune-mediated glomerular diseases that don't cause inflammation, and these are named and discussed in later frames. Inflammation of the glomeruli caused by immune-mediated reactions is called _____(1). Antibodies or antibody–antigen complexes are _____(2) from the blood and deposited in the _____(3) of the capillaries. The usual hypersensitivity mechanisms at work in these cases are either type II, which is _____(4), or type III, which is _____(5) hypersensitivity.

1. glomerulonephritis
2. filtered
3. basement membrane
4. cytotoxic
5. immune complex

14–12

Another classification of glomerular disease is metabolic disorders, which can cause glomerular disease, or **glomerulopathy.** The most well-known metabolic disorder that causes glomerulopathy is diabetes mellitus. Diabetes causes thickening and hardening of the basement membrane, which is known as **glomerulosclerosis.** The permeability, and there-fore the filtering ability of the glomeruli, is adversely affected by glomerulosclerosis. Dia-betes could also be called a multiple mechanism classification since it also causes circulatory disorders. Circulatory diseases are a third classification of glomerular disease. The circula-tory disorders that damage glomeruli include diabetic microangiopathy, atherosclerosis, hypertension, shock, and DIC. Hypoperfusion, ischemia, necrosis, and microthrombi of the kidneys are the typical results of these disorders. Diabetes causes disease of the glomeruli that is called _____(1). This is classified as a _____(2) glomerular disease. The particular injury caused by diabetes features thickening and _____(3) of the basement membranes. Glomeruli can also be damaged by dis-ease of the vessels or upset in hemodynamics, which is classified as _____(4) disorders.

1. glomerulosclerosis
2. metabolic
3. hardening
4. circulatory

14–13

The symptoms of glomerular disease present as a group called a **syndrome.** (A syndrome is a set of signs or symptoms that always occur together in a particular disease.) One syndrome is acute renal failure, which is discussed in the next section. **Nephritic syndrome** is charac-terized by generalized edema (anasarca), hypertension, hematuria [_____(1) in the urine], proteinuria [_____(2) in the urine], and hypoalbuminemia. Protein-uria is a hallmark of inflammatory glomerular disease. Normally, the junctions of the endothelial cells of the capillaries do not allow large molecules like protein to pass. If you will recall from Chapter 2, when vessels are inflamed, these junctions are opened wider or are more permeable. This allows protein, specifically albumin, and even red blood cells, to pass into the pre-urine filtrate. Loss of enough albumin into the urine decreases the amount in the blood, hence the reason for hypoalbuminemia. If you will remember from Chapter 3, albumin is responsible for the oncotic pressure that keeps fluid inside vessels. Hypoalbu-minemia will allow loss of fluid from vessels, and therefore the formation of generalized edema. **Nephrotic syndrome** presents with similar signs (edema, proteinuria, hypoalbu-

1. blood
2. protein

3. lipids
4. blood
5. lipids
6. urine

14-14

1. syndrome
2. protein
3. permeability
4. large
5. albumin
6. proteinuria
7. hematuria
8. hypoalbuminemia
9. edema

14-15

14-16

1. proteinuria
2. hematuria
3. edema
4. hypoalbuminemia

14-17

1. acute glomerulo-
   nephritis
2. poststreptococcal
   glomerulonephritis
3. group A streptococci
4. immune
5. antibodies
6. deposited
7. hypersensitivity
8. inflammatory
9. blood flow
10. juxtaglomerular

minemia) and often includes hyperlipidemia and lipiduria for reasons that are not well understood. You should be able to reason that hyperlipidemia means increased _____(3) in the _____(4), and that lipiduria means the presence of _____(5) in the _____(6).

The signs and symptoms of glomerular disease present as a specific group called a _____(1). In these syndromes, the hallmark sign of glomerular inflammation is the presence of _____(2) in the urine. The signs of nephritic and nephrotic syndrome can be explained in the following ways:

1. Inflamed vessels have an increase in _____(3), and this allows _____(4) molecules to pass into the primary filtrate and urine.
2. The loss of protein into the urine [and this protein is _____(5)] is described as _____(6).
3. The loss of red blood cells into the urine is described as _____(7).
4. Loss of a significant amount of albumin into the urine causes _____(8) in the blood.
5. Hypoalbuminemia decreases oncotic pressure so that fluid leaks into tissues and this causes the sign _____(9).

Acute glomerulonephritis is an immune-mediated inflammatory disease that can occur after an upper respiratory disease caused by some strains of group A streptococci. For this reason, it is often called **poststreptococcal glomerulonephritis.** The onset is generally a week or two after a strep throat. This disorder is seen most often in children. Today, the incidence of acute poststreptococcal glomerulonephritis is much less frequent than it was before the availability of antibiotics.

The pathogenesis of acute glomerulonephritis is as follows. During infection with streptococci, antibodies are produced against the organisms, and the antibodies bind to them. As these immune complexes in the blood pass through glomerular capillaries, they become deposited in the basement membranes. In this case, the kidneys are innocent bystanders and not a primary target of the antibodies, as they are in some diseases. The presence of the immune complexes elicits an inflammatory reaction as part of the type III or immune-complex hypersensitivity mechanism. Complement is activated, and inflammatory cells are attracted to the area. The presence of the many cells tends to block blood flow through the glomeruli. The increased permeability of the inflamed vessels is responsible for the signs of the nephritic syndrome that is seen in acute glomerulonephritis. These hallmark signs are _____(1), _____(2), _____(3), and _____(4). The blocked blood flow through the glomeruli triggers release of renin from the juxtaglomerular apparatus because these sensor cells are interpreting the hypoperfusion as systemic. The renin–angiotensin response raises blood pressure. Since systemic blood pressure is normal, hypertension results. This explains the mechanism of hypertension in nephritic syndrome.

Inflammation of the glomeruli that can follow a strep throat is called _____(1) or _____(2). The disorder can occur after an upper respiratory infection by _____(3). The cause of this inflammatory disease is _____(4) mediated. The pathogenesis is that complexes of _____(5) bound to the organisms become _____(6) in the basement membranes. Their presence causes inflammation through the type III _____(7) mechanism. The presence of many _____(8) cells block _____(9) through the glomeruli. This stimulates the _____(10) apparatus because of the local hypoperfusion. The result of the stimulation is the release of _____(11), which ultimately raises _____(12). This raised blood pressure is called _____(13). The diagnosis of acute glomerulonephritis is primary, made through the presence of the cardinal signs along with a history of streptococcal infection. Most cases of poststreptococcal glomerulonephritis are self-limiting within a few weeks. Historically, a few cases progressed to chronic glomerulonephritis and even renal failure. The best treatment is prevention with the use of antibiotics during the initial streptococcal infection.

14–18

Chronic glomerulonephritis may develop due to repeated episodes of acute glomerulonephritis. Other cases are because of progressive disease of the kidneys. The causes of these diseases include immune-mediated, where there are deposits of immune complexes in glomeruli, or attack of the basement membrane by anti-basement membrane antibodies. Immune-mediated injury causes inflammation. Another cause is idiopathic degeneration of the glomeruli, where there is no inflammatory reaction. The course of disease in the chronic form differs from that of acute glomerulonephritis. The inflammation or degeneration does not pass through an acute stage. The injury proceeds slowly and is low grade. Scarring of the glomeruli is a frequent sequela. Figure 14–4 shows the destruction and shrinking of the renal cortex after chronic glomerulonephritis. Chronic glomerulonephritis may be present for several years with periods of remission and exacerbation. One reason the exact cause of chronic glomerulonephritis cannot often be determined is because the effect on the patient is not dramatic. The condition has usually existed for some time before signs are specific enough to point to kidney disease. By then, the kidneys have suffered significant injury. Nephrotic syndrome, including hypertension, is present. The elevated blood pressure does help to make sufficient filtration of the blood possible. Many glomeruli are destroyed in the course of this disease and the remaining glomeruli are able to filter and produce urine because of the increased blood pressure. In chronic glomerulonephritis, there is long-standing _____(1) or _____(2) of the glomeruli. Inflammation accompanies injury in _____(3) cases. It is absent in cases caused by _____(4) of the glomeruli. _____(5) of the glomeruli is a result of chronic glomerulonephritis.

14–19

Eventually, in advanced stages, the kidneys are unable to concentrate the urine. This is demonstrated by the presence of a low **specific gravity.** Specific gravity is a measure of solutes dissolved in solvent, as compared to pure distilled water. A low specific gravity indicates fewer substances present in the urine, which means that the urine is abnormally dilute. The ultimate outcome of advanced chronic glomerulonephritis is fibrotic glomeruli and shrinking or contracture of the kidneys. Atrophy of the kidneys and subsequent loss of function causes renal failure and uremia.

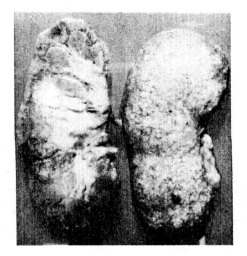

Figure 14–4. Chronic glomerulonephritis. Notice how shrunken and thinned the cortex has become. *(From Chandrasoma and Taylor,* Concise Pathology, *2nd ed., Appleton & Lange.)*

14-20

1. Lipoid nephrosis
2. children
3. hyperlipidemia
4. lipiduria
5. unknown
6. is not
7. epithelial

Some specific types of chronic glomerular diseases are described in the following frames. They are compared for you in Figure 14–5. The most common cause of nephrotic syndrome in children and adults is **lipoid nephrosis.** As the name indicates, hyperlipidemia and lipiduria are present. The cause of this disease is not known. Antibody deposits in glomeruli are *absent*. By light microscopy, the glomeruli appear normal. For this reason, lipid nephrosis is also called **minimal change disease.** The injury can be demonstrated only by electron microscopy, which shows lesions of the epithelial cells that surround the glomerular capillary membranes. The specific lesion is fusion of the foot processes of these cells. The damaged cells allow protein to escape into the urine. The basement membrane is unchanged in this disease. Corticosteroid treatment produces a good response in lipoid nephrosis. _____(1) is the most common reason for nephrotic syndrome in both _____(2) and adults. The name of this disorder is derived from the fact that _____(3) and _____(4) are features. The cause is _____(5). This _____(6) is / is not (choose one) an immune-mediated injury. The only abnormality is fusion of the foot processes of the _____(7) cells around the capillaries.

14-21

1. chronic glomerular disease
2. membranous nephropathy
3. immune
4. antigens
5. thickened
6. deposits
7. filtering
8. chronic renal failure

The second most common cause of chronic glomerular disease and nephrotic syndrome is **membranous glomerulonephritis,** also known as **membranous nephropathy.** The etiology of this disease is immune mediated. Electron microscopy shows the presence of antibody–antigen complexes deposited in thickened glomerular basement membranes. This thickening is described by the term "membranous" and it is due to massive deposits of these immune complexes. However, inflammatory cells are *absent,* which is in contrast to acute glomerulonephritis. The identity of most antigens has not been determined. A few antigens, such as the hepatitis virus, have been associated with membranous glomerulonephritis. The presence of immune complexes interferes with the filtering function of the glomeruli and increased vascular permeability allows protein to leak into the urine. The prognosis for membranous glomerulonephritis is worse than for lipoid nephrosis, since it does not respond well to any treatment. In about 40 percent of the patients, the disease progresses to chronic renal failure that requires dialysis or transplantation. Another significant cause of _____(1) is membranous glomerulonephritis, or _____(2). The cause has been determined to be _____(3) mediated; however, most _____(4) that are involved have yet to be identified. The word "membranous" describes a change in the basement membranes, which become very _____(5) because of large _____(6) of immune complexes. Their presence interferes with _____(7) by the glomeruli. Some cases of membranous nephropathy progress to _____(8).

14-22

1. autoimmune
2. antibodies

The final type of glomerular disease we will consider is **crescentic glomerulonephritis.** This is also an immune-mediated disease, specifically an autoimmune disease. Here, there are antibodies formed that target the basement membranes of the glomeruli capillaries. This is in contrast to immune complexes being filtered out of the blood and deposited in glomeruli. The damage these antibodies cause is rupture of the basement membrane. Macrophages escape through the tears in the basement membrane and accumulate in the glomerular space, therefore forming an exudate in the space. Their presence compresses the capillary bed, squeezing the loops of vessels into a crescent shape. Blood flow through the glomerular capillary bed ceases. Necrosis of the capillaries follows. This can be described as focal necrotizing glomerulonephritis. Injury to the glomeruli is severe. Urine production comes to a halt, clinically seen as **anuria** (without urine production). The patient quickly develops acute renal failure that requires dialysis or transplantation to prevent death. Several diseases can cause the formation of the anti-basement membrane antibodies and crescentic glomerulonephritis, but it is most often associated with the autoimmune disease **Goodpasture's syndrome.** Crescentic glomerulonephritis is caused by _____(1) disease in which _____(2) are formed that target and

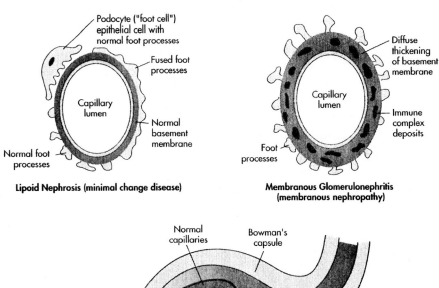

Figure 14–5. Types of chronic glomerulonephritis.

destroy the _____(3) of the glomeruli. The inflammatory cells, called _____(4), move thorough the holes in the ruptured _____(5) and build up in the glomerular space. These cells compress the loops of _____(6) into a _____(7) shape. Since blood flow ceases, death, or _____(8), of the capillaries and glomeruli follows. A clinical sign of this event is _____(9) in which there is no formation of _____(10). Death may occur due to the development of _____(11). These anti-basement membrane antibodies are most often formed in the autoimmune disease called _____(12).

3. basement membrane
4. macrophages
5. basement membranes
6. capillaries
7. crescent
8. necrosis
9. anuria
10. urine
11. acute renal failure
12. Goodpasture's syndrome

▶ PYELONEPHRITIS

14-23

We will now discuss infections of the urinary system. Urinary tract infections are abbreviated as **UTIs.** The vast majority of UTIs are caused by bacteria, as opposed to other types of microorganisms. The urinary system is susceptible to bacterial infection through two routes, which are illustrated in Figure 14–6. One is the hematogenous route. Because of the high volume of blood that passes through the kidneys, bacteria stand a good chance of being filtered out of the blood and colonizing in the kidneys. Infection of other organs and septicemia occur before hematogenous UTI. The other route is exogenous exposure because the urethral opening is external to the body, so bacteria can easily enter. Infection acquired through bacteremia is called **descending infection** because it begins in the kidneys and travels down

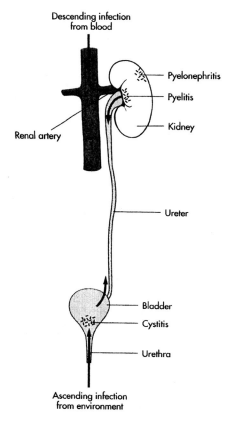

Descending infection
from blood

Pyelonephritis

Pyelitis

Kidney

Renal artery

Ureter

Bladder

Cystitis

Urethra

Ascending infection
from environment

Figure 14–6. Routes and locations of urinary tract infection.

1. urinary tract infection
2. bacteria
3. hematogenous or blood-
   borne
4. exogenous or environ-
   mental
5. descending
6. kidneys
7. ascending
8. urethra

1. pus
2. bacterial
3. kidney
4. pyelitis
5. ascending

through the system. An **ascending infection** describes one that is acquired from the environment through the urethra. It then travels up through the system. Ascending, or environmentally acquired infections, are much more common than descending, or blood-borne, infections. UTI stands for _____(1), which is usually caused by _____(2). Infection of the urinary system develops through either the _____(3) route or through _____(4) exposure. Infection caused by septicemia or bacteremia is described as a _____(5) infection because it travels down from the _____(6). Environmentally acquired infection is described as a (an) _____(7) infection because it travels up from the _____(8).

Bacterial infection of the kidneys is referred to as **pyelonephritis.** Pyelonephritis can occur alone or along with bladder infection. It may be either acute or chronic. The most common causative organisms of pyelonephritis are *E. coli* and other gram-negative enteric rods that have entered the kidneys from the bloodstream or, more commonly, from the bladder and ureters. Obstructions of the lower urinary tract predispose to these infections, as you will see when we discuss bladder infection. Streptococci and staphylococci are also causative agents. In the case of an ascending infection from the bladder, infection that reaches only as far as the renal pelvis, and not into the parenchyma, is called **pyelitis.** Unresolved pyelitis can progress to pyelonephritis. In acute pyelonephritis, the infection is suppurative because the causative bacteria are pyogenic, which means _____(1) producing. Multiple abscesses may form within the parenchyma. A severe case of acute suppurative pyelonephritis may lead to pus completely filling the renal pelvis. This is called **pyonephrosis.** Pyelonephritis is _____(2) infection of the _____(3). If the infection involves only the renal pelvis, this is called _____(4). The most common route for development of pyelonephritis is through a (an) _____(5) infection from the lower tract. Pyogenic bacteria cause the formation of pus, and so acute pyelonephritis is described as _____(6). Pyonephrosis describes a renal pelvis that is filled with _____(7).

Acute cases that are not resolved, especially those caused by obstruction of the lower tract, frequently lead to chronic pyelonephritis. The interstitial tissue (the tissue in which the tubules lie) becomes filled with inflammatory cells. As the infection persists, areas of the organ are destroyed, and fibrosis is the typical sequela. The kidney contracts with the scar tissue and becomes small, with a very irregular surface. Fortunately, in many cases the other kidney is unaffected. The clinical signs of pyelonephritis include fever and flank or back pain. Within the urine are found protein, white blood cells, and bacteria. A massive number of white blood cells in the urine is described as **pyuria,** which means pus in the urine. Pyuria is especially seen if abscesses within the kidneys rupture and release their contents into the urine. Casts may also be present in the urine. These are cylindrical molds of protein that have precipitated out in the inflamed tubules. The treatment is antibiotics, the type of which is determined by sensitivity testing after the bacteria has been cultured from the urine and identified. Any obstruction of the urinary tract must be resolved to avoid chronic pyelonephritis. In severe untreated cases, the entire kidney can fill with pus, which leads to its destruction and failure of that kidney. Chronic pyelonephritis may develop from unresolved acute cases, especially if _____(1) of the lower urinary tract exists. After a while, the kidney becomes _____(2) and _____(3) because of the shrinking or _____(4) that is associated with fibrosis. In some cases, there is the presence of a very large number of white blood cells in the urine, and this is called _____(5).

14-25

1. obstruction
2. scarred or fibrotic
3. small
4. contraction
5. pyuria

▶ CYSTITIS

Infectious inflammation of the bladder is called **cystitis.** (The word root "cyst" is descriptive of the bladder as a fluid-filled sac.) The gram-negative coliforms (especially *E. coli*), staphylococci, and streptococci are again the causative agents. Cystitis may be acute or chronic. This infection is primarily an ascending one, with bacteria gaining entry through the urethra. Cystitis is seen more frequently in women because the urethra is short, so bacteria enter the bladder more easily. Some cases of cystitis have no obvious cause. However, there are a variety of situations that predispose to bladder infection. These include medical procedures that introduce instruments into the bladder (such as catheterization), frequent sexual intercourse ("honeymoon cystitis"), pregnancy, diabetes, fecal contamination, benign prostatic hyperplasia (an obstructive condition that compresses the prostatic urethra), and obstruction of the urethra or bladder.

While fibrosis and stenosis of the urethra is one possible cause of obstruction, obstruction by bladder stones is much more common. Obstruction greatly predisposes to infection. In this case, the cystitis is secondary. Normally, bacteria that have entered the urethra are washed back out during urination. They do not have the chance to multiply and colonize the urinary tract. If a normal stream of urine can't be produced because of obstruction, the urine will stagnate in the bladder. Any bacteria present are then able to multiply and cause infection. Clinically, cystitis presents with **dysuria** (painful or difficult urination) and frequent urination, with the continuous urge to urinate. These symptoms are due to the irritation of nerve endings by inflammation. Infection of the bladder is called _____(1). It is a (an) _____(2) infection, having traveled up through the _____(3). It is seen more in women because of the _____(4) urethra. One predisposing factor in cystitis is obstruction, and this is often seen with bladder _____(5). The mechanism of infection due to obstruction is that the bacteria are not _____(6) out of the urethra by a forceful _____(7) stream. They are then able to remain and _____(8) to infectious numbers.

14-27

1. cystitis
2. ascending
3. urethra
4. short
5. stones
6. washed
7. urine
8. multiply

1. infection
2. folds
3. bacteria
4. obstruction
5. stagnant

Acute cystitis will become chronic if the infection is not effectively eliminated. The bladder stretches when full and is collapsed when empty. Because it changes in size, the interior wall contains many folds to accommodate stretching. This design creates many nooks and crannies in which bacteria can hide. The course of antibiotic treatment of cystitis must be of sufficient length so that the tissue is thoroughly penetrated and the bacteria eradicated. Obstructions that are not resolved almost always lead to chronic cystitis because there is always some pool of stagnant urine with multiplying bacteria. In these cases, the walls of the bladder become thickened in response to the chronic inflammation. Treatment of chronic cystitis caused by obstruction must include elimination of the obstruction in addition to antibiotics. In general, chronic cystitis is difficult to effectively treat, and it tends to recur in some individuals. Chronic cystitis develops when the initial _____(1) is not eradicated. One physical feature of the bladder that makes treatment difficult is the many _____(2) present in its walls. This allows a place for _____(3) to remain. The presence of a (an) _____(4) will lead to a chronic infection because there is always a small amount of _____(5) urine containing bacteria remaining in the bladder.

III. REVIEW QUESTIONS

1. d–all of the above are
   correct

2. b–glomerulonephritis

3. a–glomerulopathy
   b–glomerulosclerosis

4. d–hyperlipidemia
   g–lipiduria

1. Choose the correct statement or statements that describe the general features of glomerular disease:
   a. Circulatory disorders (disease of vessels or disruption of homeostasis) injure glomeruli because of hypoperfusion, ischemia, and necrosis.
   b. Antigen–antibody mediated diseases injure glomeruli because of immune complex deposits or direct attack.
   c. Metabolic disorders, specifically diabetes, injure glomeruli because of thickening and hardening of the basement membranes.
   d. all of the above are correct
   e. none of the above are correct

2. In immune-mediated damage of glomeruli, the injury is described as:
   a. glomerulopathy
   b. glomerulonephritis
   c. glomerulosclerosis
   d. nephritic syndrome
   e. nephrotic syndrome

3. Complete this sentence using the terms below: In general, metabolic diseases that injure glomeruli are described as a. _____, and, specifically, diabetes mellitus produces glomerular disease described as b. _____.
   chronic glomerulonephritis   nephrotic syndrome
   glomerulopathy   glomerulosclerosis
   lipoid nephropathy
   crescentic glomerulonephritis

4. Which of the following are NOT seen in nephritic syndrome (choose all that apply):
   a. hypertension
   b. proteinuria
   c. generalized edema
   d. hyperlipidemia
   e. hematuria
   f. hypoalbuminemia
   g. lipiduria

5. Please provide the terms that explain the relationship between the signs seen in nephritic syndrome:

Inflammation of glomeruli causes a (an) a. _____ in permeability, which allows b. _____ and c. _____ to escape into the filtrate and urine. The presence of these substances in the urine is called d. _____ and e. _____, respectively. The type of protein that is lost into the urine is f. _____. This can lessen the amount of this protein that is in the blood, and below normal levels is called g. _____. Because this protein provides most of the h. _____ pressure that retains fluid in vessels, its decrease allows fluid to i. _____ from vessels and produce j. _____ in the tissues.

6. Hypertension can be seen in nephritic syndrome because:
    a. inflammation of glomeruli is the stimulus that causes the juxtaglomerular apparatus to secrete renin, which ultimately raises blood pressure
    b. systemic hypoperfusion causes the stimulation of the juxtaglomerular apparatus to secrete renin, which ultimately raises blood pressure
    c. excessive renin and angiotensin are secreted from the adrenal cortex during kidney disease as a compensatory mechanism
    d. localized hypoperfusion of glomeruli causes stimulation of the juxtaglomerular apparatus to secrete renin, which ultimately raises blood pressure

7. For the following descriptions of the pathogenesis of various glomerular diseases, please provide the name of the disease being described from the list below:
    a. immune-mediated injury, specifically due to autoantibodies which are anti-basement membrane antibodies that rupture the glomerular basement membrane

    _____
    b. immune-mediated injury due to deposits of immune complexes in the basement membrane, in which the antibodies are directed against some strains of group A streptococci _____
    c. injury of unknown cause showing only slight changes of epithelial cells of the glomerular capillaries, featuring hyperlipidosis and lipiduria _____
    d. low-grade injury of glomeruli over a long period of time, caused by a variety of agents, in which scarring and destruction of glomeruli are features

    _____
    e. immune-mediated injury due to deposits of immune complexes in the basement membrane, in which inflammatory cells are NOT present and the antigen is largely unknown _____

    poststreptococcal glomerulonephritis   Goodpasture's syndrome
    nephrotic syndrome   pyelonephritis
    glomerulosclerosis   acute glomerulonephritis
    lipoid nephrosis   glomerulopathy
    crescentic glomerulonephritis   membranous nephropathy
    membranous glomerulonephritis
    chronic glomerulonephritis

8. In acute or poststreptococcal glomerulonephritis, the presence of many inflammatory cells interferes with blood flow through the glomeruli, and this causes:
    a. ischemia and necrosis of glomeruli
    b. immune complexes to be filtered out and deposited in glomerular basement membranes
    c. local hypoperfusion that stimulates the juxtaglomerular apparatus and leads to hypertension
    d. renal failure

5. a–increase; b–protein; c–red blood cells; d–proteinuria; e–hematuria; f–albumin; g–hypoalbuminemia; h–oncotic; i–escape; j–edema

6. d–localized hypoperfusion of glomeruli causes stimulation of the juxtaglomerular apparatus to secrete renin, which ultimately raises blood pressure

7. a–crescentic glomerulonephritis; b–acute glomerulonephritis or poststreptococcal glomerulonephritis; c–lipoid nephrosis; d–chronic glomerulonephritis; e–membranous glomerulonephritis or membranous nephropathy

8. c–local hypoperfusion that stimulates the juxtaglomerular apparatus and leads to hypertension

9. a–lipoid nephrosis

10. False

11. b–membranous glomeru-
lonephritis; d–crescentic
glomerulonephritis

12. b–an exudate composed of
macrophages that squeezes
the capillary loops and halts
blood flow through the capillaries

13. d–pyelonephritis

14. b–an ascending infection
from the bladder

15. a–pyuria

16. a–the ascending or exogenous route

17. c–bacteria are not removed
from the urinary tract by a
normal urine stream, so they
remain and multiply to infectious numbers

9. The most common cause of nephrotic syndrome in children and adults is:
   a. lipoid nephrosis
   b. crescentic glomerulonephritis
   c. membranous nephropathy
   d. chronic glomerulonephritis

10. True or false: Lipoid necrosis is an immune-mediated disease that causes thickening of the glomerular basement membrane. _____

11. Two glomerular diseases that carry the worst prognoses are (choose two):
    a. poststreptococcal glomerulonephritis
    b. membranous glomerulonephritis
    c. lipoid nephrosis
    d. crescentic glomerulonephritis

12. In crescentic glomerulonephritis, necrosis of the glomerular capillary bed occurs because of:
    a. the presence of many inflammatory cells that obstruct blood flow through the glomerulus
    b. an exudate composed of macrophages that squeezes the capillary loops and halts blood flow through the capillaries
    c. destruction of the capillary membranes by autoantibodies
    d. stimulation of the juxtaglomerular apparatus that causes constriction of arterioles and decreases blood flow

13. Bacterial infection of the kidney parenchyma is called:
    a. pyelitis
    b. cystitis
    c. pyonephrosis
    d. pyelonephritis
    e. pyuria

14. Pyelonephritis most often develops because of:
    a. a hematogenous or blood-borne infection
    b. an ascending infection from the bladder
    c. an extension of pyonephrosis
    d. the rupture of abscesses in the kidney

15. In acute suppurative pyelonephritis, rupture of abscesses can produce:
    a. pyuria
    b. pyelitis
    c. pyonephrosis
    d. casts in the urine

16. The most common pathogenesis of cystitis is an infection acquired through:
    a. the ascending or exogenous route
    b. the descending or hematogenous route
    c. obstruction with bladder stones
    d. none of the above

17. Obstruction of the urinary tract predisposes to infection because:
    a. bacteria become walled off and inflammatory cells cannot reach them
    b. thickening of the bladder walls in response to the irritation traps bacteria within the walls
    c. bacteria are not removed from the urinary tract by a normal urine stream, so they remain and multiply to infectious numbers
    d. there is no relationship between obstruction of the urinary tract and infection

IV. OTHER URINARY SYSTEM DISORDERS AND RENAL FAILURE ◀ SECTION

▶ METABOLIC DISORDERS

14-29

There are a variety of systemic metabolic diseases that, since they are systemic, affect several organs. This includes the kidneys. Two examples are multiple myeloma (see Chap. 9) and gout (see Chap. 8). In multiple myeloma, hypersecretion of immunoglobulins by cancerous plasma cells leads to the deposits of these proteins in the kidneys. Renal failure is the result of this infiltration. In gout, there is also deposition of substances in the kidneys. These are crystals of uric acid that damage the kidneys.

14-30

The most common and significant systemic metabolic disease that affects the kidneys is diabetes mellitus. The injury diabetes causes to the kidneys is described as **diabetic nephropathy.** As you know, diabetes causes disease of small blood vessels, and this is called _____(1). Any organ or body tissue whose vessels are diseased will also suffer. There are several pathologic changes that occur in the kidneys because of vascular changes. The arterioles that supply the glomeruli deteriorate. Their walls thicken and the lumens become narrow. This decreases blood supply to the glomeruli, which would be medically described as _____(2). The ischemia results in atrophy of tubules. Within the glomeruli, the basement membranes become thickened and hardened. This is a form of glomerulopathy called **glomerulosclerosis.** In other words, in this particular disease of glomeruli, they become hardened. The change in the permeability of the glomerular capillary bed allows protein to escape, which causes proteinuria. The degree of proteinuria is often used to assess the severity of kidney damage. These changes are slow, with onset of proteinuria about 10 to 15 years after the development of diabetes. Protein loss of 3 grams per day into the urine marks the beginning of nephrotic syndrome. Significantly more than that indicates early chronic renal failure, which becomes progressively worse over a few years. _____(3) is the most important and most common metabolic disease affecting the kidneys. The condition is called _____(4). This disease is based on the fact that _____(5) supplying the kidneys are injured. Ischemia occurs because arteriole walls become _____(6) and the lumens are _____(7). Glomerulosclerosis follows, which is _____(8) and _____(9) of the _____(10) of the glomeruli. The amount of kidney injury is estimated by the amount of _____(11) in the urine.

1. microangiopathy
2. ischemia
3. Diabetes mellitus
4. diabetic nephropathy
5. vessels
6. thickened
7. narrowed
8. thickening
9. hardening
10. basement membrane
11. protein

14-31

Additional pathology of the kidneys in diabetic nephropathy includes **papillary necrosis.** Ischemia of the medullary area can cause necrosis and sloughing of the papillae. This sloughing can cause acute obstruction of the ureters by the pieces of dead detached tissue. With urine outflow blocked, hydronephrosis results. This is swelling of the kidneys caused by backed-up urine, which will be discussed later. As is typical in diabetes, infections are prone to occur. Pyelonephritis, which is infection of the _____(1), is a complication of diabetic nephropathy. Frequent infection further damages the kidneys. Dialysis and transplantation are required in advanced cases of diabetic nephropathy to prevent death from kidney failure. Ischemia of the renal medulla can cause death of the papillae, and this is called _____(2). A complication of papillary necrosis is _____(3) of the ureters by sections of sloughed tissue. This blockage causes _____(4) of urine in the kidneys and subsequent _____(5) of the kidneys. Another complication of diabetic nephropathy is frequent bouts of _____(6) that contribute to kidney failure.

1. kidney
2. papillary necrosis
3. obstruction
4. back up
5. swelling
6. pyelonephritis or infection

Stone formation in the urinary tract is medically termed **urolithiasis** (the word root "lith" refers to stone). Another term for stones is **calculi.** Urinary stones are a common disorder. They occur more often in men than in women. Stone-like masses form from the crystallization of minerals in the filtrate and urine. The minerals precipitate or fall out of solution and the resulting crystals grow in size to become stones. Stones may lodge in the ureters or urethra, but they are most commonly found in the pelvis of the kidneys or in the bladder. Figure 14–7 illustrates these locations and two common types of stones. There are several types of stones, based on their chemical composition. The majority of these types are small, at 3 mm or less in diameter. Urinary calculi also appear in a variety of shapes such as rounded, elongated, or as crystals. Urolithiasis is classified as a metabolic disorder because abnormalities in the metabolism of various electrolytes, minerals, or amino acids are responsible for the formation. Some cases cannot be associated with a specific cause. Small stones may form if the urine becomes too concentrated because of dehydration. The formation of urinary stones is called _____(1). Urinary stones are also called _____(2). These hard masses form when minerals _____(3) out from the filtrate or urine. The most common locations for urinary calculi are the renal _____(4) and the _____(5).

The major types of calculi are calcium, struvite, uric acid, and cystine. These names reflect what the stones are made of. The most common of these four types is **calcium phosphate,** or **calcium oxalate.** These stones can develop in abnormal calcium metabolism disorders, where calcium is excreted in large amounts and the crystals precipitate out of solution in the urinary tract. It is suspected that there is a genetic predisposition to form calcium stones in these cases. Another cause can be extended bedrest, which can cause leaching of calcium from the inactive bones and subsequent increased levels of calcium in the blood. Diseases of the bones that cause loss of calcium from them and hyperparathyroidism (see Chap. 16) are

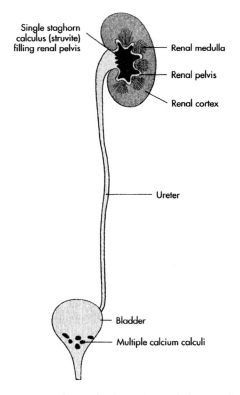

Single staghorn
calculus (struvite)
filling renal pelvis

Renal medulla

Renal pelvis

Renal cortex

Ureter

Bladder

Multiple calcium calculi

Figure 14–7. Common locations and types of urinary calculi.

other reasons for increased calcium blood levels and increased calcium excretion by the kidneys. **Struvite** calculi are made of magnesium ammonia phosphate or sulfate. Struvite stones are the second most common type of calculi. In the previous section, we said that urinary stones can be a causative factor in urinary infection and cause their recurrence. In the case of struvite stones, chronic urinary tract infection can cause the stones. They form from the excessive amount of ammonia and urea present, which are produced by bacteria. Struvite stones are larger than other types of stones, with very irregular surfaces. They may become so large that they fill the entire renal pelvis. These large mineral deposits are also known as **staghorn calculi** due to their appearance. This is one large mass (instead of several stones) that takes the shape of the renal pelvis, thereby resembling an antler or staghorn. The most common type of urinary calculi is made primarily of _____(1). The pathogenesis for their formation is the increased _____(2) of calcium by the kidneys, which allows this mineral to _____(3) out of solution into solid crystals. The kidneys excrete more calcium in cases where there is _____(4) calcium in the blood. The second most common type of stone is called _____(5) calculi. Bacterial production of _____(6) and _____(7) contribute to the formation of struvite stones, so bacterial _____(8) is a causative factor. Struvite calculi differ from other types in that they are often _____(9) solid mass that fills the _____(10), instead of multiple stones. Struvite calculi are also described by the phrase _____(11), which reflects their shape.

1. calcium
2. excretion
3. precipitate
4. increased
5. struvite
6. ammonia
7. urea
8. infection
9. one
10. renal pelvis
11. staghorn calculi

14-34

About 5 percent of urinary calculi are **uric acid** stones associated with the disease gout. In Chapter 8 we discussed the pathogenesis of gout, which included hyperuricemia. Hyperuricemia means a (an) _____(1) in the amount of uric acid in the _____(2). Some cases of uric acid stones are idiopathic and not associated with a primary disease like gout. The least common type of stone is composed of **cysteine** and is found in uncommon cases of abnormal amino acid metabolism (an inborn error of metabolism). In these cases, there is increased secretion of cysteine.

1. increase
2. blood

14-35

The clinical presentation of urolithiasis of the kidneys or ureters is that of blood in the urine, or _____(1), and sudden, severe pain. The type of pain is characterized as urinary colic. As the smooth muscle of the area contracts around the stone, it produces spasms of pain around the obstructed area. This often occurs when a small stone is passed from the renal pelvis into the ureter. Bladder stones may occur with infection, and those signs (dysuria, frequency, and urgency) usually predominate. Treatment depends on the size of the stone or stones. With the help of a dissolving medication, crystals and small stones may pass on their own with the urine stream. Larger stones may require surgical removal. A procedure called **lithotripsy** uses ultrasound shock waves to crush or pulverize stones into small enough pieces to be passed, so that surgery may not be necessary. Because urolithiasis has a tendency to recur in the same patient, medication to prevent the formation of new stones is quite helpful in its management.

1. hematuria

14-36

A stone that is impacted in a ureter and is not removed can cause unilateral **hydronephrosis.** Because of the obstruction in the passage of urine, the ureters and renal pelvis dilate proximal to, or behind, the obstruction. This swelling caused by blocked urine defines hydronephrosis. The pressure from the swelling causes pressure necrosis and the deterioration of the renal parenchyma, with subsequent loss of function. This destruction of functional tissue can be seen in Figure 14–8. Other causes of hydronephrosis (which are also obstructions) are a tumor, an enlarged prostate gland, or a congenital defect. With an enlarged prostate gland, hydronephrosis is bilateral because the obstruction is at the neck of the bladder and the urine backs up into both ureters and kidneys. The pathogenesis of hydronephrosis is _____(1) of the urinary tract, which allows _____(2) to build up within the system. Blocked urine causes _____(3) of the kidneys, _____(4) necrosis, and loss of _____(5). Depending on the site of obstruction, hydronephrosis may involve only one kidney, or be _____(6).

1. obstruction
2. urine
3. swelling
4. pressure
5. function
6. bilateral

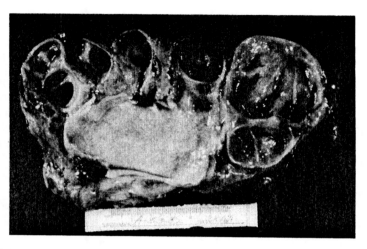

Figure 14–8. Hydronephrosis. Note the loss of kidney tissue caused by cystic swelling and pressure. *(From Mulvihill,* Human Diseases: A Systemic Approach, *4th ed., Appleton & Lange.)*

▶ CIRCULATORY DISORDERS

As would be expected, disease of blood vessels supplying the kidneys, or systemic hypertension, adversely affects these organs. Since they are not provided with a normal amount of blood, malfunction of the kidneys is the inevitable result. These disturbances in function may be either acute or chronic, depending on the cause. Circulatory disorders that cause renal insufficiency include systemic hypotension and therefore hypoperfusion, hypertension, and atherosclerosis.

1. hypotension
2. hypoperfusion
3. tubules
4. acute tubular necrosis
5. renal cortical necrosis
6. regeneration
7. function

Systemic hypoperfusion can be caused by myocardial infarction, cardiac arrest, or hypotensive shock. These conditions cause a sudden loss of arterial pressure, or acute hypotension, and therefore cause acute hypoperfusion of the kidneys. The interruption in blood flow has the greatest effect on the tubules in the cortex. If the ischemia is significant enough to destroy the tubules, the result is **acute tubular necrosis.** In severe cases, the tissue of the entire cortex may experience death, which is called **renal cortical necrosis.** Because the initial injury was due to factors outside the kidneys, failure in function can initially be classified as prerenal failure (see Frame 14–6). But the situation often becomes true renal failure. This is because even after the systemic hypotension is resolved by treating the cause, the damage to the kidneys can persist. In these cases, treatment with dialysis for a sufficient period of time allows the kidneys to rest and improves conditions for regeneration. As an epithelial-based organ like the liver, the regenerative power of the kidneys is good. If sufficient healing and regeneration of tubules can occur, kidney function can be restored. Sudden loss of arterial blood pressure is medically described as acute _____(1). This results in systemic _____(2). Decreased blood flow through the kidneys most significantly affects the _____(3). Sudden death of these structures is called _____(4). If the whole of the cortex is involved, this is called _____(5). Support of kidney function, which allows rest and healing of the parenchyma, makes _____(6) possible, which restores _____(7).

Systemic diseases of blood vessels that directly affect the kidneys are atherosclerosis and hypertension. **Hypertension** injures arteries and arterioles within the kidney. The high blood pressure causes continual contraction of these vessels and ultimately leads to thickening of the vessels. Thickened walls reduce the size of the lumens and therefore reduce blood flow. The parenchymal tissue experiences ischemia. The physical changes in the nephrons are similar to those caused by atherosclerosis and diabetes. Impaired function and possible renal failure are the sequela.

In contrast to hypertension, atherosclerosis damages the artery outside of the kidney that is the main thoroughfare for blood supply. The renal arteries, which branch off the abdominal aorta, are frequent targets of atherosclerosis. If you will remember from Chapter 9, atherosclerosis causes enough narrowing of vessel lumens that blood flow is significantly reduced. Any organ supplied by those compromised vessels suffers ischemia. In the kidneys, this ischemia damages the nephrons, particularly the glomeruli. The glomeruli harden, and this condition is described as **ischemic glomerulosclerosis.** Another term that is used to describe this damage is **nephroangiosclerosis,** which means sclerotic hardening of the nephrons and vessels. The remaining parts of the nephrons, the tubules, undergo atrophy in response to glomerulosclerosis. Multiple areas of fibrosis, which replace lost nephrons, cause the entire kidney to become scarred and shrunken. While systemic hypoperfusion causes acute renal insufficiency, hypertension and atherosclerosis cause gradual, or chronic, renal insufficiency. In hypertension, the damaged vessels are the _____(1) and _____(2) that are located _____(3) the kidneys. In atherosclerosis, the damaged vessels are the _____(4), which are the main source of blood from the aorta. In both conditions, the lumens of the vessels become _____(5), which _____(6) blood flow and therefore causes _____(7) of the kidneys. In atherosclerosis, the pathology of the nephrons, glomeruli, and vessels is described as _____(8) and _____(9). The specific pathology is _____(10) of these structures. Table 14–1 summarizes the various diseases that affect the structures of the nephron.

1. arteries
2. arterioles
3. within
4. renal arteries
5. narrow
6. reduces
7. ischemia
8. ischemic glomerulosclerosis
9. nephroangiosclerosis
10. sclerotic hardening

TABLE 14–1. CLASSIFICATIONS OF GLOMERULAR AND TUBULAR DISEASES

Disease	Features
Immune-Mediated Diseases	
Glomerulonephritis	Deposits of immune complexes in glomerular basement membrane
Acute poststreptococcal glomerulonephritis	Inflammation in response to immune complex deposits, antibodies directed against group A streptococci
Chronic glomerulonephritis	Immune complex deposits, anti-basement membrane antibodies, degeneration of glomeruli (see Chronic Glomerular Diseases, next)
Chronic Glomerular Diseases	
Lipoid nephrosis	Absence of antibody deposits, no injury to basement membrane, lesions of epithelial cells (fusion of podocyte foot processes)
Membranous glomerulonephritis or membranous nephropathy	Thickening of glomerular basement membrane due to immune-complex deposits, absence of inflammatory cells
Crescentic glomerulonephritis	Anti-basement membrane antibodies rupture glomerular basement membrane, macrophages compress capillary loops
Metabolic Diseases	
Glomerulopathy	Injury of glomerular capillary bed or basement membrane
Diabetes mellitus or diabetic nephropathy	Glomerulosclerosis (thickening and hardening) with narrowing of arterioles with ischemia
Circulatory Diseases	
Glomerulopathy	Injury of glomerular capillary bed
Systemic hypotension (heart failure, shock)	Ischemia and acute tubular necrosis, possible renal cortical necrosis
Hypertension	Thickening and narrowing of intrarenal arterioles, ischemia
Artherosclerosis	Narrowing of renal artery and ischemia, ischemic glomerulosclerosis, and nephroangiosclerosis

▶ RENAL FAILURE

14–41

Acute renal failure is sudden loss of function of the kidneys. It has a better prognosis than chronic failure. In Frame 14–38 we discussed acute tubular necrosis as the result of renal ischemia due to cardiac arrest or shock. Because of too little oxygen, these vital epithelial cells of the nephrons die. Acute tubular necrosis is also caused by toxic injury to the kidneys. There are many chemical agents that can poison the kidneys. Among those are methyl alcohol; ethylene glycol (antifreeze); heavy metals such as mercury, chloroform, carbon tetrachloride; and even some antibiotics. Whatever the cause, necrosis of renal tubules is a life-threatening event. With loss of filtering function, production of urine decreases. Decreased or insufficient urine output is called **oliguria.** Complete shutdown of the kidneys results in **anuria,** or total absence of urine production. Two waste products that are eliminated in the urine, and that build to dangerous levels in oliguria and anuria, are potassium and urea. Elevated blood potassium, or hyperkalemia, drastically affects heart function. The rate of cardiac contraction slows to below normal, which is bradycardia. With high enough potassium levels, the heart stops completely, which is asystole, or cardiac arrest. The effect of excessive blood urea nitrogen will be discussed with chronic renal failure. Retention of water and upset in other electrolyte balances contributes to the patient's demise.

14–42

1. acute renal failure
2. ischemia
3. oxygen
4. acute tubular necrosis
5. toxic
6. oliguria
7. anuria
8. potassium
9. hyperkalemia
10. heart
11. bradycardia
12. asystole
13. cardiac arrest

Abrupt loss of kidney function is described as _____(1). This can be caused by interruption in blood supply, or _____(2), which leaves insufficient _____(3) for the cells. Sudden death of the cells of the tubules is called _____(4). Another cause of acute tubular necrosis is damage from chemicals that are _____(5) to kidney cells. Acute renal failure is marked by a sudden decrease in urine output, called _____(6), or by no urine output, called _____(7). The most immediately critical value that becomes elevated in acute failure is _____(8), which is medically termed _____(9). Hyperkalemia most markedly affects the _____(10). The rate of contraction becomes abnormally slow [which is called _____(11)], or it may stop altogether (called _____(12) or _____(13)). The severity of kidney failure is monitored by testing the blood urea nitrogen (BUN) and creatinine levels. The degree of injury correlates directly with the elevation of these values. Another marker of kidney function is the creatinine clearance test, which measures the amount of creatinine cleared from the blood in 24 hours. The creatinine clearance test is a direct assessment of the glomerular filtration rate, or GFR. Because of the nature of injury in acute renal failure, dialysis and aggressive supportive therapy may allow regeneration of enough renal tubules to begin function again.

14–43

The most common type of kidney failure is **chronic renal failure,** which takes place slowly over a relatively long period of time. Acute and chronic renal failure differ in causative agents and the nature of the injury. These two different types of organ failure are compared in Figure 14–9. Chronic injury can be the result of chronic glomerulonephritis, nephroangiosclerosis (atherosclerosis), hypertension, or diabetic nephropathy. In diabetes, recurring episodes of pyelonephritis, or infection, are a contributing factor in the destruction of the kidneys. Chronic obstruction of the urinary tract and hydronephrosis are other avenues of chronic renal failure.

14–44

The signs of chronic renal failure may remain hidden for a long while. There is no sudden decrease in urine production, as in acute failure. The only specific indicators prior to the end stage of this disease are elevated levels of BUN and creatinine. Retaining these nitrogen-containing waste products in the blood is called **azotemia.** If you will remember from Chapter 13, the liver forms urea from ammonia, a protein waste product. Urea is the primary method of excretion of nitrogen from the body. Retention of urea in the body is toxic to many systems. In advanced renal failure, all of the effects of retaining wastes in the blood is called **uremia.** In uremia, or uremic poisoning, there is retention of waste products along

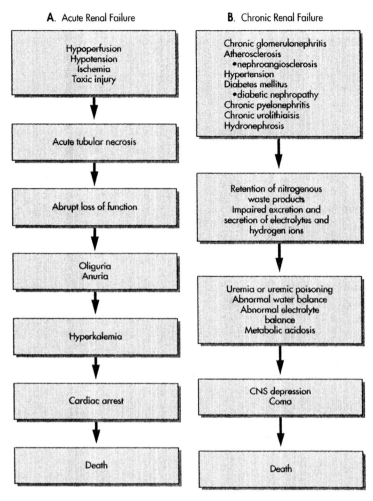

A. Acute Renal Failure

Hypoperfusion
Hypotension
Ischemia
Toxic injury

Acute tubular necrosis

Abrupt loss of function

Oliguria
Anuria

Hyperkalemia

Cardiac arrest

Death

B. Chronic Renal Failure

Chronic glomerulonephritis
Atherosclerosis
•nephroangiosclerosis
Hypertension
Diabetes mellitus
•diabetic nephropathy
Chronic pyelonephritis
Chronic urolithiaisis
Hydronephrosis

Retention of nitrogenous
waste products
Impaired excretion and
secretion of electrolytes and
hydrogen ions

Uremia or uremic poisoning
Abnormal water balance
Abnormal electrolyte
balance
Metabolic acidosis

CNS depression
Coma

Death

Figure 14-9. A comparison of the types of renal failure.

with disturbances in both water balance and electrolyte balance. In Chapter 3 you learned how vital these balances are to homeostasis. In states of significant imbalance of sodium, potassium, chloride, and calcium, all body functions are impaired. This includes muscle and nerve function. In chronic renal failure, metabolic acidosis also develops due to retention of hydrogen ions or acid in the body. As you know, pH imbalance also has significant depressing effects on muscle and nerve function. If the course of these events cannot be altered, coma and death ensue.

14-45

Gradual loss of function of the kidneys over a period of time is described as _____(1). It is more _____(2) than acute failure. There is no obvious change in _____(3) production to herald its onset. Prior to the end of the disease, the only indications are elevated levels of _____(4) and _____(5), which are _____(6)-based waste products. The presence of these elevated levels is medically termed _____(7). The effect of retaining these wastes is _____(8) to many body systems, and this is called _____(9). Imbalance in _____(10) levels significantly upsets homeostasis so that many body functions are _____(11). Because of acid retention, _____(12) also develops. Electrolyte imbalance and acidosis severely interfere with _____(13) and _____(14) function. In acute renal failure, dialysis is used temporarily if there is any hope of restoring function with regenera-

1. chronic renal failure
2. common
3. urine
4. BUN
5. creatinine
6. nitrogen
7. azotemia
8. toxicity
9. uremia
10. electrolyte
11. impaired
12. metabolic acidosis
13. muscle
14. nerve

tion of the nephrons. In chronic renal failure, the nature of the injury does not permit regeneration. Dialysis must be used regularly and permanently. Overall, the prognosis in chronic failure is poor. However, some cases may be candidates for kidney transplant.

IV. REVIEW QUESTIONS

1. c–diabetes mellitus

2. b–diabetic nephropathy

3. a–4; b–1; c–3; d–2

4. d–papillary necrosis

5. a–the formation of stone-like masses in the urinary tract

6. a–minerals; b–increased

7. a–calcium phosphate or oxalate; b–renal pelvis; c–bladder

1. The most common systemic disorder of metabolism that damages the kidneys is:
   a. gout
   b. multiple myeloma
   c. diabetes mellitus
   d. urolithiasis
   e. hypertension

2. In diabetes mellitus, microangiopathy of renal vessels is called:
   a. renal microangiopathy
   b. diabetic nephropathy
   c. glomerulosclerosis
   d. papillary necrosis

3. For the following statements that describe the pathogenesis of diabetic nephropathy, please number them in order of occurrence:
   a. _____ loss of protein into the urine
   b. _____ thickening of arteriole walls with narrowing of lumens
   c. _____ thickening and hardening of glomerular basement membranes
   d. _____ renal ischemia

4. In diabetic nephropathy, obstruction of the ureters by pieces of sloughed tissue occurs with:
   a. glomerulosclerosis
   b. renal ischemia
   c. pyelonephrosis
   d. papillary necrosis
   e. hydronephrosis

5. Urolithiasis is:
   a. the formation of stone-like masses in the urinary tract
   b. a term that means bladder stones
   c. a term that means urinary calculi
   d. the formation of minerals in the urinary tract

6. Urolithiasis occurs as a result of the precipitation of a. _____ from the urine when their levels are b. _____ or when their metabolism is abnormal.

7. The most common type of urinary calculi is a. _____, and the most common locations of urinary calculi are the b. _____ and c. _____.

renal parenchyma	ureters
cystine	calcium phosphate or oxalate
renal pelvis	bladder
struvite	urethra
uric acid	

8. Staghorn calculi are:
   a. multiple bladder stones composed of calcium
   b. a single, large struvite stone that fills the bladder
   c. multiple kidney stones composed of uric acid
   d. a single, large struvite stone that fills the renal pelvis

9. A consequence of hydronephrosis is:
   a. obstruction of ureters caused by papillary necrosis
   b. pressure necrosis of the kidneys caused by blocked urine and swelling
   c. contracture of the kidneys and shrinking caused by fibrosis
   d. acute renal failure

10. Systemic hypoperfusion, atherosclerosis, and hypertension are classified as:
    a. circulatory disorders that impair kidney function
    b. metabolic disorders that impair kidney function
    c. causes of acute renal failure
    d. causes of glomerulonephritis

11. Acute loss of arterial blood pressure can result in:
    a. glomerulosclerosis
    b. glomerulopathy
    c. nephroangiosclerosis
    d. acute tubular necrosis

12. Significant acute ischemia of the renal tubules or of the entire cortex may result in:
    a. thickening of arteriole walls and narrowing of their lumens
    b. nephroangiosclerosis
    c. acute renal failure
    d. papillary necrosis

13. List two causes of acute systemic hypoperfusion that can result in tubular or cortical necrosis: a. _____; b. _____.

14. Hypertension and atherosclerosis cause narrowing of vessel lumens. The sites of renal injury in hypertension are a. _____, while atherosclerosis affects the b. _____.

15. Nephroangiosclerosis describes the injury to the kidneys that is caused by:
    a. atherosclerosis
    b. hypertension
    c. diabetes
    d. systemic hypoperfusion

16. The major causes of acute renal failure are (choose two):
    a. ischemic glomerulosclerosis caused by atherosclerosis
    b. acute tubular necrosis caused by renal ischemia
    c. acute tubular necrosis caused by toxic injury
    d. nephropathy caused by diabetes
    e. papillary necrosis caused by diabetes
    f. acute tubular necrosis caused by hydronephrosis

17. The clinical presentation of acute renal failure is sudden change in urine output, described by the terms a. _____ and b. _____.

8. d—a single, large struvite stone that fills the renal pelvis

9. b—pressure necrosis of the kidneys caused by blocked urine and swelling

10. a—circulatory disorders that impair kidney function

11. d—acute tubular necrosis

12. c—acute renal failure

13. a—heart failure (myocardial infarction, cardiac arrest); b—hypotensive shock

14. a—arteries and arterioles within the kidneys; b—renal artery

15. a—atherosclerosis

16. b—acute tubular necrosis caused by renal ischemia; c—acute tubular necrosis caused by toxic injury

17. a—oliguria; b—anuria

18. a–cardiac arrest; b–hyper-kalemia

19. a–injury of the nephrons over a long period of time

20. d–uremia

18. The most immediate life-threatening event in acute renal failure is a. _____ caused by b. _____.

coma	uremia
hyperkalemia	metabolic acidosis
azotemia	central nervous system depression
electrolyte imbalance	cardiac arrest
water retention	water intoxication

19. The major cause of chronic renal failure is:
    a. injury of the nephrons over a long period of time
    b. cardiac arrest or shock, which causes renal ischemia
    c. acute tubular necrosis over a long period of time
    d. toxic injury
    e. urolithiasis

20. In chronic renal failure, the *toxic effects* of elevated nitrogenous waste products in the blood is called:
    a. azotemia
    b. hyperkalemia
    c. metabolic acidosis
    d. uremia
    e. anuria

SECTION ▶ V. NEOPLASIA

▶ RENAL CARCINOMA

14–46

1. malignant
2. renal cell carcinoma
3. tubules
4. renal capsule
5. metastasis

Cancer of the kidneys is relatively rare and certainly less common than cancer of the bladder. However, cancer of the kidneys is significant because it is more often malignant rather than benign. We will discuss the most common neoplasia of the kidneys, **renal cell carcinoma (RCC),** which comprises about 85 percent of the cases. The etiology of RCC is unknown, and no specific risk factors have been identified. The cells of origin from which this malignant neoplasia arises appear to be the renal tubules. The tumor grows in the cortical parenchyma and is not infiltrative. Instead, it is well defined from the normal tissue. The appearance of a renal cell carcinoma is shown in Figure 14–10. It tends to be encapsulated; however, it does grow through the renal capsule into adjacent organs. Invasion into the renal vein and vena cava provides an avenue for metastasis, which can occur before the tumor is detected. Renal neoplasia, while uncommon, is important because most cases are _____(1) instead of benign. The majority of kidney cancer is _____(2). This neoplasia most likely arises from cells of the _____(3). While well demarcated from the rest of the kidney, RCC will grow through the _____(4) and into surrounding areas. Distant _____(5) can occur before the cancer is found.

14–47

The clinical presentation of RCC is not very specific and frequently involves fever and weight loss. The most common finding is blood in the urine found only during a urinalysis exam, or microscopic hematuria. The tumor often does not manifest its presence for a long while. Many of these tumors are discovered during CT scans for other reasons. Eventually, growth of the tumor produces enlargement of the kidney and a palpable abdominal mass. Some cases present with signs of paraneoplastic syndrome, such as hypercalcemia (see Chapter 6). Surgical removal of the tumorous kidney is the treatment of choice. Tumors found early that are still small have a much better prognosis for cure.

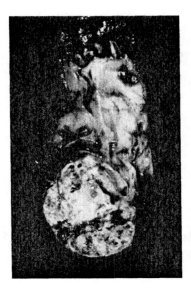

Figure 14–10. Renal cell carcinoma, showing the encapsulated, defined mass still confined to the kidney. *(From Chandrasoma and Taylor, Concise Pathology, 2nd ed., Appleton & Lange.)*

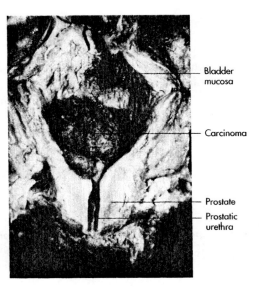

Bladder mucosa

Carcinoma

Prostate

Prostatic urethra

Figure 14–11. Carcinoma of the urinary bladder, showing a large mass which almost fills the lower bladder lumen. *(From Chandrasoma and Taylor, Concise Pathology, 2nd ed., Appleton & Lange.)*

▶ BLADDER CARCINOMA

14–48

Carcinoma of the urinary bladder is the most common neoplasia of the urinary tract. Overall, it is the fifth most common type of cancer and is found more often in men. However, the number of deaths due to renal cancer compared to bladder cancer is about the same. This is because bladder cancer causes signs and symptoms much earlier than renal cancer. The presence of a mass in the bladder causes irritation and obvious hematuria. Cytology of the cells from a urine specimen easily identifies the presence of tumor cells. Also, bladder cancer is less invasive, has less tendency to metastasize, and responds better than RCC to a combination of chemotherapy and surgery. While the exact cause of bladder cancer is unknown, the risk factor of cigarette smoking (chemical carcinogeneis) has been linked to its development. Chronic cystitis may also be a precursor in some cases. The vast majority of bladder cancer arises from transitional cell epithelium. While some tumors may be flat, many are described as papillary growths of the mucosa. This means they appear as warty, finger-like projections that protrude into the lumen of the bladder. Figure 14–11 is an example of bladder cancer as a large tumor in the bladder. Transitional cell carcinoma of the bladder is generally multifocal, that is, appearing in several locations within the bladder. Untreated cases do invade through the bladder wall and eventually metastasize to other sites.

14–49

The most common type of cancer of the urinary system affects the _____(1). The cells of origin are the _____(2). Even though it is significantly more common than renal cell carcinoma, the _____(3) rate is similar to RCC because transitional cell carcinoma of the bladder is found _____(4) than RCC. Early detection is because the _____(5), such as hematuria, are prominent and _____(6) through cytology is easy. There is a risk factor strongly suspected in bladder cancer, and this is _____(7). A common appearance of transitional cell carcinoma of the bladder is that of a mass that _____(8) into the lumen of the bladder. This growth is described as _____(9). As mentioned earlier, the clinical presentation of bladder cancer is that of lower urinary tract signs. This includes dysuria, hematuria, lower abdominal pain, and an increased incidence of infection. Cytology findings of tumor cells in the urine must be confirmed with a biopsy of the bladder mass, or suspi-

1. bladder
2. transitional epithelial cells
3. death
4. earlier
5. signs
6. identification or diagnosis
7. cigarette smoking
8. protrudes or projects
9. papillary

cious mucosa in the case of a flat lesion. Surgical removal of the tumors, chemotherapy, and immune system stimulation can produce good results. However, the final prognosis depends on the stage of detection. In some cases, the bladder must be removed completely. In cases where multiple tumors are resected and the bladder is preserved, the patient must be monitored permanently because recurrence is not uncommon.

V. REVIEW QUESTIONS

1. c–It arises from the glomerular capillary epithelial cells. e–It is locally invasive but does not metastasize.

2. d–It is relatively easily diagnosed. e–It causes early signs.

3. a–transitional cell epithelium; b–papillary projection

1. Regarding renal cell carcinoma, which of the following statements are INCORRECT (choose all that apply):
   a. It is less common than neoplasia of the bladder.
   b. It is a malignant neoplasia.
   c. It arises from the glomerular capillary epithelial cells.
   d. It is well demarcated and encapsulated but may extend outside of the kidney.
   e. It is locally invasive but does not metastasize.

2. Two reasons that bladder cancer does not cause higher death rates are (choose two):
   a. It is a relatively rare neoplasia of the urinary tract.
   b. It never metastasizes.
   c. It is benign.
   d. It is relatively easily diagnosed.
   e. It causes early signs.
   f. There are no identifiable reasons for the relatively low death rate.

3. In carcinoma of the urinary bladder, the most common cell of origin is a. _____, and the appearance is often of a b. _____.

   squamous cell epithelium   transitional cell epithelium
   ulcerated mucosa   dysplastic mucosa
   smooth muscle cells   columnar epithelium
   papillary projection   flat lesion

CHAPTER ► SUMMARY

► SECTION II

Polycystic kidney disease (PDK) is the most significant developmental defect of the urinary system. The condition is genetically transmitted as an autosomal dominant trait and involves an idiopathic obstruction of the tubules of the kidneys. The development of cysts and kidney enlargement, with resulting interference of renal function, are consequences of PDK.

► SECTION III

Glomerulonephritis is injury to the glomerulus caused by immunologic disease. The condition may be caused by antibodies toward the glomeruli (type II hypersensitivity) or antigen–antibody complexes depositing in the basement membrane of the glomerular capillaries (type III hypersensitivity). *Glomerulopathy* may result from specific metabolic disorders such as diabetes mellitus. In this condition, thickening and hardening of the renal basement membrane occurs (glomerulosclerosis), thereby adversely affecting the filtering ability of the glomeruli. Circulatory diseases such as diabetic microangiopathy, atherosclerosis, hypertension, and shock may also lead to glomerular disease. Signs and symptoms of glomerular disease present as a group called a *syndrome*. Examples of such syndromes are *acute renal failure, nephritic syndrome,* and *nephrotic syndrome.*

   Acute glomerulonephritis (poststreptococcal glomerulonephritis) is an inflammatory disease that may occur following upper respiratory bacterial infection, generally by a group A streptococcus strain (the strain which causes strep throat). The pathogenesis of acute glomerulonephritis involves deposition of bacteria–antibody immune complexes in the basement membranes of the kidneys, thereby inducing a type III autoimmune reaction. The resulting inflammation may block blood flow through the glomeruli, ultimately causing hypertension. *Chronic glomerulonephritis,* a condition in which the injury proceeds slowly and is low grade, may develop from repeated episodes of acute glomerulonephritis, from type II hypersensitive reactions, or from degeneration of the glomeruli. As the condition progresses, the kidneys become unable to concentrate the urine as the glomeruli become fibrotic. Other specific types of chronic glomerular diseases are *lipoid nephrosis* (where hyperlipidemia and lipiduria are present but glomerular antibody deposits are absent), *membranous glomerulonephritis* (where antigen–antibody complexes have deposited in glomerular basement membrane), and *crescentic glomerulonephritis* (where antibodies have targeted basement membrane capillaries, leading to severe glomerular injury, anuria, and renal failure). Crescentic glomulerulonephritis is most often associated with the autoimmune disease *Goodpasture's syndrome.*

Pyelonephritis is bacterial infection of the kidneys. The condition, which may be acute or chronic, may occur alone or along with bladder infection. *E. coli,* streptococci, and staphylococci are the most common causative agents. When an ascending infection (from the bladder to the kidneys) reaches only as far as the renal pelvis and not into the parenchyma, the condition is called *pyelitis. Acute pyelonephritis* occurs from pyogenic bacterial infection. The condition may lead to *pyonephrosis* if pus fills the renal pelvis. *Chronic pyelonephritis,* which may result from unresolved cases of the acute condition, leads to destruction of the kidney, with resulting proteinuria, pyuria, bacteria in the urine, and casts (molds of protein precipitated from inflamed tubules).

Infectious inflammation of the bladder is termed *cystitis.* The condition may be acute or chronic, and is generally due to bacterial invasion via the urethra. Cystitis is seen more frequently in women because the urethra is relatively short. Many situations may cause cystitis, including catheterization, frequent sexual intercourse, pregnancy, benign prostatic hyperplasia, and urethral obstruction (most often due to bladder stones). Unresolved bladder obstructions usually lead to chronic cystitis because of the accumulation of stagnant urine in the bladder.

▶ SECTION IV

Diabetes mellitus, which causes the condition of diabetic nephropathy, is the most common systemic metabolic disease that affects the kidneys. In *diabetic nephropathy,* glomerulosclerosis (thickening and hardening of the glomeruli basement membrane) and papillary necrosis (death and sloughing of the papillae, causing obstruction of the ureters) may occur.

Stone formation (urinary calculi) in the urinary tract is termed *utolithiasis.* In this common disorder, minerals precipitate from the glomerular filtrate and urine. The resulting calculi may lodge in the ureters, urethra, pelvis of the kidneys, or bladder. Urinary calculi appear in a variety of shapes, and are classified as calcium (composed of calcium phosphate or calcium oxalate), struvite (composed of magnesium ammonium phosphate or sulfate), uric acid (associated with the disease gout), or cysteine (from abnormal amino acid metabolism).

Some circulatory disorders may cause malfunction of the kidneys. *Systemic hypoperfusion,* leading to acute hypoperfusion of the kidneys, can be caused by myocardial infarction, cardiac arrest, or hypotensive shock. The resultant ischemia can lead to acute tubular necrosis or renal cortical necrosis. Hypertension injures renal arterioles, causing their thickening and a resultant reduced blood flow. *Atherosclerosis* may damage the renal arteries, leading to hardening of the glomeruli (*ischemic glomerulosclerosis* or *nephroangiosclerosis*), causing tubule atrophy and multiple areas of fibrosis.

Sudden loss of renal function is called *acute renal failure.* The condition may result from renal ischemia (due to cardiac arrest or shock) or certain chemical agents. Oliguria (or in the case of complete kidney failure, anuria), and the resultant hyperkalemia and uremia are signs of the disease. *Chronic renal failure* occurs over a relatively long time and may be the result of chronic glomerulonephritis, nephroangiosclerosis, hypertension, urinary tract obstruction, hydronephrosis, or diabetic nephropathy. Azotemia (elevated blood levels of nitrogenous waste products) and uremia (nitrogenous waste products in the blood, electrolyte imbalance, metabolic acidosis) are signs associated with chronic renal failure.

▶ SECTION V

Renal cell carcinoma (RCC) is the most common type of kidney cancer. The etiology of this malignant neoplasia is unknown. The cells of origin appear to be the renal tubules, and the noninfiltrative tumor grows in the cortical parenchyma. *Carcinoma of the urinary bladder* is the most common neoplasia of the urinary tract. The tumor causes irritation and hematuria. Compared to RCC, bladder cancer is less invasive, has less tendency to metastasize, and responds better to chemotherapy and surgery. Cigarette smoking has been linked to the development of bladder cancer.

The Reproductive System

▶ OBJECTIVES

SECTION II

Define all highlighted terms.

Characterize the causative agents and signs and symptoms of vaginitis, pelvic inflammatory disease, and cervicitis.

Cite the complications of pelvic inflammatory disease.

Differentiate between, describe the subtypes, and characterize the signs and symptoms of cervical carcinoma, endometrial carcinoma, leiomyoma, ovarian carcinoma, and teratoma.

Describe the condition endometriosis, and characterize the cause and signs and symptoms of the condition.

Describe the condition endometrial hyperplasia, and characterize the causes and signs and symptoms of the condition.

Describe the conditions of oophoritis and salpingitis, and characterize their causes and signs and symptoms.

Describe the causes and signs and symptoms of ovarian cysts.

Define the disorders of menstruation, and characterize the causes and signs and symptoms of each.

Describe the conditions of toxic shock syndrome and premenstrual syndrome, and characterize the causes and signs and symptoms of each.

Describe the pregnancy-associated disorders ectopic pregnancy, toxemia of pregnancy, spontaneous abortion, and puerperal sepsis. Characterize the causes and signs and symptoms of each.

Describe the neoplastic formations of the placenta.

SECTION III

Define all highlighted terms.

Describe the causes and signs and symptoms of acute mastitis.

Describe the causes and clinical presentation of fibroadenoma and fibrocystic disease.

Characterize the condition of neoplasia of the breast, and describe the causes, clinical presentation, and signs and symptoms of the disease.

SECTION IV

Define all highlighted terms.

Describe the conditions of prostatitis and benign prostatic hyperplasia, and characterize the causes, signs and symptoms, and complications of both.

Describe the condition of adenocarcinoma of the prostate, and characterize the causes and signs and symptoms of the disease.

Describe and characterize the causes and signs and symptoms of the testicular diseases orchitis, cryptorchism, seminoma, teratoma, and testicular torsion.

Describe and characterize the causes and signs and symptoms of the diseases balanitis, epididymitis, gynecomastia, and carcinoma of the male breast.

SECTION ▶ 1. ANATOMY AND PHYSIOLOGY IN REVIEW

15-1

The external reproductive structures, or the **genitalia,** of the female are the **vulva, mons pubis,** and the **clitoris.** The vulva is folds of tissue made up of a thick outside pair (the **labia majora**) and a thin inside pair (the **labia minora**). The mons pubis is the area over the pubic symphysis just above the clitoris. The clitoris is a small mound of erectile tissue that is analogous to the male penis. A secretion of lubricating fluid in preparation for sexual intercourse is produced by **Bartholin's glands.**

15-2

The internal reproductive structures of the female are the **vagina, cervix, uterus,** a pair of **fallopian tubes,** and a pair of **ovaries.** The vagina is a muscular passageway that serves as a receptacle for sperm and as the "birth canal" through which the newborn emerges from the uterus (commonly called the womb). At the proximal end of the vagina is the cervix. This doughnut shaped structure serves as the entry and exit port from the uterus. It is actually part of the neck of the uterus. While a very small opening usually exists in the center of the cervix, this opening greatly enlarges when the cervix dilates in preparation for childbirth. The body of the uterus is a strong muscular organ. It is the site of growth and development of the fetus. The inner lining of the uterus is a mucous membrane called the **endometrium.** This glandular tissue is the site of implantation of a fertilized ova. The **myometrium** is the underlying muscular layer. The smooth muscle stretches considerably and hypertrophies during pregnancy. It contracts forcibly during labor and delivery to expel the newborn child. The female reproductive system is illustrated in Figure 15–1.

15-3

The fallopian tubes are extensions of the uterus, with one on each side of the uterus suspended in the broad ligament. The fallopian tubes are passageways for the **ovum,** or egg, from the ovaries into the body of the uterus. The ends of the fallopian tubes do not directly connect with the ovaries. The finger-like or fanned-out ends of the tubes drape around the ovaries to catch released ova. The ovaries are the female **gonads,** or true sex organs. The sex organs are those that produce the sex hormones. The ovaries produce the principal female sex hormones, **estrogen** and **progesterone.** They also produce the ova, which contain half of

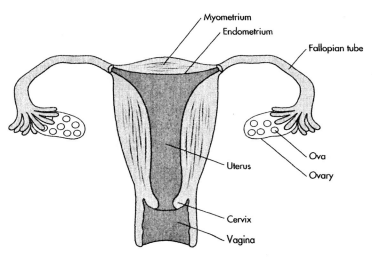

Figure 15–1. The female reproductive system.

the DNA material necessary to create a human being. All of a woman's ova (hundreds of thousands of them) are present in her ovaries when she is born. This is in contrast to sperm in a man, which are continuously generated throughout his life. The ovaries release ova only during the childbearing years. The release of eggs from the ovaries is called **ovulation.** Each ovum is surrounded by specialized cells, and together this arrangement is called a **primary follicle.**

The breasts of a woman, medically termed **mammary glands,** are secondary sex organs and function to produce and release milk to nourish the newborn. The mammary glands are made of milk glands interspersed throughout connective tissue and fat. The amount of fat in the breast has no bearing on the amount of milk that may be produced. Ducts from all of the glands meet at the nipples, through which milk is released. During pregnancy, the hormone progesterone prepares the breasts for giving milk, or **lactation.** After childbirth, the hormone **oxytocin** from the posterior pituitary gland allows the actual release of milk.

The female reproductive cycle is a series of hormonal changes that occur at monthly intervals in order to prepare the uterus for pregnancy. The cycle is called the **menstrual cycle.** The anterior pituitary gland releases gonadotropic hormones called **follicle-stimulating hormone (FSH)** and **luteinzing hormone (LH).** These hormones target the ovaries and cause them to secrete estrogen and progesterone. This second set of hormones targets the uterus and gets it ready for **pregnancy,** which is the implantation and growth of a fertilized ova, or **zygote.** The onset of the menstrual cycle is around 10 to 14 years of age. It ceases in the late forties to early fifties **(menopause).** The rigorous physical demands of pregnancy and childbirth would be very dangerous in those of advanced age, so menopause is a protective mechanism.

A brief overview of the steps of the menstrual cycle are:

1. FSH from the pituitary gland stimulates certain primary follicles in the ovaries to develop. The stimulated follicles grow and become **graafian follicles.**
2. The graafian follicles secrete estrogen into the blood. When this hormone reaches the uterus, the uterus responds with enlargement of the endometrium. The lining becomes thick and filled with blood vessels. This is in preparation to nourish the fetus.
3. About halfway through the cycle, the most mature of the graafian follicles opens and releases an ova. This release, or ovulation, is stimulated by the pituitary hormone LH.
4. After ovulation, at the previous site of the graafian follicle, a cavity or depression is left. This becomes a structure known as the **corpus luteum.** The corpus luteum will secrete progesterone, which further stimulates the endometrium to grow. These steps are illustrated in Figure 15–2.
5. Progesterone will be secreted by the corpus luteum for about another 8 to 10 days. If pregnancy occurs (if a fertilized ova has implanted itself in the endometrium), the corpus luteum will enlarge and secrete even more progesterone. The name of this hormone means "pro-gestation" or "in support of pregnancy." Fertilization of an ova actually takes place in the fallopian tubes. Then, the new zygote travels into the uterus for implantation.
6. The **placenta** is formed from parts of both the endometrium and the growing embryo. This vascular sac of membranes will house the fetus and amniotic fluid and provide nourishment through blood vessels. The placenta takes over secretion of progesterone from the corpus luteum through the remainder of pregnancy. The placenta also secretes the hormone **human chorionic gonadotropin, or HCG,** which is also required to maintain pregnancy. Detection of this hormone in the urine, which spills over from the circulation, forms the basis of pregnancy tests.
7. During pregnancy, the blood supply for the fetus consists of the umbilical artery and vein, which exchange oxygen and nutrients for carbon dioxide and other wastes. The blood supply of the fetus and mother is physically separate. The exchange takes place by diffusion through the vessel walls.

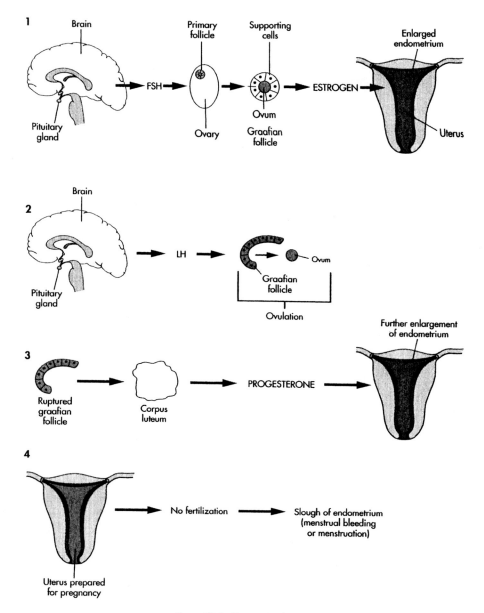

Figure 15-2. The menstrual cycle.

8. If pregnancy does not occur, the corpus luteum stops secreting hormones. The enlarged and vascular endometrium sloughs, producing the bleeding that is called menstruation.

15-8

The external reproductive structures, or genitalia, of the male are the **penis** and **testicles.** The penis is a rod-like organ composed of erectile tissue. The end of the penis is expanded and is called the **glans penis.** This is covered with a foreskin called the **prepuce.** The prepuce in newborn males is usually removed in a procedure called a circumcision. The erectile tissue of the penis contains many blood sinuses that become engorged with blood to produce an **erection.** The urethra of the male differs from the female in that it has different sections. The urethra passes through both the prostate gland and the penis. The male urethra has the double function of passing both urine and **ejaculate.** The ejaculate is seminal fluid containing sperm and is commonly known as semen.

15-9

The male reproductive system is shown is Figure 15–3. The testicles are the gonads of the male. They are housed outside of the abdomen in an outpouching of the peritoneum that is covered with skin. This sac is the **scrotum.** The secretions of the testicles, which include sperm, are released through excretory ducts called the **epididymides** (the first part of the ducts), and the **vas deferens** (the second part of the ducts). These ducts enter the abdominal cavity from the scrotum and connect with the **seminal vesicles** and the **prostate.** These structures are the accessory glands that contribute to the final production of seminal fluid, or semen. The final product is released into that section of the urethra that passes through the prostate. In the testicles are specialized cells called **Leydig cells.** These cells secrete the male sex hormone **testosterone.** Its release is also governed by the pituitary gland. The sperm are created from germ cells in ducts called **seminiferous tubules.** This process is called **spermatogenesis.** It begins at around age 13 and continues for life. Therefore, fertility in the male is possible into an advanced age. Mature sperm are stored in the epididymis and vas deferens until ejaculation. Movement of the semen is accomplished by strong muscle contractions along the ducts. During ejaculation, the sperm is mixed with fluid from both the seminal vesicles and the prostate. The mixture is discharged from the tip of the penis through the urethra. Sperm contain DNA which will fuse with the DNA of the ova during fertilization to produce the 46 chromosomes of a human being.

15-10

The prostate is a gland that encircles the neck of the urinary bladder. Because of its location, disorders of the prostate often present as urinary difficulties. Secretions of the prostate make up most of the composition of seminal fluid. Seminal fluid will contain nutrients for the sperm and prostaglandin. Prostaglandin will stimulate contractions of the uterus to help move sperm along into the fallopian tubes. Seminal fluid also has an alkaline pH to aid motility of the sperm.

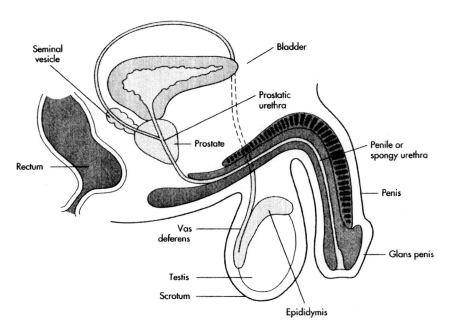

Figure 15–3. The male reproductive system.

SECTION ▶ II. DISEASES OF THE FEMALE REPRODUCTIVE SYSTEM

▶ DISEASES OF THE VULVA AND VAGINA

Vaginitis is infection of the vagina caused by a variety of microorganisms. Whatever the cause, it presents clinically as a malodorous discharge. The characteristics of the discharge vary according to the infectious agent. Additional symptoms common to most cases of vaginitis include burning and itching. Agents of venereal disease cause vaginitis. If you will recall from Chapter 5, a venereal disease is a sexually transmitted disease that primarily affects the genitals. Not all sexually transmitted diseases are venereal in nature. The best example is AIDS (see Chap. 4), which is a systemic disease. The major venereal diseases in this country are gonorrhea and syphilis (bacterial infections), herpes simplex type I (viral infection), and chlamydia (an atypical bacterial infection). These infectious states were presented in Chapter 5, and you are referred back to that chapter for review if necessary. The most common causes of infectious vaginitis are *Trichomonas* and *Candida*. Vaginitis is _____(1) of the _____(2) caused by various _____(3). Vaginitis is often caused by _____(4) disease, which is a _____(5) transmitted disease confined to the _____(6). The agents that most commonly cause vaginitis are _____(7) and _____(8).

Trichomoniasis is a common veneral disease that can be sexually transmitted by the male but generally affects women. This is vaginitis caused by the protozoa ***Trichomonas vaginalis.*** It is a minor superficial infection that is more annoying than it is pathological. It causes a foamy vaginal discharge. The microorganism is easily identified by microscopic examination of the discharge. It is treated with an antimicrobial drug such as metronidazole. The common "yeast infection" is infection by ***Candida albicans,*** which is a normal commensal of the vagina. It occasionally multiplies to infectious numbers under the right conditions. One condition is the wiping out of normal bacterial flora with antibiotics. This yeast infection also causes a superficial vaginitis with discharge. It is diagnosed by identifying the organism on a smear from the discharge. Antifungal medication easily treats this condition. Vaginitis is often caused by the protozoa _____(1), and the disease is called _____(2). It may be _____(3) transmitted by an infected _____(4), but signs are usually confined to _____(5). A yeast-caused vaginitis is produced by the microorganism _____(6). This is a normal _____(7) of the vagina but causes superficial infection if it is permitted to multiply to infectious _____(8).

Bartholin's glands of the vulva may become infected if the ducts are invaded by bacteria. The most common agents of infection are *Neisseria gonorrhoeae, Streptococcus,* and *Staphylococcus.* A complication of this infectious state is obstruction of the ducts with pus. In this case, the pus builds in the glands, causing an abscess of the glands. If this occurs, the abscess must be surgically lanced. Infection of _____(1) glands occurs if the _____(2) are invaded by _____(3). If the ducts are obstructed with _____(4), the glands may develop a (an) _____(5).

A potentially serious complication of untreated genital infection is the development of **pelvic inflammatory disease,** or **PID.** This is infection of the entire reproductive tract and includes the cervix, endometrium, fallopian tubes, and ovaries. This disease is presented under this heading because the vagina is the entryway for this **ascending** infection. PID begins as unresolved vaginitis or venereal disease. Pelvic inflammatory disease is a catch-all phrase for infection of several internal reproductive structures caused by a variety of microorganisms.

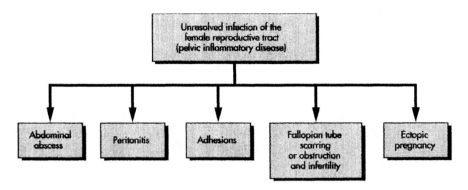

Figure 15–4. Complications of pelvic inflammatory disease.

These include the bacteria *Staphylococcus* and *Streptococcus,* viruses such as herpes simplex, and fungi. Common causes of PID include gonorrhea and chlamydial infection. In addition to venereal disease, other events leading to PID include careless abortion or delivery practices that contaminate the reproductive tract. Clinically, PID presents as lower abdominal pain, fever, nausea, and vaginal discharge. The significance of PID is potential complications in unresolved cases. These complications are abscess formation in the abdomen, peritonitis, adhesion formation, and infertility. Infertility may develop if the fallopian tubes become scarred and therefore obstructed. This will prevent the passage of ova for fertilization. Another complication is predisposition to ectopic pregnancy (see Frame–43) because fertilized ova may get caught in the inflamed tissue of the fallopian tubes. The complications of pelvic inflammatory disease are reviewed in Figure 15–4. Successful treatment of pelvic inflammatory disease requires its early and correct diagnosis. It is responsive to the proper antibiotic or other antimicrobial agent.

15–15

PID stands for _____(1), and this can be a complication of untreated _____(2) infection. PID is infectious inflammation of most structures of the internal _____(3). PID is a (an) _____(4) infection, meaning that the pathogens gain entry by moving up from the _____(5). PID may develop from pre-existing infection or from _____(6) of the reproductive tract during unclean procedures. Pelvic inflammatory disease is important because of its possible _____(7). Complications of PID include the formation of a (an) _____(8), or _____(9); infection of the abdomen, or _____(10); inability to conceive, or _____(11); and _____(12) pregnancy. Infertility is the result of _____(13) of the fallopian tubes. Ectopic pregnancy is also because of inflammation of the _____(14).

1. pelvic inflammatory disease
2. genital
3. reproductive tract
4. ascending
5. vagina
6. contamination
7. complications
8. abscess
9. adhesions
10. peritonitis
11. infertility
12. ectopic
13. scarring or obstruction
14. fallopian tubes

▶ DISEASES OF THE CERVIX AND UTERUS

15–16

Cervicitis is infectious inflammation of the cervix caused by any of the sexually transmitted infections such as gonorrhea, syphilis, herpes, and chlamydia, as well as the common agents of vaginitis (*Trichomonas* and *Candida*). The clinical presentation is also one of a vaginal discharge. Physical lesions on the cervix may be seen with the aid of an instrument called a colposcope.

Cancer of the cervix, or **cervical carcinoma,** accounts for more deaths than cancer of the vulva, vagina, and uterus all together. The death rate from cervical cancer used to be much higher, but the number of deaths has greatly decreased because of early detection by a **Pap smear.** A Pap smear involves scraping the surface of the cervix and examining the scrapings for the presence of atypical or dysplastic cells. An abnormal Pap smear is followed up with a biopsy of the cervix. The population of women who are at greater risk of developing cervical carcinoma include those who have had heavy sexual activity, those infected with venereal diseases, and heavy smokers. Of the infectious-related cases, a high number are infected with either the herpesvirus or the human papillomavirus. Both of these viruses are considered oncogenic, although a direct causative relationship has never been proven. Early detection of cervical _____(1) has greatly reduced the _____(2) rate from this cancer. Detection is accomplished through the use of the _____(3), which looks for the presence of _____(4) cells. Risk factors for cervical carcinoma include excessive _____(5) activity, _____(6) disease [especially _____(7) virus and _____(8)], and heavy _____(9).

Cervical cancer is squamous cell carcinoma and is the result of uncontrolled proliferation of the cervical epithelium. Early changes or transformation of the cells is called dysplasia or atypia. The degree of dysplasia is *graded* as mild, moderate, or severe during the cytological exam of the Pap smear. The progression of cervical carcinoma is from dysplasia, to carcinoma-in-situ, and finally to invasive cancer. Figure 15–5 is representation of the grades of cervical cancer. Fortunately, progression from the earliest stages to the invasive stage is slow, often taking up to 15 years. A local tumor may develop that can project into the vagina, or the form may be ulcerative. Invasion takes place locally, first in the pelvic reproductive structures, and then into surrounding abdominal organs. Metastasis occurs through the bloodstream or lymph channels. Routine Pap smears are the mainstay of prevention of cervical cancer, providing for early recognition and surgical removal of the neoplastic tissue. Cervical cancer is the _____(1) type because the proliferation involves the cervical _____(2). The earliest transformations of the cells are called

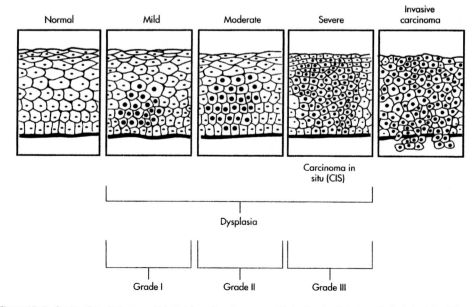

Figure 15–5. Grades of cervical cancer. *(Adapted from Chandrasoma and Taylor,* Concise Pathology, *2nd ed., Appleton & Lange.)*

_____(3) or _____(4). Characterizing the degree of dysplasia is the process of _____(5). The progression of cervical carcinoma through its stages is _____(6).

3. dysplasia
4. atypia
5. grading
6. slow

15-19

Staging of cervical cancer begins once the pre-neoplastic dysplasia has progressed to neoplasia. These stages are:

1. staging
2. 0
3. I
4. II
5. III
6. abdominal organ
7. metastasis
8. kidney failure
9. obstruction

1. Stage 0. The malignancy is of the cervical mucosa only, and is carcinoma in situ.
2. Stage I. The cancer is invasive but is still confined to the cervix.
3. Stage II. The cancer has invaded outside of the cervix but is confined to the upper vagina.
4. Stage III. The cancer has reached the lower vagina and wall of the pelvis.
5. Stage IV. Adjacent abdominal organs have been invaded, and distant metastasis may have occurred.

Clinically, the earlier cases have very nonspecific signs. These are primarily a vaginal discharge and bleeding after sexual intercourse. Late cases produce a significantly bloody discharge. Pain is not a feature of cervical cancer until it has metastasized. Because of this, without routine Pap smears, the cancer can easily go undiagnosed until it may be too late for treatment. The most common cause of death is kidney failure. Local invasion of the urinary tract produces such obstruction that urine backflow causes pressure necrosis and failure of the kidneys. Once cervical carcinoma has progressed into true malignancy, it is characterized by the process of _____(1). Carcinoma in situ is stage _____(2). Invasion of the cervix only is stage _____(3). Movement beyond the cervix characterized stages _____(4) and _____(5). Stage IV reveals _____(6) invasion with possible _____(7). The most common cause of death is _____(8) because of _____(9) of the urinary tract.

15-20

The treatment for early stages through stage II is local removal of the malignancy and radiation therapy. More radical tissue removal, such as hysterectomy, is required for stages later than II, with radiation and chemotherapy as well. The prognosis of cervical carcinoma depends entirely on the grade or stage at which it is identified. Stage 0 is curable, and this is the goal of annual Pap smears. The five-year survival rate for stage I is 85 percent and for stage II is 75 percent. After that, survival rates drop considerably, with stage III being 35 percent and stage IV only 10 percent.

▶ ENDOMETRIOSIS

15-21

Endometriosis is a disorder in which nodules of ectopic endometrial tissue are found outside of the uterus. Ectopic means an abnormal location, or found outside of the normal location. The etiology of endometriosis is unknown for certain, but the most popular belief is that bits of endometrial tissue migrate up and out of the fallopian tubes. This is believed to happen during menstruation when the tissue might be pushed up the tubes instead of passing out through the vagina. Remember that the fallopian tubes are open ended, and so the endometrial tissue may gain access to the abdominal cavity and implant there. Since the ovaries are located immediately next to the fallopian tube openings, these are the most common sites of ectopic endometrium. This endometrium is normal in the respect that it responds to hormones like the uterine endometrium. Therefore, it goes through the same cyclic changes and bleeds during the menstruation phase. Since the blood cannot pass out of the body through the vagina, a hematoma may develop. This large pocket of blood will often become walled off and become a painful blood-filled cyst on the ovary. Pain during menstruation (**dysmenorrhea**) is the most prominent clinical sign of endometriosis. Because the presence of the cyst can induce fibrosis and adhesion formation in the abdomen, endometriosis can cause infertility.

····· 15–22 ·····

1. endometrium
2. uterus
3. abdominal
4. ovaries
5. fallopian tubes
6. fallopian tubes
7. vagina
8. hormones
9. bleeding
10. cyst
11. infertility

Endometriosis is a condition where bits of _____(1) are found outside of the _____(2), in the _____(3) cavity. The most common site for ectopic endometrium is the _____(4) because of their proximity to the openings of the _____(5). The ectopic endometrium may have arrived there by movement up the _____(6) instead of out through the _____(7). These nodules of endometrium respond to _____(8) just like uterine endometrium. Therefore, there is _____(9) during menstruation. This may ultimately lead to the creation of a blood-filled _____(10) on the ovary. Manifestations of endometriosis include painful menstruation and possible _____(11). It is estimated that up to 20 percent of women of childbearing age may have some degree of endometriosis. It can only be diagnosed by seeing the nodules in the abdomen during laparoscopy, in which a tube with a light is inserted into the abdomen through a small incision. The nodules are then biopsied for a definitive diagnosis. The treatment depends on the amount of ectopic endometrium in the abdomen. For smaller amounts, hormonal therapy to suppress menstruation can be quite effective. Larger amounts, or large ovarian cysts, must be surgically removed.

▶ ENDOMETRIAL HYPERPLASIA

····· 15–23 ·····

1. hypertrophy
2. estrogen
3. progesterone
4. ovulation
5. menstruation
6. anovulation
7. proliferate, thicken, or hypertrophy
8. blood supply
9. slough

The first half of the menstrual cycle is the proliferative phase, which is dominated by estrogen from the developing follicles. Under the influence of estrogen, the endometrium becomes thickened, or undergoes hypertrophy, in preparation for pregnancy. Ovulation and the development of the corpus luteum switches hormonal control to progesterone from the corpus luteum. Under the influence of progesterone, the cycle enters the secretory phase, which ends in menstruation. If ovulation doesn't occur, this is called **anovulation.** It results in the continued influence of estrogen, which caues the ongoing proliferation or thickening of the endometrium. This defines **endometrial hyperplasia.** This cannot continue indefinitely. Eventually, the tissue becomes too large for the available blood supply to nourish it. Ischemia and necrosis occur, and the endometrium finally sloughs, with bleeding about 3 weeks after normal menstruation should have occurred. The endometrium undergoes proliferation or _____(1) because of the influence of the hormone _____(2). Normally, this control is replaced by the secretion of _____(3) from the corpus luteum. Progesterone is produced after the release of ova, which is called _____(4). This allows the cycle to progress through the secretory phase and end with _____(5). If ovulation does not occur [which is called _____(6)], estrogen continues to predominate, and the endometrium will continue to _____(7). Because the _____(8) eventually becomes inadequate to feed the tissue, the endometrium will _____(9).

····· 15–24 ·····

There are several reasons for anovulation to occur. These are:

1. The early stages of menopause in which the limited supply of ova has been exhausted. This is the most common reason for anovulation and the development of endometrial hyperplasia.
2. Extreme emotional upset, such as anxiety, which interferes with ovulation.
3. Other psychological-based disorders such as anorexia nervosa.
4. The early stages of menstruation in young girls before hormonal cycles are firmly established.
5. Excessive strenuous exercise such as might be seen in professional athletes.
6. Extreme malnourishment (since the reproductive system is viewed by nature as a "luxury" not necessary for survival, function of this sytem may be sacrificed under adverse conditions).

7. Excessive levels of estrogen. Two reasons for this are overproduction by the ovaries in the case of an ovarian tumor, and the administration of estrogen in the treatment of menopausal symptoms such as hot flashes.

A potential complication of endometrial hyperplasia is the development of uterine cancer. Endometrial hyperplasia may contain some atypical or dysplastic cells having the potential to transform into neoplastic cells. The treatment of endometrial hyperplasia should focus on identifying the cause of anovulation and resolving it. Removal of the hyperplastic tissue may be accomplished with a D&C, the dilation of the cervix and the curettage or scraping of the uterine lining. Severe cases with dysplasia often require removal of the uterus (hysterectomy).

15–25

The most common reason for the development of endometrial hyperplasia is the initial onset of _____(1). This is because _____(2) ceases if the limited supply of ova is exhausted. Exteme _____(3) states or other psychological disorders may prevent _____(4). Demands on the body such as excessive _____(5) or mal_____(6) may interfere with ova release. The presence of too much of the proliferative hormone _____(7) may cause hyperplasia. The cause for concern in this disease is the possibility of the development of _____(8) if the hyperplasia transforms into neoplasia.

1. menopause
2. ovulation
3. emotional
4. ovulation
5. exercise
6. nourishment
7. estrogen
8. uterine cancer

▶ ENDOMETRIAL CARCINOMA

15–26

Malignant neoplasia of the endometrium is the adenocarcinoma type. It arises from the epithelium of the endometrial glands in contrast to the squamous epithelial origin of cervical carcinoma. This is the most common kind of reproductive tract (not breast) cancer. It is now more common than cervical cancer because of the Pap smear. Endometrial adenocarcinoma most often strikes postmenopausal women. This is one neoplasia where hormones are thought to be part of the etiology, along with viral or chemical carcinogens. Remember that one role of estrogen is to cause proliferation of the endometrium. The incidence of high or prolonged estrogen levels and endometrial adenocarcinoma are closely associated. (Estrogen is also implicated in ovarian and breast cancer.) Risk factors for endometrial adenocarcinoma include estrogen therapy, estrogen-secreting ovarian tumors, early onset of menstruation and late onset of menopause (prolonged estrogen exposure), and lack of childbearing. In actual practice, the benefits of estrogen therapy outweigh the risk of cancer, and patients are closely monitored for its development. Malignant neoplasia arising from the endometrium is the _____(1) type because it involves the _____(2) of the endometrium. The population most often affected is _____(3) women. It is believed that a strong factor in the etiology of this cancer is _____(4), in either _____(5) amounts or for a _____(6) time.

1. adenocarcinoma
2. glands
3. postmenopausal
4. estrogen
5. excessive
6. prolonged

15–27

Endometrial cancer is also staged like cervical cancer. Stage I involves only the endometrium and so has the best cure rate. Stage II affects the myometrium (underlying muscle) and cervix. Stage III extends through the wall of the uterus but is still inside the pelvic canal. Stage IV reaches outside of the pelvis and infiltrates the gastrointestinal or urinary tract. The malignant tissue in the uterus is friable, or fragile. Therefore, it bleeds easily. This is the reason for early detection. This very visible abnormality helps in achieving the diagnosis before the cancer can metastasize. In premenopausal women, there may be small amounts of blood (spotting) in between menstrual periods or very heavy menstruation at the normal time. In postmenopausal women, any type of bleeding is highly abnormal. Abnormal vaginal bleeding in any population of women should always be investigated by a gynecologist, and an endometrial biopsy may be indicated. Endometrial cancer may also be found on a Pap smear if the malignant cells have shed from the tumor. Stage I endometrial adenocarcinoma is confined to the _____(1) only. Stage II has moved into the _____(2) and _____(3). Malignancy of the full thickness of the wall is stage _____(4). Stage IV usually invades the _____(5) or _____(6) system. Endometrial adenocarcinoma is generally found early because of the prominent sign of abnormal _____(7).

The treatment for endometrial malignancy is surgical removal of the uterus, or hysterectomy. Regional lymph nodes may also be removed if spread is suspected. Later stages require radiation as well as surgery. Chemotherapy is the approach of choice in the inoperable stage. Naturally, the prognosis depends entirely on the stage in which the cancer is found. Stage I has an excellent outcome, with an 80 to 90 percent five-year survival rate. Stage II is at about 50 percent after five years, stage III only 20 percent, and stage IV down to about 5 percent. Premenopausal or younger women tend to fare better.

▶ LEIOMYOMA

A **leiomyoma** is a benign, estrogen-dependent tumor of the uterine smooth muscle or myometrium. It has never shown a tendency to transform into a malignancy. Leiomyomas also have a fibrous tissue component, in addition to muscle. The growth of a leiomyoma is stimulated and supported by estrogen. In postmenopausal women, it shrinks or atrophies into a fibroid mass, sometimes called a fibroid tumor. Leiomyomas are fairly common, and are more so than endometrial tumors. Small leiomyomas, which are the general rule, cause no signs or symptoms. Very large muscle tumors become significant as space-occupying lesions. They cause bleeding, pressure (which causes pain and difficulty with the GI or urinary tracts), and infertility. Figure 15–6 is a photograph of several of these muscular tumors. A leiomyoma itself may be surgically removed, or a hysterectomy may be indicated. A leiomyoma is a _____(1) tumor arising from the _____(2) or _____(3) of the uterus. Its production is the result of the influence of _____(4). The only clinical significance of a leiomyoma is if it should become very _____(5) and therefore cause problems as a _____(6). The diseases of the body of the uterus are summarized in Table 15–1.

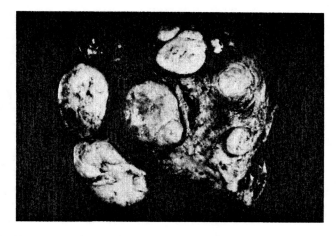

Figure 15–6. Uterine leiomyomas, showing multiple smooth muscle tumors of varying size. *(From Chandrasoma and Taylor, Concise Pathology, 2nd ed., Appleton & Lange.)*

TABLE 15–1. DISEASES OF THE UTERINE BODY

Disease	Features
Endometriosis	Nodes of endometrial tissue implanted in abdominal cavity, especially on the ovaries
	Development of hematoma
	Dysmenorrhea
	Possible infertility
Endometrial hyperplasia	Anovulation, causing continued thickening of endometrium
	Sloughing with bleeding after period of normal menstruation
	Potential for neoplastic change
Endometrial carcinoma	Cancer of the glandular cells
	May be associated with high or prolonged estrogen levels
	Abnormal bleeding
Leiomyoma	Benign tumor of uterine smooth muscle (myometrium)
	Estrogen dependent

▶ DISEASES OF THE FALLOPIAN TUBES AND OVARIES

15–30

If you will recall, pelvic inflammatory disease, or PID, is infectious inflammation of several structures in the female reproductive tract. This includes the fallopian tubes and ovaries. Inflammation of the ovaries is called **oophoritis.** Inflammation of the fallopian tubes is called **salpingitis.** The word salpinx means tube. Salpingitis is generally due to a sexually transmitted infection, or to staphylococcal or streptococcal infection. The staph and strep organisms, being pyogenic, cause purulent infection. This refers to the presence of pus. The course of infection in salpingitis is that the tubes become swollen and filled with exudate. This is a bilateral infection, meaning both tubes are affected. Acute salpingitis is where the ends of the tubes remain open, as they normally are, and the infection may spill into the abdominal cavity, leading to peritonitis. In chronic salpingitis, the ends become sealed shut because of the sticky exudate. The tubes become sacs of pus, and this is called **pyosalpinx.** There are several complications to untreated or unresolved salpingitis. An abscess may form between the ends of the tubes and the ovaries. Closure of the ends or stricture or adhesion formation within the tubes will cause infertility if ova cannot pass. The likelihood of ova getting caught in the swollen folds is increased, so ectopic pregnancy is a possibility. Salpingitis can be resolved with proper antibiotic administration.

15–31

Oophoritis is inflammation of the _____(1). Salpingitis is inflammation of the _____(2). This inflammation is usually caused by _____(3) with microorganisms. Pyogenic bacteria cause infection with _____(4) as a feature. Peritonitis can result if the _____(5) of the tubes are _____(6) and pus spills into the _____(7). If the ends become closed, the tubes are filled with pus, and this is called _____(8). Infertility and ectopic pregnancy are _____(9) of unresolved salpingitis.

1. ovaries
2. fallopian tubes
3. infection
4. pus
5. ends
6. open
7. abdominal cavity
8. pyosalpinx
9. complications

15–32

Ovarian cysts are a common condition. If you will remember, primary follicles enlarge during the proliferative stage of the menstrual cycle, and they become graafian follicles. Several graafian follicles develop, but only one ruptures and releases an ova (ovulation). The other graafian follicles usually degenerate. Sometimes, an unruptured follicle remains enlarged and fills with fluid (becomes cystic). Or a corpus luteum may fill with fluid and become a cyst. Single cysts are usually not a problem. However, if many cysts are present, this represents a disease state described as **polycystic.** Polycystic ovaries can develop if there are defects in hormonal communication between the hypothalamus and the pituitary gland. This results in inadequate release of FSH and LH, leading to abnormal development of the folli-

1. cyst
2. fluid
3. polycystic
4. estrogen
5. endometrium
6. anovulation
7. infertility

cles. Estrogen remains the dominant hormone. (Remember that progesterone is not secreted until the ruptured graafian follicle transforms into the corpus luteum.) Excessive secretion of estrogen stimulates endometrial hyperplasia, which ultimately leads to sloughing and bleeding. In polycystic ovary syndrome, the continued presence of estrogen-secreting follicles can cause hormonal imbalance. Anovulation results and causes infertility. The primary treatment is hormone medication to induce ovulation and reduce endometrial hyperplasia. An unruptured graafian follicle that does not degenerate becomes a _____(1). This is because it fills with _____(2). If many cysts are present on the ovaries, this is called _____(3) ovary syndrome. Because of their presence, the hormone _____(4) is secreted to excess. This causes hyperplasia of the _____(5) and lack of ova release, or _____(6). The end result of untreated polycystic ovary syndrome is _____(7).

15–33

Cancer of the ovaries is called **ovarian carcinoma.** There are a large variety of tumors that can arise in the ovaries. These are both benign and malignant, with benign tumors being more common. Each kind of tumor arises from one of the several types of cells found in the ovaries. Three major categories of ovarian carcinoma are recognized. The most common, comprising 70 percent of the tumors, is of the surface epithelium. The next category, making up about 20 percent, is tumors of the germ cells. The last one, at about 10 percent, is tumors of the stromal cells.

15–34

Neoplasia that develops from the epithelium of the surface of the ovaries is further subdivided into three types. The first is a **cystadenoma.** You should recognize that by the designation "adenoma," this is a benign cystic tumor. A **cystadenocarcinoma** is a complicated type of tumor. It may be benign, of low malignancy, or of high malignancy. This neoplasia is divided into two types. One is a **serous cystadenocarcinoma,** so named because the tumor secretes a clear, or serous, fluid. An example of a cystic serous tumor of the ovary is shown in Figure 15–7. The other type is a **mucinous cystadenocarcinoma,** so named because it secretes a mucous kind of fluid. The third type of epithelial-based ovarian tumor is an **endometroid adenocarcinoma.** This is not a cystic tumor, and it does not secrete any fluid. (Do not confuse this name with the endometrium of the uterus.) Endometroid adenocarcinomas are all highly malignant.

15–35

1. epithelium
2. cystadenoma
3. cystadenocarcinoma
4. serous cystadeno-carcinoma
5. mucinous cystadeno-carcinoma

To reinforce your understanding of the manifestations of ovarian neoplasia, provide the names of the tumors as they are shown here in their classifications:

1. Tumors of the _____(1) of the surface of the ovaries, which are:
   A. the benign _____(2);
   B. the variable malignancy _____(3), which can be a _____(4) or a _____(5);

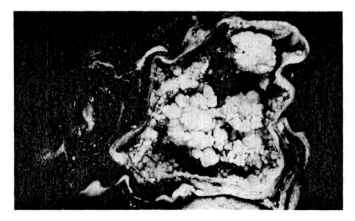

Figure 15–7. Cystic serous tumor of the ovary. *(From Chandrasoma and Taylor,* Concise Pathology, *2nd ed., Appleton & Lange.)*

C. the truly malignant _____(6).
2. Tumors of the _____(7) cells.
3. Tumors of the _____(8) cells.

6. endometroid adenocarcinoma
7. germ
8. stromal

15-36

A tumor of the germ cells is usually benign. It is called a **teratoma,** or a **dermoid cyst.** Germ cells contain the DNA and are the cells that become the embryo and then the fetus. A teratoma or dermoid cyst is a bizarre growth that is made of many body tissues, because the DNA codes for all body tissue. The material found in a teratoma includes brain, skin with oil glands, and hair (hence the name dermoid), cartilage, bone, and teeth. This is shown in Figure 15–8. A teratoma originates from stimulated oocytes which try to produce cells of the embryo. This development has to stop at a point because the other half of the DNA, provided by the sperm, is missing. A teratoma needs to be correctly diagnosed (by laparoscopy and biopsy) so that it may be surgically removed. This is to prevent malignant transformation of the mass. A teratoma, or _____(1), is a tumor of the _____(2) cells. Tumors of the germ cells produce different kinds of body tissue because they contain genetic material, or _____(3). The name dermoid cyst comes from the fact that one of the many types of tissue includes skin with _____(4). A teratoma arises when _____(5) are stimulated, but development ceases because the other half of the _____(6) from _____(7) is not present to cause formation of a true fetus.

1. dermoid cyst
2. germ
3. DNA
4. hair
5. oocytes
6. DNA
7. sperm

15-37

A tumor derived from stromal cells is also usually benign. The stromal cells are granulosa and theca cells of the primary follicles that house the ova. The normal function of these follicular cells is to secrete hormones. A stromal tumor often secretes excessive amounts of estrogen, which causes menstrual cycle abnormalities. It may also secrete androgens (male hormones), which cause virilization, or the development of some male physical characteristics. Tumors of the stromal cells are tumors of the _____(1) or _____(2) cells of the primary _____(3). These tumors often secrete either female or male _____(4).

1. granulosa
2. theca
3. follicle
4. hormones

15-38

Of the tumors just presented, the most significant ones are the adenocarcinomas. Clinically, an adenocarcinoma tends to be without symptoms for a long time. It is often not suspected until the disease is advanced. The prognosis depends on the behavior of the tumor and the point at which it is diagnosed. A benign tumor has an excellent prognosis and is curable. A tumor of low malignancy can generally be treated in time to yield a good prognosis. A high-malignancy tumor has a poor prognosis. More women die from highly malignant ovarian cancer than from cervical and endometrial cancer combined. This is largely due to late detection compared to cervical and endometrial cancer.

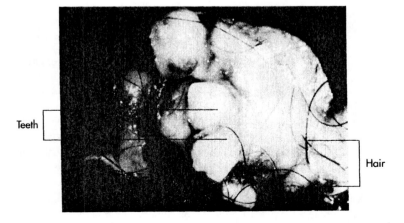

Figure 15–8. Section of a teratoma or dermoid cyst. Note the hair and teeth growing within this benign cystic tumor of the ovary. *(From Chandrasoma and Taylor,* Concise Pathology, *2nd ed., Appleton & Lange.)*

► DISORDERS OF MENSTRUATION

Amenorrhea is a lack of menstrual bleeding. Please recall that the prefix "a" means without. Amenorrhea is normal during pregnancy, lactation, and after menopause. Abnormal amenorrhea may be primary in nature or secondary. Primary amenorrhea is lack of onset of menstruation at sexual maturity. It is most often caused by improper development of the ovaries, which cannot respond to hormonal signals, or by lack of hypothalamic or pituitary hormones. Secondary amenorrhea is when menstruation stops later in life. It is defined as absence of menstruation for 12 months or longer. Secondary amenorrhea can be organic in nature (some physical cause) or it may be psychosomatic in nature. Physical causes include hormone imbalances, thyroid disease, pituitary failure, and disease of the ovaries or endometrium. Adverse conditions affecting the body such as severe systemic disease or starvation will also interfere with the reproductive cycle. Psychosomatic causes of secondary amenorrhea include extreme stress, anxiety, or depression. The absence of menstruation is called _____(1). It may be _____(2) or _____(3) in nature. Primary amenorrhea is a failure of _____(4) to begin in the young female. Secondary amenorrhea is caused later in life because of _____(5) or _____(6) causes.

Menorrhagia is blood loss during menstruation that exceeds normal. This is because of either very heavy bleeding or prolonged bleeding. Causes of excessive menstruation include endometrial carcinoma, PID, hormonal imbalance, and anovulation, which leads to endometrial hyperplasia. **Metrorrhagia** is irregular cycles or abnormal timing of menstruation. Hormonal imbalance causes the endometrium to become thickened at odd times, with later sloughing and bleeding. **Dysmenorrhea** is painful menstruation. It is most often associated with endometriosis and bleeding into the peritoneal cavity. Excessive blood loss defines _____(1). Metrorrhagia is menstruation at _____(2) times during the cycle. Painful menstruation is called _____(3).

Toxic shock syndrome (TSS) is a toxemia, or an infectious state, caused by the toxins of *Staphylococcus aureus* which enter the general circulation. Although this disease can develop in other populations, it is most often associated with the use of tampons during menstruation. It develops because of contamination of the tampons by *S. aureus* from the environment. If the tampon is left in place too long, the organism multiplies and produces a toxin. This toxin can be absorbed through the bleeding uterine wall. Older tampons of the super-absorptive variety contained synthetic fibers that supported the growth of the bacteria and toxin production. These tampons are no longer manufactured with this material. Clinically, TSS presents as a systemic illness typically associated with toxemia. Signs and symptoms include fever, nausea, and vomiting. Hypotension develops and, if it becomes severe, leads to septic shock. Treatment is aimed at controlling the shock, and antibiotics are a must. Toxic shock syndrome is a (an) _____(1) in which the bacteria _____(2) produce a _____(3) which can enter the _____(4). The bacteria are contained in a contaminated _____(5). A severe case of hypotension because of toxemia can lead to _____(6).

Premenstrual syndrome, or **PMS,** is a disorder that has only recently been validated by the medical community as having a physical basis. Previously, it was believed to be strictly psychosomatic. PMS consists of a variety of physical and emotional symptoms that begin before menstruation (at about mid-cycle) and are relieved when menstruation begins. PMS cannot be diagnosed with any tests or physical findings. It is now believed that ovarian hormones may upset the balance of neurotransmitters (chemical signals), which in turn has an adverse effect on the body. These effects are both physical and behavioral in nature. It is not known why the imbalance exists in only some women. The emotional components of PMS include hostility, irritability, anxiety, and depression. The physical maladies include

TABLE 15–2. DISORDERS OF MENSTRUATION

Disorder	Features
Amenorrhea	Absence of menstrual bleeding, primary or secondary in cause
Menorrhagia	Excessive blood loss during menstruation due to heavy or prolonged bleeding
Metrorrhagia	Irregular menstrual cycles
Dysmenorrhea	Painful menstruation usually due to endometriosis
Toxic shock syndrome	*Staphylococcus aureus* toxemia associated with contaminated tampons
Premenstrual syndrome	Hormone-induced imbalance of neurotransmitters causing physical and emotional symptoms

headache, soreness of the breasts, and abdominal bloating. There is no specific treatment for PMS. It can be alleviated with changes in the diet to exclude substances known to aggravate the condition. Salt, sugar, caffeine, and alcohol should be avoided during the second half of the menstrual cycle. Aerobic exercise, which reduces stress, and stress management techniques are also helpful. PMS stands for _____(1). The ailments of PMS are associated with the _____(2) half of the menstrual cycle. It may be due to interference with _____(3) by hormones from the ovaries. The components of PMS are both _____(4) and _____(5) in nature. You may review the disorders of menstruation by examining Table 15–2.

1. premenstrual syndrome
2. second
3. neurotransmitters
4. physical
5. behavioral or emotional

▶ DISORDERS ASSOCIATED WITH PREGNANCY

15–43

There are many disorders that can develop during pregnancy, and especially during labor or delivery. Only a few abnormalities of pregnancy will be considered here. They will be reviewed for you in Table 15–3 following Frame 15–50. An **ectopic pregnancy** is commonly known as a "tubal pregnancy." Ectopic refers to a location outside of normal, in this case, the uterus. Most ectopic pregnancies (about 95 percent) are located in the fallopian tubes. Other less common placements are in the abdominal cavity, if a fertilized ova is lost from the end of the fallopian tube, or on the ovary itself. In a tubal pregnancy, the fertilized ova implants in the fallopian tube before reaching the endometrium. This is much more likely to occur in diseased fallopian tubes. In salpingitis, the swollen, inflamed tissue is more likely to trap the ova. The passage of the ova can also be obstructed by stricture or adhesions after pelvic inflammatory disease. Endometriosis, the presence of uterine tissue on the ovary, is a reason for ectopic pregnancy of the ovary. A tubal pregnancy is medically called a (an) _____(1). This is the implantation of a _____(2) within the fallopian tubes instead of the _____(3). Other, much less common, locations for an ectopic pregnancy include the _____(4) or a (an) _____(5). A tubal ectopic pregnancy is more likely to develop if the fallopian tubes are _____(6). Two common tubal diseases are _____(7) and _____(8).

1. ectopic pregnancy
2. fertilized ova
3. uterus
4. abdomen
5. ovary
6. diseased
7. salpingitis
8. PID

15–44

As the implanted embryo develops in a fallopian tube, it reaches a point where it will rupture the tube. The associated blood vessels also burst, causing significant and possibly fatal hemorrhage into the abdomen. This generally will happen by 2 months into the development of the embryo. A good example of rupture of an ectopic tubal pregnancy is shown in Figure 15–9. Clinically, a ruptured ectopic pregnancy causes severe abdominal pain and is another reason for the presentation of an acute abdomen. Vaginal bleeding will accompany bleeding into the abdomen. Soon, systemic effects of hemorrhage will be seen as hypotension and shock develop. This condition is definitively diagnosed during laparoscopy when the rupture and hemorrhage are viewed directly. Emergency surgery is necessary to stop hemorrhage and to remove the ruptured tube and the remainder of the placental tissue. In ectopic tubal pregnancy, serious hemorrhage is due to the _____(1) of both the

1. rupture

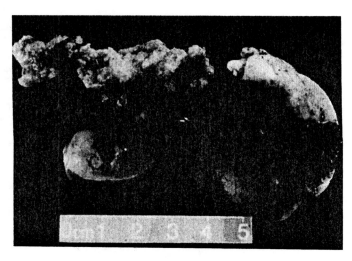

Figure 15–9. Ruptured tubal ectopic pregnancy. The developing embryo is shown on the left, and the ruptured fallopian tube is on the right. *(From Kent and Hart,* Introduction to Human Disease, *3rd ed., Appleton & Lange.)*

2. fallopian tube
3. vessels

······ 15–45 ··

1. proteinuria

_____(2) and associated blood _____(3) of the developing embryo.

In the condition **toxemia of pregnancy,** the name is misleading since this is not an infectious condition with bacterial toxins in the blood. Although the exact cause of toxemia of pregnancy is not known, it appears to be a low-grade or smoldering disseminated intravascular coagulation (DIC). One theory of cause is that the placenta may release the clotting factor thromboplastin or tissue factor. Multiple, small thrombi develop, and thrombosis especially occurs in the vessels of the kidneys, in the glomeruli. In cases of significant thrombosis, kidney failure is possible. Protein is lost into the urine by the injured kidneys. Most of the lost protein is albumin. The presence of protein in the urine is called _____(1) (see Chap. 14). Because albumin is responsible for oncotic pressure and retention of fluid in vessels, hypoalbuminemia leads to edema. Edema is another clinical feature of toxemia of pregnancy. Edema creates some degree of hypotension as fluid is lost from the vessels. In order to maintain blood pressure, the renin–angiotensin mechanism is activated. This increases the pressure too much and hypertension is created. This is often called "pregnancy-induced hypertension." A serious consequence of toxemia of pregnancy is the development of eclampsia. This is seizure activity that is life-threatening. The seizures or convulsions may lead to coma, which is followed by death.

······ 15–46 ··

1. infection
2. toxin
3. DIC
4. thromboplastin
5. glomeruli of the kidney
6. protein
7. edema
8. renin–angiotensin
9. hypertension
10. eclampsia

Toxemia of pregnancy is *not* a bacterial _____(1) with the production of _____(2) in the bloodstream. It seems to be a form of _____(3) that is activated by the release of _____(4) from the placenta. The thrombi formed during this DIC most often target the _____(5). A clinical finding of this kidney damage is the presence of _____(6) in the urine. Loss of albumin causes another clinical sign, which is _____(7). In order to combat potential hypotension because of albumin loss, the renal mechanism of _____(8) is stimulated to raise blood pressure. This often leads to pregnancy-induced _____(9). A cause of death can be excessive seizure activity and coma, which is described as _____(10). Toxemia of pregnancy generally develops during the last trimester, and women in later pregnancy are specifically monitored for this condition during frequent medical office visits. Effective means for detecting toxemia of pregnancy are checking blood pressure and testing the urine for protein. The incidence of this disorder is greater in first pregnancies and when there is more than one fetus. Women with pre-existing hypertension or kidney disease are predisposed to toxemia of pregnancy. Clinically, hypertension causes enduring headaches. The finding of the "toxemia triad" (edema, hypertension, proteinuria) is the basis for diagnosis of this disorder. The preeclampsia state, before seizure development, can be diagnosed early enough to effectively manage the condition. Management is aimed at reducing blood pressure by limiting salt intake and using diuretics, within safe boundaries for the fetus. Eclampsia requires emergency treatment with anticonvulsant drugs and the termination of the pregnancy.

15-47

A **spontaneous abortion** is commonly known as a miscarriage. This is the expulsion of the embryonic material without any outside inducement. A spontaneous abortion represents rejection by the uterus of a defective embryo. This defect is a genetic abnormality. This recognition of abnormality and expulsion takes place early in the pregnancy. It is nature's way of voiding genetic mistakes. The growth of the embryo is terminated because the chromosomes are abnormal; therefore, normal development cannot take place. Spontaneous abortion is common, affecting up to 20 percent of pregnancies. It is an isolated event, meaning that the genetic defect is confined to that ova or sperm. It is not likely to affect future pregnancies. Other less common causes of spontaneous abortion include hormonal imbalance, extreme psychological upset, infection, and inadequate circulation. The clinical presentation of a miscarriage is abdominal pain, vaginal bleeding, and the passing of placental tissue. Sometimes a D&C is necessary to remove all of the remaining products of pregnancy, to manage hemorrhage, and prevent infection (puerperal sepsis). A miscarriage is medically known as a _____(1). This is _____(2) of the early tissue of pregnancy by the uterus. The most common reason for a spontaneous abortion is that the embryo is _____(3) because of genetic abnormality of the _____(4). Genetic mistakes are confined to that individual embryo and are not likely to affect _____(5) pregnancies.

1. spontaneous abortion
2. expulsion
3. defective
4. chromosomes
5. future

15-48

Puerperal sepsis is bacterial infection of the uterus, particularly the endometrium, following childbirth or abortion. Historically, it was known as "childbed fever" and was a major cause of death because of aseptic, or dirty, conditions or techniques. Puerperal sepsis after abortion may be known as septic abortion. The tissue of the birth canal, after the trauma of delivery or abortion, is very susceptible to infection, and the bleeding vessels are a portal of entry for bacteria into the circulation. The bacteria most responsible for puerperal sepsis are *Staphylococcus* and *Streptococcus* from the environment, and *E. coli* from fecal contamination. A major complication of this uterine infection is septicemia as bacteria enter the bloodstream. A clump of bacteria in the blood (septic emboli) can cause infectious thrombophlebitis. Severe cases of septicemia can lead to septic shock and death. The clinical presentation of puerperal sepsis is fever, chills, vaginal bleeding, pain, and a malodorous, infectious discharge. The mainstay of treatment is antibiotics. Infected tissue of the uterus that has become necrotic needs to be surgically removed. Puerperal sepsis is bacterial _____(1) of the _____(2). It may develop after _____(3) or _____(4) if conditions or techniques are _____(5) or contaminated. Bacteria enter the circulation through the bleeding _____(6) of the birth canal. This leads to the dangerous complication of _____(7) and possible _____(8) in severe cases.

1. infection
2. uterus
3. childbirth
4. abortion
5. dirty
6. vessels
7. septicemia
8. fatal septic shock

15-49

The last two topics of this section deal with neoplastic formations of the placenta. They fall under the heading of "gestational trophoblastic neoplasia," which means tumors of the placenta during pregnancy. The trophoblast is the epithelial lining of the placental villi. The tumors often originate from the DNA of the sperm after abnormal fertilization. The first tumor is the **hydatidiform mole.** It is a benign condition itself but may transform into a malignancy later. This is a cystic (fluid-filled) mass of placental villi that resembles a bunch of grapes. It may be invasive or noninvasive. It may develop during an abnormal pregnancy or soon afterwards. It causes enlargement of the uterus like a normal pregnancy, but there is no fetal movement. It is diagnosed by ultrasound examination. Hydatidiform moles are usually aborted by mid-pregnancy. All tissue should be removed during a D&C to prevent progression to malignancy (choriocarcinoma). Tumors of the placenta are classified as _____(1). A benign cystic mass is called a _____(2). A hydatidiform mole causes enlargement of the _____(3), but there is no evidence of _____(4) movement. Hydatidiform moles usually end with _____(5) of the material. Any remaining tissue must be evacuated to prevent the development of _____(6).

A **choriocarcinoma** is a rare, malignant neoplasia of the placenta that will metastasize. It arises from the embryonic portion of the placenta, which is the chorion. Fifty percent of choriocarcinomas develop after a hydatidiform mole. The remainder develop in a normal placenta after delivery or in retained placental cells following an abortion. The metastasis is rapid and generally spreads to the lungs or liver. Some cases metastasize to the brain. However, the prognosis is good because the primary tumor and the metastases are very responsive to chemotherapy. The only time this is not true is in metastasis to the brain. Malignant neoplasia of the placenta is called a _____(1). The majority of cases follow the presence of a _____(2). This cancer will spread or _____(3) rapidly. Response to treatment is good except in cases of metastasis to the _____(4).

TABLE 15–3. DISORDERS OF PREGNANCY

Disorder	Features
Ectopic pregnancy	Development of an embryo outside of the uterus, most commonly in the fallopian tubes (tubal pregnancy) Tubal pregnancy predisposed by disease of the fallopian tubes Rupture of fallopian tube
Toxemia of pregnancy	Possibly a low-grade disseminated intravascular coagulation Appearance of "toxemia triad" (proteinuria, edema, hypertension) Eclampsia possible
Spontaneous abortion	Rejection of developing embryo due to genetic defect
Puerperal sepsis	Bacterial infection of uterus associated with contaminated childbirth or abortion
Gestational trophoblastic neoplasia (placental tumors)	Hydatidiform mole–benign cyst with possible neoplastic transformation Choriocarcinoma—malignant with metastasis, may develop from a hydatidiform mole

II. REVIEW QUESTIONS

1. Microorganisms associated with venereal disease that produce vaginal discharge with burning or itching best describes:
   a. cervicitis
   b. vaginitis
   c. endometriosis
   d. Bartholin's gland inflammation

2. *Trichomonas* and *Candida albicans* yeast infection are the most common causes of:
   a. vaginitis
   b. pelvic inflammatory disease
   c. cervicitis
   d. Bartholin's gland abscess

3. Choose the INCORRECT statement about pelvic inflammatory disease:
   a. It may be an ascending infection that originates as vaginitis.
   b. It may be a consequence of untreated venereal disease.
   c. It may follow contamination during delivery or abortion.
   d. It is infection of the ovaries only, which is called oophoritis.
   e. The most common complications of PID are infertility and ectopic pregnancy.

4. The Pap smear is performed primarily to detect:
   a. cervicitis
   b. pelvic inflammatory disease
   c. endometrial carcinoma
   d. endometrial hyperplasia
   e. cervical carcinoma

5. Choose the correct statement about cervical carcinoma:
   a. It is a progression through degrees of dysplasia, to carcinoma in situ, and finally to stages of invasion.
   b. The death rate is high because this cancer is difficult to detect early.
   c. Cervical carcinoma is an adenocarcinoma, affecting the glands of the cervix.
   d. The progression through the stages is rapid, which also accounts for the high death rate.

6. The best prognosis for cervical carcinoma occurs with detection and treatment during:
   a. stage 0
   b. stage I
   c. stage II
   d. stage III
   e. stage IV

7. The pathogenesis of endometriosis is best described as:
   a. infectious inflammation as part of the spectrum of PID
   b. adenocarcinoma of the glandular lining of the uterus
   c. ectopic endometrium found on the ovaries or in the abdomen
   d. hyperplasia as a consequence of anovulation

8. Dysmenorrhea (painful menstruation) associated with endometriosis is due to:
   a. abnormally strong uterine contractions
   b. bleeding into the abdomen and cyst formation
   c. abdominal fibrosis and adhesion formation
   d. migration of endometrial tissue up the fallopian tubes

9. Choose the correct statement about endometrial hyperplasia:
   a. It is due to excessive estrogen stimulation because of an estrogen-secreting tumor.
   b. It is due to excessive estrogen stimulation because of lack of corpus luteum development and progesterone secretion.
   c. It is due to excessive estrogen stimulation because of ovarian cysts.
   d. It is due to excessive estrogen stimulation because of anovulation.

10. The most common cause of endometrial hyperplasia is:
    a. the early stages of menopause
    b. excessive physical demands placed on the body
    c. extreme emotional upset or psychological disorders
    d. overproduction of estrogen by an ovarian tumor

3. d–It is infection of the ovaries only, which is called oophoritis.

4. e–cervical carcinoma

5. a–It is a progression through degrees of dysplasia, to carcinoma in situ, and finally to stages of invasion.

6. a–stage 0

7. c–ectopic endometrium found on the ovaries or in the abdomen

8. b–bleeding into the abdomen and cyst formation

9. d–it is due to excessive estrogen stimulation because of anovulation

10. a–the early stages of menopause

11. b–Early detection is due to the performance of Pap smears.

12. c–benign tumor of the uterine muscle

13. c–fallopian tubes

14. a–infertility; c–ectopic pregnancy

15. b–anovulation; c–endometrial hyperplasia

16. d–all of the above

17. b–endometroid adenocarcinoma

18. d–a variety of body tissues

19. a–amenorrhea

11. Choose the INCORRECT statement about endometrial carcinoma:
    a. It is an adenocarcinoma arising from endometrial glands.
    b. Early detection is due to the performance of Pap smears.
    c. It is suspected to be related to elevated levels of estrogen or to prolonged exposure to estrogen.
    d. The population most often affected are postmenopausal women.

12. A leiomyoma is a (an):
    a. adenocarcinoma of the uterine lining
    b. carcinoma of the uterine muscle
    c. benign tumor of the uterine muscle
    d. benign tumor of the uterine lining

13. Salpingitis is infectious inflammation of the:
    a. ovaries
    b. cervix
    c. fallopian tubes
    d. vagina

14. The two most common complications of salpingitis are (choose two):
    a. infertility
    b. peritonitis
    c. ectopic pregnancy
    d. pyosalpinx

15. Polycystic ovary syndrome results in (choose two of the following):
    a. dysmenorrhea
    b. anovulation
    c. endometrial hyperplasia
    d. endometriosis

16. Tumors of the ovaries arise from:
    a. germ cells
    b. surface epithelial cells
    c. stromal cells
    d. all of the above
    e. none of the above

17. The most malignant of the ovarian tumors is the:
    a. teratoma
    b. endometroid adenocarcinoma
    c. cystadenocarcinoma
    d. cystadenoma

18. A teratoma consists of:
    a. hyperplastic primary follicles
    b. dysplastic corpus luteum
    c. cysts surrounded by fibrosis
    d. a variety of body tissues

19. Lack of menstrual bleeding is:
    a. amenorrhea
    b. dysmenorrhea
    c. metrorrhagia
    d. menorrhagia

20. Toxic shock syndrome is:
    a. a state of eclampsia seen in toxemia of pregnancy
    b. hormonal imbalance associated with the second half of the menstrual cycle, which creates physical and behavioral abnormalities
    c. *S. aureus* infection and toxemia during tampon use
    d. another name for septic shock during puerperal sepsis

21. Choose the INCORRECT statement about ectopic pregnancy:
    a. It is implantation of a fertilized ova outside of the uterus.
    b. The most common location for ectopic pregnancy is the ovaries.
    c. Diseased fallopian tubes increases the likelihood of ectopic pregnancy.
    d. Ectopic pregnancy results in rupture and significant hemorrhage.

22. List the three clinical findings (the toxemia triad) that appear in toxemia of pregnancy:
    a. _____, b._____, c. _____.

23. The most common reason for spontaneous abortion is:
    a. contamination of the reproductive tract during childbirth
    b. hydatidiform mole
    c. excessive physical activity during the second trimester
    d. genetic defect in the embryo

24. Infection of the uterus, with possible septicemia, after a contaminated childbirth or abortion describes:
    a. endometritis
    b. toxemia of pregnancy
    c. puerperal sepsis
    d. eclampsia
    e. toxic shock syndrome

25. Hydatidiform mole and choriocarcinoma are:
    a. trophoblastic or placental tumors
    b. tumors of the fetus
    c. extensions of a teratoma
    d. tumors of the myometrium

20. c–*S. aureus* infection and toxemia during tampon use

21. b–The most common location for ectopic pregnancy is the ovaries.

22. a–proteinuria; b–edema; c–hypertension

23. d–genetic defect in the embryo

24. c–puerperal sepsis

25. a–trophoblastic or placental tumors

III. DISEASES OF THE FEMALE BREAST ◄ SECTION

► INFLAMMATORY DISEASE OF THE BREAST

15–51

Acute mastitis is inflammation of the breast caused by bacterial infection. The agents are usually *S. aureus,* which is often found on the skin, and streptococci from a newborn's mouth. Acute mastitis is found almost exclusively during lactation or breast feeding. The bacteria enter the mammary tissue through the nipples, especially if there is a crack or other injury present. Trauma caused by the baby's mouth during suckling can produce sufficient lesions for bacterial entry. If a quantity of milk remains in the breast after nursing, this milk can become stagnant and provide a good growth medium for bacteria. Clinically, acute mastitis presents with the classic signs of inflammation, swelling, heat, redness, and pain in the affected area. If an abscess should form in the tissue, pus may drain from the ducts. An abscess doesn't usually form unless the infection is not recognized and treated early. Because of the prominent discomfort, diagnosis is usually timely. Treatment consists of

1. infection
2. bacteria
3. *S. aureus*
4. streptococci
5. lactation
6. nipple
7. milk

antibiotics, local heat application, and frequent emptying of the milk to "wash out" the infection. An abscess requires surgical draining. Acute mastitis is _____(1) of the breast caused by _____(2), especially _____(3) and _____(4). It may occur during _____(5) if lesions around the _____(6) are present. Retained _____(7) in the breast contributes to the growth of the bacteria.

▶ HYPERPLASTIC DISEASE OF THE BREAST

15–52

1. benign
2. young
3. common
4. no
5. moveable
6. not

Hyperplasia in the breast is represented as proliferative states that produce a mass. The three hyperplastic conditions we will discuss are illustrated in Figure 15–10. The most common mass or lump of the breast is the **fibroadenoma.** This is a benign growth that appears as a nodule with a well-defined capsule. An important clinical feature of fibroadenoma is that it is a moveable lump. This is in contrast to a malignant state that we will discuss soon. Fibroadenoma develops in young women and is asymptomatic. An excisional biopsy both diagnoses and cures the condition. Because of its capsule, a fibroadenoma shells out easily. This is not a premalignant condition, and it tends not to recur after removal. A fibroadenoma is a _____(1) mass or lump appearing in the breast of _____(2) women. This condition is _____(3) common / uncommon (choose one). There are _____(4) signs. A characteristic feature of fibroadenoma is that it is a _____(5) lump. It does _____(6) lead to breast cancer.

15–53

A hyperplastic condition of the breasts that is considered a hormonally induced change is **fibrocystic disease,** sometimes known as **cystic hyperplasia.** Fibrocystic disease is a category that describes several proliferative changes in breast tissue as a result of the influence of estrogen and progesterone. In affected women, rising and falling levels of hormones stimulate dilation of mammary gland ducts and fibrosis. It results in fluid-filled cysts surrounded by scar tissue. Fibrocystic disease represents an inappropriate response to hormones by the breast tissue. Cysts develop because, during the secretory phase of the menstrual cycle, fluid normally accumulates in the breasts. In fibrocystic disease, the fibrosis prevents normal draining of the fluid, so the ducts become fluid-filled sacs. If the epithelium of the ducts

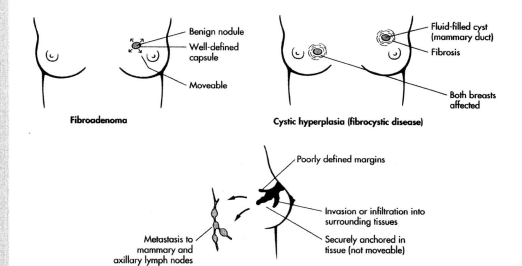

Figure 15–10. Hyperplasia in the female breast.

undergoes hyperplasia, progression to carcinoma is possible. The likelihood of this happening is directly related to the severity of hyperplasia, that is, how atypical the cells are. Most commonly, cases of fibrocystic disease are mild and produce little or no symptoms. Fibrocystic disease is a _____(1) condition of the breasts that may develop in some women in response to _____(2). It is also called _____(3). The mammary ducts become _____(4) and surrounded by _____(5). Cysts develop when _____(6) is not permitted to drain because of the restricting presence of _____(7). A situation of concern is if the epithelium of the _____(8) experiences severe _____(9), which may possibly be a precursor to _____(10).

1. hyperplastic
2. hormones
3. cystic hyperplasia
4. cystic
5. fibrosis or scar tissue
6. fluid
7. fibrosis or scar tissue
8. ducts
9. hyperplasia
10. cancer or carcinoma

15-54

Fibrocystic disease presents as uneven or lumpy areas in the breasts which feel hard and stringy. Both breasts are affected, which is an important feature in contrast to carcinoma. The areas often become tender during hormonal changes of menstruation. An initial diagnostic procedure is the fine needle aspirate. The withdrawal of fluid shows the lump to be a cyst instead of a tumor. A biopsy is required to assess epithelial hyperplasia, if any. If hyperplasia is significant, the patient is classified as higher risk for cancer and should be monitored appropriately. The actual link between fibrocystic disease and breast cancer is weak because most cases don't have significant hyperplasia. The majority of cases of fibrocystic disease don't need treatment. In hyperplastic cases, an extensive "lumpectomy" provides an excellent prognosis.

▶ NEOPLASIA OF THE BREAST

15-55

Breast cancer is the second most common cancer among women, when lung cancer is added to the statistics. Two factors considered to contribute highly to the development of breast cancer are heredity and hormones. The genetic connection is well demonstrated because if a female family member develops the cancer, the other female members are at greater risk than the general population. Hormonal influence is a significant factor if there is prolonged estrogen exposure. Examples of this are early-onset menstruation combined with late-onset menopause, or if there have been no children. Pregnancy is considered somewhat protective because estrogen is suppressed while progesterone predominates. Having other types of cancer linked to estrogen (ovarian and endometrial) also places the individual at greater risk for breast cancer. Genetic makeup and estrogen most likely combine with other common cancer factors, such as exposure to chemical carcinogens and oncogenic viruses. Breast cancer is the _____(1) most common cancer of women overall. Given two individuals exposed to the same carcinogens and viruses, the one at higher risk for developing cancer is the one with a _____(2) history of the disease [in other words, a particular _____(3) makeup], and with prolonged levels of _____(4) present in her system.

1. second
2. family
3. genetic
4. estrogen

15-56

Since it arises from the epithelium of the mammary tissue, breast cancer is a carcinoma. There are several types. The one we will discuss is the one affecting the ducts. Therefore, it is classified as an adenocarcinoma. Adenocarcinoma of the breast has poorly defined margins because of its characteristic infiltration into the surrounding tissue. The infiltration of this mass of dense tissue causes it to be fixed, which means it is not moveable like a fibroadenoma. Unchecked, mammary adenocarcinoma often progresses rapidly, and death within 2 years is likely. The spread of the cancer is through both the lymphatics and the blood. It moves first to the local lymph nodes. These are the mammary lymph nodes within the breast and the axillary lymph nodes under the arm. Once in the bloodstream, mammary adenocarcinoma most commonly metastasizes to bone, the liver, the lungs, and to the brain. Breast cancer is classified as a _____(1) because its origin is the _____(2). Carcinoma that affects the ducts (which is glandular tissue) is a (an) _____(3). Adenocarcinoma of the breast _____(4) can / cannot

1. carcinoma
2. epithelium
3. adenocarcinoma
4. cannot

5. lymph nodes
6. axillary
7. bone
8. liver
9. lungs
10. brain

15-57

1. lump or mass
2. signs
3. examinations
4. metastasis

15-58

(choose one) be moved. It spreads first to the local _____(5) of the breast and the _____(6) region. Distant metastasis is to the _____(7), _____(8), _____(9), and _____(10).

Early adenocarcinoma of the breast presents as a lump or mass long before any clinical signs develop. Advanced adenocarcinoma causes puckering of the skin and retraction of the nipple. This is because the growth extends from the chest wall through the mammary tissue and to the skin. It contracts and pulls on the superficial tissue. It may ulcerate through the skin surface, as shown in Figure 15–11. Regional lymph nodes may be swollen. The early stages are detected when lumps are found during examination, whether it is by self-examination, palpation by a physician, or by mammography. A mammogram is a specialized x-ray of the breast tissue that can identify an abnormal area before a lump can be felt. The abnormal area is seen as an increased density. This emphasizes the importance of these routine health exams, especially the self-examination. To forego these exams greatly increases the chance of metastasis. As part of the diagnosis, a fine needle aspirate (a relatively noninvasive procedure) is performed as a screening procedure. If neoplastic cells are found on the cytology, a biopsy is indicated to confirm the cancer by examining a tissue section. Early adenocarcinoma presents itself as a (an) _____(1) in the breast. At this point, clinical _____(2) are not present. It is found during routine _____(3), and these exams serve as a means of detection before _____(4) occurs.

There are a variety of treatment options available for breast cancer. The prognosis does not seem to be greatly affected by the choice of treatment protocols. Surgical removal may be in the form of a "lumpectomy" (only the tumor is excised), a simple mastectomy (the entire breast is removed), or a radical mastectomy (the breast, lymph nodes, and muscle mass are removed). Radiation or chemotherapy are used in combination, especially if a lumpectomy is performed. The prognosis depends on the stage of detection and treatment of the cancer. The 5-year survival rate for a small tumor with no metastasis is 80 percent. Larger tumors with lymph node spread yield a 40 to 65 percent survival rate. A case with metastasis has only a 10 percent survival rate. Recurrence of breast cancer is not uncommon, and this causes the 10-year survival rate to be about 50 percent overall.

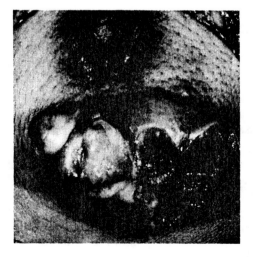

Figure 15–11. Advanced adenocarcinoma of the breast ulcerating through the skin surface. *(From Chandrasoma and Taylor,* Concise Pathology, *2nd ed., Appleton & Lange.)*

III. REVIEW QUESTIONS

1. Acute mastitis may develop:
   a. during contaminated delivery or abortion procedures
   b. during lactation if nipples are injured
   c. from hematogenous spread during puerperal sepsis
   d. during fibrocystic disease

2. The most common reason for a lump in the breast is:
   a. chronic mastitis
   b. fibrocystic disease
   c. mammary carcinoma
   d. fibroadenoma

3. Hormonally induced cyst formation of the mammary ducts, surrounded by fibrosis, best describes:
   a. mammary adenocarcinoma
   b. fibroadenoma
   c. fibrocystic disease
   d. mammary hyperplasia

4. True or false: There is a significant association between fibrocystic disease and breast cancer. _____

5. A physical characteristic of a mass that is mammary adenocarcinoma is:
   a. immobility because of infiltration
   b. mobility because of capsulation
   c. ulceration over the site early in the cause of the disease
   d. discharge from the nipple

6. Early breast cancer presents as:
   a. pain in the affected breast
   b. puckering of the skin with nipple retraction
   c. an asymptomatic lump or mass
   d. pain in a bone because of metastasis

1. b–during lactation if nipples are injured

2. d–fibroadenoma

3. c–fibrocystic disease

4. False

5. a–immobility because of infiltration

6. c–an asymptomatic lump or mass

IV. DISEASES OF THE MALE REPRODUCTIVE SYSTEM ◄ SECTION

► DISEASES OF THE PROSTATE

15–59

Prostate disease is more common than any other disease of the male reproductive system. **Prostatitis** is bacterial infection of the prostate gland that usually affects older men. If you will recall the anatomy of this gland, the secretory ducts connect to the prostatic portion of the urethra, which in turn is in connection with the urinary bladder. Microorganisms in the urethra or bladder gain direct access into the prostate through its ducts, as shown in Figure 15–12. Incomplete emptying of the bladder predisposes the prostate to invasion and infection by bacteria. This is because stagnation of urine allows bacteria to multiply to infectious numbers. Examples of specific infections are *E. coli* urinary tract infection and the sexually transmitted disease gonorrhea. Most cases of prostatitis are acute. Chronic prostatitis is only

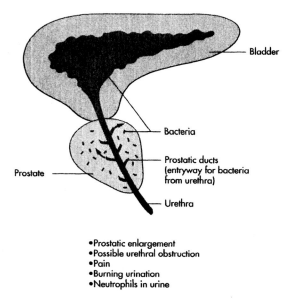

•Prostatic enlargement
•Possible urethral obstruction
•Pain
•Burning urination
•Neutrophils in urine

Figure 15–12. Prostatitis.

1. prostate
2. infection
3. prostate
4. bacteria
5. urethra
6. bladder
7. emptied
8. multiply
9. enlarged

15-60

an occasional finding and fibrosis of this gland usually accompanies the infection. The inflammation causes the prostate to enlarge to some degree and be tender when palpated. Pain and a burning sensation are present during urination. Pus may be present at the tip of the penis. Because of the prostate's location (surrounding the urethra), enlargement can compress or obstruct the urethra. This can prevent emptying the bladder and add to urine stagnation and infection. Infection of the bladder and prostate is highly suspected when leukocytes (PMNs) are found in the urine during urinalysis. The causative organism can be identified with a culture. Treatment is appropriate antibiotics. The most common reproductive disorder of men is disease of the _____(1). Prostatitis is _____(2) of the _____(3) caused by _____(4). The bacteria are present in the _____(5) or _____(6). Stagnation of urine may develop if the bladder is not completely _____(7). This allows bacteria to _____(8). The inflammation caused by the infection causes the prostate to become somewhat _____(9).

The most common disorder of the prostate is **benign prostatic hyperplasia,** or **BPH.** As the name implies, this is enlargement of the prostate (more than in prostatitis) that is not malignant. It is sometimes called benign prostatic enlargement or prostatic hypertrophy. BPH occurs fairly frequently in men over 50. The incidence increases with age. Some degree of enlargement is present in more than 90 percent of men over 70. The cause of BPH is not known. The current theory is that it is due to a hormonal imbalance that develops as men get older. There is a change in the testosterone–estrogen ratio because testosterone decreases with age while estrogen secreted by the adrenal cortex remains the same. The enlargement of the prostate is in a bumpy or nodular form. It is a combination of hyperplasia of the glands, hypertrophy of the smooth muscle, and fibrosis. The prostatic urethra becomes distorted with the changes in the gland. BPH predisposes a man to secondary prostatitis if a bladder infection develops. The most outstanding clinical feature of BPH is **dysuria,** which is painful or difficult urination. Dysuria is the foremost reason medical attention is sought in cases of BPH. The enlarged prostate compresses the urethra and interferes with normal urination. In dysuria, there is a feeling of urgency to urinate but it is difficult to initiate the process. The urine stream is weak. Stopping the stream is also difficult. Straining is sometimes necessary to empty the bladder. Attempts at urination are frequent. Dysuria and the retention of urine in the bladder are stepping stones to infection of the urinary tract and prostate. BPH stands for _____(1). It is the _____(2) common disorder of the prostate. BPH is found in older men, and the number of cases _____(3) with age. It is believed to be due to imbalance of _____(4). The uneven enlargement is described as a _____(5) form. The most obvious sign of benign prostatic hyperplasia is _____(6), which means difficulty in _____(7). This is because the enlarged gland obstructs the _____(8).

1. benign prostatic hyperplasia
2. most
3. increases
4. hormones
5. nodular
6. dysuria
7. urinating
8. urethra

⸻ 15-61 ⸻

There are several complications of BPH, a few of which have been mentioned. These complications, which are illustrated in Figure 15–13, are because of obstruction of the prostatic urethra and the neck of the bladder. They are:

1. Stagnation of urine and potential urinary tract infection.
2. Prostatitis that accompanies bladder infection.
3. Ascension of the infection to the kidneys, causing pyelonephritis.
4. Increased pressure in the urinary system because of backup of urine. This can cause dilation of the ureters (hydroureter) and the renal pelvis (hydronephrosis). Significant long-standing hydronephrosis will interfere with kidney function.

Benign prostatic hyperplasia is easily diagnosed during a rectal exam and palpation of the gland. The enlarged prostate is not painful as it is in prostatitis. The gland is firm but not hardened as it is in prostate cancer. The pattern of enlargement in BPH differs from the pattern seen in cancer. BPH can be treated medically with hormonal inhibitors. It may require surgery if significant urinary tract obstruction exists. About 10 percent of the cases require prostatectomy, or complete removal of the prostate. Other cases will benefit from resection, where enlarged portions are removed. Complications of BPH arise because of _____(1) of the urethra and neck of the _____(2). Infection can develop in the _____(3) or _____(4). The infection can travel to the kidneys, causing _____(5). Backed-up urine in the system increases the _____(6) in the system. This may enlarge the ureters [called _____(7)] or the renal pelvis [called _____(8)].

1. obstruction
2. bladder
3. urinary tract
4. prostate
5. pyelonephritis
6. pressure
7. hydroureters
8. hydronephrosis

⸻ 15-62 ⸻

The most common cancer that affects men specifically is **adenocarcinoma of the prostate.** It is the number three killer due to cancer. Most cases are diagnosed when the tumor is advanced, which accounts for the high death rate. Prostatic cancer spreads rather quickly. As with neoplasia of the female reproductive system, sex hormones are considered a contributing factor in its development. Several findings support the hypothesis of the stimulation of prostate cancer by testosterone, while other sources argue against the relationship. As in

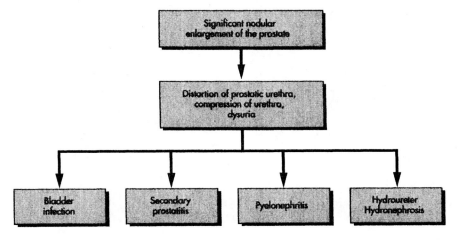

Figure 15–13. Benign prostatic hyperplasia.

1. rapidly
2. advanced
3. testosterone

15-63

1. posterior or rear
2. urethra
3. urinary
4. lumbar vertebrae
5. sacrum
6. benign prostatic
   hyperplasia

other cases of malignancy, lifestyle and environment must be considered among the causes. Prostate cancer is a major cause of death due to malignancy among men because it spreads _____(1) and is usually diagnosed when the tumor is _____(2). It is believed by some to be initiated by the hormone _____(3).

Instead of enlargement of the section of the prostate that surrounds the urethra, as in BPH, prostate cancer grows in the posterior, or rear, lobes of the gland. This is unfortunate because urinary signs are not present in early cases. The early tumor is small and confined to the prostate. It later invades locally. Regional invasion includes the pelvic organs like the bladder or rectum, as well as lymph nodes. Metastasis through the blood and lymphatics produce secondary tumors or metastases of the liver or lung, and especially the bones. The bones of the lumbar vertebral column and the sacrum are often invaded because of the vascular connections between these structures and the prostate. Common sites of metastasis of prostate cancer are illustrated in Figure 15–14. Unfortunately, the clinical presentation of prostatic adenocarcinoma is not very dramatic. Prostate cancer affects the same age group as BPH. Considering how common BPH is, many cases that develop cancer have already had prostate difficulties, so further signs may go unnoticed. Early small tumors are usually asymptomatic. The location of the growth (away from the urethra) causes no urinary signs at first. As the tumor grows and invades outside of the prostate and into the pelvic organs, the signs correspond to the system affected. Urinary invasion causes dysuria and **nocturia** (the need to urinate at night). Rectal invasion causes constipation and intestinal obstruction. Metastases of the pelvic and vertebral bones causes low back pain. Malignant tumors of the prostate tend to be located in the _____(1), of the gland. Enlargement does not initially occur surrounding the _____(2). Because of this, signs of _____(3) difficulty are not present in early cases. The bones that are frequently the site of spread include the _____(4) and the _____(5). A contributing factor to the hidden nature of prostate cancer is the pre-existence of _____(6), which may cause further signs to go unnoticed.

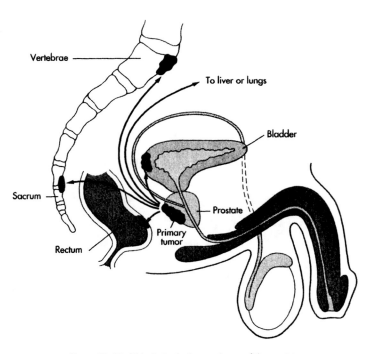

Figure 15–14. Metastasis of adenocarcinoma of the prostate.

15-64

In prostate cancer, there is a blood test that is helpful in diagnosing the condition. The enzyme acid phosphatase is found in several tissues. One type, or isoenzyme, is specific for the prostate and it is called prostatic acid phosphatase or PAP. The PAP is an indicator of prostatic activity. Malignant prostate cells secrete PAP in great amounts into the circulation. PAP is considered a serologic marker for prostate cancer. The amount of PAP in the blood has some correlation with the size of the tumor. Another serological finding is an antigen released by the tumor into the circulation. Immunologic tests using commercial antibody can detect the antigen, which is called prostate-specific antigen, or PSA. Digital rectal exam and palpation of the prostate reveals a very hard nonpainful enlargement of the posterior lobes. This enlargement can be felt in the early stages of the tumor. Therefore, routine rectal exams in older men is as important as routine breast exams in women. If the prostate is found to be enlarged, ultrasound exam using a rectal probe can help differentiate this condition from other reasons for enlargement. Any suspicious finding should be followed by a needle aspiration or biopsy.

15-65

If a malignant prostate tumor is detected early, while it is still confined to the prostate, surgical removal of the gland results in a relatively good prognosis. Cases in which there has been invasion or metastasis require radiation as well as surgical excision. Cases that are inoperable may benefit from castration to remove the source of testosterone and hopefully reduce the size of the primary tumor. Estrogen administration also inhibits the growth of the tumor. The only cases considered successfully treated are those that have not moved out of the prostate. It is not uncommon for lymph node metastasis to have occurred even in cases where it was believed to be still confined to the prostate. The five-year survival rate of prostate cancer treated when it was still confined to the prostate is around 75 percent. The rate is much lower when invasion has taken place.

▶ DISEASES OF THE TESTICLES

15-66

Inflammation of the testes is called **orchitis.** It is most often caused by infection. Infection of the testes alone, which is not part of infection of the epididymis, usually develops through hematogenous invasion. Hematogenous refers to the presence of microorganisms in the blood. Sometimes, infectious orchitis is a complication of the secondary stage of syphilis. The most common cause of infectious orchitis is the mumps virus. The mumps virus primarily targets the parotid salivary glands but will also invade the pancreas or testes. Unilateral infection of only one testicle doesn't greatly affect reproductive ability. Severe cases, where both testes are infected (a bilateral infection), can cause enough atrophy that infertility is the result. Infectious orchitis presents as swelling of the testicle, due to edema, and pain. It follows about a week after a case of the mumps. There is no specific treatment for this viral condition, and most cases resolve spontaneously. The second most common cause of testicular inflammation is "traumatic orchitis" where the inflammation is a reaction to some injury. Orchitis is _____(1) of the _____(2). Most commonly, it is due to _____(3) by the virus that causes _____(4). Infertility is only a concern in severe cases where _____(5) testes are infected. Noninfectious orchitis can result following a (an) _____(6) to the testes.

1. inflammation
2. testicles
3. infection
4. mumps
5. both
6. injury

15-67

Cryptorchism is a congenital abnormality. The testes are formed in the abdomen of the male fetus. They then descend from the abdomen into the scrotum through the inguinal canal. The canal closes behind the testes and they become enclosed in the scrotum by birth in most cases. Cryptorchism is failure of complete descent into the scrotum. Cryptorchism may be referred to as a "retained testicle." The journey of the testicle may end at any location along the route, so a retained testicle can be in the abdomen, anywhere along the inguinal canal, or at the entrance to the scrotum. Cryptorchism can affect one or both testicles. The undescended testicle is likely to atrophy or result in hypospermatogenesis (decreased production of sperm). These degenerative changes are because of the higher temperature in the abdomen compared to the relatively cool scrotal sac. If only one testicle is retained, fertility is still likely. If both are retained, the male is infertile. Cryptorchism should be treated to prevent complications. One complication is the possibility of an inguinal hernia if a portion of the intestines protrudes through the open canal into the scrotum. Another complication is the increased risk of cancer. A cryptorchid testicle is much more likely to become cancerous than a normal one.

15-68

1. testicles
2. abdomen
3. scrotum
4. retained
5. higher
6. atrophy
7. hypospermatogenesis
8. bilateral
9. inguinal hernia
10. complication
11. cancer

The diagnosis of this condition is obvious, with the testicle(s) being absent from the scrotum. Treatment is surgical fixation of the testicle in the scrotum and closure of the inguinal canal. This should be done in early infancy so that the testicle develops normally. If the testicle can't be brought down into the scrotum, it should be removed to prevent malignant transformation. In cryptorchism, one or both _____(1) have not descended from the _____(2) into the _____(3). Cryptorchism is commonly described as a _____(4) testicle. If the testicle remains in the abdomen, the _____(5) temperature leads to _____(6) or _____(7). Infertility results if the cryptorchism is _____(8) unilateral / bilateral (choose one). If part of the intestines bulge through the open inguinal canal, this is called a (an) _____(9). This condition is a _____(10) of cryptorchism. Another complication is the transformation of the testicle into _____(11).

15-69

1. testicles
2. younger
3. malignancy
4. seminoma
5. teratoma
6. malignant

Cancer of the testicles is rare, comprising only about 1 percent of male-related neoplasia. It is much less common than prostatic cancer. But when it does strike, it affects young men in the age range of about 25 to 45. Its cause is unknown. Cryptorchism, or an otherwise abnormal testicle, predisposes to malignancy. There are many types of testicular tumors that can arise from the various cell lines in the testes. We will consider only two kinds of tumors, both arising from the germ cells. The first is the **seminoma,** which is a malignancy of the seminiferous tubules. This is the most common testicular tumor and it does metastasize. The second is the **teratoma,** and it resembles the teratoma of the ovary. It arises from embryonic cells and produces a variety of both embryonic and adult tissues, like the ovarian tumor. The difference is that a testicular teratoma is malignant instead of benign. It spreads through the lymphatics and the blood. Cancer of these testes presents as an enlargement of the testes, or as a distinguishable mass. The route of metastasis of both types includes the abdominal lymph nodes, the lungs, liver, and brain. Treatment consists of surgical removal of the primary tumor and affected lymph nodes, as well as chemotherapy. Chemotherapy has greatly improved the prognosis of these tumors over the years. Radiation is also effective, especially in the case of a seminoma. The prognosis for a seminoma detected before it spreads is good, with a 90 percent 5-year survival rate. The rate is not as high for a teratoma. It can be less than a 50 percent survival rate if the tumor has metastasized. Considering neoplasia of male reproductive structures, cancer of the _____(1) is rare. Men affected with these tumors are _____(2) than the typical cancer age group. An abnormal testicle may be predisposed to _____(3). The most common testicular tumor is the _____(4). Another tumor resembles the ovarian dermoid cyst and is called a _____(5). Unlike an ovarian teratoma, this tumor is _____(6).

15-70

If you will recall from Chapter 12, a torsion is a twist or rotation of a suspended structure. A **testicular torsion** is a testicle twisted around its axis. This may occur during blunt trauma or during strenuous movement or exercise. Only certain men are prone to this condition, those with a developmental defect that allows the testicle freedom of movement. The spermatic cord and, more importantly, the blood vessels become twisted. The blood supply through the kinked vessels is cut off. After a time, infarction and necrosis of the testicle develop. Testicular torsion presents as sudden and severe pain in the scrotum. The twist must be repaired immediately by either open surgery or by manipulation from outside the scrotum. Once the danger of infarction is passed, a tacking procedure of *both* testicles should be performed to anchor them in the scrotum and prevent another torsion. Rotation of a testicle around its normal axis is called a _____(1). It also results in twisting of both the spermatic cord and the associated _____(2). This causes an interruption in _____(3) to the testicle. If the condition is sustained, _____(4) and _____(5) will result.

1. testicular torsion
2. blood vessels
3. blood supply
4. infarction
5. necrosis

▶ OTHER DISEASES OF THE MALE REPRODUCTIVE SYSTEM

15–71

Balanitis is inflammation of the glans penis (the enlarged end). It is usually due to infection acquired during sexual activity. The microorganisms most commonly causing the infection are herpesvirus or syphilis. Herpesvirus creates vesicles that rupture and become shallow ulcers. The deeper ulceration of syphilis is called a chancre. Balanitis produces redness and swelling of the glans along with the localized lesions. Treatment is directed at the causative organism. Inflammation of the glans penis is called _____(1). This is generally a (an) _____(2) caused by microorganisms most often acquired during _____(3) activity.

1. balanitis
2. infection
3. sexual

15–72

Epididymitis is inflammation of the epididymis, the tubular structure leading from the testicle to the prostate. Primary epididymitis is infection by microorganisms that are sexually transmitted. The infection ascends from the site of entry at the tip of the penis. The causative organisms of primary infection typically are *Neisseria gonorrhoeae* or *Chlamydia*. Pathogens from the urinary tract may ascend and cause a secondary epididymitis. Another cause of secondary epidiymitis is prostatitis, if the organisms travel there from the prostate. Hematogenous spread of organisms from the blood is possible, as in the case of orchitis. Epididymitis causes swelling and pain in the scrotum. A complication of significant infection is infertility if the infection is bilateral and adhesions form to block the tubules. Epididymitis is treated with antibiotics specific for the causative organism. Epididymitis is _____(1) of the _____(2) caused by _____(3) with microorganisms. Primary epididymitis is often associated with _____(4) transmitted infection. Secondary epididymitis may develop in association with infection of the _____(5) tract, or with infection of the prostate, which is called _____(6). A complication of a severe infection accompanied by scar tissue is _____(7).

1. inflammation
2. epididymis
3. infection
4. sexually
5. urinary
6. prostatitis
7. infertility

15–73

Gynecomastia is enlargement of the male breast because of proliferation of ducts and connective tissue. It should not be confused with **pseudogynecomastia,** which is enlargement because of excessive adipose tissue in obesity. Gynecomastia can be a temporary situation during the normal hormonal imbalance of puberty, or during old age when androgen levels decline. A pathologic cause of bilateral gynecomastia is the presence of increased estrogen in the male. Causes of increased estrogen include:

1. gynecomastia
2. adipose tissue
3. pseudogynecomastia
4. estrogen
5. Klinefelter's syndrome

1. Cirrhosis of the liver in which the liver cannot metabolize the small amount of estrogen normally secreted by the adrenal glands.
2. An estrogen-secreting tumor of the adrenal glands.
3. Administration of estrogen during treatment of prostate cancer.

Gynecomastia is also a feature of Klinefelter's syndrome (see Chap. 7). If the breasts of a male enlarge, this is called _____(1). It is an increase in the duct work and connective tissue, not an increase in fat, or _____(2), as seen in _____(3). Gynecomastia not related to normal hormone imbalance is generally due to an increased amount of _____(4) in the male system. It may also be due to the genetic disease _____(5).

15-74

1. worse
2. late

1. c–the prostate

2. b–benign prostatic hyperplasia

3. a–venereal disease like gonorrhea; b–urinary tract infection

4. d–all of the above

5. e–all of the above

6. b–dysuria

Carcinoma of the male breast is possible, but it is rare, accounting for only about 1 percent of all breast cancer. Male breast cancer is like female breast cancer in its histologic picture and pathogenesis. However, it carries a worse prognosis than cancer of the female breast because it is not looked for by men or during routine physical exams. Because of this, it is almost always diagnosed late. Male breast cancer, although rare, has a _____(1) prognosis than female breast cancer because it is detected _____(2) in the course of the disease.

IV. REVIEW QUESTIONS

1. The most common organ(s) in the male reproductive system affected by disease is (are):
   a. the penis
   b. the testicles
   c. the prostate
   d. the epididymis

2. The most common disorder of the prostate is:
   a. prostatitis
   b. benign prostatic hyperplasia
   c. adenocarcinoma
   d. orchitis

3. Prostatitis most commonly develops as an extension of (choose all that are correct):
   a. venereal disease like gonorrhea
   b. urinary tract infection
   c. epididymitis
   d. orchitis

4. Which of the following causes enlargement of the prostate:
   a. prostatitis
   b. benign prostatic hyperplasia
   c. prostatic adenocarcinoma
   d. all of the above
   e. none of the above

5. Diseases of the prostate may be initially distinguished from one another by the:
   a. degree of enlargement
   b. location of enlargement
   c. presence or absence of pain
   d. consistency (firm or hardened)
   e. all of the above
   f. none of the above

6. Benign prostatic hyperplasia most notably causes:
   a. urinary tract infection
   b. dysuria
   c. nocturia
   d. intestinal obstruction

7. Complications of BPH include (choose all that apply):
   a. nocturia
   b. urinary tract infection
   c. prostatic carcinoma
   d. prostatitis
   e. pyelonephritis
   f. orchitis
   g. hydroureter
   h. hydronephrosis
   i. balanitis

8. In prostatic adenocarcinoma, the typical pattern of gland enlargement is:
   a. surrounding the urethra
   b. in the anterior, or front, of the gland
   c. in the posterior, or rear, of the gland
   d. all areas of the gland

9. Early prostatic tumors cause:
   a. no noticeable signs
   b. dysuria
   c. lumbar vertebral pain
   d. nocturia
   e. intestinal obstruction

10. Inflammation of the testes is called:
    a. balanitis
    b. testiculitis
    c. epididymitis
    d. orchitis

11. The most common cause of infectious orchitis is:
    a. hematogenous spread
    b. herpesvirus
    c. mumps virus
    d. extension of epididymitis

12. A testicle that has not completed the move from the abdomen into the scrotum describes:
    a. seminoma
    b. cryptorchism
    c. testicular torsion
    d. balanitis

13. Complications of unilateral cryptorchism are (choose all that are correct):
    a. inguinal hernia
    b. testicular torsion
    c. infertility
    d. increased risk of carcinoma
    e. inguinal canal abscess

14. Choose the INCORRECT statement about cancer of the testes:
    a. It affects younger men.
    b. All tumors are benign.
    c. Overall, this is a rare neoplasia.
    d. Unlike ovarian teratoma, testicular teratoma is malignant.
    e. The seminoma is the most common testicular tumor.

7. b–urinary tract infection; d–prostatitis; e–pyelonephritis; g–hydroureter; h–hydronephrosis

8. c–in the posterior, or rear, of the gland

9. a–no noticeable signs

10. d–orchitis

11. c–mumps virus

12. b–cryptorchism

13. a–inguinal hernia; d–increased risk of carcinoma

14. b–All tumors are benign.

15. The result of sustained testicular torsion is:
    a. infertility
    b. hypospermatogenesis
    c. infarction and necrosis
    d. inguinal hernia

16. One of the most common causes of balanitis is:
    a. mumps virus
    b. gonorrhea
    c. herpesvirus
    d. *Chlamydia*

17. Primary epididymitis is infection acquired through a. _____ activity, while secondary epididymitis is associated with extension of infection from the b. _____ tract or the c. _____.

18. Increased estrogen levels in the male may cause:
    a. gynecomastia
    b. pseudogynecomastia
    c. breast cancer
    d. Klinefelter's syndrome

CHAPTER ▶ SUMMARY

▶ SECTION II

Varginitis (infection of the vagina) can be caused by a variety of microorganisms. A malodorous discharge, the characteristics of which vary according to the infectious agent, is a sign of the condition. *Trichomoniasis,* vaginitis caused specifically by the protozoan *Trichomonas vaginalis,* is a common sexually transmitted disease. Other agents that can cause vaginitis include *Candida albicans* ("yeast infection") and certain bacteria *(Neisseria gonorrhoeae, Streptococcus, Staphylococcus).*

In *pelvic inflammatory disease* (PID), the entire reproductive tract becomes infected. This can be a serious complication of untreated genital infection. PID can be caused by infectious agents (e.g., bacteria, viruses, fungi), or by medical procedures that contaminate the reproductive tract. Complications of PID include abdominal abscesses, peritonitis, ectopic pregnancy, and infertility. *Cervicitis* (inflammation of the cervix only) can be caused by any of the sexually transmitted infectious microbes.

Cervical cancer is a squamous cell carcinoma and is the result of uncontrolled proliferation of the cervical epithelium. The grade and stage of cervical cell dysplasia can be detected early by a Pap smear. A sign of cervical cancer is vaginal bleeding after intercourse and a significant bloody discharge as the cancer progresses.

Endometriosis is characterized by endometrial tissue growth at sites outside the uterus, such as the fallopian tubes, the ovaries, and the abdominal cavity. Endometriosis can cause a hematoma, which may develop into a cyst. *Dysmenorrhea* (painful menstruation) is the most prominent symptom of endometriosis. Left untreated, the condition can lead to fibrosis and infertility.

In the absence of ovulation *(anovulation), endometrial hyperplasia* may occur as the result of continued estrogen-induced thickening of the endometrium. When the endometrial tissue overthickens, ischemia and necrosis can occur, causing sloughing and bleeding. Several factors can cause anovulation, including emotional distress, anorexia nervosa, entry into menopause, excessive exercise, malnourishment, or excessive levels of estrogen. Uterine cancer is a potential complication of endometrial hyperplasia.

The most common type of reproductive tract cancer is *malignant neoplasia of the endometrium.* This form of adenocarcinoma arises from the epithelium of the endometrial glands, and most often strikes postmenopausal women. Hormones, viruses, and chemical carcinogens are thought to contribute to the etiology of endometrial cancer. The neoplasia is staged like cervical cancer. A *leiomyoma* is an estrogen-dependent benign tumor of the myometrium that does not transform into a malignancy. In postmenopausal women, the leiomyoma can atrophy into a fibroid tumor.

Oophoritis and *salpingitis*, two signs of pelvic inflammatory disease, are inflammation of the ovaries and fallopian tubes, respectively. Salpingitis, which may be acute or chronic, is generally due to a microbial infection. Left untreated, salpingitis can cause ectopic pregnancy or infertility. An *ovarian cyst* forms when an unruptured graafian follicle or a corpus luteum becomes filled with fluid. *Polycystic ovary syndrome* may develop as a result of hormone miscommunication between the hypothalamus and the pituitary glands.

Cancer of the ovaries includes a large variety of carcinomas. Neoplasia that arises from the epithelial cells of the ovaries are classified as *cystadenoma* (a benign cystic tumor), *cystadenocarcinoma* (which may be benign or of high malignancy), or *endometroid adenocarcinoma* (a malignant, noncystic tumor). A *teratoma* is a benign tumor of the germ cells in which brain tissue, skin, hair, cartilage, bone, and teeth are found. This form of tumor originates from oocytes attempting to develop into embryonic cells. Stromal cell tumors, which are usually benign, may cause menstrual cycle abnormalities due to their secretion of estrogen.

Amenorrhea is the absence of menstrual bleeding. A normal situation during pregnancy, lactation, and menopause, amenorrhea may be either primary (lack of onset of menstruation at puberty) or secondary (cessation of menstruation). Primary amenorrhea is most often caused by improper development of the ovaries or by the lack of hypothalamic or pituitary hormones. Secondary amenorrhea may be psychosomatic or due to a physical cause, such as hormone imbalance or disease of the ovaries. *Menorrhagia* is abnormally excessive menstrual blood loss. The condition can be caused by endometrial carcinoma, PID, or endometrial hyperplasia. *Metrorrhagia*, characterized by irregular menstrual cycles, is due to hormonal imbalance. *Dysmenorrhea* (painful menstruation) is generally associated with endometriosis and bleeding into the peritoneal cavity.

Toxic shock syndrome (TSS) is an infectious state caused by toxins produced by *Staphylococcus aureus*. TSS is most often associated with staph-contaminated tampons being retained too long, thereby allowing for overgrowth and entry into circulation of the bacteria. Fever, nausea, vomiting, hypotension, and septic shock are characteristic of the disease. *Premenstrual syndrome* (PMS) is a condition that begins approximately midway through the menstrual cycle. The precise cause of PMS is unknown, although it is believed that ovarian hormones upsetting the balance of the body's neurotransmitters may play a role. Hostility, irritability, anxiety, and depression are characteristics of PMS. The condition is not experienced by all women.

Many disorders can develop during pregnancy. An *ectopic pregnancy* ("tubal pregnancy") is the occurrence of a pregnancy outside the uterus. Most ectopic pregnancies occur in the fallopian tubes, which can eventually rupture the tube. In *toxemia of pregnancy,* multiple small blood clots cause thrombosis in the vessels of the kidneys. While the exact cause of the condition is unknown, placental release of thromboplastin or tissue factor is suspected. A *spontaneous abortion* ("miscarriage") is the expulsion of embryonic material without outside inducement, usually in response to a genetically abnormal embryo. The spontaneous abortion occurs early in the pregnancy and does not affect subsequent pregnancies. Bacterial infection of the uterus following childbirth or abortion is called *puerperal sepsis* ("childbed fever"). Bacteria generally associated with this condition are *Staphylococcus, Streptococcus,* and *E. coli.* Fever, chills, and vaginal bleeding are characteristic signs of the disease. Left untreated, septic shock and death are possible.

Tumors of the placenta during pregnancy are characterized as *gestational trophoblastic neoplasia*. Such a tumor is the *hydatidiform mole,* a cystic mass of placental villi. This tumor is benign but may transform into a malignancy, which may be invasive or noninvasive. A *choriocarcinoma* is a malignant neoplasia of the placenta which will metastasize. The neoplasia can develop after a hydatidiform mole, in normal placenta after delivery, or in placental cells following an abortion.

► SECTION III

Acute mastitis is inflammation of the breast caused by bacterial infection. The condition occurs almost exclusively during breast feeding, when bacteria enter the mammary tissue through the nipples. Swelling, heat, redness, and pain are characteristic symptoms of the condition. *Hyperplasia in the breast* is most often a *fibroadenoma,* a moveable, encapsulated, benign nodule. Fibroadenoma develops in young women and is asymptomatic. *Fibrocystic disease* (cystic hyperplasia) describes several types of proliferative changes in breast tissue induced by estrogen and progesterone. Fluid-filled cysts surrounded by scar tissue are characteristic of the condition. These present as "lumpy" areas in both breasts. Generally, fibrocystic disease does not require treatment.

Breast cancer (neoplasia of the breast) is of the carcinoma type. Genetics and hormones likely contribute to this common form of cancer. Cancer specifically affecting the ducts is classified as an adenocarcinoma. Infiltration into the surrounding tissue causes the tumor to be immoveable. Early signs of the disease are a lump in the breast, which when the cancer progresses, leads to retraction of the nipple and swelling of regional lymph nodes. Routine examinations are critical for early detection of breast cancer.

► SECTION IV

Prostate disease is the most common type of disease affecting the male reproductive system. *Prostatitis,* an acute condition that generally affects older men, is caused by bacterial infection that invades the prostate by way of the urethra or urinary bladder. *Benign prostatic hyperplasia* (BPH) is a nonmalignant enlargement of the prostate. The cause of BPH is unknown, but it is thought to be due to a hormonal imbalance that develops as men age. Several complications of BPH can occur, including secondary prostatitis, urinary tract infection, kidney infection, and kidney dysfunction. *Adenocarcinoma of the prostate* is the most common cancer that affects men specifically. The cancer, which originates in the rear lobes of the prostate, eventually invades the bladder, rectum, and lymph nodes. Metastasis produces secondary tumors in the liver, lungs, or bones. Signs and symptoms of prostate cancer include nocturia, intestinal obstruction, and lower back pain. Sex hormones, lifestyle, and environmental factors are considered among the causes of the disease.

Orchitis (inflammation of the testicles) is most often caused by infection via hematogenous (blood-borne) invasion. The most common cause of the condition is the mumps virus. The infection can be unilateral or bilateral. Infection of both testes can cause infertility. *Cryptorchism,* a congenital abnormality, is the failure of one or both testicles to descend into the scrotum during fetal development. The "retained testicle(s)" may be situated in the abdomen, in the inguinal canal, or at the entrance to the scrotum. Left uncorrected, the condition can lead to infertility, an inguinal hernia, or cancer.

Seminoma, the most common form of testicular tumor, is malignancy of the seminiferous tubules. A *testicular teratoma,* like an ovarian teratoma, produces a variety of tissues. A testicular teratoma, however, is malignant instead of benign. A testicle which has become twisted around its axis is a *testicular torsion.* The condition can occur as the result of a blunt trauma or heavy exercise. If unrepaired, it can lead to infarction and necrosis of the testicle. *Balanitis* (inflammation of the glans penis) is usually due to infection (e.g., herpesvirus or syphilis) acquired during sexual activity. Inflammation of the epididymis *(epididymitis)* may be due to sexually transmitted infection (primary epididymitis) or infection by pathogens from the urinary tract, prostate, or blood (secondary epididymitis).

Gynecomastia is enlargement of the male breast because of proliferation of ducts and connective tissue. The condition is generally caused by a hormonal imbalance due to cirrhosis of the liver, an estrogen-secreting tumor, or estrogen therapy. *Carcinoma of the male breast* is similar to female breast cancer in pathogenesis. The condition is rare but has a worse prognosis than female breast cancer.

The Endocrine System

▶ OBJECTIVES

SECTION II

Define all highlighted terms.

Describe the condition of hyperpituitarism. Characterize the causes and signs and symptoms of prolactinoma, somatotropic adenoma, and corticotropic adenoma.

Describe the conditions of hypopituitarism and panhypopituitarism, and characterize their causes and signs and symptoms.

SECTION III

Define all highlighted terms.

Describe the condition of hyperthyroidism. Characterize the causes, signs and symptoms, and complications of adenomatous goiter, Graves' disease, toxic nodular goiter, and Hashimoto's disease.

Describe the conditions of hypothyroidism and thyroid aplasia, and characterize the causes and signs and symptoms of the diseases.

Describe the condition of goiter, and characterize the causes and signs and symptoms of the types of goiter.

Describe the forms of thyroid gland neoplasia.

Describe the conditions of hyperparathyroidism and hypoparathyroidism, and characterize their causes and signs and symptoms.

SECTION IV

Define all highlighted terms.

Describe the general condition of hyperadrenalism, and characterize the causes and signs and symptoms of the forms of the condition.

Describe the conditions of hypercortisolism, hyperaldosteronism, and adrenogenital syndrome. Characterize the causes and signs and symptoms of the forms of each disease.

Describe the condition of hypoadrenalism, and characterize the causes and signs and symptoms of primary (Addison's disease) and secondary adrenal cortical insufficiency.

Describe the conditions of pheochromocytoma and neuroblastoma.

SECTION ▶

I. ANATOMY AND PHYSIOLOGY IN REVIEW

The term **"endocrine"** refers to a substance secreted from a gland directly into the circulation without the use of ducts (secretion through ducts is termed exocrine). The substances are chemicals called **hormones,** and they have very specific effects on organs or body parts some distance from the gland of origin. The endocrine system is made up of glands (the organs of this system) that create and release hormones. Many body processes are regulated by hormones. They can be thought of as chemical "on/off switches." They act as chemical messengers to send signals or communications. The glands of the endocrine system are the pituitary, thyroid, parathyroid, adrenals, islets of Langerhans in the pancreas, and the sex glands, or gonads. The glands located in the body are governed by the pituitary gland located in the brain. The pituitary gland is regulated by the hypothalamus, a specialized area in the brain.

Hormones, which are generally steroids or proteins, affect either whole body function or target a specific organ. Secretion or release of hormones from glands is directed according to need. The need for hormone release is generally signaled by low levels of the hormone. This is called a **positive feedback mechanism.** Adequate levels are the signal for suppression of release. This is the **negative feedback mechanism.** Positive feedback stimulates secretion, and negative feedback prevents release, as shown in Figure 16–1. The amount of hormones in the blood must be carefully controlled and this is accomplished through the feedback mechanisms. Diseases of the endocrine system fall into two general categories, **hypersecretion** (too much of a hormone in circulation) and **hyposecretion** (not enough of a hormone in circulation). Abnormal levels of a hormone upsets the delicate balance of control that is necessary for a state of health.

The **pituitary gland,** also called the **hypophysis,** is considered the master gland since its hormones control the body's glands and their hormones. It is a tiny structure at the base of the brain. It hangs off from the hypothalamus by a stalk and rests in a bony depression of the skull. This depression is the **sella turcica,** and it protects this vital gland. The pituitary gland is divided into two separate sections, each section secreting different hormones. The front section is the **anterior pituitary,** also known as the **adenohypophysis.** The rear section is the **posterior pituitary,** also called the **neurohypophysis.** The anterior pituitary is directly connected to the hypothalamus through blood vessels. The hypothalamus releases hormones called **releasing factors** that strictly control the activity of the anterior pituitary. Such tight control is necessary because the pituitary, in turn, will direct hormone secretion from body glands by the secretion of **trophic hormones,** which means causing a change.

Some of the hormones the anterior pituitary gland manufactures and releases are:

1. **Growth hormone (GH),** or **somatotropin,** which stimulates growth and development of all of the tissues of the body. Most of this growth takes place by puberty. After adult size is reached, levels of growth hormone decrease, but it is still important to promote tissue repair and regeneration.
2. **Thyroid-stimulating hormone (TSH),** or **thyrotropin,** which stimulates the thyroid gland to secrete hormones that regulate metabolism.
3. **Adrenocorticotropic hormone (ACTH),** which stimulates the cortex of the adrenal glands to release their hormones.
4. **Gonadotropins,** which are **FSH** and **LH.** If you will recall from Chapter 15, FSH causes the creation of graafian follicles from primary follicles, and therefore estrogen secretion. LH causes ovulation and therefore progesterone secretion. In the male, FSH and LH stimulate secretion of male hormones by the testes. **Prolactin** is another pituitary sex hormone that stimulates milk production by the mammary glands.

Positive Feedback

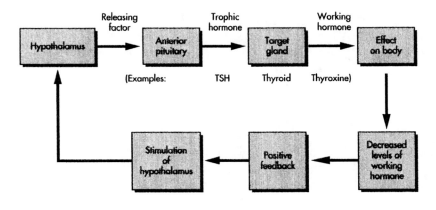

Negative Feedback

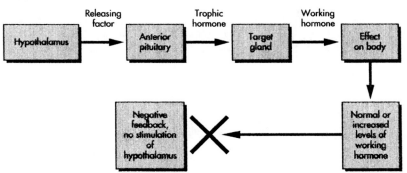

Figure 16–1. Hormone release according to feedback mechanisms.

16–5

The posterior pituitary, or neurohypophysis, is so named because hormones are released from nerve cells where the hormones are stored. The hormones are *not* manufactured by the posterior pituitary but are made by the hypothalamus. They are sent to the posterior pituitary for storage only and are secreted as needed. These hormones are:

1. **Oxytocin,** which causes the uterus to contract during labor and delivery, and vessels to contract afterwards to decrease hemorrhage. Oxytocin is also responsible for milk "letdown" or release from the mammary glands.
2. **Antidiuretic hormone (ADH),** which prevents too much water loss through the kidneys. Retaining the normal amount of water in the body supports normal blood pressure, and so this hormone is also called **vasopressin.** ADH was discussed in Chapter 3.

Examine Figure 16–2 to understand the relationships presented in the last few frames.

16–6

The **thyroid gland** is composed of two lobes on either side of the trachea just beneath the larynx, or Adam's apple, in the upper neck. The two lobes are connected by a strip of tissue called the isthmus. The structure of the thyroid gland is mainly follicles or sacs with capillaries running among them. A follicle is a ring of hormone-synthesizing cells that secrete the hormones into a center mass of colloidal material for storage until needed. The predominant hormones are **thyroxine** and **triiodothyronine.** They are protein based and incorporate iodine. The primary use of this mineral in the body is in the synthesis of thyroid hormones. In the blood, thyroid hormones combine with plasma proteins to form **T4** and **T3,** respectively. Tests to determine thyroid gland activity measure levels of T4 and T3, which may be

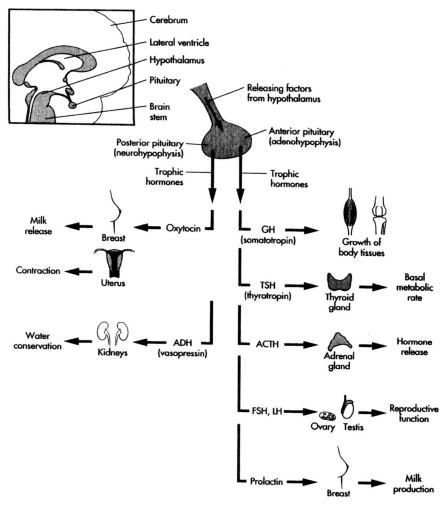

Figure 16–2. Hormones of the pituitary gland.

normal, increased, or decreased. Release of thyroid hormones (often collectively just called thyroxine) is controlled by TSH from the anterior pituitary gland. Low levels are the signal to the pituitary to release TSH, which will stimulate the thyroid to secrete thyroxine (positive feedback). Adequate or high levels will signal the pituitary to stop releasing TSH (negative feedback).

16-7

Thyroxine governs the **basal metabolic rate (BMR),** which is the use or consumption of oxygen by cells at rest. Remember that oxygen consumption results in energy production (ATP), heat generation, and waste production. The metabolism of cells, and therefore the rate of oxygen use with heat and energy production, is stimulated by thyroxine. When the metabolism of the body is increased, the heart and circulatory system must respond to provide more oxygen and remove more carbon dioxide and wastes. The increased blood flow requires an increased cardiac output. The rate of breathing or respiration must also increase to provide oxygen for circulation. Body temperature also increases because of the increased heat generated by stimulated metabolism. Since cells need glucose to fuel metabolism, absorption of carbohydrates from the intestines also increases. To review, the effects of thyroid hormones are an increase in metabolism, heart rate, respiration, body temperature, and intestinal absorption.

The **parathyroid glands** are four nodular areas located on the thyroid gland, with two nodules on each thyroid lobe. Their hormone is called **parathormone** or **parathyroid hormone.** This substance is vital in the regulation of calcium and phospate metabolism. In particular, it regulates levels in the blood. The majority of calcium (about 99 percent) is found in bone. The tiny amount in circulation plays crucial roles in nerve condition, muscle contraction, and blood clotting (see Chap. 3). When blood calcium levels are decreased, parathyroid hormone stimulates release of calcium from the bone and its absorption from the intestines. It also decreases calcium excretion by the kidneys. This causes calcium levels to increase to normal, at which time negative feedback inhibits further release of parathyroid hormone. Figure 16–3 illustrates the structure and function of the thyroid and parathyroid glands.

There are a pair of **adrenal glands,** which lie one on top of each kidney (adrenal means upon the kidneys). There are two sections of each adrenal gland. The outer layers are the cortex, while the inner layers are the medulla. Each section secretes its own hormones. The cortex manufactures and secretes three types of steroid hormones. These are:

1. **Mineralocorticoids,** of which the primary hormone is **aldosterone.** As you learned in Chapter 3, aldosterone regulates levels of salt or the sodium balance of the body. It causes sodium to be retained by the kidneys and potassium to be excreted. (You have probably noticed several references to Chapter 3, which presented homeostasis. That is because hormones are the primary caretakers of electrolyte balance.)
2. **Glucocorticoids,** of which the primary hormone is **cortisol,** or **hydrocortisone.** This is very similar to the cortisone ("steroids") used to treat noninfectious inflammatory conditions. Glucocorticoids play many roles in normal metabolism and overall body function. This includes a vital part in carbohydrate, protein, and fat metabolism.
3. **Sex hormones,** which are the androgens of the male and estrogen of the female.

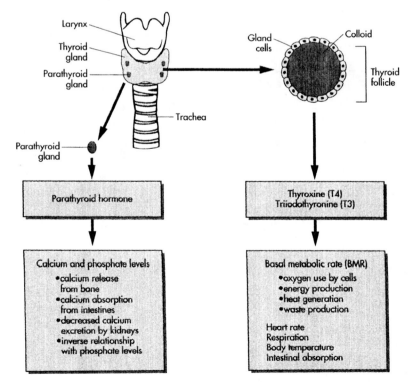

Figure 16–3. Structure and function of the thyroid and parathyroid glands.

16–10

The medulla of the adrenal glands secretes **epinephrine,** or **adrenalin.** This hormone is released in times of severe stress to help the body meet the demands of the situation. It results in increased available energy and strength. It is called the "fight or flight" hormone. It stimulates increased cardiac output, blood pressure, blood glucose levels, and blood flow to muscles. The "jump start" effect of epinephrine is useful as a treatment in cases of shock or cardiac arrest. Please refer to Figure 16–4 for the structure and function of the adrenal glands.

16–11

In some texts, the disease diabetes mellitus is presented as an endocrine disease, since insulin is a hormone. In other texts, this disease may be found in the chapter dealing with diseases of the pancreas, since insulin is produced by the islets of Langerhans in the pancreas. In this text, it was presented in Chapter 8 on metabolic diseases, since diabetes represents a gross abnormality in carbohydrate and fat metabolism.

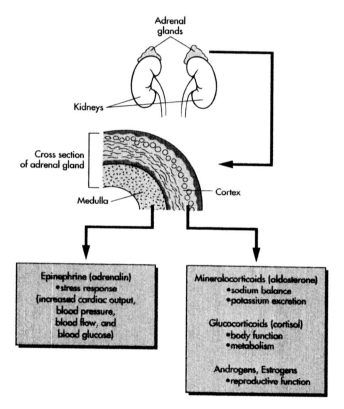

Figure 16–4. Structure and function of the adrenal glands.

II. DISEASES OF THE PITUITARY GLAND ◄ SECTION

► HYPERPITUITARISM

16-12

Diseases of the pituitary gland are not very common. The first disorder we will consider is **hyperpituitarism,** or excessive secretion of one or several of the trophic hormones. Since the hormones of the pituitary target the glands and therefore hormones of the body, over-secretion of trophic hormones causes excessive stimulation of target glands and over-secretion of the working hormones. The working hormones, such as cortisol or thyroxine, then overexert their effect on body tissues. In hyperpituitarism, the specific hormones that are oversecreted depend on which pituitary cells are affected, since specialized cells each create a different hormone. The cause of hyperpituitarism is a tumor of the gland. In general, a tumor of a gland is called a (an) _____(1). The adenomas of the pituitary are named according to the cell type that is neoplastic. Pituitary adenomas are generally benign, and their early surgical removal is because of the signs they cause. There are also nonfunctioning adenomas, which means there are tumors that secrete only a minimal amount of hormone. The significance of a nonfunctional adenoma is that it may cause difficulty as a space-occupying lesion. It may grow to the point where it compresses the optic nerves and interferes with vision. Hyperpituitarism is _____(2) secretion of _____(3). This in turn causes overstimulation of the _____(4) in the body and oversecretion of their _____(5). Hyperpituitarism is caused by the presence of a neoplastic growth called a (an) _____(6). They are named according to the _____(7) that has proliferated.

1. adenoma
2. excessive
3. trophic hormones
4. target glands
5. working hormones
6. adenoma
7. cell type

16-13

The most common pituitary tumor affects the cells that manufacture prolactin, so the tumor is called a **prolactinoma.** The predominant signs of a prolactinoma in women is amenorrhea, anovulation, and milk production, or lactation, when the woman is not pregnant. In men, the signs are nonspecific and usually include loss of libido and impotence. A tumor of the cells that secrete growth hormone is called a **somatotrophic adenoma.** If a somatotrophic adenoma develops before puberty, the growth plates at the ends of the long bones have not yet closed and so are still responsive to stimulation. Excessive growth hormone, or somatotropin, prevents sealing of the growth plates and causes excessive growth in height. This condition is called **gigantism,** and the individual may reach a height of 8 feet. In adults, excessive growth hormone causes the condition **acromegaly.** This is thickening and enlargement of the bones at the end of the extremities (the hands and feet) and the bones of the face. Adults with acromegaly do not become very tall but have large hands and feet and broad, coarse facial features, as shown in Figure 16–5. Growth hormone also stimulates the enlargement of most of the soft tissue of the body. Internal organs, such as the heart, enlarge. It also causes metabolic disturbances. A **corticotropic adenoma** is a tumor of the cells that make ACTH. Therefore, the tumor produces too much ACTH, and this leads to overstimulation of the adrenal cortex to secrete glucocorticoids. This causes a disorder called Cushing's disease, which will be discussed in Frame 16–40.

16-14

The most common pituitary tumor is called a _____(1) because it is of the cells that secrete _____(2). A somatotrophic adenoma leads to too much secretion of _____(3). The effects of excessive levels of growth hormone depend on the _____(4) of the patient. In children, the condition is called _____(5) because they _____(6) several feet taller than normal. In adults, it is called _____(7), and it results in enlargement of the _____(8) of the hands, feet, and face. It also causes enlargement of internal _____(9) and interferes with normal _____(10). Treatment of pituitary tumors consists of surgical removal if possible (access to the pituitary gland is

1. prolactinoma
2. prolactin
3. growth hormone
4. age
5. gigantism
6. grow
7. acromegaly
8. bones
9. organs
10. metabolism

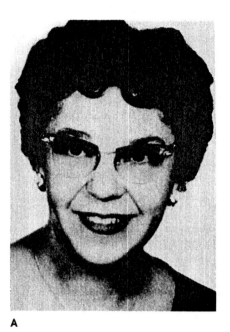
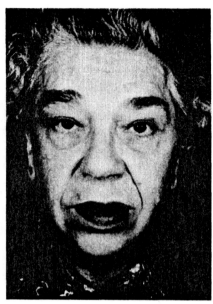

A   **B**

Figure 16–5. Facial features in acromegaly. **A.** Before development of acromegaly. **B.** After development of acromegaly. *(From Kent and Hart,* Introduction to Human Diseases, *3rd ed., Appleton & Lange.)*

through the nose). Radiation may be successful in shrinking the tumor. In acromegaly, removal greatly improves metabolic difficulties, but bony enlargement is permanent.

▶ HYPOPITUITARISM

16-15

1. hypopituitarism
2. target glands
3. atrophy
4. working hormones
5. injury
6. destruction
7. panhypopituitarism

Just as oversecretion of pituitary trophic hormones affects body glands, undersecretion does as well. Absence of pituitary trophic hormones causes widespread failure of the body's glands, which require stimulation to function. If target glands are not properly stimulated to secrete their hormones, the glands will **atrophy,** or wither away. For instance, lack of TSH (thyroid-stimulating hormone) will lead to thyroid gland atrophy, insufficient thyroid hormones, and hypothyroidism. **Hypopituitarism** is undersecretion of pituitary trophic hormones. Pituitary insufficiency is caused by some kind of injury to the gland, which produces destruction of the functioning cells. Examples of injuries that cause such destruction are ischemia, infarction, trauma, infection (encephalitis or meningitis), hemorrhage, and tumors. In **panhypopituitarism,** all of the glandular anterior cells have been destroyed by the injury ("pan" means all). Other types of pituitary insufficiency may be limited to specific cells and their trophic hormones. Lack of sufficient production and secretion of pituitary trophic hormones is called _____(1). It will lead to understimulation of the _____(2) of the body and allow the glands to _____(3). In turn, the glands of the body will not release their own _____(4), and this causes specific disorders. Hypopituitarism is caused by some _____(5) that results in _____(6) of the glandular cells. If all of the cell types are destroyed, this is called _____(7).

In hypopituitarism, the signs will depend on which trophic hormones are lacking, if not all. Lack of thyroid stimulation and insufficient thyroxine causes a decrease in basal metabolism rate with lethargy and cold intolerance (hypothyroidism). Lack of adrenal stimulation causes cortisol insufficiency with resulting interference in nutrient metabolism and sodium or salt balance (Addison's disease). Insufficient gonadal stimulation causes impaired sexual development in children and amenorrhea or loss of libido in adults. You will understand and appreciate these effects more once we discuss some of these disorders in the next two sections.

1. child
2. panhypopituitarism
3. growth hormone
4. gigantism

Panhypopituitarism in children leads to the opposite of gigantism. These children experience **pituitary dwarfism.** Growth cannot be stimulated if growth hormone is lacking. While mental development is usually normal, these children become adults who are both physically and sexually underdeveloped. Besides being of very small stature, these individuals have extremities and heads that are out of proportion with the trunk of the body. Pituitary dwarfism occurs when a _____(1) has the disease _____(2). Lack of normal growth and development is because of insufficient levels of _____(3). This condition is the opposite of _____(4).

If the injury affects the posterior pituitary, it results in insufficient amounts of antidiuretic hormone. This causes the disease diabetes insipidus, which was presented in Chapter 3. Disease of the hypothalamus can also cause diabetes insipidus since ADH is actually manufactured there. ADH prevents too much water loss by making the kidneys resorb a certain amount of fluid. Its lack leads to the excretion of a large volume of a dilute urine, which is called polyuria. To prevent dehydration, the body responds with excessive thirst and drinking, or polydipsia. Treatment of hypopituitarism is by replacement therapy, where the missing hormones are administered as medication. Thyroxine, cortisol, and the sex hormones may be replaced this way. Growth hormone is very effective to prevent dwarfism, and ADH is also effective in diabetes insipidus.

II. REVIEW QUESTIONS

1. In the disease state hyperpituitarism, the *end result* is:
   a. oversecretion of trophic hormones from the pituitary
   b. overstimulation of the target glands of the body
   c. oversecretion of working hormone from target glands
   d. overexertion of the effects on the body by working hormones

2. The general cause of hyperpituitarism is:
   a. excessive stimulation by releasing factors from the hypothalamus
   b. a functional adenoma
   c. a functional carcinoma
   d. idiopathic hyperplasia of the anterior pituitary

3. A somatotrophic adenoma of the anterior pituitary secretes excess
   a. _____ hormone, which produces b. _____ in children and
   c. _____ in adults.

1. d–overexertion of the effects on the body by working hormones

2. b–a functional adenoma

3. a–growth; b–gigantism; c–acromegaly

4. Hyperpituitarism may cause secondary hyperadrenalism by the secretion of too much
   a. _____. This secondary disease of the adrenals is known by the common
   name b. _____.
   a. TSH
   b. Conn's syndrome
   c. prolactin
   d. Cushing's syndrome
   e. Addison's disease
   f. ACTH

5. Choose the INCORRECT statement about hypopituitarism:
   a. target glands atrophy from lack of trophic hormone stimulation
   b. hypopituitarism generally results from injury that causes destruction of the glandular cells
   c. panhypopituitarism causes secondary hyperactive states of the target glands of the body
   d. hypopituitarism is undersecretion of pituitary trophic hormones

6. Panhypopituitarism in children causes:
   a. gigantism
   b. dwarfism
   c. cretinism
   d. acromegaly

7. Diabetes insipidus is the result of:
   a. lack of ACTH from the diseased anterior pituitary
   b. lack of ACTH from the diseased posterior pituitary
   c. lack of ADH from the diseased anterior pituitary
   d. lack of ADH from the diseased posterior pituitary

SECTION ▶ **III. DISEASES OF THE THYROID AND PARATHYROID GLANDS**

▶ HYPERTHYROIDISM

Hyperthyroidism is hyperactivity of the thyroid gland and therefore hypersecretion of thyroxine and overstimulation of the basal metabolic rate. There are several causes of hyperthyroidism, all of which result in enlargement of the thyroid. In one cause, hyperactivity is the result of a functional (hormone-producing) tumor. The enlargement is in nodular fashion. The general term for an enlarged thyroid gland is **goiter.** Clinically, it is seen as a bulge of various sizes in the neck. In the case of a functional tumor, it is called an **adenomatous** (glandular) **goiter.** Oversecretion of thyroxine by the tumor causes the signs and symptoms of hyperthyroidism, which are many. They are the result of the acceleration of the normal effects of thyroxine. The signs and symptoms include nervousness, irritability, fatigue, muscle weakness, tremors (shaky hands), tachycardia and rapid pulse, heat intolerance, profuse sweating, and weight loss in spite of increased appetite. Calories are burned at a tremendous rate and the passage of food through the digestive tract is accelerated. If the tumor reaches a significant size, it becomes problematic as a space-occupying lesion if it compresses the trachea or esophagus. Overactivity of the thyroid gland causes the disease _____(1), where there is excessive secretion of _____(2). This results in too much stimulation of the _____(3). All of the normal effects of thyroxine are _____(4). Hyperthyroidism causes _____(5) of the gland itself. The general term for thyroid enlargement is _____(6). One cause of hyperthyroidism is a _____(7) that is functional, which means it secretes _____(8).

16–20

The most common cause of hyperthyroidism is **Graves' disease.** It is also the most severe form of hyperthyroidism. The population most frequently affected is young women. There may be some genetic basis for the disease. The goiter or enlargement in this case is not due to a tumor. Instead of a nodular type of swelling, as in adenomatous goiter, it is a diffuse swelling. The etiology of Graves' disease has not been proven, but it is generally accepted to be an autoimmune disease. Autoantibodies are formed against antigens in the thyroid. These antigens are the TSH receptors, where TSH from the anterior pituitary gland connects with the thyroid cells to stimulate them. In this case, the autoantibodies displace TSH and bind to the antigens in its place. The antibody–antigen complex then continuously stimulates the follicular cells to produce and release thyroxine. The supposed autoimmune basis of this hyperactivity is supported by the histologic finding of heavy lymphocyte infiltration of the thyroid. The thyroid gland hypertrophies in response to the constant stimulation. Since the glandular tissue is functional, hypersecretion of thyroxine and clinical hyperthyroidism results. Graves' disease is the most _____(1) cause of _____(2). In addition, it is the most _____(3) kind of hyperthyroidism. It is most likely a (an) _____(4) disease, in which _____(5) are formed against _____(6) in the thyroid. The antigens are the _____(7) receptors, and so they are the site of stimulation of the gland. In this case, the thyroid is continuously stimulated by the _____(8) complexes and secretes far too much _____(9).

16–21

As was mentioned in Frame 16–20, the effects of Graves' disease can be quite severe. While the appetite can be voracious, weight loss is pronounced to the point of cachexia. Diarrhea is common since water resorption is decreased because of the speed of passage of material through the digestive tract. The water loss of diarrhea combines with heavy sweating to threaten dehydration. Excessive thirst, or polydipsia, is a compensatory mechanism. The facial appearance of a patient with Graves' disease is very recognizable. Edema and swelling of soft tissue behind the eyes causes them to bulge out in a "pop-eyed" appearance. This protrusion is called **exophthalmos.** It produces a startled look and a staring effect, as shown in Figure 16–6. In really severe cases, the eyelids cannot close and there is pressure on the optic nerves. The most significant consequence of Graves' disease is its effects on the heart. Over time, the accelerated metabolic activity and heart activity can lead to heart failure. This is called **thyrotoxic myopathy.**

16–22

Another cause of hyperthyroidism is **toxic nodular goiter.** This is not due to a tumor but is a hyperplastic nodular enlargement whose cause is unknown. An unknown cause is described as _____(1). Hyperthyroidism may also be caused by **Hashimoto's disease,** which is also more common in women. The gland enlargement is due to massive infiltration by immune cells (T lymphocytes and plasma cells). In this case of goiter, the hyperthyroidism is short lived and mild. It is followed by a return to normal thyroxine levels (which is called **euthyroid**) and then to hypothyroidism (see Frame 16–24). This is also considered an autoimmune disease, with autoantibodies that target the TSH receptors. However, the difference from Graves' disease is that after initial stimulation and hypersecretion, the antibodies destroy the follicles, which is the reason for later hyposecretion. The cause of toxic nodular goiter is _____(2). The cause of Hashimoto's disease is _____(3) disease. Autoantibodies target the _____(4) receptors and cause mild _____(5). Initial stimulation is replaced by _____(6) of follicles, which causes _____(7)secretion of thyroxine. An overview of hyperthyroidism is shown in Figure 16–7.

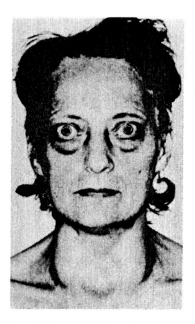

Figure 16–6. Exophthalmos in Graves' disease. The eyes are bulging and pop-eyed, with a staring expression. The enlarged thyroid gland causes swelling of the neck. *(From Mulvihill,* Human Diseases: A Systemic Approach, *4th ed., Appleton & Lange.)*

16–23

There are several approaches to the treatment of hyperthyroidism. Antithyroid medication suppresses gland function by interfering with the production of thyroxine. Parts of the thyroid gland may be destroyed by the use of radioactive iodine, which is administered and then picked up by the gland for use in hormone production. Surgical removal of the entire gland (thyroidectomy) requires hormone replacement therapy afterwards on a permanent basis. Removal of part of the gland (partial thyroidectomy), in theory, leaves enough tissue for normal thyroxine production.

▶ HYPOTHYROIDISM

16–24

1. hypothyroidism
2. thyroxine
3. myxedema
4. injury
5. hyperthyroidism
6. removal
7. radiation or radioactive iodine

Hypothyroidism is just the opposite of hyperthyroidism. There is underactivity of the gland and hyposecretion of thyroxine. Adults with severe hypothyroidism are sometimes described as having **myxedema.** Myxedema is swelling due to fluid and to abnormal deposits of mucoproteins. Myxedema, or severe hypothyroidism, most commonly affects middle-aged women. Secondary hypothyroidism, which is not common, is due to disease of the pituitary gland and subsequent hypopituitarism. There is inadequate TSH secretion and inadequate thyroid stimulation. Primary hypothyroidism is more common and may be caused by injury to the thyroid gland, atrophy of the gland, or iodine deficiency. Of these causes, the most common reason for the development of hypothyroidism is gland injury caused by treatment for hyperthyroidism. Surgical removal of the gland, or a large part of it, as well as destruction by radiation (radioactive iodine), often leaves the patient without enough functioning thyroid to remain euthyroid, or normal. This is called iatrogenic (treatment-induced) hypothyroidism. Administration of thyroxine is required for the life of the patient. Since iatrogenic hypothyroidism is so effectively treated, the outcome is actually better than leaving hyperthyroidism untreated. Insufficient thyroid gland activity is called _____(1). In this condition, there is not enough secretion of _____(2). Severe cases in adults are described as _____(3). Primary hypothyroidism is most commonly caused by _____(4) to the thyroid gland during treatment for _____(5). The reasons for injury to the thyroid include surgical _____(6) of much of the gland or destruction by _____(7).

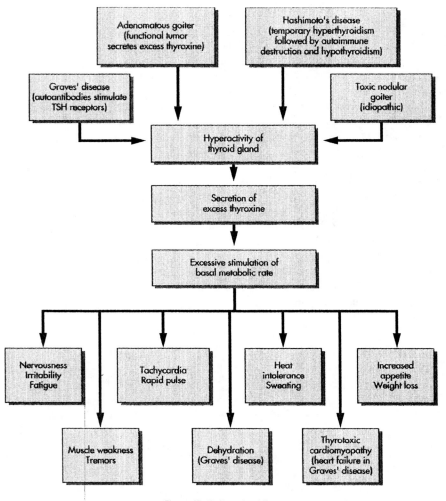

Figure 16–7. Hyperthyroidism.

16–25

Iodine deficiency is rare in this country because iodine is an additive in table salt. More about iodine deficiency will be discussed under the general topic of goiter (see Frame 16–28). Atrophy of the thyroid gland is of two main causes. The first is idiopathic, in which the cause of the atrophy is unknown. The second is Hashimoto's disease. Hashimoto's disease is also called **autoimmune thyroiditis** because this is an immune-mediated inflammation. This is an autoimmune disease that destroys thyroid follicles, causing hypothyroidism. Initially, this disease produces gland enlargement and mild hyperthyroidism. Later, the gland shrinks because of contraction of fibrotic tissue during healing attempts. The shrinking and atrophy result in inadequate secretion of thyroxine. Hashimoto's disease is usually diagnosed in the later stages when the patient has entered hypothyroidism. One cause of atrophy of the thyroid gland is unknown, which is called _____(1). Another is Hashimoto's disease, which is also called _____(2) because this is a (an) _____(3) disease. The inflammation is caused by destruction of the gland by _____(4)antibodies. In the later stages, the gland _____(5) because of _____(6), and there is inadequate secretion of _____(7). This causes the condition of _____(8).

1. idiopathic
2. autoimmune thyroiditis
3. autoimmune
4. auto
5. shrinks
6. fibrotic contraction
7. thyroxine
8. hypothyroidism

Clinical presentations of hypothyroidism, especially myxedema, include bloating of the face, puffy eyelids, minimal sweating, cold intolerance, **somnolence** (excessive sleeping), sluggish mental and physical responses, bradycardia, slow circulation, weight gain, and constipation. Interference in circulation is in part responsible for the characteristic edema of significant hypothyroidism. Constipation results from a decrease in passage time of material in the digestive tract. You will note that the presentation of hypothyroidism is the opposite of the signs we discussed for hyperthyroidism. Treatment for hypothyroidism consists of thyroxine replacement, usually for the life of the patient. Please refer to Figure 16–8 for an overview of hypothyroidism.

There is a congenital defect in which **thyroid aplasia** exists. Aplasia means without form or development. Essentially, it is the absence of a functioning thyroid gland. In the fetus, there may be abnormal formation or complete failure of formation of the thyroid. This may be a random defect or caused by a lack of iodine in the mother. The hypothyroidism caused by this congenital insufficiency of thyroxine is called **cretinism.** Thyroxine is necessary for all normal development processes, so the child suffers from dwarfism (physical stunting) and cretinism (mental retardation). The short stature and severe mental deficiency is accompanied by abnormal facial features (including a slack mouth and thick, protruding tongue), absence of sex organ development, and several metabolic disturbances. Early diagnosis and

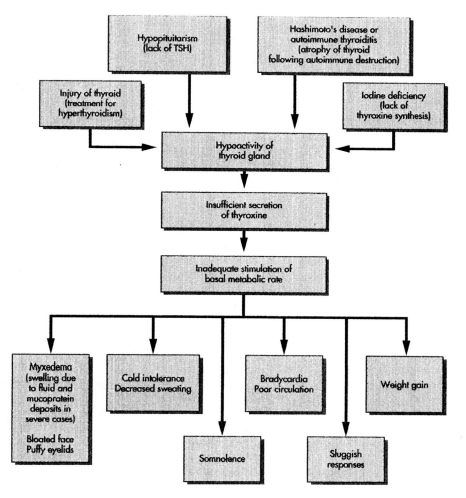

Figure 16–8. Hypothyroidism.

lifelong thyroxine replacement therapy greatly improve the prognosis for relatively normal development. Even mild cases of hypothyroidism in babies should be identified with blood tests and treated with thyroxine. Thyroid aplasia is a _____(1) defect in which there is lack of normal formation of the _____(2). This results in the condition of _____(3) in infants, which is specifically called _____(4). This term is applied to the mental _____(5) the child suffers. There is also dwarfism, which is lack of _____(6) development, as well as _____(7) disturbances.

1. congenital
2. thyroid gland
3. hypothyroidism
4. cretinism
5. retardation
6. physical
7. metabolic

► GOITER

Having already been introduced to the term goiter, you know that it means _____(1) of the thyroid gland. *Both* overstimulation (hyperactivity) and understimulation (hypoactivity) will cause enlargement of the thyroid. The association between hyperactivity and enlargement is easy to understand. More and more follicles respond to the stimulation and secrete thyroxine. The association between hypoactivity and enlargement is because of hyperplasia of the tissue in an attempt to make up for insufficient thyroxine levels. TSH from the anterior pituitary is secreted continuously as part of the positive feedback mechanism. In addition, the negative feedback signals don't kick in because normal thyroxine levels are not reached. Not all goiters represent a functional disturbance (either a hyper- or hypoactive state). Some enlargements are nonfunctional mass lesions or non-neoplastic growths. Whatever the cause, goiters present as a swelling in the neck ranging anywhere from a slight bulge to a very large round mass. Enlargement of the thyroid gland, or _____(2), can be caused by both _____(3), and _____(4), of the gland. A goiter may be due to an abnormal activity state, which is a _____(5) disturbance, or to a nonfunctional _____(6) lesion. A goiter appears as a _____(7) in the neck of various sizes.

1. enlargement
2. goiter
3. overstimulation, or hyperactivity
4. understimulation, or hypoactivity
5. functional
6. mass
7. swelling

One cause of nonfunctional goiter is iodine deficiency. The condition has several names, which are **diffuse colloidal goiter, nontoxic** (nonfunctional) **goiter,** and **endemic goiter.** The term "endemic goiter" comes from the fact that certain areas of the country and of the world have an iodine deficiency in the soil and water. Endemic goiter is much more likely to be seen where the diet is not supplemented with iodine. This condition is common in some parts of the world. The term "diffuse colloidal goiter" relates to the fact that the center of the thyroid follicles are made of colloid, a protein, and synthesized thyroxine is secreted into the colloid for storage. In the absence of enough iodine, and insufficient thyroxine, too much colloid is produced, which causes the gland to swell. However, the reason this goiter is usually not associated with hypothyroidism is because enough hormone is able to be produced to prevent signs. The thyroxine levels in iodine deficiency goiter are often normal or just slightly low. There may be no other signs other than swelling in the neck. Occasionally, there may be so much swelling that the goiter causes problems as a space-occupying lesion, which may require surgical reduction in size. Otherwise, the usual treatment is dietary iodine supplement.

Iodine deficiency causes a _____(1) goiter. The description "endemic goiter" is related to deficiency of iodine in the _____(2) and _____(3) in some parts of this country and the world. It is usually a problem only if the diet is not supplemented with _____(4). The phrase "diffuse colloidal goiter" describes the effect of the deficiency, which causes follicles to swell because excessive _____(5) has been produced. Hypothyroidism is generally not seen in nontoxic goiter because sufficient levels of _____(6) can still be produced. Another cause of nontoxic goiter falls into the ever-present idiopathic category. In this case, the enlargement is due to the presence of swollen nodules instead of the diffuse swelling in iodine deficiency. **Idiopathic nodular goiters** are euthyroid (neither hyper- nor hypothyroid)

1. nonfunctional
2. soil
3. water
4. iodine
5. colloid
6. thyroxine or hormone

and are a problem only as large space-occupying lesions in the neck. Figure 16–9 shows various presentations of goiter.

▶ NEOPLASIA OF THE THYROID GLAND

16-31

Neoplasia of the thyroid gland is fairly common, but the majority of the growths are benign. They are small, well-encapsulated nodules that do not produce any signs or disease even as a space-occupying lesion. They are nonfunctional adenomas that don't require treatment. Malignant thyroid neoplasia is rare. The affected population is often younger women. The risk factors for thyroid cancer have not been identified as they have been for some cancers. Thyroid cancer is a carcinoma that arises from the follicular cells. It is divided into four types, based on the histology of the tumor. The most common type is **papillary thyroid carcinoma.** This type makes up over 80 percent of the cases. It is typically a low-grade malignancy and is nonfunctional, so hyperthyroidism does not exist. Initial spread is to local lymph nodes, and distant metastasis does not occur until very late in the disease. With sur-

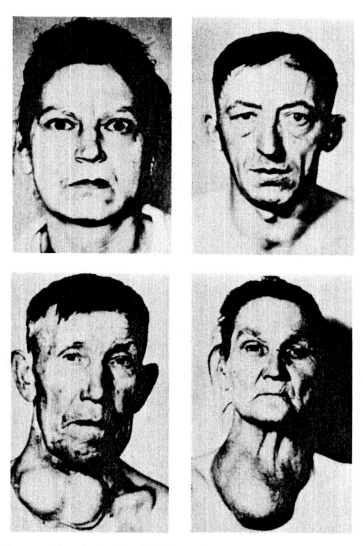

Figure 16–9. Various presentations of goiter. *(From Mulvihill,* Human Diseases: A Systemic Approach, *4th ed., Appleton & Lange.)*

gical removal and hormone replacement therapy, the prognosis is very good, with an approximate 80 percent 10-year survival rate. Neoplasia affecting the thyroid gland is _____(1) common / uncommon (choose one), and most of the tumors are _____(2). They do not cause any _____(3) and do not need _____(4). Malignant cases are one of _____(5) types, the most common being _____(6). The grade of malignancy is _____(7), and the tumor is not _____(8). Because it is a low-grade malignancy, distant _____(9) does not develop until much later in the disease.

1. uncommon
2. benign
3. signs
4. treatment
5. four
6. papillary thyroid carcinoma
7. low
8. functional
9. metastasis

► HYPERPARATHYROIDISM

16-32

Since the parathyroid glands regulate blood calcium and phosphate levels through parathyroid hormone, abnormalities in function create high or low levels of blood calcium and phosphate. As with other endocrine system disturbances, diseases of the parathyroid glands is seen as hyper- or hypoactivity. **Hyperparathyroidism** is hyperactivity of the parathyroid glands that results in increased secretion of parathyroid hormone. Primary hyperparathyroidism arises from a disturbance in the glands. Most cases are due to benign neoplasia, an adenoma. In this instance, only the affected gland is enlarged. Some primary cases are due to hyperplasia of the glands, in which instance all four glands are enlarged. A very few cases are due to malignant carcinoma. Secondary hyperparathyroidism arises from a disturbance outside of the glands. Most cases are due to chronic renal failure. Secondary cases look just like primary hyperplasia because all four glands are enlarged. In renal failure, too much phosphate is retained and too much calcium is lost. This lowers blood calcium and so causes continuous stimulation of the glands to secrete parathyroid hormone to raise the levels of calcium. A significant vitamin D deficiency can also lead to low calcium and secondary hyperparathyroidism.

16-33

The parathyroid glands govern levels of _____(1) and _____(2) present in the _____(3), so disease of these glands causes _____(4) levels of these electrolytes. Hyperactivity and hypersecretion of _____(5) describes the disease _____(6). Abnormalities within the glands is _____(7) hyperparathyroidism. Abnormalities elsewhere in the body that affect the glands is _____(8) hyperparathyroidism. Most primary cases are because of _____(9) neoplasia, called a (an) _____(10). Secondary cases are most often due to _____(11) failure. Secondary hyperparathyroidism is because of continual _____(12) of the glands because of low blood _____(13).

1. calcium
2. phosphate
3. blood
4. high or low
5. parathyroid hormone
6. hyperparathyroidism
7. primary
8. secondary
9. benign
10. adenoma
11. renal or kidney
12. stimulation
13. calcium

16-34

Hyperplastic, or enlarged, parathyroid cells secrete excessive parathyroid hormone. This hormone raises blood calcium by causing its release from bone (resorption), decreasing its excretion by the kidneys, and helping in formation of active vitamin D for calcium absorption from the intestines. These activities raise calcium levels to normal, or else maintain them at normal. Therefore, too much parathyroid hormone creates high blood calcium levels, or **hypercalcemia.** Since phosphate levels are kept opposite to calcium, this also causes low phosphate, or **hypophosphatemia.** (The levels are opposite because equal levels may lead to formation of calcium phosphate crystals and their precipitation in the body.) Excessive levels of parathyroid hormone creates _____(1) and _____(2) in the blood because of the action of this hormone. It draws calcium from the _____(3), keeps it in the body through the _____(4), and promotes its absorption from the _____(5).

1. hypercalcemia
2. hypophosphatemia
3. bones
4. kidneys
5. intestines

The clinical presentations of both primary and secondary hyperparathyroidism are the same and relate to the effects of hypercalcemia. Loss of calcium from the bone (decalcification) causes bone to lose its normal rigidity and become rubbery. It may become deformed through bending. Such weakened bone is susceptible to pathologic fracture, although this is seen only in advanced cases. (A pathologic fracture is a break, not because of trauma but because of weakness from disease.) This decalcification may be seen on x-ray of certain bones. The hypercalcemia, created by all three mechanisms of increase, leads to precipitation of the calcium in the body and deposits of calcium in soft tissues. Calcium in soft tissue makes it hard, as it does in bones. Walls of several organs may become affected, as well as blood vessels. The most notable site of deposit is in the kidneys where it interferes with normal function. Formation of kidney stones, nephrolithiasis, is the most common presentation in this disease. Another significant consequence of hypercalcemia is interference in muscle contraction and depression of nerve impulse conduction. This creates weakness, which also affects the heart. Cardiac arrhythmias are not uncommon because of abnormal nerve impulses. Other signs are related to interference in function by deposits of calcium in organs. The signs and symptoms of hyperparathyroidism are due to the effects of _____(1). Please refer to Figure 16–10 for a summary of hyperparathyroidism.

Primary hyperparathyroidism because of an adenoma is treated surgically, with the removal of only the neoplastic gland. In cases of hyperplasia, primary or secondary, generally three of the glands are removed. Leaving one hyperactive gland can usually maintain normal calcium–phosphate homeostasis. Secondary hyperplasia should be approached by treating the primary cause, such as kidney transplant for failing kidneys. This often will normalize the glands enough so that surgical removal is not necessary.

▶ HYPOPARATHYROIDISM

In **hypoparathyroidism,** hypoactivity of the parathyroid glands leads to insufficient secretion of parathyroid hormone. This is a rare disorder that can be congenital, genetic, or autoimmune in nature. The most common reason for hypoparathyroidism is removal of the parathyroid glands during treatment for hyperthyroidism (removal of the thyroid or thyroidectomy), or during neck surgery for cancer. Complete removal of all four parathyroid glands is an unintentional complication of such surgery. Their location, embedded in the thyroid gland, can make it difficult to spare them. Insufficient parathyroid hormone produces **hypocalcemia.** There is not enough normal bone resorption to release calcium, and not enough retention by the kidneys. Hypoparathyroidism results in hyposecretion of _____(1). The most common cause of hypoparathyroidism is inadvertent removal of _____(2) during treatment of _____(3) or some other neck surgery. Inadequate parathyroid hormone causes _____(4) because there is not enough release of _____(5) from the _____(6) or retention by the _____(7).

You know that blood calcium plays a vital role in nerve impulse conduction and muscle contraction (see Chap. 3). In hypocalcemia, there is sensitized neuromuscular excitability that causes the muscles to become spastic. The sustained contractions that are seen are called **hypocalcemic tetany.** A common presentation is contraction of the fingers that make the hand look claw-like. Nerve function varies between depression and hyperexcitability. The tetany results from overstimulation of the muscles, which is also described as increased irritability. In severe cases, there may be cardiac arrest, convulsions, or laryngeal spasm and suffocation. Emergency treatment for hypocalcemia is intravenous administration of calcium. Hormone replacement therapy with parathyroid hormone is required on a long-term basis. The signs seen in hypocalcemia are related to the effect this electrolyte has on _____(1) and _____(2) function. Spastic muscular contractions in this disorder are described as _____(3).

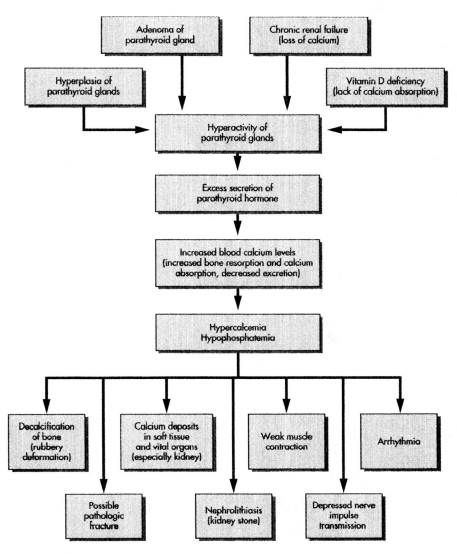

Figure 16–10. Hyperparathyroidism.

III. REVIEW QUESTIONS

1. The *end result* of hyperthyroidism is:
   a. overstimulation of the basal metabolic rate
   b. the production of a goiter
   c. hyperactivity of the thyroid gland
   d. hypersecretion of thyroxine

2. In hyperthyroidism, oversecretion of thyroxine causes:
   a. an adenomatous goiter
   b. Graves' disease
   c. acceleration of metabolism
   d. depression of metabolism

1. a—overstimulation of the basal metabolic rate

2. c—acceleration of metabolism

3. b–Graves' disease

4. d–autoimmune disease

5. b–overstimulation of follicles by autoantibodies bound to TSH receptors

6. c–heart (thyrotoxic myopathy)

7. a–severe hypothyroidism

8. b–iatrogenic injury of the thyroid gland during treatment of hyperthyroidism

9. e–iodine deficiency is a more common cause than states of atrophy

10. 1. e–thyroid aplasia
    2. g–formation
    3. h–dwarfism
    4. c–cretinism

3. The most common cause of hyperthyroidism is:
   a. adenomatous goiter
   b. Graves' disease
   c. Hashimoto's disease
   d. diffuse colloidal goiter

4. In the most severe form of hyperthroidism, the cause is generally accepted to be:
   a. a functional tumor
   b. iodine deficiency
   c. idiopathic nodular goiter
   d. autoimmune disease

5. In Graves' disease, hypersecretion of thyroxine is most likely due to:
   a. overstimulation of follicles by TSH from the anterior pituitary
   b. overstimulation of follicles by autoantibodies bound to TSH receptors
   c. overproduction of thyroxine by a functional adenoma
   d. excessive iodine in the diet

6. The most significant consequence of Graves' disease is its effects on the:
   a. thyroid (adenomatous goiter)
   b. basal metabolic rate
   c. heart (thyrotoxic myopathy)
   d. eyes (exophthalmos)

7. Myxedema is a condition of excessive swelling due to fluid accumulation and mucoprotein deposits that is seen in cases of:
   a. severe hypothyroidism
   b. severe hyperthyroidism
   c. Hashimoto's disease
   d. Graves' disease

8. Primary hypothyroidism is *most commonly* caused by:
   a. autoimmune-mediated injury of the thyroid gland
   b. iatrogenic injury of the thyroid gland during treatment of hyperthyroidism
   c. hypopituitarism and inadequate TSH secretion
   d. iodine deficiency

9. Choose the INCORRECT statement about causes of primary hypothyroidism:
   a. atrophy of the thyroid may be idiopathic
   b. atrophy of the thyroid may be due to autoimmune destruction
   c. autoimmune destruction is called autoimmune thyroiditis
   d. autoimmune destruction is also called Hashimoto's disease
   e. iodine deficiency is a more common cause of primary hypothyroidism than atrophy

10. A congenital form of hypothyroidism is due to 1. _____. This means there is lack of 2. _____ of the thyroid gland. Infants who are afflicted with this defect, if untreated, will suffer from physical stunting, or 3. _____, and mental retardation, or 4. _____.
   a. thyroxine
   b. myxedema
   c. cretinism
   d. goiter
   e. thyroid aplasia
   f. gigantism
   g. formation
   h. dwarfism

11. Enlargement of the thyroid, or goiter, may be caused by (choose all that are correct):
    a. autoimmune destruction
    b. understimulation of the thyroid gland
    c. idiopathic atrophy
    d. overstimulation of the thyroid gland

12. Hypothyroidism caused by iodine deficiency may be described as:
    a. endemic goiter
    b. nontoxic goiter
    c. diffuse colloidal goiter
    d. any of the above
    e. none of the above

13. Which of the following statements most accurately describes neoplasia of the thyroid gland?
    a. It is common and most tumors are small and benign.
    b. It is rare and most tumors are malignant.
    c. It is common and most tumors are benign but cause injury as a large space-occupying lesion.
    d. It is common and most tumors are malignant.

14. Disturbance in function of the parathyroid glands generally results in abnormal levels of
    1. _____ and 2. _____ in the blood.
    a. sodium
    b. calcium
    c. glucose
    d. phosphate
    e. cortisol

15. Hyperparathyroidism causes 1. _____ and 2. _____, while hypoparathyroidism causes 3. _____ and 4. _____.
    a. hypophosphatemia
    b. hypercortisolism
    c. hypoglycemia
    d. hypercalcemia
    e. hyperglycemia
    f. hypocalcemia
    g. hypernatremia
    h. hyperphosphatemia

16. Chronic renal failure causes:
    a. primary hyperparathyroidism
    b. secondary hyperparathyroidism
    c. primary hypoparathyroidism
    d. secondary hypoparathyroidism

17. True or false: In chronic renal failure, excessive loss of calcium and retention of phosphate produces blood levels of these electrolytes that stimulate the parathyroid glands. _____

18. Parathyroid hormone raises blood calcium through:
    a. bone resorption to release calcium
    b. kidney loss of calcium through the urine
    c. intestinal loss of calcium through the stool
    d. all of the above

11. b–understimulation of the thyroid gland; d–overstimulation of the thyroid gland

12. d–any of the above

13. a–it is common and most tumors are small and benign

14. 1. b–calcium
    2. d–phosphate

15. 1. d–hypercalcemia
    2. a–hypophosphatemia
    3. f–hypocalcemia
    4. h–hyperphosphatemia

16. b–secondary hyperparathyroidism

17. True

18. a–bone resorption to release calcium

SECTION ▶ IV. DISEASES OF THE ADRENAL CORTEX AND MEDULLA

▶ HYPERADRENALISM

16-39

The cortex of the adrenal glands produces three corticosteroid hormones—glucocorticoids, mineralocorticoids, and androgens. These hormones are secreted by three different zones of specific cells—the zona glomerulosa, zona fasciculata, and zona reticularis. Each different zone may be affected by hyperplasia or neoplasia, or they may be affected all together. Each hypersecretion of these steroid hormones causes a different syndrome. Therefore, the syndromes may be seen separately or together, depending on which cortex zone is hyperactive. Hyperactivity of one or more zones, and oversecretion of hormone, defines **hyperadrenalism.**

16-40

1. cortisol
2. hypercortisolism
3. steroid
4. outside
5. pituitary
6. ACTH
7. within
8. tumor
9. hyperplasia
10. ACTH
11. paraneoplastic

In a disorder called **Cushing's syndrome,** or **hypercortisolism,** there is excess production of the glucocorticoids, especially cortisol. This hormone most closely resembles the steroid drugs used as medication. Cortisol is the body's natural steroid. There are several causes of endogenous Cushing's syndrome. These include:

1. Hyperpituitarism, in which a pituitary tumor secretes excessive ACTH. This causes continuous stimulation of the adrenal cortex to secrete glucocorticoids. The adrenal glands undergo hyperplasia in response to the stimulation and increased workload. This is **secondary hyperadrenalism,** because the stimulus originates outside of the adrenal glands. Secondary hyperadrenalism was historically called **Cushing's disease** to distinguish it from other causes of hypercortisolism.
2. A functional (hormone-secreting) tumor of the cortex, in which cortisol is secreted to excess. The tumor may be an adenoma or a carcinoma. There are also cases of idiopathic hyperplasia where the gland becomes enlarged and overactive for no apparent reason. A tumor or idiopathic hyperplasia causes **primary hyperadrenalism** because the stimulus originates from within the adrenal gland.
3. Paraneoplastic syndrome, in which a carcinoma tumor somewhere else in the body secretes hormone-like compounds, in this case, ACTH. This is most commonly seen in some forms of lung cancer.

In Cushing's syndrome, there is too much secretion of the glucocorticoid hormone _____(1). This condition is also called _____(2). This hormone is very like _____(3) medications. In secondary hyperadrenalism, the stimulus for cortisol secretion is coming from _____(4) of the glands. It is generally because of a tumor in the _____(5) gland that secretes too much _____(6). In primary hyperadrenalism, the stimulus is coming from _____(7) the glands. It is generally due to a _____(8) of the glands or to _____(9) of the glands. Some forms of cancer may secrete substances closely resembling _____(10), and this is called _____(11) syndrome.

16-41

The *most common* cause of hypercortisolism is **iatrogenic hyperadrenalism.** This is very different from other causes because it is *not* due to overactivity of the adrenal glands. The cause is exogenous, or coming from outside the body. In fact, the glands have shut down to a large extent. You know that iatrogenic means treatment induced. In these cases, corticosteroids have been administered to treat a disease. Steroids decrease both inflammation and immune activity. Disorders responsive to steroid treatment include hypersensitivity such as asthma, and autoimmune diseases such as autoimmune hemolytic anemia, rheumatoid arthritis, and systemic lupus erythematosus. Many skin diseases are also treated with steroids. Suppression of the immune response to decrease rejection of a transplant or graft also requires the use of steroids. This cause of hypercortisolism is also called **exogenous Cushing's syndrome.** This disorder is illustrated in Figure 16–11. In addition to creating high

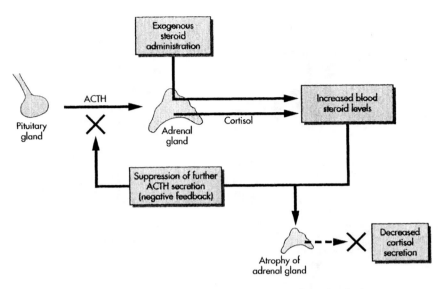

Figure 16–11. Exogenous Cushing's syndrome (iatrogenic hyperadrenalism).

blood levels of cortisol-like drugs, exogenous steroids also cause atrophy of the adrenal glands. The pituitary gland is inhibited from secreting ACTH by high steroid blood levels (the negative feedback mechanism). Absence of ACTH means absence of adrenal gland stimulation and atrophy of the glands. The exogenous steroids have replaced the body's production of cortisol. The most common reason for the development of hypercortisolism is _____(1). It is also called _____(2) Cushing's syndrome. This means that the cortisol-like hormones are coming from _____(3) of the body as a form of _____(4) for some disease. Steroids are used in the treatment of _____(5) and _____(6) disorders. The medication replaces the body's production of _____(7) because the pituitary gland is inhibited by _____(8) feedback and does not secrete ACTH. This leads to _____(9) of the adrenal glands because their function is not needed.

1. iatrogenic hyperadrenalism
2. exogenous
3. outside
4. treatment
5. inflammatory
6. immune-mediated
7. cortisol
8. negative
9. atrophy

16-42

The actions of cortisol in the body include a vital role in carbohydrate and fat metabolism, and in helping the body deal with physical stress. It raises the blood glucose level and raises the level of circulating fats or lipids from body stores. It also causes retention of sodium. Lower levels of steroids dampen the inflammatory response, a fact taken advantage of in treatment. High levels suppress the immune system, which are also used in treatment protocols. The drawback of immune suppression is susceptibility to infection. The clinical presentation of Cushing's syndrome, both endogenous and exogenous, is related to the actions of steroids. A central obesity develops from elevated blood lipids, and the fat is deposited in a characteristic pattern. A fat pad develops on the back between the shoulders, and this is described as a "buffalo hump." Fat deposits and rounding of the face give rise to the description of "moon face." The abdomen protrudes. These features are shown in Figure 16–12. Capillary fragility leads to easy bruising. Retention of sodium and water leads to hypertension. Elevated lipid levels creates atherosclerosis. Osteroporosis develops and the weakened bones are susceptible to pathologic fracture. Raising of the blood glucose causes diabetes, often called adrenal diabetes. Other disturbances include increased body hair (hirsutism), fatigue and muscle weakness, and mental imbalances, sometimes leading to psychosis. Wound healing is poor, and suppressed immune function combined with hyperglycemia makes the patient very susceptible to frequent infection. In iatrogenic Cushing's syndrome, all these harmful effects are considered *less* harmful than allowing the patient to suffer the primary disease without the benefits of steroid therapy. The actions of cortisol on the body include raising blood _____(1) and circulating _____(2), as

1. glucose
2. lipids or fats

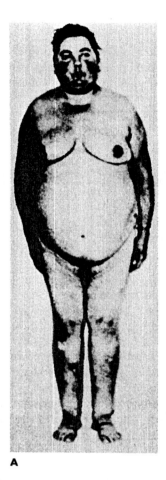 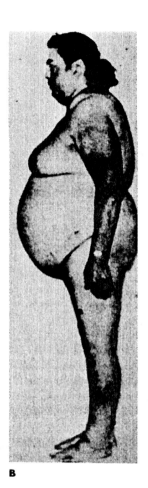

A   B

Figure 16–12. A. The appearance of Cushing's syndrome. Note the round, red face ("moon face"); stock neck; and marked central obesity with protruding abdomen. **B.** A side view shows the fat pads above the collarbone and on the upper back, producing the characteristic "buffalo hump." *(From Mulvihill,* Human Diseases: A Systemic Approach, *4th ed., Appleton & Lange.)*

3. sodium
4. inflammatory
5. immune

16–43

well as increasing retention of _____(3). It also decreases both the _____(4) and _____(5) response depending on its levels.

The treatment of noniatrogenic hypercortisolism is directed toward the cause. A tumor of the pituitary gland or adrenal glands may be surgically removed or reduced in size with chemotherapy or radiation. A hyperplastic adrenal gland may also be removed. Medication to destroy parts of a hyperplastic gland can also be helpful in idiopathic cases. Hormone replacement therapy may be given depending on the amount of functional tissue remaining. In iatrogenic cases, removal of the exogenous steroids produces a good response since the pituitary and adrenal glands were never diseased. However, because of adrenal gland atrophy, it is *vital* that the patient is weaned off of the medication gradually so that positive feedback kicks in and pituitary secretion of ACTH stimulates the adrenal glands to secrete cortisol again. Sudden withdrawal of steroid medication creates an emergency, life-threatening condition described as acute adrenal insufficiency, which is described in Frame 16–50.

Depending on which zones of the adrenal cortex are hyperactive in disease, the following two syndromes may occur to some extent with Cushing's syndrome, which is the most common of the three syndromes. **Conn's syndrome** is also called **primary hyperaldosteronism** because it is hypersecretion of the mineralocorticoid aldosterone. This is a rare disease by itself and is due to a tumor (an adenoma) of the aldosterone-secreting zone of the cortex. It also develops in some cases of hyperplasia of the cortex. You know from Chapter 3 that aldosterone is the "salt keeper" of the body. Excessive aldosterone causes **hypernatremia,** or high sodium levels, because of sodium retention by the kidneys. It also causes **hypokalemia,** or low potassium levels, as more potassium is lost through the kidneys. Sodium retention, and therefore water retention, leads to hypertension. The patient is excessively thirsty because of increased salt in the body, and so polydipsia results. Increased drinking leads to increased urination, or polyuria. Removal of the adrenal gland resolves the hypertension and associated signs. Excessive levels of aldosterone is called _____(1), or _____(2). Hyperaldosteronism causes increased sodium levels in the body, called _____(3), and decreased potassium levels, called _____(4). Sodium retention, and therefore _____(5) retention, leads to increased blood pressure, or _____(6). Poly_____(7) and poly_____(8) are also effects of hyperaldosteronism.

1. Conn's syndrome
2. primary hyperaldosteronism
3. hypernatremia
4. hypokalemia
5. water
6. hypertension
7. dipsia
8. uria

Secondary hyperaldosteronism is more common than the primary state. In kidney disease, renin may be secreted in excess. This increases production of angiotensin, which stimulates secretion of aldosterone and results in sodium and water retention. This is a normal mechanism for maintaining or increasing blood pressure when necessary. Therefore, secondary hyperaldosteronism is most often associated with renal disease, although heart failure and liver cirrhosis can also cause overproduction of aldosterone. _____(1) hyperaldosteronism is more common than primary because it is caused by _____(2) disease. The normal mechanism that supports _____(3) is enhanced because of excess _____(4) secretion by the kidneys. Renin ultimately leads to increased secretion of _____(5) by the adrenal glands. Hypertension results from increased retention of _____(6) and _____(7).

1. Secondary
2. kidney
3. blood pressure
4. renin
5. aldosterone
6. sodium
7. water

In **adrenogenital syndrome,** the zone that produces androgens (male sex hormones) is affected by a functional tumor or hyperplasia. This is a rare disease whose signs most dramatically affect females. There is **virilization,** or development, of male characteristics. The breasts atrophy, the clitoris enlarges, menstruation ceases, facial hair develops, and the voice deepens. This syndrome can also be found as a rare congenital disorder, as an inborn error of steroid and androgen metabolism. Female children experience virilization, and male children experience very premature and enhanced sexual development. In adults, treatment is directed toward the cause of adrenal overproduction of androgens. In children, cortisol administration blocks overproduction of androgens. Females with excessive androgen production develop male characteristics, and this is known as _____(1). It is seen in _____(2) syndrome when this zone of the adrenal cortex is affected by a _____(3) or _____(4). This syndrome can also occur as a _____(5) defect.

1. virilization
2. adrenogenital
3. tumor
4. hyperplasia
5. congenital

► HYPOADRENALISM

An inadequate secretion of hormones from the adrenal glands defines **hypoadrenalism.** It is often called **primary adrenal cortical insufficiency.** Lack of sufficient gland activity stems from one of two problems, either destruction of the gland by disease (which is most common) or neoplasia. Injury to the gland caused by disease can be autoimmune in nature. For this reason, some cases are referred to as **autoimmune adrenalitis,** which is inflammation caused by the activity of autoantibodies directed against glandular tissue. Infection can also

1. inadequate
2. hormones
3. adrenal glands
4. primary adrenal cortical insufficiency
5. destruction
6. disease
7. neoplasia
8. autoimmune
9. infection

cause enough deconstruct to result in gland insufficiency. Historically, tuberculosis was a common infectious cause of injury. Other infections that target the adrenal glands include histoplasmosis and meningococcal septicemia, commonly called Waterhouse–Friderichsen syndrome. Neoplasia of the adrenals may be a primary malignant tumor, which is rare, or a secondary metastasis from the breast or lungs. Hypoadrenalism is _____(1) secretion of _____(2) from the _____(3). This is also known as _____(4). Insufficiency may be caused by _____(5) of the glands from either _____(6) or _____(7). Two causes of disease are _____(8)-mediated inflammation and _____(9).

16–48

1. hypopituitarism
2. pituitary gland
3. ACTH

Secondary adrenal cortical insufficiency is caused by hypoactivity of the pituitary gland, which is called _____(1). Here, decreased ACTH levels do not produce normal stimulation of the adrenal glands. The secretion of both aldosterone and glucocorticoids is affected. Due to lack of adequate cortisol, secondary insufficiency can result in the same life-threatening crisis seen in primary insufficiency, which is discussed with the clinical presentation of hypoadrenalism. Secondary adrenal cortical insufficiency is the result of hypopituitarism, which is insufficient activity of the _____(2). The adrenal glands are not adequately stimulated because of a decrease in _____(3).

16–49

1. Addison's disease
2. cortisol
3. stress
4. metabolism
5. autoimmune
6. idiopathic adrenal cortical atrophy
7. immunosuppressed
8. steroid
9. atrophy

Primary adrenal cortical insufficiency causes the clinical syndrome called **Addison's disease.** Addison's disease represents a lack of normal cortisol blood levels. Since the steroid cortisol enables the body to handle physical stress and maintain normal metabolism, these mechanism are greatly reduced in Addison's disease. Of the causes of this state, listed in Frame 16–47, autoimmune destruction is the most common. In autoimmune adrenalitis, heavy infiltration with immune cells (lymphocytes and plasma cells) is seen histologically. However, because immune-mediated destruction has not been definitively proven, this cause of Addison's disease is called idiopathic adrenal cortical atrophy by some sources. While infection is not as common a cause of injury as it once was, it is still seen in immunosuppressed patients (those with cancer, on chemotherapy, or with AIDS). Another cause of Addison's disease may be iatrogenic, that is, the sudden withdrawal of heavy doses of steroids. Remember that iatrogenic Cushing's disease leads to atrophy of the adrenal glands because it inhibits positive feedback and stimulation by ACTH. Removal of the steroid medication leaves the patient unable to immediately produce his or her own cortisol because of the atrophy. Clinically, primary adrenal insufficiency is called _____(1). In this disorder, there is not enough _____(2) present in the blood. Mechanisms that deal with _____(3) and maintain normal _____(4) are hindered by this lack. The most common cause of Addison's disease is probably _____(5)-mediated destruction, although this state is sometimes called _____(6) to reflect uncertainty about the true cause. Infectious causes are generally seen in _____(7) patients. An iatrogenic cause of Addison's disease may be the abrupt ending of _____(8) treatment, because such treatment leads to _____(9) of the adrenal glands.

16–50

There are many clinical signs and symptoms associated with adrenal cortical insufficiency, all because of inadequate cortisol and aldosterone. These include hyperpigmentation of the skin (due to lack of inhibition of a pituitary hormone by cortisol), fatigue, weakness, weight loss, depression, and GI disturbances. The excessive loss of sodium, and therefore water loss, creates dehydration and hypotension with frequent fainting spells (syncope). Hypoglycemia (due to decreased cortisol), hyponatremia, and hyperkalemia (due to decreased aldosterone) create significant metabolic disturbances. In untreated cases, abnormalities in these electrolyte levels may cause cardiac arrest and death. The lack of the ability to tolerate stress greatly interferes with a normal lifestyle. An **addisonian crisis** is acute adrenal insufficiency that results from significant stress or infection. The body is unable to cope with the stress because of lack of cortisol. Hypotension, hypoglycemia, and electrolyte imbalances become life-threatening. Vomiting and diarrhea develop, which worsens dehydration, hypotension, and electrolyte imbalances. A coma usually precedes death. Treatment of Addison's disease is required to maintain life. Hormone replacement therapy includes corticosteroids, such as prednisone, which must be given on a regular schedule for the life of the patient. An addisonian crisis requires emergency treatment with intravenous administration of corticosteroids along with glucose and sodium in fluids. Please refer to Table 16–1 for an overview of diseases of the adrenal cortex.

▶ PHEOCHROMOCYTOMA

16–51

The last disorders of this chapter concern the adrenal medulla, the inner section of the adrenal glands. The most important cause of disease of the medulla is tumors. In adults, the most common adrenal medulla tumor is the **pheochromocytoma.** Even so, this is still a rare disease. A pheochromocytoma is benign but functional, which means it secretes _____(1). This tumor is often relatively large by the time it is diagnosed. Even though it is rare, its significance lies in the fact that if it is the cause of hypertension, its diag-

1. hormones

TABLE 16–1. DISEASES OF THE ADRENAL CORTEX

Disease	Causes	Features
Hyperadrenalism		
Hypercortisolism (Cushing's syndrome)	Exogenous steroids	Excess production of cortisol
	Functional tumor	Abnormal fat deposits
	Idiopathic	Capillary fragility
	Hyperplasia	Hypertension
	Hyperpituitarism	Atherosclerosis
	Paraneoplastic syndrome	Osteoporosis
		Diabetes
		Weakness
		Psychosis
		Immune suppression
		Poor healing
		Frequent infection
Primary hyperaldosteronism (Conn's syndrome)	Tumor	Sodium retention
	Hyperplasia	Hypertension
		Polydipsia/polyuria
Secondary hyperaldosteronism	Kidney disease	Potassium loss
		Disturbances in nerve transmission and muscle contraction
Adrenogenital syndrome	Tumor	Virilization of females
	Hyperplasia	Premature sexual development of males
Hypoadrenalism		
Primary adrenal cortical insufficiency (Addison's disease)	Gland injury (autoimmune adrenalitis or infection)	Decreased production of cortisol
		Hyperpigmentation
	Tumor	Weakness
	Iatrogenic (withdrawal of steroid treatment)	Weight loss
		Depression
		Dehydration
		Hypotension
		Hypoglycemia
		Hyponatremia
		Hyperkalemia
Secondary adrenal cortical insufficiency	Hypopituitarism	Possible cardiac arrest
		Addisonian crisis
		Acute, severe insufficiency
		Coma
		Death

2. pheochromocytoma
3. benign
4. functional
5. epinephrine
6. norepinephrine
7. vessels
8. constriction
9. pressure
10. hypertension

nosis and surgical removal cures the hypertension. Therefore, some effort to investigate this possible cause should be made in cases of hypertension. If you will remember, the adrenal medulla secretes the vasoactive chemicals epinephrine and norepinephrine. These chemicals are classified as catecholamines. A pheochromocytoma secretes these substances to excess. The vasoconstrictive action of these hormones decreases the vessel lumens, thereby raising blood pressure. Over time, excess levels of these catecholamines also cause heart disease. The prognosis of pheochromocytoma is excellent because these well-encapsulated tumors are easily removed, which allows hemodynamics to return to normal. The most common tumor of the adrenal medulla in adults is the _____(2). This tumor is _____(3) benign / malignant (choose one) and secretes hormones, so it is a _____(4) tumor. The hormones it secretes are the catecholamines _____(5) and _____(6). The activity of these hormones affects the blood _____(7). They cause _____(8) of the vessels, which raises blood _____(9). Therefore, a pheochromocytoma causes a state of _____(10).

NEUROBLASTOMA

16–52

1. children
2. malignant
3. metastasize
4. transformation
5. neuroblasts

A **neuroblastoma** is a malignant tumor of the adrenal medulla in children. It arises from the embryonic fetal precursor cells of the medulla, the neuroblasts. These cells do not differentiate into normal medullary cells but instead undergo malignant transformation. A neuroblastoma is found in newborns and in children under the age of 5. It grows quickly and metastasizes rapidly, often by the time of diagnosis. If it is diagnosed soon enough, even with metastasis, modern cancer treatment greatly improves the prognosis over what it has been historically. A neuroblastoma is a tumor of the adrenal medulla found in _____(1). In contrast to the benign pheochromocytoma of adults, a neuroblastoma is _____(2) and it does spread, or _____(3). A neuroblastoma results from the malignant _____(4) of cells called _____(5).

IV. REVIEW QUESTIONS

1. a–hypercortisolism
   b–hyperaldosteronism
   e–adrenogenital syndrome

2. c–It is part of paraneoplastic syndrome in some cases of carcinoma.

3. b–iatrogenic hyperadrenalism

1. Hyperadrenalism is overactivity of the adrenal glands, which may be seen as (choose all that are correct):
   a. hypercortisolism
   b. hyperaldosteronism
   c. adrenal cortical insufficiency
   d. Addison's disease
   e. adrenogenital syndrome

2. Choose the *correct* statement about hypercortisolism:
   a. It is part of primary hyperadrenalism in cases of hyperpituitarism.
   b. It is part of secondary hyperadrenalism in cases of a functional cortical tumor or idiopathic hyperplasia.
   c. It is part of paraneoplastic syndrome in some cases of carcinoma.
   d. It is known by the common name Addison's disease.

3. The most common cause of hypercortisolism is:
   a. Cushing's syndrome
   b. iatrogenic hyperadrenalism
   c. idiopathic hyperplasia
   d. hyperpituitarism

4. Iatrogenic hyperadrenalism is (choose all that apply):
   a. due to exogenous steroids administered to treat certain diseases
   b. due to endogenous steroids secreted by a functional cortical tumor
   c. also called exogenous Cushing's syndrome
   d. also called endogenous Cushing's syndrome

5. Iatrogenic hyperadrenalism leads to atrophy of the adrenal glands because:
   a. negative feedback mechanisms (high cortisol levels) suppress pituitary release of ACTH
   b. positive feedback mechanisms (low cortisol levels) suppress pituitary release of ACTH
   c. the adrenal glands are injured by treatment for certain diseases
   d. negative feedback mechanisms (low cortisol levels) stimulate pituitary release of ACTH

6. The effects of cortisol of the body are to (choose all that are correct):
   a. raise blood glucose
   b. lower circulating fats
   c. decrease sodium retention
   d. lower blood glucose
   e. suppress the inflammatory response
   f. raise circulating fats
   g. increase the immune response
   h. increase sodium retention
   i. increase the inflammatory response
   j. decrease the immune response

7. The action of aldosterone is to (choose all that are correct):
   a. increase sodium retention
   b. decrease sodium retention
   c. increase potassium loss
   d. decrease potassium loss

8. In hyperaldosteronism or Conn's syndrome:
   a. decreased aldosterone causes hypernatremia and hypokalemia
   b. increased aldosterone causes hypernatremia and hypokalemia
   c. decreased aldosterone causes hyponatremia and hyperkalemia
   d. increased aldosterone causes hyponatremia and hyperkalemia

9. The most common manifestation of hyperaldosteronism is:
   a. a primary state caused by a functional adenoma of the cortex
   b. a primary state caused by hyperpituitarism
   c. a secondary state caused by kidney disease
   d. a secondary state caused by hyperpituitarism

10. Virilization in females is the result of:
    a. Conn's syndrome
    b. adrenogenital syndrome
    c. Cushing's syndrome
    d. Addison's disease

4. a–due to exogenous steroids administered to treat certain diseases; c–also called exogenous Cushing's syndrome

5. a–negative feedback mechanisms (high cortisol levels) suppress pituitary release of ACTH

6. a–raise blood glucose; e–suppress the inflammatory response; f–raise circulating fats; h–increase sodium retention; j–decrease immune response

7. a–increase sodium retention; c–increase potassium loss

8. b–increased aldosterone causes hypernatremia and hypokalemia

9. c–a secondary state caused by kidney disease

10. b–adrenogenital syndrome

11. a–neoplastic destruction of the gland; c–autoimmune destruction of the gland; e–infectious injury of the gland

12. a–Addison's disease

13. d–atrophy of the adrenal gland

14. b–addisonian crisis

15. 1. g–benign
    2. e–medulla
    3. f–adults
    4. a–malignant
    5. e–medulla
    6. b–children

16. c–hypertension

11. Primary adrenal cortical insufficiency may result from (choose all that apply):
    a. neoplastic destruction of the gland
    b. hypopituitarism
    c. autoimmune destruction of the gland
    d. chronic renal disease
    e. infectious injury of the gland

12. Adrenal cortical insufficiency is commonly called:
    a. Addison's disease
    b. Cushing's syndrome
    c. adrenogenital syndrome
    d. Conn's syndrome

13. Iatrogenic hyperadrenalism will lead to primary adrenal cortical insufficiency if treatment is stopped suddenly because of:
    a. destruction of the adrenal cortex by the steroid treatment
    b. destruction of the adrenal medulla by the steroid treatment
    c. atrophy of the pituitary gland
    d. atrophy of the adrenal gland

14. In adrenal cortical insufficiency, a state of emergency which may lead to death is called:
    a. adrenal collapse
    b. addisonian crisis
    c. cortical failure
    d. hypoadrenalism shock

15. A pheochromocytoma is a 1. _____ tumor of the adrenal 2. _____ in 3. _____. A neuroblastoma is a 4. _____ tumor of the adrenal 5. _____ in 6. _____.
    a. malignant
    b. children
    c. metastasis
    d. cortex
    e. medulla
    f. adults
    g. benign

16. A pheochromocytoma causes:
    a. hyperglycemia
    b. hypernatremia
    c. hypertension
    d. hyperkalemia

CHAPTER SUMMARY ▶

▶ SECTION II

Excessive secretion of one or more of the pituitary trophic hormones is called *hyperpituitarism*. The condition results in an overexertion of the effects of the pituitary-dependent hormones, such as cortisol and thyroxine. Hyperpituitarism is caused by a functional (i.e., hormone-secreting) tumor of the gland, characterized as a *prolactinoma* (the tumor affects the prolactin-producing cells), a *somatotropic adenoma* (affecting the growth hormone-producing cells), or a *corticotropic adenoma* (affecting the ACTH-producing cells). *Gigantism, acromegaly,* and *Cushing's disease* are conditions resulting from functional pituitary tumors.

Undersecretion of one or more of the pituitary hormones *(hypopituitarism)* leads to eventual atrophy of other glands. This condition is generally caused by an injury (e.g., ischemia, infarction, trauma) to the pituitary. In *panhypopituitarism,* all of the anterior pituitary cells have been destroyed by an injury. Panhypopituitarism in children results in the condition of *pituitary dwarfism.*

▶ SECTION III

In the condition of *hyperthyroidism,* oversecretion of thyroxine by the thyroid gland leads to a general overstimulation of the basal metabolic rate. Causes of the condition, all of which result in the enlargement of the thyroid *(goiter),* include a functional tumor, Graves' disease, toxic nodular goiter, and Hashimoto's disease. A functional tumor of the thyroid, defined as an *adenomatous goiter,* leads to the signs and symptoms of hyperthyroidism, such as irritability, tremors, tachycardia, and weight loss. *Graves' disease,* the most severe form of hyperthyroidism, is characterized by a diffuse swelling of the thyroid. This condition is considered an autoimmune disorder, since autoantibodies against thyroid antigens are present. Dehydration, polydipsia, exophthalmos, and thyrotoxic myopathy are signs and symptoms of the disease. In *toxic nodular goiter,* hyperplastic nodular enlargement is detected. *Hashimoto's disease,* also an autoimmune condition, is characterized by infiltration, and eventual destruction, of the thyroid by immune cells.

Underactivity of the thyroid gland is defined as *hypothyroidism,* or, in its most severe form, *myxedema* (swelling due to fluid accumulation and to abnormal deposits of mucoproteins). *Secondary hypothyroidism* is generally due to inadequate thyroid-stimulating hormone (TSH) secretion by the pituitary gland. Primary hypothyroidism may be caused by thyroid injury or atrophy, or by iodine deficiency. Injury to the thyroid can occur during treatment for hyperthyroidism *(iatrogenic hypothyroidism). Hashimoto's disease,* also known as *autoimmune thyroiditis* because of the immune-mediated destruction of the gland, is a cause of thyroid atrophy. *Thyroid aplasia,* a congenital defect in which there is an absence of a functioning thyroid gland, results in *cretinism,* a condition in which the affected child suffers from dwarfism, mental retardation, abnormal facial features, absence of sex organ development, and several metabolic disturbances.

Both overstimulation and understimulation of the thyroid gland will cause *goiter* (enlargement of the thyroid). *Diffuse colloidal goiter* (also known as nontoxic goiter or endemic goiter) results from a deficiency of dietary iodine. This form of goiter generally is not associated with hypothyroidism since the gland is still able to produce adequate levels of thyroxine. In *idiopathic nodular goiter,* swollen nodules are present in the thyroid. No deficiency of thyroxine production is associated with this condition.

Most *thyroid neoplasias* are small, benign nodules. The rarely occurring *malignant* thyroid neoplasias are carcinomas that arise from the follicular cells. Four types, based on the tumor histology, are recognized. The most common of these is *papillary thyroid carcinoma,* a low-grade, nonfunctional malignancy.

Hyperparathyroidism, or hyperactivity of the parathyroid glands, is usually due to benign neoplasia. Excessive parathyroid hormone is secreted in the condition, resulting in *hypercalcemia* (high blood calcium) and *hypophosphatemia* (low blood phosphate). As a result, bones lose their rigidity and may become deformed, calcium deposits in various tissues (e.g., kidneys, blood vessels), muscle contraction and nerve conduction are affected, and cardiac arrhythmias can occur. Hypoparathyroidism may be congenital, genetic, or autoimmune. In this condition, an abnormally low blood calcium level (hypocalcemia) causes *hypocalcemic tetany,* a situation characterized by sustained, spastic muscle contractions. Hypoparathyroidism, and the resulting hypocalcemia, can lead to cardiac arrest, convulsions, or suffocation.

▶ SECTION IV

Three different hormone families (glucocorticoids, mineralcorticoids, and androgens) are secreted by three different zones (the zona glomerulosa, the zona fasciculata, and the zona reticularis, respectively) of the adrenal cortex. Hyperactivity of one or more zones defines the condition of *hyperadrenalism.*

In *Cushing's syndrome* (also called *hypercortisolism),* there is an excess production of the glucocorticoids. This condition can be caused by hyperpituitarism, a functional tumor of the adrenal cortex, paraneoplastic syndrome, or, most commonly, by corticosteroid treatment of a disease (defined as iatrogenic hyperadrenalism or exogenous Cushing's syndrome). Because cortisol increases glucose, lipid, and sodium levels in the blood, hypercortisolism can lead to obesity, capillary fragility, hypertension, atherosclerosis, diabetes, and other physical and mental disturbances.

Hypersecretion of the mineralocorticoid aldosterone defines *Conn's syndrome* (also called *primary hyperaldosteronism).* This rare disease is due to an aldosterone-secreting tumor of the adrenal cortex. Because aldosterone causes sodium retention, and therefore water retention, by the kidneys, hypertension is a sign of the disease. In *secondary hyperaldosteronism,* more common than the primary condition, sodium and water retention are the result of excess renin secretion by the kidneys. Secondary hyperaldosteronism is, therefore, generally associated with renal disease. In *adrenogenital syndrome,* the adrenal zone that produces androgens is affected by a functional tumor, resulting in virilization in females (atrophy of the breasts, clitoral enlargement, amenorrhea, development of facial hair, deepening of the voice) and premature and enhanced sexual development in males.

Hypoadrenalism (also called *primary adrenal cortical insufficiency*) is characterized by the inadequate secretion of adrenal hormones. The condition results from adrenal destruction by a disease (autoimmune or infectious) or from neoplasia. *Addison's disease* is the result of primary adrenal cortical insufficiency. *Secondary adrenal cortical insufficiency* is caused by inadequate secretion of ACTH by the pituitary, resulting in inadequate secretion of aldosterone and glucocorticoids by the adrenal gland.

A *pheochromocytoma* is a benign, functional tumor of the adrenal gland. The tumor secretes the hormones epinephrine and norepinephrine to excess, causing hypertension and, over time, heart disease. A *neuroblastoma* is a malignant tumor of the adrenal medulla in children. The tumor, which grows quickly and metabolizes rapidly, arises from the embryonic fetal precursor cells of the medulla.

CHAPTER 17

The Musculoskeletal System

▶ OBJECTIVES

SECTION II

Define all highlighted terms.

Describe the hereditary bone diseases osteogenesis imperfecta, achondroplasia, and osteopetrosis, and characterize the signs and symptoms of each.

Describe the metabolic bone diseases osteoporosis, osteomalacia (rickets), Paget's disease, and osteitis fibrosa cystica. Characterize the causes and signs and symptoms of each.

Describe the causes of ischemic bone disease. Characterize the signs and symptoms of aseptic bone necrosis and Legg–Calvé–Perthes disease.

Describe the infectious bone diseases suppurative and nonsuppurative osteomyelitis, and characterize the causes and signs and symptoms of each.

Characterize and cite the complications of the types of bone fractures: simple, incomplete, complete, closed, compound, complicated, comminuted, compression, stress, greenstick, and pathologic.

Describe the process of fracture healing.

Describe the benign and malignant forms of bone neoplasia, and characterize the cells of origin, suspected causes, and signs and symptoms of each.

SECTION III

Define all highlighted terms.

Characterize the forms of arthritis synovitis, gout, infectious arthritis, Lyme disease, osteoarthritis, and rheumatoid arthritis. Cite the causes and signs and symptoms of each form.

Describe the signs of the disease ankylosing spondylitis.

Describe the joint disorders sprain, whiplash, strain, subluxation, luxation, and carpal tunnel syndrome. Characterize the causes and signs and symptoms of each.

Describe the condition of intervertebral disk herniation.

SECTION IV

Define all highlighted terms.

Describe the forms of muscular dystrophy: limb–girdle, facioscapulohumeral, myotonic, and Duchenne's. Characterize the causes and signs and symptoms of each.

Describe the cause and signs and symptoms of myasthenia gravis.

Describe the condition myositis. Characterize the causes and signs and symptoms of infectious and immune-mediated myositis.

Describe the causes and signs and symptoms of myopathy and neurogenic muscle disease.

Cite the most common form of muscle neoplasia, and describe the properties of the tumor.

1. ANATOMY AND PHYSIOLOGY IN REVIEW

Bone tissue contains two major types of cells, the **osteoblasts** and the **osteoclasts**. Together, these are called **osteocytes** (literally, "bone cells" since "osteo" refers to bone, and you know that "cyte" means cell). Bone is not as metabolically active as much of the soft tissue cells of the body, but it is certainly not as inert as it appears. While the hard matrix is inert, the cells within are constantly making changes within the bone (remodeling) and responding to the body's needs. Osteoblasts form the substance we call bone, and osteoclasts resorb or break down bone to release its minerals. Osteocytes live within a hardened extracellular matrix called **osteoid**. Osteoid is collagen that has become calcified (turned into bone). Calcification is the deposit of calcium phosphate mineral into the base matrix. Calcium phosphate crystals are in a form called **hydroxyapatite**.

The bones of the extremities (arms and legs) are long and round while those of the trunk (pelvis and ribs) and skull are short and flat. Long bones have a **cortex**, or outer part, and a **medulla**, or hollow center. This center is also called the **medullary cavity**. The bone marrow is found in the medullary cavity. **Red marrow** is found in the ends of long bones and in some flat bones. Red marrow is the site of hematopoiesis, or the production of blood cells. **Yellow marrow** is found in the shaft of long bones and is largely fat. There are several patterns and types of bone. An **osteon** is the basic unit of arrangement of cells and matrix in compact bone of the cortex. **Compact** bone is very dense and makes up the outer cortex of the shaft of long bones. At the ends of long bones, and inside along the medullary cavity, is **cancellous**, or **spongy**, bone which is not as dense. Spongy bone also makes up the short and flat bones of the skeleton. The arrangement of bone elements in spongy bone is in spicule-like formations called **trabeculae**. Osteocytes are found on the inside surfaces of compact bone and in trabeculae. The medullary cavity is lined with a membrane called **endosteum**. The outside surface of bones is covered with a membrane called the **periosteum**. The periosteum contains various types of cells, nerves, and blood vessels which supply the bone with nutrients. Nerves in the periosteum are responsible for feeling bone pain. The periosteum also serves as a site of attachment for tendons of muscles.

The long bones have several distinct parts. The center shaft is called the **diaphysis**. Toward the ends are the growth plates, or **physes**. This is also referred to as the **epiphyseal plate**. At the very end, or on top of the physis, is the **epiphysis** ("epi" means upon or above). The epiphysis is covered with articular cartilage, meaning the cartilage of the joints. The area of the growth plate and the end of the diaphysis together are called the **metaphysis**. It is this area that is the most metabolically active during growth. The components of a long bone are shown in Figure 17–1.

Growth or bone formation in long bones is through a process called **endochondral ossification**. This means turning cartilage into bone. "Chondr" refers to cartilage, and ossification is calcification. (Calcification, the deposition of calcium, will turn any tissue bone-hard as we have studied in some pathologic states.) The cartilage is in the growth plates. Cartilage is also collagen-based, although it is a different type of collagen from osteoid. The cartilage serves as a framework for new bone formation. Cartilage cells (**chondrocytes**) die, and the remaining matrix becomes calcified by deposits of hydroxyapatite. The majority of this transformation and growth takes place by puberty. In adults, most new bone formation occurs during the healing of fractures and in some arthritic and neoplastic states. Flat bone formation is accomplished through **intramembranous ossification**, which doesn't use cartilage as a base structure. Fibrous tissue is turned into osteoid and then mineralized, meaning that hydroxyapatite or calcium phosphate crystals are deposited. Both mechanisms of bone formation involve the calcification of collagen fibers, either in cartilage or a fibrous matrix. The initial calcification of the collagen meshwork is disorganized. Its appearance under the

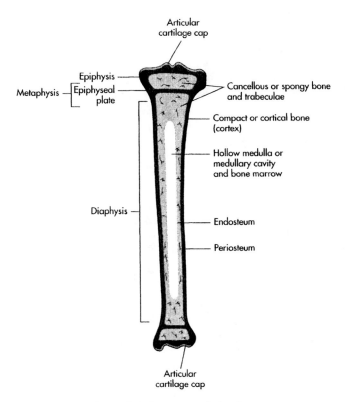

Figure 17–1. Cross-section of a long bone.

microscope is described as **woven** bone. Once the fibers are organized in a pattern in which they are parallel to each other, it is described as **lamellar** bone. Lamellar bone has the appearance of growth rings in a tree trunk. New bone is formed by osteoblasts. They synthesize osteoid collagen and cause mineralization or ossification of the collagen to produce bone. Osteoclasts break down or resorb existing bone to release calcium and phosphate into the circulation to maintain normal levels of these electrolytes. Bone is also remodeled or changed by osteocytes to accommodate the pull of muscles and gravity.

17–5

There are over 200 bones in the human skeleton and the function of this system can be divided into two categories, mechanical and metabolic. Mechanically, the skeleton provides protection of the internal organs of the trunk and head. It provides a structural framework for and support of the soft tissue of the body. Bones furnish the attachments for contracting muscles and therefore make movement possible. Metabolically, bones are the main source of blood cell production. They are also a reservoir for calcium and phosphate stores. Ninety-nine percent of the total body store of these minerals are found in the skeleton. Bone is responsible for furnishing that 1 percent level of calcium in the blood that is necessary for nerve conduction, muscle contraction, cardiac rhythm, and blood clotting. Blood levels of calcium are maintained by the bone's response to signals from PTH and calcitonin. In addition to these hormones from the parathyroid and thyroid glands, bone also responds to vitamin deficiencies, corticosteroids, estrogen and androgens, and growth hormone.

17–6

The term **articular** applies to joints. To articulate means to join parts together. A joint is made up of the ends of two bones held together by a tough, fibrous capsule. The bone ends are covered with cartilage. There is a small space between the two ends and a small amount of lubricating fluid coating the surfaces. The purpose of a joint is to allow a wide range of movement (called the range of motion) between the parts of the skeleton. The joints of the extremities that allow a great deal of movement are called **synovial** joints. A synovial joint

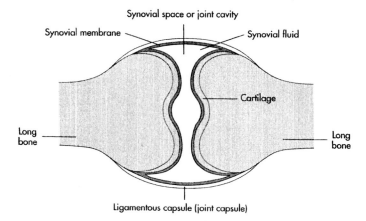

Figure 17-2. A synovial joint.

is illustrated in Figure 17–2. The skull and trunk have joints called **synarthroses** that do not allow much movement. In synovial joints, the exterior connective capsule is made of **ligaments.** A ligament is the fibrous connective tissue that connects bone to bone. The inside of a joint is lined with **synovial membrane** that secretes a clear, thick **synovial fluid.** This fluid provides lubrication during movement and nourishment for the cartilage cells, or chondrocytes. The joint surfaces are the caps of cartilage on the epiphyses of the two bones. The space between them is the **synovial space,** or **joint cavity. Bursae** are pouches of synovial fluid around some of the most moveable joints, such as the shoulder, that ease friction during motion.

17-7

Smooth muscle is so named because it is not striated like skeletal muscle. Smooth muscle is found in the walls of internal organs, the bronchi, and the blood vessels. Smooth muscle causes constriction, dilation, and other movement of these structures. It is called involuntary muscle because it is not under conscious control. It is controlled by the nervous system, chemical mediators, and hormones. **Cardiac muscle** is arranged in branch-like fashion and is found only in the heart. The branched configuration allows for faster and more efficient conduction of nerve impulses in heart muscle. The remainder of our review will center on **skeletal muscle.** This type of muscle is under voluntary control and is responsible for movement. Muscle cells make up **muscle fibers** that are **striated.** Striations are named for the way they appear microscopically. They look like fine bands. These bands are created by the overlapping of the contractile filaments (actin and myosin) in the fiber. A muscle is made of many bundles of muscle fibers, as shown in Figure 17–3. A fiber is made of many bundles of **myofibrils.** The fibers are bundled together in groups called **fascicles** and enclosed in a connective tissue sheath called the **perimysium.** Fascicles are separated from each other by branches of the **epimysium,** which is the connective tissue that encloses the entire muscle. Muscles are attached to bones by stringy bands of connective tissue called **tendons.**

17-8

A muscle cell is very long and runs the entire length of a muscle. There are many nuclei along the length of the cell to maintain its needs. Muscle cells are one of the more specialized cells of the body, like neurons. Unfortunately, this means that there is little ability to regenerate new muscle after an injury. Muscle is one of the poorer healing tissues of the body. (An advantage to this is that little proliferation of muscle cells means that neoplasia of muscle is rare.) Muscle cells contain **actin** and **myosin,** which are protein filaments that contract and relax. The actin and myosin filaments lie parallel to each other in rows and slide back and forth on each other to produce contraction and relaxation. The contraction of these proteins is in response to motor nerve stimulation.

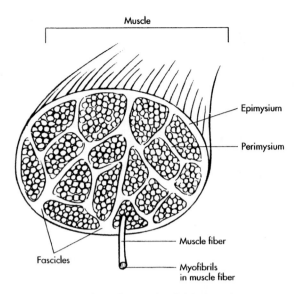

Figure 17–3. Cross-section of skeletal muscle.

The axon of a motor nerve contacts the muscle fiber at the **neuromuscular junction,** or **NMJ.** The NMJ consists of the nerve ending, a tiny space, and the neuromuscular plate on the muscle fiber. This is illustrated in Figure 17–4. The tiny space between the axon and muscle fiber is called the **synapse.** The nerve axon releases **acetylcholine,** or **ACh,** which is a neurotransmitter or specialized chemical messenger. It is released in vesicles or tiny packets and travels across the synapse and binds to receptors on the muscle fiber. This causes depolarization of the muscle's membrane and a contraction (shortening) results. Repolarization and relaxation occurs when **cholinesterase,** an enzyme, breaks down ACh and stops its message to contract. A muscle and its peripheral nerve are considered a single unit since loss of innervation leads to muscle atrophy or paralysis.

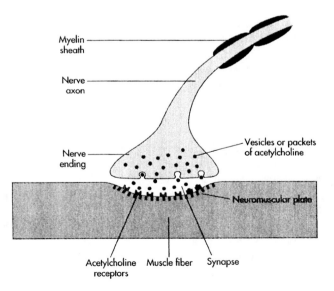

Figure 17–4. A neuromuscular junction.

The contraction and relaxation of skeletal muscles allow for movement, respiration, and maintenance of an upright posture. (Movement also requires the skeleton and nerves.) The work performed by muscles generates a large part of body heat, so they contribute to temperature homeostasis. Muscles also serve as a reservoir of glycogen for energy. In times of reduced food intake, the protein in muscle may be used as a nutrient source.

SECTION ▶ # II. DISEASES OF BONE

▶ DEVELOPMENTAL ABNORMALITIES

Developmental abnormalities of bone are not common. Our discussion will be limited to a few generalized genetic diseases. There are no specific treatments for generalized genetic bone diseases, only management of the signs and symptoms. Two localized genetic abnormalities that affect the skeletal system are clubfoot and congenital hip dysplasia. These were presented in Chapter 7 on genetic diseases. The disease **osteogenesis imperfecta** literally means deficient or imperfect formation of bone. This is a hereditary defect in the production of bony tissue. The particular abnormality lies in the collagen that is to become osteoid. Since the basis for the osteoid (the collagen) is defective, the end product (the bone) will also be defective. The resulting cortex of bone is thin. Osteogenesis imperfecta that is congenital, or present at _____(1), can be so severe that the baby is born with fractures. During childhood, growth is abnormal, deformities are present, and fractures occur frequently. Adults with a less severe form of the disease are more susceptible to fractures from relatively slight trauma. The kind of collagen that precedes osteoid is also found elsewhere in the body, so problems outside of the skeletal system are likely. Extreme forms of the disease may result in death before or just after birth. Osteogenesis imperfecta is a _____(2) disease in which there is _____(3) formation of _____(4). The primary defect lies in the _____(5) from which osteoid is made. The most severe congenital form may show as _____(6) in a newborn. Abnormalities may not be confined to the _____(7) system, but may be generalized.

Achondroplasia is another hereditary disease where the bone formation is defective. The particular cause is abnormality in the process of endochondral ossification. The cartilage in the growth plates, which forms the basis for this process, is disorganized to the point where normal formation and growth are impaired. Endochondral ossification occurs in long bones and is responsible for growth. Therefore, achondroplasia leads to dwarfism. This is specifically called **achondroplastic dwarfism.** The extremities, which undergo endochondral ossification, are greatly affected. The trunk, which undergoes intramembranous ossification and doesn't rely on cartilage, is relatively unaffected. Because of this, achondroplastic dwarfs have very short arms and legs, with a relatively normal trunk. The legs often are deformed (bowed) because of the weight of a relatively heavy trunk. _____(1) is defective bone formation because of an abnormality in _____(2) ossification. The _____(3) in the growth plates does not allow for normal formation and therefore _____(4) is impaired. This affects the _____(5) bones of the _____(6) because they grow by endochondral ossification. The trunk is generally not affected because these bones grow by _____(7). The overall result of achondroplasia is very short stature, or _____(8).

17-13

Osteopetrosis is a genetic bone disease where bone formation is greater than resorption or removal. It is believed that the osteoclasts do not remodel the osteons to withstand the pressure of weight as they should. Osteoclasts create a balance between too much bone formation and not enough resorption. Without their proper function, too much bone is formed. The resulting matrix is thick and stone-like (the Latin word "petrus" means stone). Because of its appearance microscopically, osteopetrosis is also called **marble bone disease.** Even though it is thick and hard, it is also brittle and susceptible to fractures. The thickening of the cortex invades the space of the medullary cavity, leaving less room there for the cells of hematopoiesis. Anemia may result. Outward thickening puts pressure on the periosteum and the vessels and nerves in this membrane. The pressure can impair blood supply to some degree and cause pain. Bone formation at a greater rate than bone removal describes the disease _____(1). This results in too much _____(2). It is thought this is because the _____(3) are not functioning properly. The word element "petrosis" refers to a Latin term that describes the bone being like _____(4). Inward thickening encroaches on the space of the _____(5) and can interfere with blood cell production, or _____(6). Outward thickening can put pressure on the _____(7), along with its _____(8) and _____(9).

1. osteopetrosis
2. bone formation
3. osteoclasts
4. stone
5. medullary cavity
6. hematopoiesis
7. periosteum
8. vessels
9. nerves

▶ METABOLIC BONE DISEASE

17-14

As the title implies, metabolic bone disease is some abnormality in the metabolism of bone. This frequently is related to levels of some hormones, vitamins, minerals, age, and lifestyle. Probably the most common bone disease in this country, of any cause, is **osteoporosis.** It is a disease that primarily affects the elderly, with more women affected than men. The bone that is present is *normal* in respect to the percentages of matrix and mineralization. There is just *less* total bone mass. Osteoporosis is a loss of bone mass as a result of thinning. A deficiency of bone is termed **osteopenia** ("penia" means decreased or deficient). Both dense cortical bone and cancellous bone are lost. The cortex becomes thin, and the spicules in the trabeculae of spongy bone become narrowed. Figure 17–5 compares a histologic section of normal bone with the thinned bone of osteoporosis. Some thinning of bone is a natural age-related process. After a certain age, resorption becomes slightly greater than formation, so there is a net loss of bone mass with each year. This loss most significantly affects those populations that had less bone to begin with. Women have less bone mass than men. Therefore, age-related thinning is most dramatic in women as compared to men, and even more so in small-framed or small-boned women. People who exercise a great deal will have more bone mass because hypertrophy in response to exercise occurs in bone as well as muscle. Therefore, this population is ahead of the aging game in respect to osteoporosis. Osteoporosis is _____(1) of bone, specifically because the bones become _____(2). There is _____(3) total bone mass, but what bone is present is _____(4) in its composition. Bone deficiency is called _____(5). There is a loss in both _____(6) and _____(7) types of bone. A decrease in total bone mass is a normal change that accompanies _____(8). This is because resorption becomes greater than new bone _____(9). Thinning of bones will most significantly affect populations that have _____(10) initial bone mass.

1. loss
2. thin
3. less
4. normal
5. osteopenia
6. cortical
7. cancellous or spongy
8. aging
9. formation
10. less

17-15

Symptomatic osteoporosis is most frequently seen in postmenopausal women. For some unknown reason, estrogen is necessary for normal bone density. Lack of estrogen, combined with a relatively slight initial bone mass, makes elderly women targets for this disease. Osteoporosis is also seen in elderly men with enough bone loss. Other cases of thinning are related to disuse atrophy, such as with prolonged bedrest or paralysis. Muscle mass also declines in these cases which symbolize the "use it or lose it" axiom. Prolonged steroid ther-

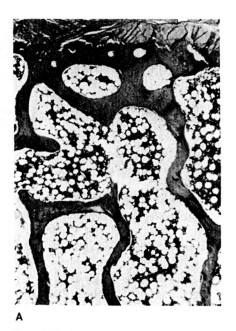 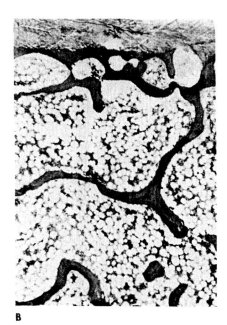

A   **B**

Figure 17–5. A comparison of normal bone with osteoporosis. **A.** Normal bone. Note the thickness and amount of trabeculae of cancellous bone, and the density of the cortex on the left. **B.** Osteoporosis in an 80-year-old. Note the very thin and decreased trabeculae, and the less dense cortical bone on the left. *(From Kent and Hart,* Introduction to Human Disease, *3rd ed., Appleton & Lange.)*

1. estrogen
2. density
3. disuse atrophy

.... 17–16 ....

1. thinner
2. vertebrae
3. hip
4. femoral head
5. disability
6. healing

apy, genetic predisposition, and lack of exercise are other causative factors. Postmenopausal women are more at risk for osteoporosis because of lack of _____(1), which appears to be required for healthy bone _____(2). Loss of mass because of lack of use is called _____(3). This is another reason for thinning bones.

The parts of the skeleton that are naturally thinner than the rest, such as the vertebrae, suffer the most from osteoporosis. Vertebral disease is shown by compression fractures, pain in the spine, shortening of height, and a bending or hunching over. This is such a common sign in elderly women that it is informally called "widow's hump." The worst complication of osteoporosis is hip fracture, specifically fracture of the femoral head. This can, and often does, occur with any type of fall. These fractures heal very poorly, and about 25 percent never heal at all. This leads to permanent disability. There is no treatment for osteoporosis since the amount of bone never returns to normal through any treatment. Prevention, particularly in susceptible populations, is vital. Calcium and vitamin D should be more than adequate in the diet or else supplemented. Hormone replacement therapy (estrogen) for postmenopausal women has been shown to be very helpful in prevention. Men with low levels of testosterone should also be supplemented. Weight-bearing exercise is effective in helping to maintain bone mass. Bones that are most affected by loss of mass are _____(1) than other bones to begin with. Bones of the spine, or the _____(2), cause many signs and symptoms of osteoporosis. The most debilitating effect is fracture of the _____(3), in particular, fracture of the _____(4). This may lead to permanent _____(5) because of the poor rate of _____(6).

.... 17–17 ....

Osteomalacia and **rickets** are essentially the same bone disease, but they are labeled differently according to the population they affect. The word element "malac" means soft, specifically a morbid (disease-associated) softening. This is a softening of the bones that is not common in this country. It is due to lack of sufficient calcium and phosphorus deposits in bone because of lack of vitamin D. The condition is called osteomalacia in adults and rickets when it affects the growing bones of children. The total bone mass is normal, that is, there is enough bone present, but the osteoid or bone tissue itself is abnormal. The abnormality is a softening to the point of becoming rubbery or pliable. Since calcium phosphate deposits give bone its hard character, insufficient deposition or mineralization produces inadequate hardening. The bones are composed of more collagen matrix than osteoid. The cause of decreased mineralization is inadequate vitamin D through a variety of causes such as:

1. Malnutrition. Insufficient vitamin D in the diet decreases mineralization.
2. Impaired vitamin D synthesis in the skin. This is caused by insufficient exposure to sunlight.
3. Malabsorption. In this case, either all nutrient absorption is impaired in intestinal disease, or fat absorption is hindered in biliary or pancreatic disease (vitamin D is fat soluble and must be absorbed with fat).

A deficiency in vitamin D leads to inadequate absorption of calcium and phosphate from the intestine, so this creates a secondary deficiency of these minerals.

17-18

Osteomalacia means _____(1) of the bones in _____(2). Rickets is softening of the bones in _____(3). The bones become soft because of lack of _____(4), which leads to decreased amounts of the minerals _____(5) and _____(6), because vitamin D is necessary for their _____(7) from the intestines. The bones become soft because there is not enough _____(8), or deposition of calcium phosphate in the collagen, to create hard osteoid. In children, rickets causes stunted growth. Untreated cases result in deformity, especially of the weight-bearing bones like the legs. The softened leg bones will often bow under the weight of the trunk. The spine becomes abnormally curved, and there is improper tooth formation. Both children and adults are susceptible to fractures.

1. softening
2. adults
3. children
4. vitamin D
5. calcium
6. phosphorus
7. absorption
8. mineralization

17-19

Paget's disease may be a genetic disorder, but the actual cause is unknown. This could also be classified as a hyperplastic condition because the underlying pathology is overproduction of bone. It is also known as **osteitis deformans.** The normal processes of bone formation and resorption are greatly accelerated, and the end result is very thickened bones. There are three phases. First, resorption is increased, leaving the bones softened and porous. Then, new formation equals resorption. Last, osteosclerosis, or excessive hardening, develops because of a disorganized proliferation that results in overgrowth of osteoid. Clinically, individuals with this disease are susceptible to fracture and experience some bone pain. Because the skull is so thickened, pressure is exerted on cranial nerves, causing headache, dizziness, and other neurological signs. The significance of Paget's disease is that it is a likely forerunner of bone cancer, which is not a common disease.

17-20

Hyperparathyroidism causes a metabolic bone disease known as **osteitis fibrosa cystica.** Parathyroid hormone, or PTH, is a very significant hormone in terms of response by bone. Therefore, excessive PTH will definitely upset the normal metabolism of bone. You know that PTH causes calcium to be released from bone stores to maintain plasma levels of calcium. (Calcium is required for _____(1) conduction, _____(2) contraction, _____(3) rhythm, and blood _____(4).) Excessive PTH causes too much release of calcium and depletes bone of this necessary mineral. PTH increases the activity of the resorbing osteoclasts and causes osteolysis of bone. The bone becomes porous and decalcified, or demineralized. The demineralized areas are replaced with fibrous tissue, and occasionally cysts may develop. The decalcification causes weakness, bending, and deformity of the skeleton. There is bone pain with increased susceptibility to fractures. Significant events occur outside of the skeletal system, and these relate to excessive plasma levels of calcium, which would be called _____(5). Hypercalcemia leads to deposits of calcium in soft tissue. This most notably affects the kidney, where stone, or calculus, formation can cause obstruction and interfere with kidney function. Osteitis fibrosa cystica is a bone disease that is secondary to the condition _____(6). Excessive levels of the hormone _____(7) will cause

1. nerve
2. muscle
3. cardiac
4. clotting
5. hypercalcemia
6. hyperparathyroidism
7. PTH

8. calcium
9. bone
10. demineralization
11. fibrous
12. weak
13. kidneys

excessive release of _____(8) from _____(9) stores. This leaves the bones in a state of _____(10). The demineralized areas fill with _____(11) tissue. The bones become _____(12) from lack of calcium. This all leads to hypercalcemia, which often results in calcium deposits in soft tissue, especially the _____(13). The features of metabolic bone disease are summarized in Table 17–1.

► ISCHEMIC BONE DISEASE

17-21

1. blood supply
2. infarction
3. more
4. metaphysis
5. aseptic bone necrosis
6. avascular necrosis
7. children
8. fracture

Impairment of a bone's blood supply will cause ischemia and often lead to bone infarction. Blood supply to bones is not as plentiful as it is in other tissues, so disruption of an artery has greater effects. There is less collateral circulation, or alternative routes of supply. The area of a long bone that has the most blood supply is the metaphysis, which contains the epiphyseal growth plate. The arteries that supply bone are called nutrient arteries. In the past, the majority of cases of ischemia and necrosis were because of bacterial infection. Therefore, the condition was called septic necrosis. Today, infarction is usually associated with other causes, and noninfectious cases are called **aseptic bone necrosis,** also known as **avascular necrosis.** Aseptic bone necrosis is most often seen in children with fractures near the metaphysis. (The incidence of fracture is higher in children than adults because of their activities.) Because of the location of the break, the infarct occurs around the growth plates, also known as the ossification centers in growing bones. The metaphyseal area is at greatest risk for infarction because it is the area of a long bone that has the greatest metabolic activity and therefore the greatest need for adequate blood supply. Ischemia of bone develops because of interruption in _____(1). This often leads to _____(2). Bone is _____(3) more / less (choose one) susceptible to infarction than soft tissue. The area of a long bone most hurt by ischemia and infarction is the _____(4). Infarction *not* caused by infection is called _____(5) or _____(6). Bone infarction is most often seen in _____(7) who have a _____(8) near the metaphysis.

17-22

In addition to fractures that involve the nutrient arteries, a less common cause of infarction and necrosis is emboli which lodge in the nutrient arteries. Examples of emboli include tumor cells, nitrogen bubbles in decompression syndrome, thrombi, fat in alcoholic hepatic lipidosis, masses of bacteria, and clumps of abnormal red cells in sickle cell anemia. The elderly are also targets for ischemic bone disease, especially in cases of osteoporosis and resulting fracture of the femoral head. There are many cases that are idiopathic. These also

TABLE 17–1. FEATURES OF METABOLIC BONE DISEASE

Disease	Features
Osteoporosis	Normal osteoid (percentages of matrix to mineralization) Decreased total bone mass (osteopenia) Thin bones
Osteomalacia	Decreased mineralization of osteoid due to insufficient calcium and phosphorus deposits Normal total bone mass Soft bones in adults
Rickets	Same pathogenesis as osteomalacia Soft bones in children
Paget's disease (osteitis deformans)	Overproduction of osteoid Thick bones
Osteitis fibrosa cystica	Hyperparathyroidism Depletion of calcium from bones with fibrous tissue replacement and cyst formation Weakened decalcified bones

are seen more in children. They go by many names according to the researcher who identified the particular disease. The most well known is probably **Legg–Calvé–Perthes disease.** This is idiopathic avascular necrosis of the femoral head. Besides fractures, a less common cause of bone necrosis is _____(1), which obstruct the _____(2). Many cases are of unknown origin, or are _____(3), and occur in _____(4). Legg–Calvé–Perthes disease is idiopathic _____(5) involving the _____(6).

17–23

1. emboli
2. nutrient arteries
3. idiopathic
4. children
5. avascular necrosis
6. femoral head

Clinically, aseptic bone necrosis heals slowly and signs may be absent. In Legg–Calvé–Perthes disease, or in fractures of the neck of the femur, the pressure of bearing weight can cause disintegration and collapse of the avascular femoral head. This can severely compromise the integrity of the hip joint and lead to osteoarthritis.

▶ INFECTIOUS BONE DISEASE

17–24

Bacterial infection of bone is called **osteomyelitis.** This infection is usually a secondary complication, as you will see when the causes are presented. **Suppurative osteomyelitis** is bone infection caused by pus-producing bacteria. Another term for pus-producing or suppurative would be _____(1). Suppurative osteomyelitis can be acute or chronic. It is seen most frequently in children (because of the incidence of fracture and surgery) and often affects the metaphysis or epiphyseal growth plate in long bones. **Nonsuppurative osteomyelitis** is caused by bacteria that don't cause pus and will be briefly discussed later. Acute suppurative osteomyelitis is most commonly caused by *Staphylococcus aureus,* a pyogenic (pus-producing) bacteria. The organisms gain access during trauma such as a compound or open fracture, during surgery to repair a fracture, from infection in soft tissue next to bone, and even from skin infections in children. *S. aureus* may enter bone through the nutrient artery during bacteremia. This would be classified as _____(2) spread. Osteomyelitis is _____(3) of bone. In cases where the bacteria produce pus, it is called _____(4). The most common cause of suppurative cases is _____(5), which is a pyogenic organism. The bacteria enter bone during trauma such as an open _____(6) or during _____(7), or may enter from adjacent _____(8) infection. Hematogenous spread is infection that has entered from the _____(9) during _____(10).

1. purulent
2. hematogenous
3. bacterial infection
4. suppurative osteomyelitis
5. *S. aureus*
6. fracture
7. surgery
8. soft tissue
9. bloodstream
10. bacteremia

17–25

The events of acute suppurative osteomyelitis are as follows:

1. Inflammation of the area causes the typical signs of heat, swelling, and pain. Because it is infectious in nature, fever and chills are common.
2. The presence of purulent exudate under the periosteum creates great pressure because the underlying bone is rigid and there isn't any "give" under the pressure. This can severely compromise blood supply as vessels are squeezed shut. Ischemia usually leads to necrosis of the bone and in the marrow cavity.
3. Following the path of least resistance, the pus will spread further along under the periosteum, raising it and snapping small vessels. This causes more tension in the area and more impairment of blood supply. The necrosis worsens and moves along the bone shaft. Most cases today are recognized by this stage and treated with antibiotics to halt the progression of events. If it is not treated, and in cases prior to effective antibiotics, the events continue.
4. Loss of blood supply to an area of bone and necrosis results in a piece of dead bone, which eventually detaches and floats freely in the exudate. This dead bone is called a **sequestrum,** meaning it is sequestered, or cut off, from the rest of living bone. Once it is formed, a sequestrum is viewed by the body as a foreign body and further inflammation develops in response. It also acts as a **nidus,** which is a continual source of infection and inflammation as bacteria continue to thrive and multiply in the piece.

Ischemia and necrosis can result from purulent infection because _____(1) underneath the _____(2) causes enough pressure that _____(3) are squeezed or collapse. This may spread under the periosteum and cause more _____(4) to be damaged. This resulting loss of blood supply causes _____(5) of the bone. A small piece of necrotic, or _____(6), bone breaks off, and this piece is called a _____(7). The response to a sequestrum is more _____(8). It also serves as a continued source of infection, and this is called a _____(9).

Cases that are not stopped by treatment beyond this point enter the stage of chronic suppurative osteomyelitis. The events continue as:

5. Pressure from the pus or exudate eventually ruptures the periosteum, leaving a hole for drainage. The draining material tracks through muscle, subcutaneous tissue, and breaks through the skin to create a **fistulous tract.** A **fistula** is an unnatural opening to the outside from a site within the body. Pus drains from the fistula.
6. In chronic inflammation in soft tissue, a pyogenic membrane is formed around the area in an attempt to wall off an abscess (see Chap. 2). In chronic suppurative osteomyelitis, new bone is formed over the area for the same purpose. The new bone lies over the area of the sequestrum like an outer wrapper. The new encasing bone is called an **involucrum,** and its Latin origin means wrapper.
7. Cases still untreated at this point may lead to death by way of toxemia and septic shock.

The complications of untreated acute and chronic suppurative osteomyelitis are shown in Figure 17–6. Chronic suppurative osteomyelitis is heralded by the presence of a hole in the skin that drains _____(1). This is because the exudate has ruptured the _____(2) and pushed out through the soft tissue. The hole is called a _____(3), and its path from the inside is called a _____(4). An involucrum then forms, which is _____(5) bone that encloses the area of the _____(6) in an attempt to wall off the infection.

Overall, bone is not as easily infected as soft tissue. However, once infected, a cure is more difficult because of the relatively limited blood supply of bone. Antibiotics reach and penetrate target tissue through blood supply, and so in bone this is not as easily done as in soft tissue. It is more difficult to produce therapeutic levels of drugs in bone than in soft tissue. Treatment should initially consist of intravenous administration of antibiotics that penetrate bone best, followed by prolonged oral administration. Often, surgical drainage and debridement are necessary to remove the sequestrum and necrotic tissue.

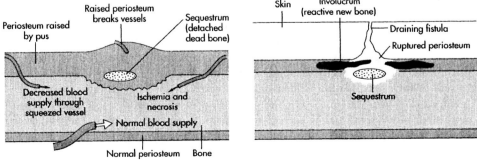

Acute Suppurative Osteomyelitis   **Chronic Suppurative Osteomyelitis**

Figure 17–6. Complications of untreated suppurative osteomyelitis.

Nonsuppurative osteomyelitis may be caused by the organisms of tuberculosis and syphilis. Syphilitic osteomyelitis is rare today because the *Treponema* don't infect bone until the late stages and most cases are treated by then. Tuberculosis of bone, also uncommon today because of detection and treatment, doesn't cause purulent inflammation. It is a quiet, smoldering infection that destroys bone, just like it creates cavitations, or holes, in lung tissue. There is little reactionary new bone formation. Caseous abscesses are also formed, as they are in the lungs. Historically, TB of bone most often affected the spine, causing a variety of signs called Pott's disease.

► FRACTURES OF BONE

A **fracture** is a break in bone usually (but not always) caused by mechanical force or trauma. There are several types or classifications of fractures. Some of these types are illustrated in Figure 17–7. A **simple** fracture is a single line of disruption or break. It may be an **incomplete** fracture, which involves only one side of the bone or one cortex. An incomplete fracture doesn't extend completely through and the bone is still in one piece. A **complete** break involves both sides, or extends completely through both cortices. A complete fracture results in the bone's being in at least two pieces. Most simple fractures are **closed;** that is, the skin over the break is intact. A **compound** fracture is where the skin over the break is open, so that bone ends are exposed to the environment. This is also called an **open** fracture. Compound fractures are almost always complete by their nature. What often tears the skin is the sharp edges of bone cutting through tissue. Two serious complications are hemorrhage, if an artery is cut in the process, and infection because of exposure to the environment. Bone infection is called _____(1). Osteomyelitis is especially a concern in cases where the wound is contaminated with dirt or debris. A fracture that has become infected is called a **complicated** fracture. A disruption or break in the continuity of a bone is called a _____(2). A single break is called a _____(3) fracture. If it is through only one side, this is a _____(4) fracture. If it is through both sides, it is a _____(5) fracture. A closed fracture is where the _____(6) over the break has not been opened. If the skin has been pierced and the fracture ends exposed, this is called a _____(7), or _____(8), fracture. Two concerns in a compound fracture are _____(9) and _____(10).

1. osteomyelitis
2. fracture
3. simple
4. incomplete
5. complete
6. skin
7. compound
8. open
9. hemorrhage
10. infection

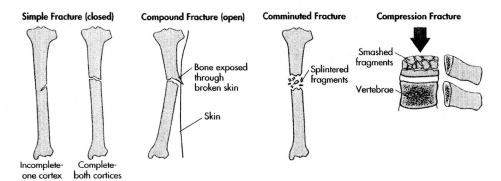

Figure 17–7. Types of fractures.

1. comminuted
2. compression
3. vertebrae
4. stress
5. greenstick
6. bends
7. pathologic
8. spontaneous

In a **comminuted** fracture, the break has created several pieces or fragments of bone. The bone may be described as being splintered. This type is often the most difficult to repair surgically. Instead of just realigning the ends, the bone must be rebuilt and gaps created by destroyed pieces must be grafted with spongy bone. A **compression** fracture generally occurs in diseased vertebrae such as in osteoporosis. Instead of being pulled apart as in other fractures, the bone is smashed together. A **stress** fracture is tiny linear (line-like) cracks, generally occurring in the anterior tibia due to jolting exercise. Stress fractures are most often seen in athletes or enthusiastic runners. A **greenstick** fracture is most often seen in children whose bones bend more than break. The cortex opposite the bend often breaks. A **pathologic** fracture, also called a **spontaneous** fracture, is a break that occurs under normal strain or pressure, or with only slight trauma. The bone fractures because it has become weakened by bone disease. The most common causes of pathologic fractures are osteoporosis and metastatic (secondary) bone cancer. In fact, a pathologic fracture is a red flag to look for the presence of neoplasia elsewhere in the body. A bone that has been splintered into many pieces has undergone a _____(1) fracture. A bone that has been pushed together from either end describes a _____(2) fracture, which is usually seen in the _____(3). Tiny cracks associated with strenuous exercise is a _____(4) fracture. Children often experience _____(5) fractures if one side of the bone _____(6) instead of breaks. A bone that is so weak from disease that it breaks under normal wear and tear describes a _____(7), or _____(8), fracture.

1. hematoma
2. granulation
3. fibrous cartilage
4. trabeculae of spongy bone
5. scaffold
6. across
7. capillaries
8. callus
9. cortical

The healing of a fracture follows several principles discussed in Chapter 2 on healing. Fracture healing is generally described as a **union.** First is a hematoma or clot formation between the two realigned and stabilized ends. Granulation tissue then forms and matures into fibrous cartilage and trabeculae of spongy bone. This manner of maturation is orchestrated by the osteoblasts that are present. The cartilage, spongy bone, and delicate new capillaries grow across the gap using the remaining granulation tissue as a scaffold or support. All of the granulation tissue eventually reorganizes into a bony **callus,** which unites the two ends. This is later remodeled into dense cortical bone. The healing of bone follows the lines of soft tissue healing in that first a _____(1) is formed. This is replaced by _____(2) tissue. Osteoblasts cause the granulation tissue to mature into _____(3) and _____(4). The remaining granulation tissue serves as a _____(5) to support the growth of the early bone material _____(6) the gap, along with new _____(7). The two ends are fused together when the material finally reorganizes into bony _____(8). This is later remodeled into _____(9) bone.

Specific management of fractures is required for these stages to progress to complete healing. It is also important to handle fractures in a manner that prevents simple closed fractures from becoming compound fractures. The ends of the bone must be **reduced,** or realigned, as closely together as possible. When we spoke of the gap that must be bridged in healing, it is on a microscopic level, and a properly reduced fracture doesn't look like it has a gap. Compressed and impacted are two terms that describe how tightly the two ends are placed together. After this, absolute immobilization must be achieved. Complete stability is required to allow the elements to grow across the gap. It is especially important not to disrupt the delicate granulation tissue scaffold or snap the fragile new vessels. Immobilization may be achieved with casts in some simple fractures. Larger, more complex breaks require surgical techniques such as intramedullary pins, plates and screws, and wires to stabilize the site. Removal of necrotic tissue and replacement of interfering soft tissue are also necessary.

There are a few complications in the healing of bone. In a **delayed union,** healing is poor or is slowed because of a variety of factors. Fractures in the elderly often take much longer to heal for many reasons. Vitamin deficiencies (specifically D) and mineral deficiencies (specifically calcium or phosphate) produce delayed union. Infection at the site, or osteomyelitis, can cause either delayed union or no union at all. Failure of the two ends to unite is called a **nonunion.** Poor healing that is specifically caused by too much movement at the fracture site (that is, not enough stability) can lead to a **fibrous nonunion.** This is where a fibrous scar develops instead of a callus. Osteoblasts in the granulation tissue have acted like fibroblasts under the influence of the instability. Once scar tissue bridges the gap, it cannot be turned into bone, so this represents lack of bony union. A true **nonunion** develops when some soft tissue has wedged between the bone ends and no bridging across the gap occurs at all, not even by scar tissue. It is physically impossible for the scaffold material to develop across the gap. If the two ends of a fracture take longer than normal to unite, this is called a _____(1). Lack of uniting in a normal fashion describes a _____(2). A fibrous nonunion is where _____(3) takes the place of the bony callus. It is caused by too much _____(4) at the site of the break, which disrupts the healing process. Complete lack of bridging by any material is a _____(5), and this will occur if _____(6) physically interferes with growth across the gap.

1. delayed union
2. nonunion
3. scar tissue
4. instability
5. nonunion
6. soft tissue

▶ NEOPLASIA OF BONE

Primary tumors of bone are very uncommon compared to cancer of the rest of the body. The most common of this neoplasia is of the blood-forming cells in the medullary cavity, or cells of the bone marrow. Cancer of the various types of white blood cell precursors are the leukemias we studied in Chapter 9. Cancer of the B lymphocytes, specifically plasma cells, is multiple myeloma. This was also presented in Chapter 9. Two prominent features of bone tumors are pathologic fractures and pain. In soft tissue tumors, or carcinomas, pain is usually a later development. In bone tumors, pain is an early feature. This is because the pressure of new proliferating material is great because it is growing on rigid, unyielding bone. **Benign** tumors of bone are named according to the cells of origin. An **osteoma** originates from bone-producing cells. This is the most common benign bone tumor. A **chondroma** is a benign growth of cartilage cells. Occasionally, a chondroma may transform into a malignant chondrosarcoma. A **fibroma** originates from fibroblasts. Benign tumors cause little problem and present as a swelling or bump on or within the bone. Pain may or may not be present, depending on its size and location. Painful benign growths that have grown large enough to apply pressure to nerves in the periosteum are surgically removed. In this instance, the growth is a problem as a space-occupying lesion like soft tissue growths. The two main signs of a bone tumor are _____(1) and _____(2). In contrast to soft tissue cancer, pain appears _____(3) in the course of the disease. The most common benign bone tumor is the _____(4) of bone cells. Cartilage cells may give rise to a _____(5) and fibroblasts to a _____(6).

1. pain
2. pathologic fracture
3. early
4. osteoma
5. chondroma
6. fibroma

Malignant bone tumors have the term **"sarcoma"** in their name because that is the nomenclature for neoplasia of connective tissue origin. The most common and most malignant of the primary bone cancers is **osteosarcoma,** also known as **osteogenic sarcoma.** The cells of origin are the osteoblasts that produce osteoid or bone matrix. The overproduction of osteoid and bony spicules forms a large, painful mass, which is shown in Figure 17–8. The most common location for osteosarcoma is the metaphysis of long bones, especially in the legs around the knee. Osteosarcoma most often affects young people (teenagers and those in their early 20s). Older adults who develop this cancer usually do so as a sequela to Paget's disease. Death from this malignancy is a result of metastasis to the lungs. The prognosis for this

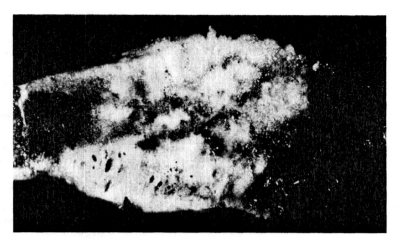

Figure 17–8. Osteosarcoma, showing the solid destructive mass in the metaphysis of the fibula. *(From Chandrasoma and Taylor, Concise Pathology, 2nd ed., Appleton & Lange.)*

1. osteosarcoma
2. osteogenic sarcoma
3. malignant
4. osteoblasts
5. mass
6. knee
7. young
8. lungs

disease is fair to good. The five-year survival rate following proper treatment is up to 60 percent. Chemotherapy is used to shrink the tumor and the remainder is surgically removed. Chemotherapy and radiation is required in any case of metastasis. The most common primary malignant bone tumor is the _____(1), or _____(2). It is also the most _____(3). It arises from the cells called _____(4). The common presentation is a large, painful _____(5) often located around the _____(6). The population affected are _____(7) people, and death is due to metastasis to the _____(8).

17–37

1. chondrosarcoma
2. maturity
3. prognosis
4. trunk

A **chondrosarcoma** is malignant neoplasia of cartilage cells, specifically the chondroblasts. This cancer can be graded since the tumor is made up of cells in different stages of maturity. Tumors of cells that are the most mature, or differentiated, yield the best prognosis. Chondrosarcomas are most frequently located in the bones of the trunk, such as the vertebrae, pelvis, and ribs. The prognosis of this cancer depends entirely on its grade, meaning how primitive the cells are, and on its location (whether it can be removed). Chondrosarcoma is unresponsive to chemotherapy. Malignancy of chondroblasts is called a _____(1). Cells in various stages of _____(2) allow this cancer to be graded. This is important in determining the probable outcome, or _____(3). Chondrosarcomas most often affect the bones of the _____(4).

17–38

1. giant cell
2. lysis
3. air
4. bubbles
5. knee
6. benign

In a **giant cell tumor,** the cells are large and multinucleated and probably originate from osteoclasts. Mononuclear cells are also present in the tumor. In osteosarcoma, osteoblasts produce excessive bone and therefore a mass. In giant cell tumor, since osteoclasts function to resorb bone, it is not surprising to find cysts in the bone as areas are destroyed by lysis. On x-ray, these cysts have been described as looking like air sacs or bubbles. Giant cell tumors most often form in the epiphysis of long bones, also near the knee. Many cases are benign. About 10 to 15 percent are malignant in the sense of uncontrolled proliferation by mononuclear cells and metastasis. The prognosis is good with removal of the tumor, unless it displays highly malignant characteristics. About half of the treated cases develop new tumors after removal of the original lesion. A bone tumor of osteoclasts and mononuclear cells is the likely basis of a _____(1) tumor. The lesion in a giant cell tumor is one of _____(2) of the bone instead of bony growth. The resulting cysts appear as _____(3) sacs or _____(4) on x-ray. Giant cell tumors frequently develop around the _____(5) like osteosarcomas. Most cases are _____(6) but some are malignant.

Ewing's sarcoma is a malignant tumor arising from the most primitive or undifferentiated cells of bone. It is assumed to be of the stem cells of the medulla. The location of a Ewing's sarcoma is in the diaphysis of long bones, which corresponds to the location of the medullary cavity. This cancer does invade or spread locally. It moves from the medulla out through the cortex and into soft tissue. New bone formation under the periosteum produces spicules that create a "sunburst" appearance on x-ray. Ewing's sarcoma affects a population slightly younger than in osteosarcoma (children and into the teen years). This malignancy does metastasize to the lungs. The prognosis is fair, with about a 30 percent 5-year survival rate. Ewing's sarcoma most likely originates from primitive or _____(1) cells of the _____(2) cavity. Its location corresponds to the location of the medulla, which is the _____(3) of long bones. Local spread, or _____(4), moves the cancer out through the _____(5) and into _____(6). Characteristic appearance on x-ray is because of _____(7) of new bone growth.

17-39

1. undifferentiated
2. medullary
3. diaphysis
4. invasion
5. cortex
6. soft tissue
7. spicules

By far, the most common type of bone cancer overall is **secondary bone neoplasia,** or **metastatic bone cancer.** Cancer due to metastases in bone is 10 times more common than primary bone cancer. Secondary bone metastases arise from spread of carcinoma at a distant site. The most common carcinomas that spread to bone are of the breast, prostate, lung, kidneys, and thyroid. The most common location for bone metastases are the flat bones of the trunk which have the most blood supply. This is because of the route of spread of the primary cancer, through the blood. Clinically, secondary bone cancer is very painful. Secondary tumors are usually found at many sites, instead of one as in a primary tumor. These multiple tumors destroy the bone. The bone destruction leads to a high incidence of pathologic fracture. Spontaneous bone fracture is an important signal to look for cancer elsewhere in the body, if it hasn't already been diagnosed. The most common kind of bone cancer is _____(1), or _____(2) bone cancer. Metastatic bone cancer develops as a result of metastasis by a _____(3) elsewhere in the body. The most common sources of secondary bone cancer are the kidneys, thyroid, _____(4), _____(5), and _____(6). Bone metastases usually end up in the bones of the _____(7) and at _____(8) sites. Destruction of bone causes pain and _____(9) fracture.

17-40

1. secondary bone neoplasia
2. metastatic
3. carcinoma
4. breast
5. prostate
6. lungs
7. trunk
8. multiple
9. pathologic

II. REVIEW QUESTIONS

1. Bone formation that is so defective that a baby may be born with fractures occurs in:
   a. achondroplasia
   b. osteopetrosis
   c. osteogenesis imperfecta
   d. marble bone disease

2. A developmental abnormality affecting the endochondral ossification centers of long bones and causing extreme shortening of the extremities describes:
   a. achondroplasia
   b. osteogenesis imperfecta
   c. osteopetrosis
   d. marble bone disease

3. The most common disease of bone in this country is:
   a. osteopetrosis
   b. osteoporosis
   c. osteomyelitis
   d. osteomalacia

1. c–osteogenesis imperfectica

2. a–achondroplasia

3. b–osteoporosis

4. Osteopenia is a a._____ amount of bone, resulting in a decrease in total bone b._____. A small amount of osteopenia is due to c._____. Larger amounts leading to a disease state is called d._____.

1. increased	6. osteoporosis
2. decreased	7. osteitis deformans
3. mineralization	8. vitamin D deficiency
4. aging	9. aseptic bone necrosis
5. mass	

5. Which of the following is NOT a factor in the development of osteoporosis (choose all that are correct)?
   a. weight-bearing exercise
   b. sex
   c. aging
   d. adequate calcium in the diet
   e. menopause
   f. lack of exercise
   g. estrogen replacement therapy
   h. initial bone mass

6. The most debilitating complication of osteoporosis is:
   a. spinal deformity
   b. hip fracture
   c. vertebral compression fracture
   d. avascular necrosis of the femoral head

7. Lack of vitamin D, and therefore calcium absorption, causes softening of bones as seen in (choose all that are correct):
   a. rickets
   b. osteopetrosis
   c. osteitis fibrosa cystica
   d. osteomalacia

8. Excessive loss of calcium from bone and hypercalcemia is seen in the bone disease a._____, and this is secondary to b._____.

1. osteogenesis imperfecta	4. osteitis deformans
2. kidney disease	5. hyperparathyroidism
3. hypoparathyroidism	6. osteitis fibrosa cystica

9. Trauma or blockage of the nutrient arteries of bone can lead to:
   a. septic bone necrosis
   b. osteomyelitis
   c. aseptic bone necrosis
   d. pathologic fracture

10. Idiopathic avascular necrosis in Legg–Calvé–Perthes disease affects the:
    a. medullary cavity in the diaphysis of long bones
    b. intervertebral disks
    c. metaphysis of any extremity
    d. head of the femur

11. Osteomyelitis is:
    a. ischemic bone disease
    b. infectious bone disease
    c. metabolic bone disease
    d. developmental bone disease

12. Osteomyelitis does NOT develop as:
    a. a complication of a compound fracture
    b. a result of hematogenous spread
    c. ingestion or inhalation of *Staphylococcus aureus*
    d. secondary to adjacent soft tissue infection

13. In osteomyelitis, a small section of dead, detached bone is:
    a. a sequestrum
    b. a fistula
    c. a nidus
    d. an involucrum

14. A sequestrum forms as a result of:
    a. pus production
    b. ischemia and necrosis
    c. new bone production
    d. rupture of the periosteum

15. Pus draining from a fistula that overlies a bone infection indicates:
    a. acute suppurative osteomyelitis
    b. nonsuppurative osteomyelitis
    c. chronic suppurative osteomyelitis
    d. any of the above

16. Please match the types of fracture in the left column with their descriptions in the right column:
    a. simple   1. _____ bone ends exposed to the environment
    b. complete   2. _____ bone has been pushed together
    c. compound   3. _____ one side of bone has bent
    d. comminuted   4. _____ a single line of breakage
    e. pathologic   5. _____ bone has been shattered
    f. greenstick   6. _____ both sides or cortices have been broken
    g. compression   7. _____ a result of weakness from disease

17. List two complications of a compound fracture:
    a._____ b._____

18. The term to describe a fracture that will not heal is:
    a. reduced
    b. callus
    c. union
    d. nonunion

19. Spontaneous fracture and bone pain are most often associated with:
    a. neoplasia
    b. osteomyelitis
    c. osteoporosis
    d. avascular necrosis

11. b–infectious bone disease

12. c–ingestion or inhalation of *Staphylococcus aureus*

13. a–a sequestrum

14. b–ischemia and necrosis

15. c–chronic suppurative osteomyelitis

16. 1. c–compound
    2. g–compression
    3. f–greenstick
    4. a–simple
    5. d–comminuted
    6. b–complete
    7. e–pathologic

17. a–hemorrhage
    b–osteomyelitis or infection

18. d–nonunion

19. a–neoplasia

20. The most common and malignant primary bone neoplasia is:
 a. chondrosarcoma
 b. Ewing's sarcoma
 c. osteosarcoma
 d. giant cell tumor

21. The most common type of malignant bone neoplasia is:
 a. osteosarcoma
 b. metastatic bone neoplasia
 c. osteogenic sarcoma
 d. Ewing's sarcoma

SECTION ► III. DISEASES OF JOINTS

► ARTHRITIS

You know what the suffix "itis" means. "Arthr/o" refers to a joint. Therefore, the term "arthritis" literally means _____(1) of a _____(2). In joint inflammation, the irritation usually involves the synovial membrane, or joint lining, first. This is because the synovium covers all surfaces of the joint. This is called **synovitis.** Because the synovium normally produces synovial fluid, during synovitis there is an increase in the amount of fluid in a joint. Depending on the nature of the inflammation, the increased synovial fluid may mix with exudate. Arthritis may be caused by trauma, infection (see Frame 17–42), possible autoimmune activity (see Frame 17–46), or age-related degeneration (see Frame 17–43). **Gout** is arthritis caused by deposits of tophi crystals in joints that are formed in hyperuricemia or increased uric acid in the blood. Crystal deposits cause severe inflammation, crippling pain, and eventual deformity of the joint. Gout was presented in Chapter 7 as a multifactorial genetic disease, and in Chapter 8 as a disorder of metabolism (the metabolism of uric acid). In arthritis, the first structure to become inflamed is the _____(3), and this is referred to as _____(4). This irritation causes an increase in the production of _____(5).

Infectious arthritis can develop through a variety of mechanisms, although bacterial infections are not a common joint disorder. First, there can be direct introduction of bacteria into a joint during a penetrating injury, during surgery, or during arthrocentesis (the removal of joint fluid). Second, there can be spread of infection from nearby bone or soft tissue. And third is hematogenous spread during sepsis, which means the bacteria arrived in the joint from the _____(1), and their presence in the blood is called _____(2). Probably the most common infectious arthritis is **Lyme disease.** Lyme disease is caused by a spirochete organism called *Borrelia burgdorferi.* This organism is harbored in deer ticks and is transmitted by their bites. The symptoms of Lyme disease are generalized illness and skin rash, followed by arthritis of various joints in a shifting pattern (migratory or moving arthritis). The inflammation spreads from joint to joint through the mechanism of bacteremia; therefore, this would be called _____(3) spread. Lyme disease is easily cured with correct diagnosis through blood tests and appropriate antibiotics. Arthritis due to the presence of microorganisms in a joint is called _____(4) arthritis. Bacteria may gain entry into a joint through direct _____(5), through spread from adjacent _____(6) or _____(7) infection, or from the _____(8). *Borrelia burgdorferi* is a spirochete that causes an infectious arthritis called _____(9). Bacteremia during Lyme disease is responsible for a _____(10) pattern of arthritis.

The majority of the elderly population have some degree of **osteoarthritis.** This chronic disease is the arthritis of old age and is the type most thought of when the term arthritis is heard. Its cause is the degeneration associated with age, so it is also called **degenerative joint disease,** or **DJD.** Osteoarthritis, or DJD, is the most common affliction of joints. Joints that have been subjected to continued use trauma, such as repeated movements or activities, are more susceptible to DJD. The more wear and tear, the greater the chance of osteoarthritis. The wear involves the articular cartilage that covers the bone ends in the joint. Increased stress on a joint surface speeds the development of DJD. DJD is also more likely to develop in injured joints, or in those which are congenitally deformed. Osteoarthritis is joint inflammation caused by _____(1), which goes along with old _____(2). It is also referred to as _____(3). The most common disorder of joints is _____(4). Joints that have been subjected to _____(5) are susceptible to DJD.

1. degeneration
2. age
3. degenerative joint disease
4. osteoarthritis, or DJD
5. stress

The signs and symptoms of osteoarthritis are directly related to pathologic changes in the joint, which are shown in Figure 17–9. First, the articular cartilage wears down, becoming thin and soft. Bits may flake off into the joint (called fragmentation). This leaves denuded or exposed areas of bare bone, which is very painful. In advanced cases, the eroded cartilage becomes calcified. The underlying bone degenerates and small fluid-filled cysts are formed. As the condition progresses, nodules of new bone called **spurs** are formed around the perimeter of the joint. This is called "lipping." The bone spurs are also called **osteophytes.** The protruding presence of osteophytes causes inflammation and pain in the surrounding soft tissue. This is called **periarticular** (around the joint) **inflammation.** Fibrosis of the area commonly develops. If an osteophyte breaks off and is freely floating in the joint, this is referred to as a **joint mouse.** The first occurrence in the development of DJD is the wearing and thinning of the _____(1). Flaking off, or _____(2), of the cartilage leaves painful bare areas of exposed _____(3). Small bumps of new bone called _____(4) form around the periphery of the joint. New bone spurs are also called _____(5), and if they break free and fall into the joint space, the term _____(6) is applied to them. The presence of osteophytes causes _____(7) inflammation and usually _____(8) of the surrounding soft tissue.

1. articular cartilage
2. fragmentation
3. bone
4. spurs
5. osteophytes
6. joint mouse
7. periarticular
8. fibrosis

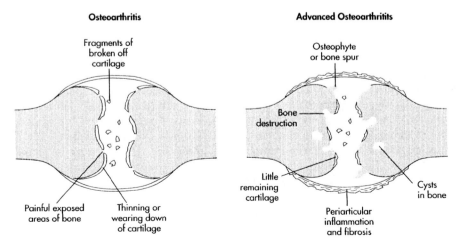

Figure 17–9. Osteoarthritis (degenerative joint disease).

17-45

Clinically, the prominent features of osteoarthritis are pain and loss of mobility or stiffness. Swelling and increased heat in the area are common. In advanced cases with periarticular changes, deformity results in some degree of disability. **Crepitus** is present, which is a crackling noise associated with the movement of rough surfaces on each other. (The rough surfaces are the denuded bone with its loss of cartilage.) Pain and stiffness are most prominent after a period of resting. Therefore, osteoarthritis is worse in the morning and is somewhat relieved by movement in which the joint warms out of the stiffness. The number of joints that are affected varies with the individual. The most common joints that are affected are the hips, knees, spine, feet (the weight-bearing joints), and the hands. DJD of the spine often occurs in conjunction with spondylosis, a degeneration of intervertebral disks in older adults. Obesity worsens arthritis of weight-bearing joints.

17-46

1. women
2. autoimmune
3. inflammation
4. joints
5. IgM
6. rheumatoid factor
7. auto

Rheumatoid arthritis is a chronic inflammatory disease of the joints and other parts of the body that affects more women than men, and is seen more in younger women. Rheumatoid arthritis is more crippling than osteoarthritis. This is a systemic disease with several abnormalities outside of the joints. Individuals with rheumatoid arthritis experience fatigue, weight loss, fever, and anemia, among other complaints. Rheumatoid arthritis is suspected to be autoimmune in nature, with possibly a genetic predisposition. Its autoimmune nature is likely because of the presence of an abnormal IgM, a proven autoantibody, that targets another antibody, IgG. This IgM autoantibody (an antibody against an antibody) may be tested for and has been named **rheumatoid factor.** Rheumatoid arthritis is a systemic disease of predominantly young _____(1) which is probably _____(2) in nature. It causes chronic _____(3) of both the _____(4) and other body structures. An abnormal antibody of the _____(5) type has been identified and named _____(6). Since this IgM targets the body's own IgG antibodies, it is classified as an _____(7)antibody.

17-47

The antibody–antigen complexes (autoIgM–IgG) are thought to be deposited on the synovial membrane of some joints. Their presence causes an intense inflammatory reaction, or synovitis. Inflammatory cells, such as neutrophils, and exudate containing the cells' lytic enzymes fill the joint space. If you will recall from Chapter 2, the enzymes and chemical mediators of inflammation are capable of tissue damage themselves, and in a confined space like a joint, the damage can be extensive. There is no chance for these chemicals to be diluted out in surrounding soft tissue. The synovial membrane becomes thickened, further filling the joint space. The inflammation spreads to the articular cartilage and the enzymes erode and destroy it. A layer of granulation tissue forms from the inflamed synovium, and this tissue is called a **pannus.** The pannus covers the exposed bone surfaces. The damaged joint surfaces are replaced with fibrotic tissue, or become scarred. The scar tissue frequently runs from one free joint surface to another like adhesions in the abdomen. In severe cases, this connection of the surfaces by scar tissue causes loss of all movement. The joint becomes fused or frozen. Fusion of a joint and loss of movement is called **ankylosis.** Osteoporosis develops in bone closest to the ankylosed joint because of disuse atrophy. The joint destruction of rheumatoid arthritis is shown in Figure 17–10. Severe cases of rheumatoid arthritis demonstrate inflammatory lesions in other parts of the body, such as the lungs, muscle, heart, and eyes. Vasculitis may be present in organs and cause further damage through ischemia.

17-48

1. antibody–antigen complexes
2. synovial membrane
3. inflammatory
4. cells
5. lytic enzymes
6. exudate
7. enzymes
8. chemical mediators
9. pannus

The pathogenesis of rheumatoid arthritis is believed to be due to the deposits of _____(1) on the _____(2) of joints. This creates an intense _____(3) reaction, complete with the presence of the _____(4) of inflammation and their _____(5). Inflammatory fluid, or _____(6), fills the joint space. Much damage to joint surfaces is caused by lytic _____(7) and other _____(8). The thickened synovial membrane develops into granulation tissue that covers the joint surfaces, and this is called a _____(9). The joint

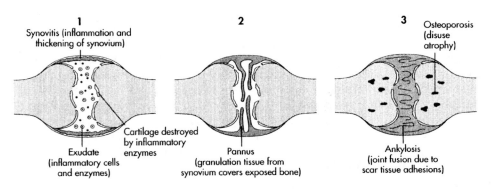

Figure 17-10. Stages of rheumatoid arthritis.

may become fused because of the presence of _____(10) tissue that prevents movement. A frozen joint is described as experiencing _____(11). Disuse of the joint leads to _____(12) of surrounding bone.

10. scar
11. ankylosis
12. osteoporosis

17-49

The severity of rheumatoid arthritis ranges from mild stiffness to joint deformity and anky-losis of several joints. The hands are most often affected and show an ulnar deformity, or bending laterally toward the ulna. Clinically, along with systemic disorders, there is joint pain, loss of movement, and deformity. Age, x-rays, and blood tests for the rheumatoid fac-tor help to distinguish this disease from osteoarthritis. Corticosteroids are helpful in this dis-order, both from an anti-inflammatory aspect and because steroids decrease immune activity. The goal of treatment is to reduce deformity and ankylosis. Some ankylosed joints may be replaced surgically.

17-50

Another fusion disorder of joints is **ankylosing spondylitis.** You know that ankylosing means fusion. The word element "spond" means spine. Therefore, ankylosing spondylitis is inflammatory fusion of the spine because of arthritis of the vertebral joint spaces. Occa-sionally, the sacroiliac joints are involved. The lesions in the vertebral joints resemble rheumatoid arthritis, and the inflammation later leads to ankylosis. This disorder occurs in young men. It has a familial tendency, and in most cases the individual has the HLA-B27 antigen. Inheritance of the HLA-B27 antigen seems to accompany the development of this disorder. Ankylosing spondylitis causes spinal deformity that leads to disability. The fusion causes a very stiff spine, commonly called a "poker back." The ligaments associated with the intervertebral disks become calcified, contributing to the rigidity. Ankylosing spondylitis is _____(1) of the _____(2) caused by the effects of _____(3) in the _____(4) joints. Seen most often in young _____(5), its development is associated with the presence of the _____(6) antigen. This disorder is sometimes commonly called _____(7) because of the extreme _____(8) of the spine.

1. inflammatory fusion
2. spine
3. arthritis
4. vertebral
5. men
6. HLA-B27
7. poker back
8. stiffness

▶ OTHER DISORDERS OF JOINTS

17-51

Other disorders of the joints are often due to traumatic injury, whether it is true trauma or excessive strain on a joint. A **sprain** is a slight injury, or tear, to the ligaments of a joint. It usually results from twisting or bending beyond the normal range of motion. Other soft tissue (tendons, muscle, blood vessels) can also be injured by the same movement. A rup-tured vessel bleeds and causes swelling and bruising of the area. Swelling and pain are the most common reactions to the injury. These reactions are typical of inflammation. A twisted ankle is the most common example of a joint sprain, with rupture of the ligaments on the

1. sprain
2. twisting
3. bending
4. strain
5. joint capsule
6. slight
7. luxation
8. dislocation

outside, or lateral, side of the ankle. When the sprain involves the ligaments of the vertebrae in the neck, this is commonly called a **whiplash** injury. You should not confuse a sprain with a **strain,** which is torn muscle tissue or tendon. A strain is commonly called a "pulled muscle." A **subluxation** is a partial tear in the joint capsule that allows the bones of the joint to become slightly out of place or misaligned. A subluxation is commonly called a partial dislocation. A **luxation** is complete rupture of the joint capsule with the bones significantly out of alignment. This is commonly called a dislocation. Slight injury to the joint ligaments is called a _____(1). It is commonly caused by excessive _____(2) or _____(3). A pulled muscle is medically termed a _____(4). A subluxation is a small tear in the _____(5) which results in _____(6) misplacement of the bones of a joint. A ruptured capsule with gross misplacement of the bones is a (an) _____(7), commonly called a _____(8).

17-52

1. injury
2. motion, movement, or activity
3. inflammation
4. median nerve

Carpal tunnel syndrome is injury to the wrist and hand due to long-term repetitive movement (the same motion over and over with the wrists bent at an angle). Carpal tunnel syndrome results in damage to the median nerve by pressure from inflammation. When inflammation in the area of the carpal tunnel puts pressure on the nerves, it interferes with nerve impulse conduction. Other joints may be affected but the wrist is most commonly affected. The most well-known motions that produce this syndrome are computer keyboard strokes, although other repeated activities can cause it. Pain from the area may extend up the arm. Numbness and tingling from impaired nerve impulses precede outright pain. The symptoms become worse at night. This condition is alleviated or relieved with rest from the causative motions. Splinting the wrist helps to decrease the inflammation, along with anti-inflammatory medication or steroids. Severe cases require surgery to relieve the pressure on the median nerve. Carpal tunnel syndrome is _____(1) of the wrist joint because of continued _____(2) that is always the same. The injury results in the typical response of _____(3). This applies pressure to the _____(4), which results in the symptoms.

17-53

Chronic low back pain is an extremely common and debilitating complaint that has many causes. Pinpointing the exact cause is often frustrating and unsuccessful. Mankind's upright posture puts strain on the vertebral column daily. Factors that add to the strain are poor posture, abdominal obesity, and lumbar and abdominal muscle weakness. The most common cause of acute, severe low back pain is **intervertebral disk herniation.** This is commonly known as a "slipped disk" and is often associated with sudden motion or excessive weight bearing. In between the vertebrae of the spine are spongy, cartilaginous pads (the disks) that act as shock absorbers and increase the flexibility of the spine. Their cushioning nature can easily be compromised by injury or degeneration. A weakened disk is more susceptible to herniation. You know from Chapter 12 that a herniation is a bulge in soft tissue that protrudes into another area. The fibrous walls of a disk (the annulus fibrosus) can break down and allow the inner soft material (the nucleus pulposus) to protrude outward to various degrees. An incomplete herniation is protrusion of the material. A complete herniation is rupture and spillage of the material (a slipped disk). The most common location of a slipped disk is in the lumbar spine or lower back.

17-54

1. intervertebral disk herniation
2. slipped disk
3. cartilaginous
4. herniation
5. incomplete
6. complete

Pain in the lower back that is severe and occurs abruptly is most commonly caused by _____(1), commonly known as a _____(2). The disks are spongy, _____(3) pads that absorb the shock of walking and running. A diseased or injured disk may bulge outward, and this is called a _____(4). Protrusion of various degrees describes a _____(5) herniation. Rupture of the disk describes a _____(6) herniation. As the disk material pushes out or spills out, it applies pressure on the nerves exiting the spinal cord, or on the cord itself. This causes pain in the area of herniation and in the area innervated by the compressed nerve. It often involves the sciatic nerve, which runs down the back of the leg. Pain of this nerve is called **sciatica.** The pain is felt in the buttock and down the back of the leg. Muscle weakness (paresis) may exist depending on the amount of injury to the nerve. Muscle spasm always accompanies the pain, and the resulting tension worsens the pain. Spraining of the ligaments around the affected vertebral joint also contributes to pain. Treatment for disk disorders is extremely varied and depends on the cause of the injury and the extent of damage. Some cases need only rest, anti-inflammatory medication, and heat treatment followed by muscle strengthening exercise. Other cases require traction or surgical intervention.

If you will recall, bursae are sacs of synovial fluid around joints that move a great deal and they help to decrease friction. If a bursa becomes inflamed, this is described as **bursitis.** Bursitis most often occurs in the shoulder joint, one of the most moveable joints of the body. It is caused by excessive motion, injury to the bursa, or other stress on the joint such as repetitive activity. Bursitis is very painful and interferes with movement of the joint. It is treated like other traumatically induced inflammation of joints, with supportive therapy. Bursitis is _____(1) of the _____(2) around a joint. The prominent clinical features of bursitis are _____(3) and interference in joint _____(4).

1. inflammation
2. bursae
3. pain
4. movement

III. REVIEW QUESTIONS

1. The most common of these afflictions of joints is:
   a. luxation
   b. ankylosis
   c. arthritis
   d. strain

2. Increased synovial fluid in an inflamed joint is due to:
   a. pannus
   b. synovitis
   c. osteophytes
   d. periarticular inflammation

3. The most common joint affliction in the elderly is:
   a. osteoarthritis
   b. infectious arthritis
   c. rheumatoid arthritis
   d. ankylosing spondylitis

4. List in order of occurrence these pathologic changes in osteoarthritis:
   a. _____ periarticular inflammation
   b. _____ articular cartilage thinning
   c. _____ joint mouse formation
   d. _____ cartilage fragmentation
   e. _____ osteophyte formation

5. Which of the following is NOT true of rheumatoid arthritis?
   a. It is considered an autoimmune disease.
   b. It is a systemic disease.
   c. The autoantibody is called rheumatoid factor.
   d. It causes fusion of the intervertebral joints in the spine.

1. c–arthritis
2. b–synovitis
3. a–osteoarthritis
4. a–4; b–1; c–5; d–2; e–3
5. d–It causes fusion of the intervertebral joints in the spine.

6. a–4; b–3; c–1; d–5; e–2

7. b–young men with the HLA-B27 antigen

8. c–intervertebral disk herniation

9. b–rupture of a disk with spillage of the inner material

6. List in order of occurrence these events of rheumatoid arthritis:
   a. _____ thickened, inflamed synovium produces a layer of granulation tissue called pannus
   b. _____ exudate containing inflammatory cells, lytic enzymes, and chemical mediators destroy joint surfaces
   c. _____ antibody–antigen complexes deposit on the synoval membrane
   d. _____ fibrosis may causes ankylosis in severe cases
   e. _____ synovitis

7. Ankylosing spondylitis is most often seen in:
   a. elderly men with the HLA-B27 antigen
   b. young men with the HLA-B27 antigen
   c. postmenopausal women
   d. young women with rheumatoid factor in their circulation

8. The most common cause of acute severe low back pain is:
   a. lumbar and abdominal muscle weakness
   b. abdominal obesity
   c. intervertebral disk herniation
   d. subluxation of the lumbar vertebrae

9. A slipped disk is the common term for:
   a. slight protrusion of the inner material of a disk
   b. rupture of a disk with spillage of the inner material
   c. luxation of a vertebral joint
   d. sciatica

SECTION ▶ # IV. DISEASES OF MUSCLE

▶ MUSCULAR DYSTROPHY

······ 17–56 ······

1. genetic
2. inherited
3. degeneration
4. atrophy
5. myocytes or muscle cells
6. disabled

Muscular dystrophy is a group of genetic, or inherited, muscle diseases in which the myocytes (muscle cells) are defective. The muscle fibers undergo degeneration that is genetically predestined. Muscular dystrophy is progressive; that is, once the degeneration begins, it continues along a known course, causing the individual to become worse with time. The primary pathology is that of muscular atrophy, or wasting away. Therefore, it follows that there is loss of function which in this case is normal movement and coordination. There are several types of dystrophy, each affecting patients at different ages from childhood to adult. The severity of each form varies, and some forms affect other body systems. Affected individuals with more severe forms eventually are completely disabled. Two of the types of dystrophy are named for the muscle groups they involve. These are **limb–girdle dystrophy** (legs and pelvis) and **facioscapulohumeral dystrophy** (face, shoulders, and arms). These forms are not common, and the symptoms are relatively mild. **Myotonic dystrophy** is more common. Along with muscle atrophy there is also mental degeneration. **Myotonia** is present, and this means that the muscle groups do not relax right away after contraction. The hands demonstrate this when the patient grips an object and is unable to let go. Myotonic dystrophy is a systemic disease also affecting the heart and causing diabetes. The life span is often shortened in these patients. The cause of muscular dystrophy is _____(1), or _____(2). The basic abnormality is that the muscles undergo _____(3) and _____(4) because the _____(5) are defective. In severe forms of muscular dystrophy, the patient loses all function of the muscles and becomes _____(6).

The most common, well-known, and most severe form is **Duchenne's muscular dystrophy.** This is an X-linked, or sex-linked, recessive genetic disease. Because it is X-linked, only _____(1) males / females (choose one) are affected. This disease develops at a very young age. (A mild form of the same type of dystrophy is called **Becker's dystrophy.**) In Duchenne's dystrophy, the underlying lesion is a defective protein in the muscle cell membrane. This protein is responsible for the integrity of the cell, so the cells are compromised in their basic structure and are unable to function normally. The muscle groups degenerate and become weak, too weak in fact to support weight. Muscle fibers degenerate and die, and the remaining cells are abnormal. Fibrosis (scar tissue) and adipose (fat) deposits fill in the gaps caused by necrosis and loss of the myocytes. A photomicrograph of dystrophic muscle can be seen in Figure 17–11. Replacement of muscle fiber by this material obviously leads to decreased function, since scar tissue in muscle is about as functional as it is in the heart after an MI. Regeneration of the lost tissue is poor, which is typical of muscle healing. On a larger scale, this disease results in whole muscle groups with lost muscle fibers and replacement of the fibers with nonfunctional connective tissue (scarring). Duchenne's muscular dystrophy is the most _____(2) and most _____(3) form of the dystrophies. The inheritance of this disease is through the _____(4) recessive gene mechanism. The basic pathology is a defective _____(5) found in the muscle cell _____(6). When this protein is not normal, the basic _____(7) of the cell is sacrificed and function is abnormal. Muscle fibers break down or _____(8) and then _____(9). Muscle tissue lost through degeneration and necrosis is replaced with _____(10) and _____(11). These infiltrates have none of the original _____(12) of muscle tissue.

1. males
2. common
3. severe
4. X- or sex-linked
5. protein
6. membrane
7. structure
8. degenerate
9. die
10. fibrosis
11. fat
12. function

Clinically, the signs of Duchenne's dystrophy appear in very young boys just a few years old. It begins as great weakness in the legs and hips. Both rising from a squatting position and walking become extremely difficult. The legs become very uncoordinated. Deformities of the legs and spine develop because normal muscle function is necessary to exert forces on bones that influence their development. The boy becomes disabled and is usually confined to a wheelchair in just a few years. The respiratory muscles are also affected, causing dyspnea, which means difficult _____(1). Poor respiratory function makes the patient very susceptible to frequent bouts of pneumonia. Often, there is weakness of the muscles of

1. breathing

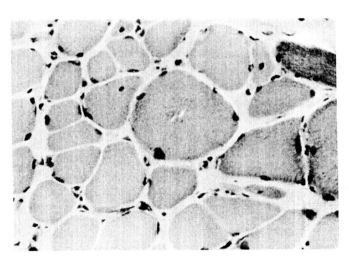

Figure 17–11. The appearance of dystrophic muscle fascicles. Note the excessive amount of fibrosis or connective tissue among the fascicles, and the marked variation in size of individual fascicles. *(From Kent and Hart,* Introduction to Human Disease, *3rd ed., Appleton and Lange.)*

the heart, leading to heart failure. When combined with the pathology of other body systems, early death by about age 20 is inevitable. There is no treatment for Duchenne's dystrophy, other than supportive therapy, and there is no cure.

▶ MYASTHENIA GRAVIS

Myasthenia gravis is also a progressive disease with muscle weakness during activity and atrophy later. It is a defect at the biochemical level that is most likely autoimmune in cause. This is because there is an antibody in the circulation that targets the acetylcholine (ACh) receptors at the neuromuscular junction (NMJ). Therefore, instead of being a disease of purely muscle fibers or nerves, this disorder affects the NMJ where the nerve impulses are received by the muscle fibers. The autoantibody causes degeneration in this area and greatly interferes with nerve impulse conduction. Some sources say that the autoantibody destroys ACh, which is the neurotransmitter, while others contend that the antibody binds to the ACh receptor sites and prevents ACh from binding. Either way, muscle weakness results from impaired reception of nervous stimulation. Muscle contraction and strength is directly dependent upon proper nerve impulse conduction and reception by the muscle. The source of the autoantibody is believed to be the thymus gland, which is enlarged in many cases of myasthenia gravis. The cause of myasthenia gravis is considered to be _____(1) in nature. This is because a (an) _____(2) against the _____(3) receptors at the _____(4) are found in the blood. The autoantibody prevents normal nerve impulse conduction by either _____(5) ACh, or binding at the _____(6), preventing _____(7) from binding and completing the impulse. Since the nerve impulse is not conducted to the muscle fibers, _____(8) of the muscles results.

The onset of myasthenia gravis is insidious (slow or gradual and unnoticed at first). Any activity causes depletion of muscle strength. Fatigue quickly sets in. The muscles eventually atrophy from lack of nervous stimulation. Myasthenia gravis affects all muscle groups. Normal movement (walking, even eating) becomes extremely difficult. The facial and eye muscles are involved early in the course of the disease. The respiratory muscles also weaken to the point of failure, and respiratory failure is generally the cause of death in untreated cases. The primary treatment is administration of an anticholinesterase medication. Cholinesterase is an enzyme that breaks down ACh at the NMJ after it has performed its function of carrying impulses across the synapse. This is a normal, necessary destruction of ACh. Its breakdown stops the impulse and allows the muscle fiber to relax. Anticholinesterase removes the enzyme that removes ACh, thus allowing ACh to build up and remain at the receptors until a normal impulse can be conducted. This medication is not a cure but greatly relieves the symptoms and prolongs life. Removal of an enlarged thymus is also helpful. The effects of myasthenia gravis can be reduced with a medication that destroys _____(1), which is a (an) _____(2) that normally destroys _____(3). This allows enough ACh to remain at the NMJ until a nerve _____(4) can be conducted.

▶ OTHER DISEASES OF MUSCLE

Myositis, as the name implies, is an inflammatory disease of muscle. It is generally called **polymyositis** ("poly" means many) because several muscle groups are usually involved. Inflammation caused by infection with a microorganism is classified as **infectious myositis.** The most common muscle infections are caused by:

1. Pyogenic bacteria. *Staphylococcus aureus* during bacteremia and septicemia can lodge in muscle and produce an abscess.

1. myositis
2. polymyositis
3. infection
4. microorganisms
5. infectious myositis

2. Anaerobic bacteria. *Clostridium perfringens* during gas gangrene of infected wounds (see Chap. 5) causes necrosis.
3. Viruses. Coxsackievirus is best known for muscle invasion. Viral myositis causes pain, and pain of muscle is called **myalgia.** Coxsackievirus has a predilection for the heart, causing **viral myocarditis.**
4. Parasites. *Toxoplasma gondii* is a protozoal infection of muscle acquired from infected cats, and *Trichinella* is an intestinal worm from undercooked pork that lodges in muscle.

Disease of muscle that is inflammatory in nature is called _____(1) or _____(2). It may be caused by _____(3) with several types of _____(4), in which case it is specifically called _____(5).

17-62

1. antibodies
2. antigens
3. hypersensitivity
4. inflammation
5. ANA or antinuclear antibodies
6. nuclei

Another classification of myositis is **immune-mediated myositis.** It is the action of antibodies against antigens, often during a hypersensitivity reaction, that causes inflammatory injury to muscle. Many of these patients have ANAs (antinuclear antibodies) in their blood. These are autoantibodies that target the nuclei of various cells of the body. Some of the disease states that cause immune myositis include:

1. Systemic lupus erythematosus. In this systemic autoimmune disease (see Chap. 4), type III hypersensitivity mechanisms predominate. Immune complexes deposit in vessel walls in muscle and many other tissues. The resulting vasculitis compromises whatever tissue is supplied by the injured vessels. In the muscle, atrophy develops.
2. Sarcoidosis. This is a cell-mediated type IV hypersensitivity leading to granuloma formations in muscle, which are infiltrated with epithelioid cells and giant cells (see Chap. 2).
3. Immune polymyositis. Chronic inflammation of muscle results from infiltration by immune cells (plasma cells and lymphocytes) in this autoimmune disease. Muscle fibers are destroyed by the infiltration, and fibrosis replaces the resulting necrosis.

Immune-mediated myositis responds well to corticosteroids and other immunosuppressive drugs. In immune-mediated myositis, the injury to muscle occurs because of the action between _____(1) and _____(2). These are often classified as _____(3) reactions. The injury causes _____(4) of the affected muscle tissue. Often there is the presence of _____(5), in the circulation, and these are antibodies that try to destroy the _____(6) of many body cells.

17-63

Myopathy literally means muscle disease and is a very general, nondescriptive term. A myopathy may be primary as a congenital disorder, or acquired later in life secondary to a systemic disease. Congenital myopathy is rare and is usually a result of a genetic error in the metabolism of lipids or glycogen. Some of these myopathies are confined to muscle; others are systemic diseases. Overall, affected children have extreme muscle weakness and limpness. They may not be able to raise their head when lifted and appear like a rag doll. This has led to the common description "floppy infant syndrome." Acquired myopathies are secondary diseases of the muscle, generally seen as weakness caused by disease of some other body system. The most common metabolic disease that affects muscles is diabetes. You know that diabetes causes microangiopathy (disease of small vessels), and this creates chronic ischemia in muscle. The abnormal carbohydrate and lipid metabolism that accompanies diabetes also impairs muscle function because muscle has such a relatively high metabolic rate and great need for these nutrients. Endocrine disease, specifically thyroid disease, affects muscle. In hyperthyroidism, the greatly accelerated basal metabolic rate quickly depletes muscle stores of glycogen, leaving them without an energy source. In hypothyroidism, the depressed basal metabolic rate causes sluggishness of muscle function. Malignant neoplasia, which creates paraneoplastic syndrome, can cause muscle weakness through several mechanisms.

The term that means disease of muscle is _____(1). This term _____(2) does / does not (choose one) describe the cause of the disease. Most primary myopathies are _____(3), or present at birth. The limpness and weakness of affected babies has led to the description _____(4). Most secondary myopathies are _____(5), or develop later in life as a result of a primary _____(6) disease. The most common metabolic disease that impairs muscle function is _____(7) because of microangiopathy and therefore chronic _____(8) of the tissues. Upset in levels of hormones from the _____(9) gland disturb muscle function, as well as some cancers through _____(10) syndrome.

In **neurogenic muscle disease,** since muscle function depends completely on nerve stimulation, disease of neurons leads to wasting of muscle, or **neurogenic atrophy** (wasting originating from disease of the nerves). Lack of normal innervation, or stimulation from nerve impulses, creates disuse atrophy of muscles similar to that seen from immobilization. Nonuse of muscle for any reason leads to withering of its mass. In neurogenic muscle disease, the nerve impairment may involve the upper motor neuron (UMN) of the brain, or the lower motor neuron (LMN) of the spinal cord. The UMN connects the brain to the spinal cord, and the LMN connects the spinal cord to the muscles as the peripheral nerves. Any of the many causes of both upper and lower motor neuron injury can lead to muscle atrophy. Examples of these injuries include trauma, stroke, infections, and toxins. Most common is diabetic neuropathy, or nerve disease due to microangiopathy and ischemia. The degree of atrophy in skeletal muscle, which ranges from individual fibers to an entire fascicle, depends on how much nerve tissue is injured. The muscle fibers usually atrophy in groups because they are all innervated by the same nerve axon. The worst case scenario is trauma to the spinal cord or brain that leaves entire muscle groups paralyzed. Muscle will recover only if it is reinnervated, which isn't likely since central nervous system regeneration is practically nonexistent. Fortunately, peripheral nerve damage is more common and the prognosis is a little better. Peripheral nerves that are transected (cut completely through) have some chance of very slow regeneration, especially if surgically repaired. Re-establishing muscle function is possible in these cases with proper physical therapy.

Neurogenic atrophy means that the muscles are _____(1) away because of lack of _____(2) from injured or diseased _____(3). This muscle disorder as a whole is called _____(4). The muscles atrophy because they are not _____(5), similar to immobilization. The nerve injury that causes neurogenic muscle disease may be found in the _____(6) or _____(7) motor neurons. The metabolic disease that produces nerve damage because of small vessel disease and ischemia is called _____(8). Whenever a nerve is damaged, the muscle fibers atrophy in _____(9) because they are all connected to the same nerve _____(10). Recovery of muscle fibers requires reinnervation by nerves, which is least likely in trauma of the _____(11) or _____(12). The causes and features of diseases of muscle are reviewed for you in Table 17–2.

▶ NEOPLASIA OF MUSCLE

Neoplasia of muscle tissue is very rare, and this is related to the property of muscle in which the cells do not readily proliferate. While this property does not allow speedy healing, it also dampens the chances of cell transformation and proliferation. There are a variety of both benign and malignant muscle tumors. The most common and clinically significant is the **rhabdomyosarcoma.** Given this name, you should be able to recognize that this neoplasia is _____(1) benign / malignant (choose one). Rhabdomyosarcoma is a malignant cancer that arises from skeletal muscle cells and occurs most frequently in children

TABLE 17–2. CAUSES AND FEATURES OF MUSCLE DISEASES

Disease	Cause	Features
Duchenne's muscular dystrophy	Genetic, X-linked inheritance	Degeneration of muscle fibers due to defective protein Fibrosis replaces muscle fibers Weakness leading to complete disability with failure of heart and respiration
Myasthenia gravis	Autoantibodies prevent reception of ACh neurotransmitter (autoimmune disease)	Weakness and fatigue due to lack of stimulation by nerves Atrophy Respiratory failure
Myositis (polymyositis)	Infection Immune-mediated hypersensitivity Autoimmune disease	Inflammation of muscle groups due to injury by causative agent
Acquired myopathy	Secondary to diabetes	Weakness due to microangiopathy, ischemia, and insufficient nutrients
	Secondary to hyperthyroidism or hypothyroidism	Weakness due to depleted energy stores or decreased BMR
	Secondary to malignant neoplasia	Weakness due to paraneoplastic syndrome
Neurogenic muscle disease	Secondary to nerve disease, especially diabetic neuropathy	Wasting or atrophy due to lack of stimulation by nerve impulses

(although it may be seen in adults). The tumor can be located in almost any muscle group. It does demonstrate the typical malignant properties of local invasion and metastasis to the lungs. The prognosis depends on the size and location of the tumor, that is, whether or not it can be completely removed. Complete removal is usually curative, while incomplete removal requires chemotherapy and radiation to yield a 40 percent 5-year survival rate. Neoplasia of muscle is _____(2) common / rare (choose one) because muscle cells do not readily _____(3). The most significant malignancy of muscle is the _____(4).

2. rare
3. proliferate
4. rhabdomyosarcoma

IV. REVIEW QUESTIONS

1. Genetically programmed degeneration of muscle fibers with progressive atrophy best describes:
   a. muscular dystrophy
   b. myasthenia gravis
   c. neurogenic muscle disease
   d. myositis
   e. myopathy

1. a–muscular dystrophy

2. The most common and severe form of muscular dystrophy is:
   a. Becker's dystrophy
   b. myotonic dystrophy
   c. Duchenne's dystrophy
   d. limb–girdle dystrophy

2. c–Duchenne's dystrophy

3. b–it is a sex-linked recessive inheritance

4. b–fibrosis; d–adipose tissue

5. b–the neuromuscular junction

6. d–blockage of nerve impulse conduction by an autoantibody that displaces ACh from its receptors

7. b–a medication that interferes with cholinesterase allows ACh to build up at the receptors

8. a–myositis

9. b–secondary myopathy; c–neurogenic muscle disease

10. d–neurogenic muscle disease

3. Duchenne's muscular dystrophy occurs in boys because:
   a. it is a direct inheritance of a defective gene from the father
   b. it is a sex-linked recessive inheritance
   c. it is associated with the HLA-B27 antigen, which only males inherit
   d. females who inherit this gene are stillborn

4. In Duchenne's muscular dystrophy, lost muscle fibers are replaced with (choose all that apply):
   a. nonfunctional skeletal muscle fibers
   b. fibrosis
   c. necrosis
   d. adipose tissue
   e. smooth muscle fiber

5. Myasthenia gravis is a disorder of:
   a. nerve axons
   b. the neuromuscular junction
   c. skeletal muscle fibers
   d. acetylcholine production

6. The mechanism of disease in myasthenia gravis is:
   a. an autoantibody that destroys the ACh receptors
   b. blockage of nerve impulse conduction due to degeneration of nerve axons
   c. failure of response to nerve impulses by degenerating muscle fibers
   d. blockage of nerve impulse conduction by an autoantibody that displaces ACh from its receptors

7. In myasthenia gravis, a nerve impulse may be received by muscle fibers if:
   a. corticosteroids decrease the activity of the autoantibody
   b. a medication that interferes with cholinesterase allows ACh to build up at the receptors
   c. a medication that interferes with ACh allows cholinesterase to build up at the receptors
   d. corticosteroids decrease the activity of ACh

8. Inflammatory disease of muscle is called:
   a. myositis
   b. myopathy
   c. neurogenic atrophy
   d. dystrophy

9. Diabetes can cause (choose all that apply):
   a. secondary myositis
   b. secondary myopathy
   c. neurogenic muscle disease
   d. primary myopathy
   e. paraneoplastic syndrome

10. Muscular atrophy resulting from lack of nerve impulses and disuse best describes:
    a. secondary myopathy
    b. rhabdomyosarcoma
    c. muscular dystrophy
    d. neurogenic muscle disease

► SECTION II

Osteogenesis imperfecta ("imperfect formation of bone") is a hereditary defect in the production of bone tissue, caused by abnormally formed collagen. Abnormal growth, deformities, and frequent fractures are signs of the condition. *Achondroplasia,* another hereditary disease, results from abnormal formation, growth, and ossification of the cartilage of the long bones. The condition leads to *achondroplastic dwarfism,* in which the affected individual has very short arms and legs with a relatively normal trunk. *Osteopetrosis* (marble bone disease) is a genetic condition where bone formation is greater than resorption, resulting in thickened, yet brittle, bone. Thickening of the cortex invades the medullary cavity of the bones, which leaves less room for the hematopoietic stem cells. Anemia is a possible complication of osteopetrosis.

In *osteoporosis,* there is less than normal bone mass (osteopenia), yet the composition of the bone is normal. The cortex becomes thin and the spicules in the trabeculae of spongy bone become narrowed. Since estrogen is necessary for normal bone density, post-menopausal women are most often affected with the disease. Prolonged bedrest, paralysis, steroid therapy, and lack of exercise may also lead to osteoporosis. The thinner bones (e.g., the vertebrae) are most susceptible to the effects of osteoporosis. *Osteomalacia* (called *rickets* when it affects children) is softening of the bones due to insufficient deposition of calcium and phosphorus in bone because of a lack of vitamin D. In contrast to osteoporosis, the bone tissue is abnormal. Causes of osteomalacia include malnutrition, impaired vitamin D synthesis in the skin, and malabsorption. *Paget's disease (osteitis deformans),* the cause of which is unknown, is characterized by excessively thickened bones due to overgrowth of osteoid. Affected individuals are susceptible to fracture and experience bone pain, headache, and dizziness (due to increased pressure on cranial nerves). Paget's disease is considered a forerunner of bone cancer.

Osteitis fibrosa cystica is a metabolic disorder caused by excessive production of parathyroid hormone (PTH), which leads to an increase in the activity of bone-resorbing osteoclasts. Bone becomes porous and decalcified, which causes skeletal weakness and deformity, bone pain, and increased susceptibility to fractures. *Aseptic bone necrosis* (avascular necrosis) results from noninfectious (i.e., no infectious particle is associated) bone infarction. The condition often occurs in children with fractures near the metabolically active metaphysis, or it may result from emboli that lodge in the nutrient arteries. Many cases are idiopathic. *Legg–Calvé–Perthes disease,* for example, is idiopathic avascular necrosis specifically of the femoral head.

Suppurative osteomyelitis is bone infection by pus-producing bacteria. The condition is most frequently seen in children and may be acute or chronic. *Nonsuppurative osteomyelitis* is bone infection by non-pus-producing bacteria. *Acute suppurative osteomyelitis* is most commonly caused by *Staphylococcus aureus,* which gains access to the bone from trauma, surgery, or infection of the soft tissues next to bone. Inflammation, ischemia, and necrosis of the bone are events associated with the condition. Left untreated, the disease can progress to *chronic suppurative osteomyelitis,* where the draining tissue creates a fistulous tract to the outside of the body. An *involucrum* (area of new bone formed around the site of infection) may form in an attempt to wall off the infection. Toxemia, septic shock, and death may ensue.

A *fracture* (a break in bone) may be classified as *simple* (a single line of disruption or break), *incomplete* (only one side of the bone is involved), or *complete* (extending completely through the bone). Fractures may be *closed* (the skin over the break is intact) or *compound* (the skin over the break is open, exposing the bone ends to the environment). A *complicated* fracture is a compound fracture that has become infected. In a *comminuted* fracture, the break has created bone fragments. This type of fracture is the most difficult to treat surgically. A *compression* fracture occurs when two bones (usually diseased vertebrae) are forcefully compressed. A *stress* fracture, which generally occurs in the anterior tibia from jolting exercise, is tiny linear cracks in the bone. A *greenstick* fracture, in which the bones bend more than break, is most often seen in children. A *pathologic* (spontaneous) fracture is a break that occurs under normal pressure or only slight trauma. Osteoporosis and bone cancer are the most common cause of pathologic fractures. Healing of a fracture involves the initial formation of a hematoma between the broken ends, followed by fibrous cartilage and trabeculae formation. A *callus* unites the two ends of bone. A *delayed union* is poor healing of a fracture, and may be caused by vitamin D and mineral deficiency. Delayed union is often seen in the elderly. Failure of the two ends of the bone to unite is a *nonunion,* a condition that develops when soft tissue interferes with bridging across the break gap. A *fibrous nonunion,* where a fibrous scar develops instead of a callus, may result from too much movement at the fracture site.

The most common form of bone neoplasia is of the blood-forming cells in the bone marrow. *Leukemia* and *multiple myeloma* are examples of such diseases. An *osteoma,* which originates from the bone-producing cells, is the most common benign bone tumor. A *chondroma* is a benign growth of cartilage cells. A *fibroma* originates from fibroblasts. These tumors generally cause little problem, and pain may or may not be present. The most common malignant bone tumor is *osteosarcoma* (osteogenic sarcoma), in which overproduction of osteoid forms large masses on the metaphyses of long bones. Osteosarcoma most often affects young people. Death is the result of metastasis to the lungs. A *chondrosarcoma* is malignant neoplasia of the chondroblasts, most often located in the vertebrae, pelvis, or ribs. In a *giant cell tumor,* the cells are large and multinucleated, and probably originate from osteoclasts. In this form of cancer, which may be malignant or benign, areas of the bone have been destroyed by lysis, resulting in cyst formation. *Ewing's sarcoma* is a malignancy arising from the stem cells of the medulla. The cancer is located in the diaphyses of long bones, and it metastasizes to the lungs. *Secondary bone neoplasia* (metastatic bone cancer) is the most common type of bone cancer. The most common carcinomas that spread to bone are those of the breast, prostate, lung, kidneys, and thyroid. Secondary bone tumors are generally found at numerous sites where they destroy the bone tissue, resulting in a high incidence of pathologic fracture. As such, spontaneous bone fracture is an important sign of possible neoplasia elsewhere in the body.

▶ SECTION III

Arthritis (joint inflammation) can be caused by trauma, infection, autoimmune activity, or age-related degeneration. The condition usually begins as *synovitis,* or inflammation of the joint lining. This increases the amount of fluid in the affected joint, which may mix with exudate. *Gout* is arthritis caused by deposits of tophus crystals in joints, which leads to severe inflammation, extreme pain, and joint deformity. *Infectious arthritis,* a relatively uncommon condition, may occur from bacterial contamination of a joint (e.g., from a wound, surgery, or arthrocentesis), or from bacterial spread from nearby tissue or from blood. *Lyme disease,* caused by the spirochete *Borrelia burgdorferi* and transmitted by the deer tick, is the most common form of infectious arthritis.

Osteoarthritis (also called degenerative joint disease, or DJD) is the arthritis of old age. The majority of the elderly have some degree of the disease. DJD occurs most frequently in individuals whose joints have been subjected to repeated movements. Signs and symptoms of the disease include fragmentation of bone into the joint, erosion and calcification of the cartilage in the joint, the formation of *bone spurs* (nodules of new bone formed around the perimeter of the joints, also called osteophytes), inflammation, pain, and loss of mobility. *Rheumatoid arthritis,* a condition more crippling than osteoarthritis, is suspected to be autoimmune in nature. Rheumatoid factor, an abnormal IgM autoantibody that targets an IgG antibody, is found in patients with the disease. The IgM–IgG complexes are thought to deposit in the synovial membrane of joints, inducing inflammation and synovial tissue destruction. A layer of granulation tissue (pannus) forms to cover the exposed bone surfaces, and damaged joint surfaces form scar tissue, leading to immobilization of the joint *(ankylosis).* Osteoporosis may develop, and inflammatory lesions may form in other parts of the body. *Ankylosing spondylitis* is inflammatory fusion of the spine due to arthritis of the vertebral joint spaces. This condition, which occurs mainly in young men, leads to spinal deformity ("poker back").

A *sprain* is a slight trauma to the ligaments of a joint, which usually results from bending the joint beyond the normal range of motion. Swelling, bruising, and pain (from localized inflammation) are signs and symptoms associated with a sprain. A *whiplash* is a sprain that involves the ligaments of the neck. A *strain* ("pulled muscle") is torn muscle or tendon tissue. A *subluxation* ("partial dislocation") is a partial tear in a joint capsule that allows the bones of the joint to become misaligned. A *luxation* ("dislocation") is a complete rupture of a joint capsule, causing significant misalignment of the bones. *Carpal tunnel syndrome* is injury to the wrist and hand from repetitive, long-term movement, such as typing. Inflammation results in interference with nerve impulse transmission. Pain, numbness, and tingling are symptoms of the condition. The most common cause of low back pain is *intervertebral disk herniation* ("slipped disk"). This condition is most often associated with sudden motion or excessive weight bearing. It may be incomplete (the inner soft material of the disk protrudes from the disk) or complete (the material spills from the herniated disk). As the material protrudes or is spilled, it may compress the sciatic nerve (sciatica). *Bursitis,* a condition that most often involves the shoulder joint, is due to inflammation of the bursae (sacs of synovial fluid around joints). It is caused by excessive or repetitive motion or by trauma.

▶ SECTION IV

Muscular dystrophy is a group of inherited muscle diseases that are both degenerative and progressive, and which lead to loss of normal movement and coordination. Several types of dystrophy are recognized, *limb–girdle* (which affects the muscles of the legs and pelvis), *facioscapulohumeral* (which affects the muscles of the face, shoulders, and arms), *myotonic* (in which myotonia is accompanied by mental degeneration), and *Duchenne's,* which is the most common and most severe form of the condition. The pathology of Duchenne's, an X-linked recessive disease that develops in affected males at a young age, involves a defective protein in the muscle cell membrane which leads to abnormal functioning of the muscles. Muscles weaken and degenerate, and scar tissue and fat deposits replace necrotic muscle tissue. Affected individuals are usually confined to a wheelchair at an early age.

Like muscular dystrophy, *myasthenia gravis* is a degenerative and progressive disease of the muscles. In this autoimmune condition, an antibody targets the acetylcholine (ACh) receptor at the neuromuscular junction, leading to impaired impulse conduction at the muscle tissue and, ultimately, atrophy of the muscles. The source of the autoantibody is thought to be the thymus gland. The onset of the disease is gradual, and easy fatigue is a common symptom. Left untreated, the condition can lead to respiratory failure.

Myositis (polymyositis) is an inflammatory disease of the muscles. *Infectious myositis* can be caused by bacterial, viral, or parasitic infection. Inflammatory injury to muscles that occurs during a hypersensitivity reaction is defined as *immune-mediated myositis.* Conditions that cause immune-mediated myositis include systemic lupus erythematosus, sarcoidosis, and immune polymyositis. *Myopathy* ("muscle disease") may be primary (a congenital disorder) or secondary (due to a systemic disease) in nature. *Congenital myopathy,* in which the affected child has extreme muscle weakness, is rare. Secondary, or acquired, myopathies are generally due to a metabolic disease such as diabetes or an endocrine imbalance. *Neurogenic muscle disease* is caused by nerve impairment of the upper neuron of the brain or the lower motor neuron of the spinal cord. The result of such impairment is neurogenic atrophy, or wasting of the muscles due to disease of the nerves. Trauma, stroke, infections, and toxins can cause neurogenic muscle disease.

Because muscle cells do not readily proliferate, neoplasia of muscle tissue is very rare. The most common muscle neoplasia is *rhabdomyosarcoma,* a malignant cancer arising from skeletal muscle cells. The tumor invades locally and may metastasize to the lungs. Complete removal of the tumor is usually curative.

The Central Nervous System and Major Sensory Organs

▶ OBJECTIVES

SECTION II

Define all highlighted terms.

Outline the causes of CNS developmental defects. Characterize the causes and signs and symptoms congenital hydrocephalus and cerebral palsy.

Describe the degenerative diseases multiple sclerosis, Parkinson's disease, Huntington's disease, amyotrophic lateral sclerosis, and Alzheimer's disease. Characterize the suspected cause and signs and symptoms of each.

SECTION III

Define all highlighted terms.

Characterize the signs and symptoms of the infectious diseases meningitis and encephalitis, and list the causative agents of both diseases.

SECTION IV

Define all highlighted terms.

Describe the conditions cerebrovascular disease and cerebrovascular accident. Characterize the causes of both, and the types and signs and symptoms of the conditions.

Define and describe the conditions intracranial hemorrhage, epidural hematoma, subdural hematoma, and subarachnoid hemorrhage.

Distinguish between the brain traumas concussion and contusion. Describe the signs and symptoms of both.

SECTION V

Define all highlighted terms.

Outline the differences between benign and malignant CNS tumors, and between primary and secondary CNS tumors.

Define and describe the types and characteristics of glioma, meningioma, and neuroma.

Describe the causes, signs and symptoms, and manifestations of the disorders epilepsy and coma.

Define all highlighted terms.

Describe the forms of injury that can occur to the eye.

Describe the conditions of conjunctivitis, hordeolum, photophobia, and keratitis. Characterize the causes and signs and symptoms of each.

Describe the effects on the eye caused by the diseases hypertension and diabetes mellitus. Characterize the causes and signs and symptoms of the conditions hypertensive retinopathy and diabetic retinopathy.

Describe the causes, types, and signs and symptoms of glaucoma and cataract.

Describe the abnormalities and the causes of the vision disturbances myopia, hyperopia, presbyopia, and astigmatism.

Describe the causes and signs and symptoms of the neoplasias retinoblastoma and melanoma.

Define all highlighted terms.

Describe the causes, signs and symptoms, and complications of the conditions otitis media, cholesteatoma, otosclerosis, and Ménière's disease.

SECTION ▶   **I. ANATOMY AND PHYSIOLOGY IN REVIEW**
18-1

The central nervous system is made up of the **brain** and **spinal cord.** The brain has three major parts, the cerebrum, the cerebellum, and the brain stem. The **cerebrum** forms the bulk of the brain and performs most of the voluntary functions one associates with the brain. The outer portion is the cortex, and it is composed of **gray matter,** which is the bodies of the nerve cells or neurons. Cerebral cortical neurons are responsible for the functions of intelligence, emotions, thought, and sensory and motor functions. The **white matter** of the cerebrum is the axons of the cerebral cortical neurons. Axons are long processes that extend from the body of the neuron and carry messages in the form of electrical impulses. Axons of the central nervous system are covered with a lipid envelope called a **myelin sheath.** This sheath greatly facilitates the transmission of nerve impulses. The axons of the cerebral white matter connect to neurons in other parts of the brain and the spinal cord. Axons of neurons in the spinal cord connect with skeletal muscle. Deep within the cerebral white matter are the **basal ganglia.** These are groups of neuron bodies among the white matter axons that assist in governing body position and movement.The **cerebellum** is a small portion of the brain to the rear of the cerebrum. The cerebellum is responsible for coordinating movement. The **brain stem,** which is composed of the midbrain, pons, and medulla, controls autonomic functions such as heart rate and respiration. All of these structures of the brain are encased and protected by the bony **skull.**

18-2

Both the brain and spinal cord are covered with a three-layered membrane called the **meninges.** The pia mater is the delicate inside layer lying over the brain and spinal cord, the arachnoid is the middle layer, and the dura mater is the tough outer layer. There are four hollow spaces within the brain called the **ventricles.** The ventricles contain structures known as the choroid plexus. The choroid plexus of the ventricles manufacture **cerebral spinal fluid,** or **CSF.** This fluid is found in between the nerve tissue and the meninges. CSF bathes and cushions the brain and spinal cord, as well as providing a medium for metabolic exchanges and excretion of waste. Once the CSF has run its course, it is absorbed into the venous system.

18-3

The spinal cord is a continuation of the brain stem. It is encased in protective bone known as the **vertebrae,** which make up the vertebral column. The spinal cord is a two-way street of communication to and from the brain. Within the spinal cord are ascending and descending nerve tracts. The spinal cord is the connection between the brain and the rest of the body. It is also covered by the same meninges, which are continuous from the brain. Figure 18–1 depicts the major structures of the central nervous system.

18-4

The circulation of the brain is provided by arterial blood though the carotid arteries in the neck, which perfuse most of the cerebrum. The posterior portions of the brain (the cerebellum and brain stem) are perfused by vertebral arteries. The vessels connect at the base of the brain in a rounded circuit called the **circle of Willis.** A vital function of this configuration is that it provides a great deal of collateral circulation (detours) in the event of blockage of a major artery. The capillary beds of the brain differ from those in the rest of the body. They create the **blood–brain barrier,** which means they are not as permeable to many substances as are capillaries in the rest of body. This is an important protective function because it keeps substances from entering the brain. The blood–brain barrier is created by specialized endothelial cells and by cells called astrocytes that help endothelial cells control the passage of molecules.

18-5

The major cells of the central nervous system are the astrocytes, the neurons, and oligodendroglia. In addition to assisting with the blood–brain barrier, the **astrocytes** provide structural support for the nervous parenchyma. As the equivalent of connective tissue, they proliferate after injury to form a **glial scar,** which contains no collagen. The **neurons** are the basic unit of the central nervous system. They are the nerve cells of the gray matter that generate and conduct messages and instructions known as nerve impulses. At one end of a neuron are **dendrites,** which are short and multiple. Dendrites are the afferent (incoming) processes through which impulses enter from other neurons. At the other end of the neuron is the **axon,** which is very long and singular. Axons are the efferent (outgoing) processes through which nerve impulses exit the neuron. This is always a one-way process. The tiny

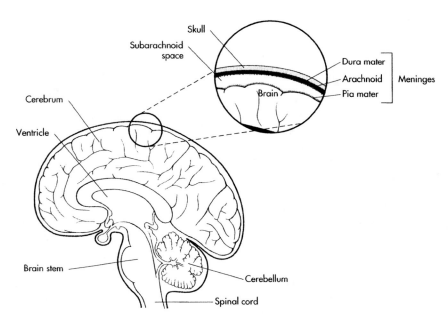

Figure 18–1. The central nervous system.

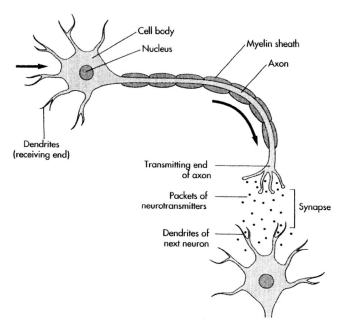

Figure 18–2. A neuron.

space in between the axon of one neuron and the dendrites of the next neuron is called a **synapse.** The structure of a neuron is shown in Figure 18–2. Sensory neurons process input from the internal and external environment and convey these messages to the brain. Motor neurons conduct messages from the brain to skeletal muscle, glands, and other structures to cause a response. The **oligodendroglia** are the cells that manufacture the myelin sheath that covers neural axons.

18–6

The **autonomic nervous system** is that system that helps control the internal environment, so it is crucial to homeostasis. Some of the homeostatic mechanisms governed by the autonomic nervous system include blood pressure, heart rate, temperature, sweating, gastric acid production, and intestinal motility. The motor neurons of the autonomic nervous system affect smooth muscle and cardiac muscle, rather than voluntary skeletal muscle. This system is composed of the sympathetic and parasympathetic nervous systems, which work in opposite manners of each other to create balance. Stress is one thing that activates the sympathetic system to create the "fight or flight" mode, while the parasympathetic system directs "business as usual." The autonomic nervous system is largely directed by the hypothalamus.

18–7

The purpose of the central nervous system, or CNS, is to function as an intricate communication system that regulates and controls body processes and responds to sensory input (vision, hearing, touch, smell, pressure, temperature, and pain). This communication is accomplished by nerve impulses that are electrical in nature. Impulses cross or jump synapses as packets containing a chemical messenger. This transmitter substance is released from an axon ending, crosses the synapse, and binds to receptors on dendrites. The impulse then speeds through the neuron and is passed along over the next synapse.

18–8

The sensory portion of the CNS receives messages about the environment from sensory neurons in skin and muscles. The most basic response is a **reflex arc** where information is received into and directed back out of the spinal cord. An example is jerking your hand back from a flame. More complex responses require that information travel to the brain for processing. Sensory impulses are sent to specific sections of the brain for interpretation and response instructions. The motor portion of the CNS is also assigned to specific sections of the brain and is responsible for directing voluntary movement. Because nerve fibers from one side of the body cross over in the medulla to reach the other side of the brain, one side of the brain controls the opposite side of the body. This is illustrated by the fact that a stroke affecting the right hemisphere of the brain impairs function of the left side of the body.

.... 18-9 ....

The CNS processes sensory information through the input of the senses, which include vision, hearing, taste, touch, temperature, pain, and pressure. The major sensory organs of the CNS are the eyes and ears. The visual pathways include the eyeballs (called the **globes**), optic nerves, the tracts of these nerves, and the occipital lobe of the brain, which interprets the nerve impulses as vision. The auxiliary structures of the eyes include the body depressions in the skull called **orbits,** which house and protect the eyes. The eyes move due to contraction of the **extraocular muscles** at their sides. The eyelids protect the eyes at their anterior surface. **Lacrimal glands** secrete **tears,** which keep the cornea moist. Tears contain **lysozyme,** which is an antibacterial enzyme.

.... 18-10 ....

The globes have three main parts. The first is the white fibrous layer called the **sclera.** On the front, or anterior, side of the globe the sclera becomes the **cornea.** This is the clear layer that permits entry of light into the eye and assists in light refraction. (Refraction of light is bending so as to direct it to a specific area.) Under the sclera is the vascular layer which is made up of the **choroid, ciliary body,** and **iris.** The choroid provides blood supply. The iris is pigmented and is responsible for eye color. The iris can dilate or constrict in response to environmental light and impulses from the autonomic nervous system. The dilation or constriction changes the size of the **pupil,** the aperture, or hole, in the center of the iris. The ciliary body secretes **aqueous humor,** the fluid of the anterior chamber inside the globe. The aqueous humor is a means of supplying nutrition for the cornea, which has no vessels. The fluid drains out through tiny ducts. The smooth muscle of the ciliary body changes the shape of the lens so that rays of light can be refracted normally.

.... 18-11 ....

The third layer is the **retina,** located at the posterior of the globe. The retina contains the nerve cells called **rods** and **cones.** The rods distinguish light from dark and detect shape and movement. The cones provide color vision. The axons of these neurons form the **optic nerve,** which transmits visual input to the brain. The **lens** of the eye is located behind the iris. It divides the inside into anterior and posterior chambers. The lens is anchored by the smooth muscle ligaments of the ciliary body. The lens plays a major role in light refraction so that light rays strike the retina. Behind the lens in the posterior chamber is the gelatinous **vitreous humor,** which provides the shape and intraocular pressure of the globe. The structure of the eye is shown in Figure 18–3.

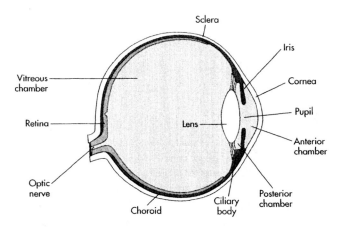

Figure 18–3. The eye.

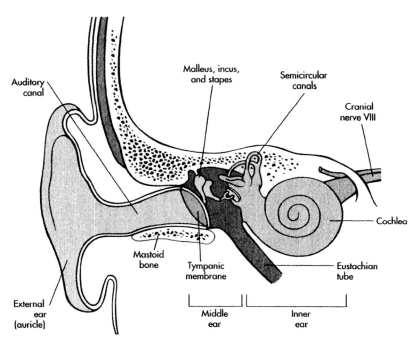

Figure 18–4. The ear.

The three parts of the ear are the **external ear,** the **middle ear,** and the **inner ear,** which are shown in Figure 18–4. The external ear consists of the cartilaginous **auricle** and the **auditory canal,** through which sound waves travel to the middle and inner ear. The auricle collects and directs sound waves into the canal. At the end of the canal is the eardrum, or **tympanic membrane.** The eardrum marks the end of the external ear. On the other side, the middle ear houses the auditory bones called the **malleus,** the **incus,** and the **stapes.** These tiny bones are a pathway that connects sound vibrations from the eardrum to the semicircular canals. In this manner, they transmit sound impulses. The **eustachian tube** is also in the middle ear. This tube serves as a pressure outlet for the ears, and the other end opens in the pharynx or throat. In the inner ear are the **semicircular canals,** the **cochlea,** and **cranial nerve VIII.** The semicircular canals function in maintaining equilibrium, and the cochlea is the main organ of hearing. Impulses from the semicircular canals and cochlea are transmitted to the temporal lobes of the brain through the cranial nerve.

SECTION ▶ **II. DEFECTS IN DEVELOPMENT AND DEGENERATIVE DISEASES**

▶ DEVELOPMENTAL DEFECTS

Developmental defects are those that occur in the forming embryo or fetus. Malformation of the brain or spinal cord, or biochemical defects, may lead to severe consequences for the individual since the central nervous system is the control center of the body. The consequences affect both quality of life and life span. The cause of many developmental disorders is idiopathic. Some are due to defective genes or chromosomes. The disorder Down's syndrome, which was discussed in Chapter 8, is one example of a defective chromosome. If you will recall, it is medically termed trisomy 21 because there are three of the chromosome 21, instead of the normal pair. Spina bifida is another developmental disorder that was presented in Chapter 8. This relatively common malformation affects the vertebrae and spinal cord. In the various forms of this disease, parts of the vertebrae (the posterior arches and spines) are missing, allowing spinal fluid, meninges, and even the spinal cord to bulge through the gap. Developmental errors or malformation due to specific factors can create severe retardation and helplessness in some individuals. Other individuals may be impaired but relatively functional. Some of these specific factors include infection of the developing CNS, alcohol or other drugs, trauma, and hypoxia.

18-14

A severe developmental defect is **anencephaly.** The word root "ceph" refers to head or brain, so joined with the prefix "a," you can guess that anencephaly loosely means _____(1). Indeed, anencephaly is a malformation in which the infant is born with most if not all of the forebrain missing. Obviously, this condition is incompatible with life and the child is generally stillborn or dies immediately after birth. Anencephaly is attributed to failure of skull formation, and so the unprotected brain is destroyed in utero.

1. without brain

18-15

Congenital hydrocephalus is another phrase whose meaning you should be able to determine. Again, looking at the word root "ceph," and knowing that "hydro" refers to water, congenital hydrocephalus means _____(1) on the _____(2). In this condition there is an excess of cerebral spinal fluid (CSF). Hydrocephalus may be acquired later in life due to a space-occupying lesion of the brain that blocks CSF outflow. In the congenital disorder, there is stenosis, or closure, of the ducts within the ventricles that drain the fluid out of the ventricles after its formation. This stenosis represents a failure of the ducts to open. The ventricles enlarge from the pressure of the excess CSF. After the ventricles swell, the entire head enlarges. Congenital hydrocephalus has a characteristic appearance in a newborn. The sutures of the skull have not yet closed, so this allows the skull to expand and the head to enlarge. (In older children and adults the skull cannot expand. Lack of expansion creates tremendous intracranial pressure that must be relieved to prevent significant brain injury and herniation through the foramen magnum.) Congenital hydrocephalus develops because of lack of opening of _____(3) in the ventricles. This causes excess _____(4) to build up in the ventricles, leading to their _____(5) and enlargement of the entire _____(6).

1. water
2. brain
3. ducts
4. spinal fluid
5. enlargement
6. head

18-16

Cerebral palsy is a CNS disorder that is due to destruction or injury of brain tissue, rather than defective development. Cerebral palsy is a general term applied to impaired CNS function because of early injury, rather than a specific disease. The injury occurs anywhere from the second half of the pregnancy (after the brain is formed) to months after birth. The most significant cause of cerebral palsy is lack of oxygen to the brain. This is most likely to happen during long and difficult deliveries or in premature infants with respiratory distress. CNS infection such as meningitis can also cause cerebral palsy. The degree of abnormality in the affected child depends on the severity of injury. Both mental retardation and motor impairment can be seen, again, depending on the injury. Motor impairment may include **paresis** (weakness) and **ataxia** (incoordination). Since the injury creates a certain amount of damage, and then the insult is over, cerebral palsy is *not* a progressive disease. That means the impairment remains the same and does not get worse with time. Cerebral palsy represents impairment of _____(1) function because it has suffered some _____(2) early in life. The injury of most consequence is insufficient _____(3) to the brain. The amount of dysfunction depends on the _____(4) of the injury. Cerebral palsy may affect either _____(5) or _____(6) capabilities. Since it does not worsen, cerebral palsy is not a _____(7) disease.

1. central nervous system
2. injury
3. oxygen
4. severity
5. mental
6. motor
7. progressive

▶ DEGENERATIVE DISEASES

18-17

1. worse
2. myelin
3. axons
4. white
5. demyelinating

A **degenerative** disease is one that gets progressively worse with time. There is no turning back and there is no cure. The first degenerative disease we will discuss is **multiple sclerosis,** or **MS.** MS is classified by some sources as an autoimmune disease because studies have shown the presence of immune cells in early lesions in the brain. The presumed antigen is myelin. A virus or immune response to a virus is also suspected. The exact cause of MS is unknown. Multiple sclerosis is a demyelinating disease that destroys the myelin sheath of CNS neural axons in a random fashion. It is assumed that the oligodendroglia cells, which manufacture myelin, are also destroyed since they are absent from the histological picture. The lesions of MS are found in the white matter of the CNS since neural axons make up the white matter. The destruction of the myelin leaves hardened (sclerosed) plaques along lesions in the brain and spinal cord. Because multiple sclerosis is a degenerative disease, it gets _____(1) with time. The basic pathology in this disease is destruction of the _____(2) that covers CNS neural _____(3). Therefore, the lesions are found in the _____(4) matter of the brain and spinal cord. A term that describes the destruction of myelin is _____(5).

18-18

1. paresis
2. ataxia
3. slowly
4. myelin sheath
5. sensory
6. motor
7. slowly
8. incapacitated

Since the myelin sheath is responsible for the speed and efficiency of nerve impulse conduction, in MS nerve impulses travel relatively slowly. Deficits in nerve function become apparent as more and more axons become compromised. Because myelin destruction can occur anywhere in the white matter of the brain or spinal cord, symptoms and their severity differ greatly from patient to patient. Clinically, MS is a chronic debilitating disease with both sensory and motor impairment. Symptoms include blurry vision, loss of sensation, weakness [medically called _____(1)], loss of coordination [medically called _____(2)], muscle tremors, difficulty speaking, and urinary incontinence because of loss of sphincter muscle control. MS generally affects adults before the age of 50. The degeneration is slow. Those who become incapacitated from weakness, which are the majority of cases, take many years to become wheelchair bound or bedridden. There is no specific treatment for multiple sclerosis. In multiple sclerosis, nerve impulses travel _____(3) because the _____(4) normally speeds them along. Function of both the _____(5) and _____(6) systems are impaired. MS progresses _____(7), and most individuals become completely _____(8) over many years.

18-19

1. degeneration
2. basal ganglia
3. involuntary
4. dopamine
5. shaking palsy
6. rigid
7. face
8. bradykinesia

Parkinson's disease is a degeneration of the basal ganglia, neurons in the midbrain which help to control involuntary movement. It is considered to be a result of lack of dopamine production. Dopamine is an important chemical transmitter. The cause of Parkinson's disease is idiopathic, with possible hereditary factors. The onset of signs is gradual and the progression of the disease is slow. This crippling disorder affects older adults and is sometimes called "shaking palsy." The three main features are tremors (shaking), rigidity of the muscles, and **bradykinesia,** which means slow movement. The signs include hand tremors, nodding of the head, and poor postural reflexes resulting in falling. Extreme muscle stiffness creates a rigid, mask-like facial appearance. Voluntary movement is difficult and slow. Posture becomes bent over, creating a characteristic shuffling walk to maintain balance. A small percentage of patients experience dementia. Parkinson's disease is a result of _____(1) of the _____(2) which govern _____(3) movement. It is thought to be due to a deficiency in _____(4) production. A common phrase that describes this disease is _____(5) because of the presence of muscle tremors. In addition to tremors, the muscles are _____(6) and this causes a mask-like appearance of the _____(7). Movement is difficult and also slow, which is medically described as _____(8). Treatment of Parkinson's disease includes physical therapy, with specific exercises to cope with impaired movement, and avoidance of stress, which worsens the disorder. Since dopamine deficiency underlies this disease, replacement therapy with L-dopa is effective in improving symptoms in at least half of the cases. L-dopa is not a cure, and some pre-existing conditions make the drug contraindicated.

Huntington's disease is also called **Huntington's chorea.** This progressive disease is genetically based. It is an autosomal dominant inheritance pattern, so if either parent has the disease, all of the children have a 50 percent chance of developing the disorder. Huntington's disease is familial; that is, it occurs in families. It is caused by a defective gene on chromosome 4. The underlying pathology is atrophy of parts of the cerebral cortex, with loss of other nerve cell nuclei. The onset of Huntington's disease is not until middle age but once it manifests, progression is rapid. Both motor function and mental capacity are affected. There are rapid, jerky, involuntary movements that earned the disease its name (the term chorea describes the spastic movements). This is due to loss of control caused by abnormal nerve impulse transmission. Loss of speech accompanies muscle spasms. Personality changes and a failing memory occur early in the course of the disease. Dementia, or mental incompetence, is present later and it progresses to mental incapacitation within a few years. There is no treatment for Huntington's disease. Testing for the defective gene and genetic counseling help afflicted individuals make reproductive choices. The cause of Huntington's disease is _____(1). A defective _____(2) on chromosome 4 has been identified. Children of Huntington's patients have a _____(3) chance of developing the disease. The jerky, spastic involuntary movements in Huntington's are described by the term _____(4). Patients ultimately end with _____(5) incapacitation.

18–20

1. genetic
2. gene
3. 50 percent
4. chorea
5. mental

Amyotrophic lateral sclerosis, or **ALS,** is more commonly known as **Lou Gehrig's disease.** It was initially named after the prominent athlete in whom it was first described. The cause of this rare disease is unknown. A small percentage of the cases are familial, with a defective gene identified on chromosome 21 (the abnormal chromosome in Down's syndrome). AML features a progressive wasting of muscles of the extremities, with extreme weakness and ultimate death. The pathology points to a loss of motor neurons in the spinal cord, the midbrain, and some of the cranial nerves. It is older adults (50 to 60) who develop symptoms, which include difficult movement, muscle atrophy of the arms and legs, **dysphonia** (difficulty speaking), and **dysphagia** (difficulty swallowing). The mental faculties are not affected. The respiratory muscles become very weak, leading to a poor cough reflex and the potential for aspirating material into the lungs. Death occurs in a few years after onset as a result of respiratory failure. Lou Gehrig's disease is medically known as _____(1). A prominent feature of this disease is _____(2) of the muscles of the _____(3) and extreme _____(4). The intellect is _____(5) affected. Death occurs because of _____(6) failure.

18–21

1. amyotrophic lateral sclerosis
2. wasting
3. extremities
4. weakness
5. not
6. respiratory

The last disorder we will consider is also of unknown cause. This is **Alzheimer's disease,** which is prominent among those of advanced age. It is an age-related degeneration. Alzheimer's disease results in a loss of mental capabilities, so it is classified as a dementia. The population affected are almost always in their 70s or older. The incidence of this disease greatly increases with age, with up to 50 percent of those 85 years or older having some degree of dementia. The only certain pathological findings to date are atrophy of parts of the cerebrum and loss of neurons. A few cases that may be familial have revealed the presence of amyloid that may have caused brain injury. The prominent features of Alzheimer's disease are loss of short term memory, personality change, and failure to recognize surroundings and family members or friends. The dementia is progressive and interferes greatly with normal activities. Most cases end as completely dysfunctional and bedridden. Since there are several organic causes of dementia (such as metabolic disease, drugs, chronic alcoholism, infection, and tumors), these causes must be ruled out before arriving at a diagnosis of Alzheimer's disease. Alzheimer's is a disease that usually affects people _____(1) years old or older. It is classified as a dementia because there is loss of _____(2) capacity. It seems to be related to _____(3) of the cerebral cortex and neuron loss. The dementia worsens, or _____(4), to even-

18–22

1. 70
2. mental
3. atrophy
4. progresses

TABLE 18–1. DEVELOPMENTAL AND DEGENERATIVE DISEASES OF THE CENTRAL NERVOUS SYSTEM

Disease	Features
Developmental Defects	
Down's syndrome	Extra chromosome 21
Spina bifida	Malformation of the vertebrae with herniation of various tissue
Anencephaly	Absence of forebrain
Congenital hydrocephalus	Ventricles and head enlarged due to excess spinal fluid
Destructive Lesions	
Cerebral palsy	Injury of the CNS late in pregnancy or in newborns, causing impaired function
Degenerative Diseases	
Multiple sclerosis	Demyelination of neural axons, causing impaired nerve transmission
Parkinson's disease	Lack of dopamine production, causing abnormal involuntary movement (shaking palsy and bradykinesia)
Huntington's disease	Genetic atrophy of cerebral cortex with spastic movements (chorea) and eventual mental incapacitation
Amyotrophic lateral sclerosis (Lou Gehrig's disease)	Extreme atrophy and weakness of the extremities, normal mental function, respiratory failure
Alzheimer's disease	Age-related degeneration of mental capacity (dementia) ending in total dysfunction

tual dysfunction. Developmental, destructive, and degenerative diseases of the CNS are reviewed in Table 18–1.

II. REVIEW QUESTIONS

1. What do embryonic CNS infection, hypoxia, and alcohol all have in common?
   a. Any of these will cause trisomy 21.
   b. All of these must be present to cause spina bifida.
   c. All of these are specific factors that may cause CNS developmental defects.
   d. Any of these will cause idiopathic malformation.

2. Which of the following CNS disorders is NOT progressive?
   a. cerebral palsy
   b. multiple sclerosis
   c. congenital hydrocephalus
   d. amyotrophic lateral sclerosis

3. Failure of duct opening in fetal ventricles allows cerebral spinal fluid to accumulate, causing enlargement of the head. This best describes:
   a. anencephaly
   b. congenital hydrocephalus
   c. cerebral palsy
   d. multiple sclerosis

4. Define the term "degenerative" as it relates to disease:

_____

5. Atrophy of the cerebral cortex, with associated loss of mental function, in very old adults best describes:
   a. amyotrophic lateral sclerosis
   b. Alzheimer's disease
   c. multiple sclerosis
   d. Huntington's disease

6. Extreme atrophy of muscle of the extremities, severe weakness, and death due to respiratory failure is seen in:
   a. Parkinson's disease
   b. Huntington's chorea
   c. amyotrophic lateral sclerosis
   d. multiple sclerosis

7. Demyelination, or destruction of myelin sheath, of neural axons is the underlying pathology in:
   a. multiple sclerosis
   b. Lou Gehrig's disease
   c. Alzheimer's disease
   d. Parkinson's disease

8. Inadequate production of dopamine is associated with:
   a. amyotrophic lateral sclerosis
   b. Parkinson's disease
   c. cerebral palsy
   d. Huntington's disease

9. The cause of Huntington's chorea is:
   a. idiopathic
   b. due to autoimmune destruction
   c. a defective gene
   d. age-related degeneration

5. b–Alzheimer's disease

6. c–amyotrophic lateral sclerosis

7. a–multiple sclerosis

8. b–Parkinson's disease

9. c–a defective gene

III. INFECTIOUS DISEASES ◄ SECTION

18-23

The major forms of infection of the central nervous system include encephalitis (brain infection), myelitis (spinal cord infection), and meningitis (infection of the meninges). There are several microorganisms that can cause infection of the CNS. Some of these organisms target the CNS in preference over other tissue. The most common organisms to infect the CNS are bacteria, viruses, fungi, and protozoa. The pathogens may gain access to the CNS through:

1. The blood (which would be called _____(1) spread).
2. By traveling through the nerves.
3. From infected adjacent structures (the middle ear, sinuses, or upper respiratory tract).
4. Through animal or insect bites.
5. Directly during trauma.

Bacteria, viruses, fungi, and protozoa gain access by hematogenous spread. Bacteria enter through wounds and spread from nearby sites of infection (sinusitis, pharyngitis, or otitis media). Some viruses spread through peripheral nerves or can enter the bloodstream from the bites of vectors.

1. hematogenous

▶ MENINGITIS

18-24

1. meninges
2. cover
3. secondary
4. respiratory

Meningitis is infectious inflammation of the membranous covering of the CNS, the meninges. It is the soft tissue of the two inner layers (the pia mater and arachnoid) that become infected by the pathogens. Bacteria cause meningitis in different populations. Meningitis may be a primary disease, or secondary due to extension of infection of the upper or lower respiratory tract. The bacteria that most commonly cause meningitis and the affected populations are:

1. *Escherichia coli* in newborns.
2. *Hemophilus influenzae* in young children.
3. *Streptococcus pneumoniae* and *Neisseria meningitidis* in adolescents and adults.

You studied all of these pathogens in Chapter 5 on infectious disease. If you will recall, *Neisseria* meningitis can occur in epidemics because of its airborne route of spread. Common fungal causes of meningitis in immunosuppressed patients (especially AIDS cases) include *Candida albicans* and *Cryptococcus neoformans*. Meningitis is infection of the _____(1) which _____(2) the brain and spinal cord. Meningitis may be primary or _____(3), if it has spread from an infection of the _____(4) tract.

18-25

1. purulent exudate
2. neutrophils
3. protein
4. common
5. diagnose
6. lymphocyte

Acute bacterial meningitis, which is generally due to pyogenic bacteria, produces a purulent exudate that fills the subarachnoid space. The pus may cover the entire surface of the brain in severe cases. Occasionally, the bacteria may cause an abscess within the brain parenchyma. As a space-occupying lesion, this can be deadly. Acute viral meningitis is probably more common than bacterial, but it is harder to diagnose. Several of the upper respiratory viruses have been implicated in these cases, including influenza and the mumps virus. Clinically, acute meningitis presents as high fever (which can easily lead to convulsions in a child), chills, severe headache and neck pain (due to swelling of the meninges and pressure by exudate), and rigidity of the neck muscles. Spasm of the neck muscles and avoidance of movement to reduce pain create the rigidity. Untreated cases usually lead to coma. In bacterial meningitis, analysis of the CSF reveals the presence of many neutrophils, high protein (from the exudate), low glucose (due to use of it by the bacteria), and bacteria may be cultured from the specimen. Viral infections are associated with the presence of lymphocytes in the CSF. Prompt diagnosis and treatment with antibiotics usually resolve these cases, but meningitis can easily be fatal if not treated. A feature of acute meningitis due to pyogenic bacteria is the presence of _____(1) in the subarachnoid space. This is supported by CSF findings that show the presence of the inflammatory cells called _____(2) and high amounts of _____ (3). Meningitis due to viruses may be more _____(4) than bacterial cases but are more difficult to _____(5). The type of cell seen in the CSF with viral infections is the _____(6).

18-26

1. neurosyphilis
2. tertiary
3. syphilis
4. fibrosis
5. contracture

In the past, chronic meningitis was often a manifestation of neurosyphilis, the third, or tertiary, stage of syphilis (see Chap. 5). The meninges become infiltrated with immune cells (lymphocytes and plasma cells), and fibrosis is a feature as a result of attempts at healing. Contracture of this scar tissue often results in compression of the nerve roots exiting the brain. Brain ischemia and loss of neurons lead to the motor weakness (paresis) and the mental disturbances associated with neurosyphilis. Historically, tertiary syphilis was a significant cause of insanity. Other causes of chronic meningitis include tuberculosis and fungi, especially *Cryptococcus neoformans*. Fibrosis, contracture, and compression of nerve roots are also features in these cases because the reaction to chronic inflammation is the same. In chronic meningitis, the development of acquired hydrocephalus is possible if drainage of CSF is prevented. A prominent historical cause of chronic meningitis was _____(1), which represents the _____(2) stage of _____(3). In reaction to chronic inflammation, scarring, or _____(4), and shrinking, or _____(5), accompany the infection. Fibrotic contracture of the meninges generally causes _____(6) of nerve roots. If ducts that drain CSF become closed off, _____(7) can result.

6. compression
7. acquired hydrocephalus

▶ ENCEPHALITIS

18–27

Widespread infectious inflammation of the brain is called **encephalitis.** Most cases are caused by viruses. The virus invades neurons and causes infiltration of the brain parenchyma by lymphocytes. Occasionally, the spinal cord may also be involved in the infection. In a child, viral encephalitis can be secondary to childhood viruses such as chickenpox, measles, and mumps. Encephalitis can also be a result of a mosquito bite. An insect that transmits infectious agents by biting the victim is called a _____(1). Viral enceph-alitis that is transmitted in this manner (by a mosquito vector) is often associated with seasonal epidemics. Some of these infections have specific names such as St. Louis, equine, and Venezuelan encephalitis. *Toxoplasma gondii* is a protozoon that causes encephalitis in newborns. The child is infected through the mother while in utero. Toxoplasmosis is also a significant cause of encephalitis in AIDS patients. Fungi, such as *Candida* and *Cryptococcus,* frequently produce encephalitis in AIDS or other severely immunosuppressed patients. Herpes simplex type I (oral) has been isolated in some cases of encephalitis. Sources disagree as to how prevalent this is. Besides the typical clinical presentation seen in CNS infection (fever, headache, possibly delirium), lethargy is a prominent feature. Lethargy refers to mental drowsiness, which is so extreme in some forms of encephalitis that it has been called the "sleeping sickness." Lymphocytes can be found in the CSF, and often there is a specific serologic test for the antibodies against the suspected virus. There is no specific treatment for viral encephalitis because there are few effective antiviral drugs. Therefore, the prognosis is unpredictable and varies from case to case. The outcome ranges from complete recovery to nerve or mental impairment or death.

1. vector

18–28

Encephalitis is _____(1) inflammation of the _____(2). The most common causative pathogens are _____(3). If encephalitis is the result of vector transmission, this means it has been transmitted by the _____(4) of a (an) _____(5). Vector-transmitted viral encephalitis often occurs in episodes called _____(6). Other, more common causes of encephalitis today include infection in AIDS patients due to a protozoon that causes _____(7), and fungi such as _____(8) or _____(9). Encephalitis has been called the _____(10) because it can produce significant lethargy. On a final note, in Chapter 4 we discussed AIDS dementia complex (ADC) as the result of CNS infection in AIDS patients. ADC is seen in the terminal stages of HIV infection. This is also called AIDS-related encephalopathy. It may be a combination of meningitis, encephalitis, or even brain abscesses. CNS infection is a common cause of death in these patients, second to pneumonia. Most cases are due to *Toxoplasma* or *Cryptococcus.* The damage caused by these organisms is increased by toxic secretions from HIV-infected cells in the brain. You may review the major infectious diseases of the CNS by referring to Table 18–2.

1. infectious
2. brain
3. viruses
4. bite
5. insect
6. epidemics
7. toxoplasmosis
8. *Candida*
9. *Cryptococcus*
10. sleeping sickness

TABLE 18–2. MAJOR INFECTIOUS DISEASES OF THE CENTRAL NERVOUS SYSTEM

Disease	Features
Acute meningitis	
Bacterial	Purulent exudate in subarachnoid space, covering surface of the brain; possible abscess; neutrophils in CSF
Viral	May follow upper respiratory infection or childhood virus infection; lymphocytes in CSF
Chronic meningitis	Neurosyphilis (tertiary stage of syphilis), fibrosis and contracture around nerve roots, mental derangement, possible acquired hydrocephalus; *Cryptococcus neoformans* also a causative agent
Encephalitis	Viral infection of the brain, often transmitted by a mosquito vector, or as secondary infection of childhood viruses; *Toxoplasma, Candida,* and *Cryptococcus* also causative agents

▶ OTHER INFECTIOUS DISEASES

Myelitis is infectious inflammation of the spinal cord. It is most often caused by viruses. A disease of historical significance is polio, or poliomyelitis, which affected children and caused severe crippling. The poliovirus affects the gray matter of the spinal cord, destroying motor neurons and causing paralysis. Often, this paralysis included the muscles of respiration. Only artificial respiration could prolong life. Polio has been eliminated because of effective immunization programs. The original vaccine (the Salk vaccine) consisted of an intramuscular injection. The later oral vaccine (the Sabin vaccine) is just as effective but also eliminates carrier states and prevents transmission of the virus.

Rabies is a rare CNS infection (encephalomyelitis), but it is significant because of its invariably fatal outcome. The reservoir for the rabies virus is wild animals (notably the fox, wolf, skunk, raccoon, and bat). It may be transmitted to domestic animals or household pets. The human population is at risk through bites from infected or rabid animals. The virus is transmitted through the saliva of the animal. From the bite wound, the virus enters the fibers of peripheral nerves and travels through them to the brain. The incubation period for rabies is long, 1 to 2 months, but it does depend on how close the wound is to the spinal cord or brain. The signs of rabies include fever, mental derangement, rage, seizures, and paralysis. Muscle spasms of the throat make it impossible to swallow water, and the aversion to water in this infection is called **hydrophobia.** Because water cannot be swallowed, the victim exhibits profuse salivation. The onset of signs means that the infection has reached the brain and death is inevitable. There is no treatment for rabies. Bite wound cases are managed by confining the biting animal (if domestic) for 10 to 12 days for observation. If no CNS signs develop in the animal by the end of the isolation period, the animal is considered free of rabies. If any signs do develop, or if the animal cannot be confined, the bite victim must be immunized against the virus. Victims of wounds on the neck or head should be immunized right away. If possible, a wild animal should be caught and brain tissue submitted to a reference laboratory for rabies testing. A positive test includes the finding of viral inclusions (Negri bodies) in the neurons of the brain tissue.

Tetanus is an infection discussed in Chapter 5 under the topic of diseases caused by bacterial toxins. This infection of nerve tissue is commonly called **lockjaw.** It is the result of the poison released by the bacteria *Clostridium tetani. C. tetani* spores inhabit soil contaminated with animal feces. The spores germinate and grow in deep puncture wounds or in necrotic tissue because of the anaerobic nature of the bacteria. *C. tetani* secretes a toxin that moves through nerves and adheres to receptors on motor neurons. It also enters the spinal cord. The adherence to the receptors activates the neurons, which in turn activate muscle groups, causing rigid paralysis. Along with the rigidity are muscle spasms and convulsions. The rigidity includes the muscles of mastication, or jaw muscles. The mouth cannot be opened. Swallowing becomes impossible. Death occurs if respiratory muscles become paralyzed. Management of tetanus is aimed at prevention. The toxin must be inactivated before it reaches the spinal cord. Tetanus antitoxin is the first vaccine given, with tetanus toxoid boosters given if it has been more than 5 years since the last immunization.

Reye's syndrome is an encephalopathy ("brain disease") that can develop in some children after certain viral infections, such as Epstein–Barr virus, influenza, or chickenpox. The exact mechanism or pathogenesis of Reye's syndrome is unknown. The use of aspirin in these viral cases is suspected as a factor by some sources. Reye's syndrome causes swelling of the cerebrum with a subsequent dangerous rise in the intracranial pressure. The affected child exhibits neurological symptoms including mental confusion, seizures, and possible coma. Most cases resolve with proper supportive therapy and measures to decrease intracranial pressure.

III. REVIEW QUESTIONS

1. Which of the following is NOT a route of infection in infectious disease of the CNS?
   a. hematogenous
   b. open wound
   c. spread from adjacent structure
   d. fomites
   e. through nerves
   f. vectors

2. The organism that causes acute meningitis in epidemics is:
   a. *Streptococcus pneumoniae*
   b. *Escherichia coli*
   c. *Neiserria meningitidis*
   d. *Hemophilus influenzae*

3. Acute meningitis that is accompanied by a purulent exudate is caused by:
   a. pyogenic bacteria
   b. viruses
   c. protozoa
   d. fungi

4. Fibrosis and contracture of scar tissue with possible compression of nerve roots is a feature of:
   a. acute bacterial meningitis
   b. chronic meningitis
   c. acute viral meningitis
   d. acquired hydrocephalus

5. Infectious inflammation of the brain is:
   a. meningitis
   b. myelitis
   c. encephalopathy
   d. encephalitis

6. The majority of cases of encephalitis are caused by:
   a. vectors
   b. viruses
   c. bacteria
   d. mosquitos

7. The role of vectors in the spread of encephalitis is:
   a. to contaminate food with their feces
   b. to infiltrate lymphocytes in brain parenchyma
   c. to pass a virus from their saliva into a bite wound
   d. to act as infectious fomites

8. *Toxoplasma gondii, Candida albicans,* and *Cryptococcus neoformans* are common agents of encephalitis in:
   a. AIDS patients
   b. the general population
   c. children
   d. the elderly

1. d—fomites

2. c—*Neisseria meningitidis*

3. a—pyogenic bacteria

4. b—chronic meningitis

5. d—encephalitis

6. b—viruses

7. c—to pass a virus from their saliva into a bite wound

8. a—AIDS patients

682

9. d–a prominent feature is
lethargy

9. Encephalitis is sometimes called the "sleeping sickness" because:
   a. the onset of signs begin while the patient is asleep
   b. a prominent feature is coma
   c. delirium may be present
   d. a prominent feature is lethargy

SECTION ▶ IV. VASCULAR DISEASE AND TRAUMA

▶ VASCULAR DISEASES OF THE BRAIN

---- 18–33 ----

1. cerebrovascular disease

Diseases affecting the blood vessels supplying the brain are the most common cause of brain lesions. Disease of these vessels is called **cerebrovascular disease,** or **CVD.** Cerebrovascular disease leads to a **cerebrovascular accident,** or **CVA.** A cerebrovascular accident is the injury that results from cerebrovascular disease. The clinical presentation, or what is seen as a result of a CVA, is what we commonly call a **stroke.** A stroke represents an acute neurological deficit due to vascular occlusion or bleeding. CVD leads to a CVA because of blockage of an artery by a thrombi or emboli, or because of rupture of an artery due to hypertension, arteriosclerosis, or aneurysm. The relationships between cause and effect in cerebrovascular disease are shown in Figure 18–5. A CVA is a very common cause of crippling and death. The number one and two causes of death in this country are ischemic heart disease and respiratory tract infection, respectively, with stroke being the third most common cause. The underlying pathology of many cases of CVD is atherosclerosis of the arteries of the brain. Complications of atherosclerosis, such as thromboembolism, add to the incidence of CVA and stroke. When the arteries supplying the brain are diseased, this is known as _____(1). The damage that occurs to brain func-

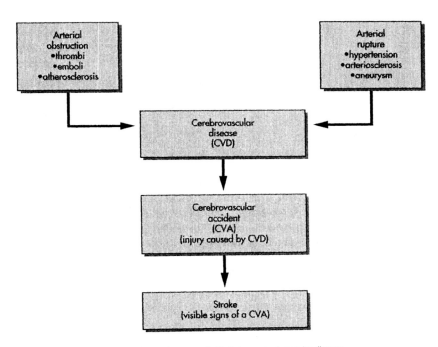

Figure 18–5. Causes and effects in cerebral vascular disease.

tion as a result of CVD is called a _____(2). The signs of a CVA are called a _____(3). The most common cause of injury to the brain is _____(4). The two major reasons for a CVA are _____(5) of an artery or _____(6) of an artery.

2. cerebrovascular accident
3. stroke
4. cerebrovascular disease
5. occlusion
6. rupture

-- 18-34 ------

Atherosclerosis of cerebral arteries is generally seen in two forms, **diffuse ischemia of the cerebrum** and **cerebral infarct.** Widespread ischemia of brain tissue is directly proportional to the degree of spread of atherosclerosis. Remember that atherosclerosis causes narrowing of vessels and therefore a decrease in blood supply to the normally perfused area. It follows that areas of ischemic necrosis will result. Impairment of mental function is also proportional to the amount of necrosis of brain tissue. This is known as **infarct dementia.** Other causes of systemic ischemia (hypotensive shock, heart failure) are also implicated in cerebral ischemia and mental deterioration. The amount of atherosclerosis affecting cerebral vessels will dictate the amount of _____(1) of brain tissue. Ischemia results from _____(2) of vessel lumens and a decrease in _____(3). Infarct dementia describes deterioration of _____(4) function because of areas of _____(5) in the brain.

1. ischemia
2. narrowing
3. blood supply
4. mental
5. necrosis

-- 18-35 ------

A **cerebral infarct** is the result of sudden and complete obstruction of a major cerebral artery. This is usually the middle cerebral artery, the largest cerebral artery. It is a direct extension of the carotid artery in the neck. A cerebral infarct is the most common cause of stroke. The middle cerebral artery supplies the motor control sections of the cerebrum, so the signs of this type of stroke relate mainly to motor function. The most common reason for this CVA is occlusion of the atherosclerotic artery by a thrombus (thrombosis). Remember that clot formation on the ulcerated surface of an atherosclerotic plaque is common. Thrombi that originate elsewhere in the body can reach the middle cerebral artery through the carotid artery. When a thrombus lodges in the brain (thromboembolism), it produces the same results. The most common causes of thromboembolism leading to cerebral infarct are cardiac in origin. These may be the aftermath of a myocardial infarction or due to endocarditis. In cerebral infarct, all of the brain tissue supplied by the blocked artery suffers death if the obstruction remains for any length of time. Function is lost immediately. The area becomes necrotic within a few days and the loss of tissue leaves a cavity that becomes cystic. Edema around the infarct causes significant swelling and increased intracranial pressure so that the severity of signs and the likelihood of death are increased. Swelling of the brain is always a major concern since the skull leaves no room for expansion and increased pressure results. Any neurological deficits resulting from the CVA, or stroke, are permanent since dead neurons do not regenerate. Astrocytes, the fibroblasts of the brain, proliferate to form a glial scar to patch the area. Figure 18–6 is of a cross-section of brain containing an infarcted and cystic area.

-- 18-36 ------

Complete occlusion of a major cerebral artery causes a _____(1). This is the most common reason for the signs of a CVA, or a _____(2). Blockage of an artery by a thrombus, which is called _____(3), is generally the cause of cerebral infarction. The clot may form at the site of a (an) _____(4) atherosclerotic plaque or it may form in other parts of the body. In this second case, the occlusion is called a _____(5) because the thrombus has traveled as an embolism. Edema in response to necrosis causes _____(6) of the brain, and this raises the _____(7). Neurons do not _____(8), so neurologic impairment is permanent. The clinical presentation of stroke in survivors will depend on which areas of the cerebrum have undergone infarction, and this depends on which arteries were blocked. The most common site of occlusion, the middle cerebral artery which supplies the motor control area, causes weakness of one side of the body **(hemiparesis)** or paralysis of one side of the body **(hemiplegia).** The side of the body opposite the hemisphere where the infarction occurred is generally affected because nerve tracts from brain hemispheres cross over to the other side as they course through the brain stem. Loss of sensation of the affected side, loss

1. cerebral infarct
2. stroke
3. thrombosis
4. ulcerated
5. thromboembolism
6. swelling
7. intracranial pressure
8. regenerate

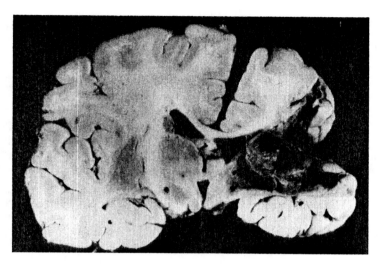

Figure 18–6. Cerebral infarction, which shows a cystic area that collapsed when the brain was cut. *(From Chandrasoma and Taylor,* Concise Pathology, *2nd ed., Appleton & Lange.)*

of parts of the visual field, and impairment of speech (**aphasia**) are also seen. Edema and high intracranial pressure are responsible for stupor and coma. These conditions usually improve with treatment if the patient has survived the episode. It is critical that the swelling be decreased or controlled with the use of hyperosmolar drugs. These are dehydrating agents that draw water out of the brain tissue and decrease pressure. Following a stroke, physical therapy is the most important supportive measure to help victims cope with their disability.

The other type of cerebrovascular accident is rupture of an artery. This is most commonly associated with hypertension. This causes an **intracerebral hemorrhage,** or bleeding within the brain. Hypertension damages vessels by causing arteriosclerosis and therefore weakening of the vessels. Because they are hard and brittle, they are susceptible to bursting. The overall result is a stroke because that area of the brain undergoes infarction due to sudden and complete loss of blood supply. Edema and swelling also accompany intracerebral hemorrhage, which is shown in Figure 18–7, and intracranial pressure rises. In addition to CVD

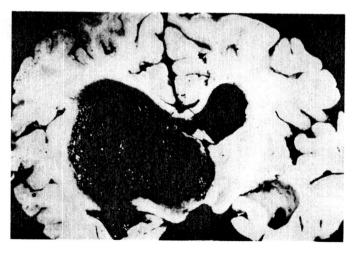

Figure 18–7. Intracerebral hemorrhage caused by rupture of an aneurysm. Note the compression of the brain by the large hematoma. *(From Chandrasoma and Taylor,* Concise Pathology, *2nd ed., Appleton & Lange.)*

and CVA, intracerebral hemorrhage can be caused by various types of trauma. In survivors, signs mimic stroke caused by occlusive cerebral infarct. Stroke because of intracerebral hemorrhage also causes severe pressure-related headache and loss of consciousness. Many cases of intracerebral hemorrhage CVA are fatal. Intracerebral hemorrhage is when an artery _____(1), causing _____(2) in the brain tissue. The most common cause of rupture is _____(3). This is because high blood pressure hardens and weakens _____(4), so they are more likely to rupture. The loss of blood supply to an area of the brain causes _____(5) of the area. The presence of edematous fluid along with the blood from the artery causes intracranial _____(6) to rise.

1. ruptures
2. bleeding
3. hypertension
4. arteries or vessels
5. infarction
6. pressure

18–38

Intracranial hemorrhage is bleeding within the skull. The various locations are shown in Figure 18–8. The hemorrhage may be within the brain itself (intracerebral hemorrhage as just discussed) or outside of the brain within the skull. Those hemorrhages outside of the brain include:

1. **Epidural hematoma.** This is bleeding in between the skull and the dura mater (outer layer) of the meninges. The term epidural means upon ("epi") the dura ("dural"). The area between the skull and the dura is a potential space that normally has no appreciable free space present. Therefore, a space-occupying lesion like a hematoma or pocket of blood exerts significant pressure that can cause coma and death. Epidural hematoma results from tearing a meningeal artery during trauma.
2. **Subdural hematoma.** This is bleeding in between the arachnoid layer of the meninges and the dura mater. Subdural means under ("sub") the dura. Subdural hematoma occurs due to rupture or tearing of the meningeal veins that cross this space. This is most often associated with blunt trauma that causes sudden impact of the skull. There is often less hemorrhage in a subdural hematoma because pressure in veins is less than in arteries. However, a large hematoma may develop and worsen the prognosis.

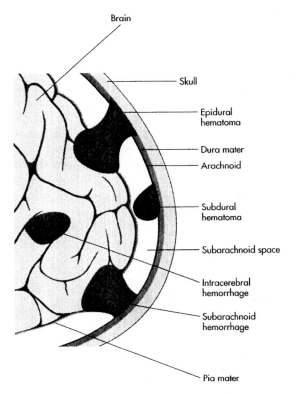

Figure 18–8. Locations of intracranial hemorrhage.

3. **Subarachnoid hemorrhage.** This is bleeding under the arachnoid layer, upon the pia mater and brain surface. This type of bleeding can be associated with a contusion (see Frame 18–41). Another cause is rupture of a congenital berry aneurysm in the circle of Willis. You have learned that an aneurysm is a weakened area of the wall of an artery that causes it to bulge and be susceptible to bursting. The rupture of a berry aneurysm is usually spontaneous but can be precipitated by hypertension. Sudden loss of consciousness accompanies the rupture, and subarachnoid hemorrhage is often fatal. Varying amounts of neurologic damage are likely in survivors.

18-39

1. intracranial hemorrhage
2. intracerebral hemorrhage
3. epidural hematoma
4. artery
5. trauma
6. pressure
7. subdural hematoma
8. vein
9. subarachnoid hemorrhage
10. aneurysm
11. ruptures

Bleeding anywhere within the skull is called _____(1). If the bleeding is within the brain itself, this is referred to as _____(2). Hemorrhage between the skull and dura mater is a (an) _____(3). An epidural hematoma generally results from rupture of a meningeal _____(4) during _____(5). The high pressure of the bleed from an artery can create a space-occupying lesion that applies a great deal of _____(6) on the brain. Hemorrhage in between the dura and arachnoid layers is called a _____(7). This is due to the rupture of a meningeal _____(8). Bleeding on the brain surface, under the arachnoid, is described as _____(9). A congenital defect called a (an) _____(10) of the circle of Willis can cause subarachnoid hemorrhage if the aneurysm _____(11).

▶ TRAUMA OF THE BRAIN

18-40

Brain trauma is also a major cause of disability and death, although not as common as CVD. Automobile accidents probably account for the majority of head trauma cases. Acts of violence and falls are other reasons for head trauma. The final injury to the brain during some of the following types of trauma may not be immediate. In cases of hemorrhage, it may take a short while for enough blood to accumulate to a critical state. This is the primary reason for monitoring head trauma victims for at least 24 hours. As with other types of cerebral injury, edema and swelling with increased intracranial pressure pose the same threats to the life of the victim.

18-41

The features of brain trauma are summarized in Table 18–3. A **concussion** is the simplest and mildest form of brain trauma. There is usually loss of consciousness and motor reflexes, but there is no structural injury or physical lesion of the brain. Consciousness is regained in a short while and severe headache, dizziness, and nausea are common. Loss of memory surrounds the traumatic event. Concussion is self-limiting and recovery is complete. Monitoring of the victim is necessary to ensure that the injury is not worse than a concussion. A **contusion** is a bruise of the brain surface created during an impact or blunt trauma. Small vessels rupture and bleed. With this bleeding are the complications of edema and raised pressure. The side of the brain that sustained the impact creates a contusion called a *coup lesion,* and bruising occurs here. The reactive jerking motion of the brain

TABLE 18–3. TRAUMA OF THE BRAIN

Injury	Features
Concussion	No physical injury to the brain, mildest type of trauma
Contusion	Bruising of the brain at site of injury (coup lesion) and on opposite side due to impacting skull (contrecoup lesion), potential for brain damage or death
Epidural hematoma	Tearing of meningeal arteries with significant hemorrhage, often seen in skull fracture
Subarachnoid hemorrhage	Cutting of cerebral arteries by bone fragments in skull fracture
Subdural hematoma	Tearing of meningeal veins with less hemorrhage
Penetrating injury	Damage of brain parenchyma, hemorrhage, skull fracture impaction, infection

causes it to hit the skull on the opposite side, causing a *contrecoup lesion* due to small hemorrhages. Contusions are much more severe than concussion, and brain damage or death is a possibility. Injury to the brain that causes no physical damage is called a _____(1). A concussion resolves on its own, or is _____(2). A contusion is a _____(3) of the brain surface. This bruise is from vessel _____(4) and bleeding. A coup lesion develops at the _____(5) of impact and further trauma on the opposite side is called a (an) _____(6). A contrecoup lesion occurs because the brain is thrown forward in the skull and then it _____(7) the opposite side of the skull.

1. concussion
2. self-limiting
3. bruise
4. rupture
5. site or side
6. contrecoup lesion
7. hits

18-42

Epidural and subdural hematomas occur when trauma tears larger blood vessels. Recall that epidural hematomas are associated with tears of the dural arteries, and subdural hematomas with tears of meningeal veins. Epidural hemorrhages are seen in fractures of the skull where the sharp bone fragments cut the arteries. Skull fracture is also a cause of subarachnoid hemorrhage. Arterial rupture (epidural hematoma) is more life-threatening than venous rupture (subdural hematoma) because of increased arterial pressure. In epidural hematomas, the accumulation of blood is more rapid and so is the increase in intracranial pressure. Lifesaving measures must include surgical removal of the hematoma and tying off of the vessels.

18-43

Penetrating injury of the brain is most commonly due to gunshots. In addition to massive trauma of brain tissue caused directly by the bullet, fractured pieces of bone or splinters are driven into the wound and impacted. Infection is a major concern in survivors because this is an open wound. Infection of the brain is called _____(1). Survivors may also have permanent neurologic impairment or develop epilepsy (seizures).

1. encephalitis

IV. REVIEW QUESTIONS

1. Which of the following is the correct relationship?
   a. A stroke describes pathology of vessels of the brain, which manifest as signs commonly called CVD.
   b. A CVA describes pathology of vessels of the brain, which manifest as signs commonly called a stroke.
   c. CVD describes pathology of vessels of the brain that causes an injury or a stroke. The signs of a stroke are commonly called a CVA.
   d. CVD describes pathology of vessels of the brain that causes an injury or CVA. The signs of a CVA are commonly called a stroke.

2. Which of the following are the major reasons for CVA (choose two):
   a. occlusion of an artery in the brain
   b. epidural hematoma
   c. concussion
   d. rupture of an artery in the brain
   e. cerebral infarct

3. Complete obstruction of a major cerebral artery causes:
   a. diffuse ischemia of the cerebrum
   b. cerebral infarct
   c. cerebral thromboembolism
   d. intracerebral hemorrhage

1. d–CVD describes pathology of vessels of the brain that causes an injury or CVA. The signs of a CVA are commonly called a stroke.

2. a–occlusion of an artery in the brain; d–rupture of an artery in the brain

3. b–cerebral infarct

4. d–cerebral infarct

5. b–thrombosis of an athero-sclerotic artery

6. c–edema, swelling, and increased intracranial pressure

7. a–hypertension

8. a–in between the dura mater and the arachnoid layer of the meninges; b–within the brain; c–in between the skull and the dura mater, the outer layer of the meninges; d–under the arachnoid layer, on the pia mater and the brain surface

9. b–subdural

10. d–subarachnoid hemorrhage

11. a–contusion

12. c–skull fracture

4. The most common cause of stroke is:
    a. hypertension
    b. diffuse ischemia of the cerebrum
    c. arterial rupture
    d. cerebral infarct

5. The most common reason for stroke due to cerebral infarct is:
    a. aneurysm
    b. thrombosis of an atherosclerotic artery
    c. hypertension
    d. subarachnoid hemorrhage

6. A significant consequence of several types of CVA is:
    a. coma
    b. hemiplegia
    c. edema, swelling, and increased intracranial pressure
    d. infarct dementia

7. The most common reason for arterial rupture and intracerebral hemorrhage is:
    a. hypertension
    b. aneurysm
    c. trauma
    d. arteriosclerosis

8. For these types of intracranial hemorrhage, list the location of the bleeding:
    a. subdural:_____
    b. intracerebral:_____
    c. epidural:_____
    d. subarachnoid:_____

9. The type of intracranial hemorrhage that is *least* severe, because it involves rupture of veins, not arteries, is:
    a. epidural
    b. subdural
    c. intracerebral
    d. subarachnoid

10. Rupture of a berry aneurysm causes:
    a. intracerebral hemorrhage
    b. epidural hematoma
    c. subdural hematoma
    d. subarachnoid hemorrhage

11. Coup lesions and contrecoup lesions are associated with the brain trauma called:
    a. contusion
    b. concussion
    c. subdural hematoma
    d. epidural hematoma

12. Epidural and subarachnoid hemorrhage are generally associated with:
    a. mild impact injury
    b. blunt trauma
    c. skull fracture
    d. the aftermath of a concussion

V. NEOPLASIA OF THE CENTRAL NERVOUS SYSTEM AND OTHER DISORDERS ◀ SECTION

▶ NEOPLASIA

Cancer of the central nervous system is rare compared to other types of cancer, but it is significant because the death rate is very high. Malignant tumors are very infiltrative, making adequate removal impossible. The patient dies before metastasis has a chance to occur. Death due to the malignant nature of a tumor is not surprising, but even a benign tumor inside the skull is significant because of the increase of intracranial pressure and compression of the brain. Depending on its location, a benign tumor can compress an area that controls vital functions like respiration. Removal of a benign tumor can also be difficult depending on its location. Because of these factors, a tumor that is classified as benign histologically may still be considered malignant. In the younger population (children and young adults) brain tumors are more prominent than other types of cancer. In children, leukemia is the most common malignancy and brain tumors are second.

Secondary tumors, or metastases, occur about as frequently as primary tumors. Half of the cases of brain tumors are due to metastasis. Malignancy of any type could spread to the brain but the type with the most predilection for the brain are primary tumors of the breast, lung, and malignant melanoma. Of the primary brain tumors, 90 percent are either of glial cells (75 percent) or meninges (15 percent). Table 18–4 outlines these tumors of the CNS. Primary lymphoma of the brain is seen in AIDS patients. The etiology of CNS neoplasia is idiopathic, as with many kinds of malignancy. No specific lifestyle or risk factors have been implicated as increasing the likelihood of CNS neoplasia. Research is focusing on possible genetic causes, such as changes in chromosomes, changes in tumor suppressor genes, or familial incidence of other types of cancer. The signs of a brain tumor cause both physical and psychiatric disturbances. These include severe headache, seizures, lethargy, coma, delirium (confusion), personality and behavioral changes, and dementia. Even though it is rare, neoplasia of the CNS is of great importance because of the high _____(1) associated with it. Malignant tumors have a tendency to _____(2) deeply into the surrounding tissue, so _____(3) is impossible. _____(4) occurs before the tumor spreads. Characteristics of benign tumors cause them to be considered _____(5) as far as behavior. Fifty percent of brain tumors are _____(6) tumors that have _____(7), to the brain.

1. death or mortality rate
2. infiltrate
3. removal
4. Death
5. malignant
6. secondary
7. spread, or metastasized

A **glioma** is a malignant tumor that arises from the glial cells. Glial cells are supportive cells, not neurons. These cells are the astrocytes, oligodendroglia, and ependymal cells of the ventricles and spinal cord canal. The majority of gliomas (80 percent) arise from astrocytes and are classified as **astrocytic gliomas.** There are two forms of astrocytic gliomas. The first is the **astrocytoma.** This tumor is less malignant because initially it is slow growing and the cells are well differentiated. The **glioblastoma multiforme** is a highly malignant tumor that grows rapidly and is composed of very anaplastic cells. The invasive and destructive nature of a glioblastoma is shown in Figure 18–9. The glioblastoma is the most common tumor of the central nervous system. It most often affects the geriatric population. **Oligodendrogliomas** and **ependymomas** are less common and will not be discussed. The prognosis of a glial tumor depends on its location and its degree of malignancy (rate of growth and cellular anaplasia). A glioblastoma is always fatal regardless of its location. Tumors of the CNS support cells are called _____(1). They are generally histologically classified as _____(2). Most gliomas are classified as _____(3). Of these, the less malignant form is the _____(4), while the highly malignant tumor is the _____(5). The most common tumor arising within the central nervous system is the _____(6). The worst prognosis is associated with a _____(7).

1. gliomas
2. malignant
3. astrocytic gliomas
4. astrocytoma
5. glioblastoma multiforme
6. glioblastoma multiforme
7. glioblastoma multiforme

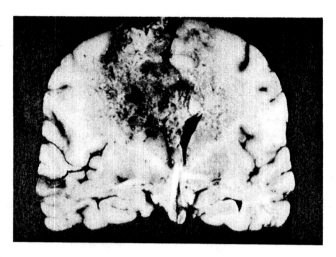

Figure 18–9. A glioblastoma multiforme. Note the extensive infiltration and poor margins of the tumor, accompanied by destruction of brain tissue. *(From Chandrasoma and Taylor,* Concise Pathology, *2nd ed., Appleton & Lange.)*

18–47

1. meninges
2. second
3. benign
4. good
5. removed
6. base

The second most common tumor of the central nervous system is a **meningioma.** As the name implies, it arises from the meninges, specifically the dura mater. Meningiomas are benign, well encapsulated, and slow growing. They do not infiltrate into the brain which assists their removal. Compare the isolated appearance of a meningioma in Figure 18–10 with the glioblastoma in Figure 18–9. The degree of disorder caused by a meningioma depends on where it is located. The most common site is on the dorsum, or top of the cerebrum. It grows outside of the brain and so applies pressure to the surface. A meningioma may cause motor impairment or seizures. Other locations of a meningioma include the base of the brain or along the spinal cord. Many cases carry a good prognosis because of the ease with which the tumor can be shelled out or removed. However, a meningioma at the base of the brain is difficult to remove because of the vessels and nerves coursing through the area, so the prognosis in this case is worse. A meningioma is neoplasia of the _____(1), and it is the _____(2) most common tumor of the CNS. A meningioma is classified as _____(3). The prognosis is _____(4) for this tumor because it is easily _____(5). The exception to this is when the tumor is found at the _____(6) of the brain.

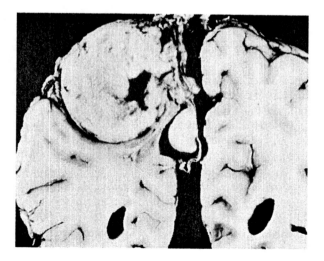

Figure 18–10. A meningioma. Note the well-defined margins and lack of infiltration as compared to Figure 18–9. The isolation is due to the capsule and nature of the tumor. *(From Kent and Hart,* Introduction to Human Disease, *3rd ed., Appleton & Lange.)*

TABLE 18–4. TUMORS OF THE CENTRAL NERVOUS SYSTEM

Neoplasia	Features
Glioma (75% of CNS tumors)	Central nervous system, support cells
Astrocytic glioma (80% of gliomas)	Astrocytes
Astrocytoma	Less malignant
Glioblastoma multiforme	Most malignant, highest mortality rate, most common
Oligodendroglioma	Oligodendroglia cells
Ependymomas	Ependymal cells
Meningioma (15% of CNS tumors)	Meninges, well encapsulated, benign
Neuroma	CNS neurons
Schwannoma	Schwann cells of neural axons
Neurofibroma	Benign tumor of neurofibroblasts
Neurofibrosarcoma	Malignant tumor of neurofibroblasts

18–48

1. neuromas
2. benign
3. schwannomas
4. neurofibroblasts

Another type of benign tumor is the **neuroma.** This is a tumor of the nerve cells, specifically of the cells associated with the axons. A **schwannoma** arises from schwann cells while a **neurofibroma** originates from neurofibroblasts. Schwannomas can be located on cranial nerves or spinal nerves. Neurofibromas are often multiple in nature and found on the peripheral nerves as part of a condition called neurofibromatosis. The malignant form of this neoplasia is the **neurofibrosarcoma,** which is rare. It is thought to represent transformation of a previously benign neurofibroma. In general, tumors of the nerve cells are called _____(1), and they are classified as _____(2). Schwann cells give rise to _____(3) while neurofibromas are produced from _____(4).

▶ OTHER DISORDERS OF THE CENTRAL NERVOUS SYSTEM

18–49

1. contractions
2. excited
3. irritated
4. impulses or electrical discharges
5. seizure

A **convulsion** is involuntary contraction of skeletal muscle which often occurs in a series. It is a result of excitation or irritation of neurons that innervate voluntary muscle. A convulsion represents an abnormal "setting off" of the nerve cells, and they react by transmitting impulses or electrical discharges in a random, abnormal fashion. There are many causes of convulsions. They include chemical imbalances, drugs, uremia, toxemia of pregnancy, encephalitis, meningitis, and high fevers in children. A specific type of convulsion is a **seizure** seen in the disorder **epilepsy.** Disturbances in electrical activity occur within the brain, causing muscle contractions and mental effects. The majority of cases of epilepsy are idiopathic in cause. Heredity is suspected in some cases. Brain trauma can create permanent foci of abnormal discharges from the brain because of the presence of a glial scar. A tumor can also produce epileptic seizures. A convulsion is a series of involuntary muscle _____(1) because the neurons have been _____(2) or _____(3). During a convulsion, abnormal _____(4) are emitted and so the muscles react. In the disease epilepsy, the convulsion is called a _____(5).

······ 18-50 ······

1. petit mal
2. consciousness
3. collapse
4. severe
5. loss
6. collapse
7. aura

In children and some adults, epilepsy may manifest as the **petit mal** form. This is a mild seizure with very brief loss of consciousness, during which time the individual appears dazed. Twitching is mild and there is no collapse. The more severe form of epilepsy is the **grand mal.** Here, there is loss of consciousness that causes collapse, with dramatic involuntary movements (thrashing and shaking) that are classically recognized as seizures. Excessive salivation and loss of bladder control are also features. The individual is groggy and disoriented afterwards. The duration and frequency of grand mal seizures vary. An interesting note about grand mal epilepsy is that the individual usually knows in advance when a seizure is approaching. The signals that make up this warning are collectively called an **aura.** An aura includes an "out of body" feeling along with blurred vision and tingling sensations. Epilepsy is managed by preventing injury to the individual during seizures, and with anticonvulsant drugs such as Dilantin. Dilantin decreases the frequency of seizures and is very effective in controlling epilepsy. The mildest form of epilepsy is called a _____(1). During a petit mal, there is unrecognizable loss of _____(2) and the individual does not _____(3). A grand mal is the _____(4) form of epilepsy. There are both obvious _____(5) of consciousness and _____(6). The warning signs that precede a seizure are called a (an) _____(7).

······ 18-51 ······

1. failure
2. brain
3. vital
4. stem
5. motor
6. mental

A **coma** represents generalized failure of brain function. Many of the diseases we have discussed can lead to this failure if they are severe enough. A coma produces a vegetative state in which only vital functions are maintained by the involuntary section of the brain, the brain stem. Motor and mental function of the cerebral cortex are absent. The prognosis, regarding whether or not the coma will be reversible, depends of the nature and extent of the injury. A state of "brain death" is highly controversial to determine, and both legal and ethical issues enter into the medical criteria. A coma is _____(1) of higher level _____(2) function. Only _____(3) functions continue to keep the patient alive, and this is accomplished by the brain _____(4). There are no _____(5) or _____(6) capabilities at all.

V. REVIEW QUESTIONS

1. a–Primary brain tumors are much more common than metastases, or secondary tumors.

2. True

3. b–glioblastoma

4. a–glioblastoma; b–meningioma

1. Which of the following statements about cerebral neoplasia is INCORRECT?
   a. Primary brain tumors are much more common than metastases, or secondary tumors.
   b. A benign tumor can be considered malignant in regards to its behavior and effects.
   c. Death generally occurs before metastasis of the tumor.
   d. The comparative rarity of cerebral tumors is overshadowed by the high death rate.

2. True or false: The most common malignancy of the brain arises from glial or supportive cells instead of neurons. _____

3. Of the astrocytic gliomas, the most malignant is the:
   a. astrocytoma
   b. glioblastoma
   c. oligodendroglioma
   d. neuroma

4. The most common tumor of the CNS is the a. _____, while the second most common tumor is the b. _____.

   neuroma   oligodendroglioma
   glioblastoma   ependymoma
   meningioma   astrocytoma

5. Benign in nature, well encapsulated, slow growth, and ease of removal are typical characteristics of:
   a. neurofibrosarcoma
   b. meningioma
   c. neuroma
   d. schwannoma

6. In epilepsy, the warning signs that signal an oncoming seizure is called a (an):

   _____

7. Loss of consciousness, collapse, and uncontrollable thrashing describe:
   a. petit mal epilepsy
   b. an aura
   c. grand mal epilepsy
   d. idiopathic epilepsy

5. b–meningioma

6. aura

7. c–grand mal epilepsy

VI. DISEASES OF THE EYE ◀ SECTION

······ 18–52 ······

As people get older, diseases of the eye become more common. These problems often relate to diabetes, atherosclerosis, and hypertension, which are all circulatory disorders. Glaucoma and cataracts are also age-related. Several of the conditions we will discuss can lead to blindness. Infections and allergic responses can affect any age. The eyes are susceptible to these insults because of their exposure to the environment. The most common eye problems are disturbances in vision, or a decrease in the ability to see clearly. Visual disturbances are not a true pathological state; that is, there is no physical lesion that can be demonstrated histologically. They are due to impaired function because of abnormal light refraction.

▶ **INFLAMMATORY AND CIRCULATORY DISORDERS**

······ 18–53 ······

Infection of the eyes by pathogens can affect several structures. The less common infections that we will not discuss, and the affected structures, include iridocyclitis (iris), scleritis (sclera), blepharitis (eyelid), dacryocystitis (lacrimal gland and duct), uveitis (entire vascular layer), retinitis (retina), optic neuritis (optic nerve), and endophthalmitis (interior of the posterior chamber). Several of these infections represent superficial infections that have descended into deeper layers. This is uncommon since superficial infections are obvious and easily treated. Superficial infections have a very good prognosis, while untreated ulcerative infections of those deeper layers may lead to blindness.

······ 18–54 ······

Superficial infections and inflammations, which are much more common, include conjunctivitis and keratitis. **Conjunctivitis** is infectious or allergic inflammation of the pink tissue surrounding the anterior external surface of the globe. Conjunctiva lines the inside of the upper and lower eyelid. Conjunctivitis is commonly called "pink eye" because the inflamed tissue around the eye becomes very red because of hyperemia. Hyperemia means increased _____(1) in an area. This hyperemia can also be described as vascular congestion. Swelling accompanies the redness. Pathogens capable of causing conjunctivitis are bacteria, viruses, *Chlamydia*, and fungi. Allergens can also cause conjunctivitis. Conjunctivitis may be primary (occurring alone) or be secondary to upper respiratory infection. Bacterial conjunctivitis can be secondary to viral or allergic conjunctivitis since compromised tissue is always susceptible to bacterial invasion. Pyogenic bacteria produce purulent exudate, and pus may fill the eyelid pockets. Conjunctivitis

1. blood supply

2. conjunctivitis
3. infection
4. allergy
5. pink eye
6. upper respiratory
   infection
7. bacterial
8. photophobia

18-55

1. cornea
2. ulcers
3. Photophobia
4. herpesvirus
5. scarring

18-56

may present as a stye, or infected gland of the eyelid, medically called a **hordeolum.** Blepharitis and dacryocystitis may be complications of conjunctivitis. **Photophobia** may accompany this inflammatory condition. Photophobia is intolerance to light, commonly described as the light hurting one's eyes. Inflammation of the pink tissue surrounding the exterior of the eye is called _____(2). The inflammation may be due to either _____(3) or _____(4). Hyperemia, or vascular congestion, has earned this condition the common name of _____(5). Conjunctivitis may be primary, or secondary to _____(6). Viral and allergic conjunctivitis may lead to secondary _____(7) conjunctivitis. Conjunctivitis can lead to avoidance of light because of sensitivity, and this is called _____(8).

Keratitis is infection of the cornea and it most often manifests as painful ulcers. Tearing and photophobia can be pronounced because of the pain. The most common reason for keratitis in this country is herpesvirus infection. As in other types of herpes infection, tiny vesicles, or blisters, develop and then erode into ulcers. These lesions can produce tiny scars in the cornea after healing. The majority of cases are not so severe that the ulcer erodes through the cornea or that the scars cause disturbance in vision. However, so that you are familiar with the appearance of a corneal scar, Figure 18–11 shows significant scarring of the cornea in a case of chronic keratitis. In Chapter 5 we discussed the disease trachoma, which is conjunctivitis caused by *Chlamydia.* In trachoma, severe keratitis is possible with so much scarring that blindness results. This is rarely seen in this country, but trachoma is a prominent cause of blindness around the world. Keratitis is infection of the _____(1). It usually causes painful _____(2) on the cornea. _____(3) is more prominent than in conjunctivitis due to the discomfort. A common cause of keratitis is _____(4) infection. A sequela of keratitis can be the presence of _____(5) on the cornea after healing.

Inflammation of the eyes may be caused by trauma, which can be either physical injury or chemical burns, or irritation. Physical injuries are superficial, blunt, or penetrating. Blunt injury is associated with impact or jerking motions of the head and may cause hemorrhage within the eye. A hematoma that forms on external surfaces is obvious. Intraocular hemorrhage can be determined by examining the inside of the globe with an ophthalmoscope. Bleeding within the eye is reported by the patient as blurred, reddish vision. The most serious type of intraocular hemorrhage is that which can occur behind the retina. The pocket of blood can detach the retina, causing blindness. Retinal detachment is the lifting of the retina with subsequent tearing of the capillaries and neuron connections. Blunt trauma can also tear

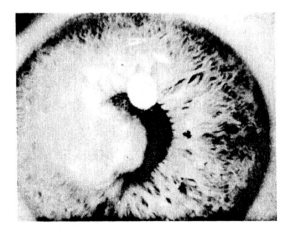

Figure 18–11. Severe scarring of the cornea, following recurrent herpes keratitis. *(From Chandrasoma and Taylor,* Concise Pathology, *2nd ed., Appleton & Lange.)*

the filamentous ligaments that secure the lens, causing dislocation of the lens and possible glaucoma (see Frame 18–61). A frequent result of blunt trauma is _____(1) within the eye. The bleeding may be seen on the surfaces, or require ophthalmoscopic examination if it is _____(2). Bleeding behind the _____(3) can lift it or cause _____(4), which results in _____(5).

1. hemorrhage or hematoma
2. intraocular, or inside the eye
3. retina
4. detachment
5. blindness

18–57

Superficial abrasions generally affect the conjunctiva or cornea. A variety of mechanical insults, such as sharp objects or foreign bodies, can abrade or scratch the external surfaces. This causes inflammation, tearing, and pain. A sharp object can penetrate the eye and produce significant consequences. As a result of the puncture, fluid is lost from within the globe and it may collapse. The damage may be permanent, and infection is a concern. Chemical irritation causes superficial abrasions of the sclera and cornea. An ulcer often develops, and infection is a possibility. Deep ulcers may erode to the point of penetration into the anterior chamber. Severe burns of the cornea can cause significant scarring and greatly interfere with vision. A badly damaged cornea may require transplantation. Scratching of the conjunctiva or cornea is seen in _____(1). Penetration can occur by a _____(2). Possible collapse of the globe is related to _____(3) that is lost during the puncture. The most common manifestation of chemical injury is a (an) _____(4) on the cornea. Penetration can occur if a deep ulcer _____(5) through the cornea. The aftermath of severe corneal burns is _____(6).

1. superficial abrasions
2. sharp object
3. fluid
4. ulcer
5. erodes
6. significant scarring

18–58

Circulatory disturbances that affect the vessels of the eye are usually complications of systemic vascular disease. The most significant of these conditions are hypertension and diabetes. You have learned that hypertension damages vessels, and the delicate vessels of the eye are no exception. Diabetes, if you will remember from Chapter 8, produces disease of tiny vessels, which is called microangiopathy. Figure 18–12 outlines the damage suffered by the eyes, particularly the retina, in systemic vascular disease.

18–59

Vascular disease of the eye, specifically the retina, caused by hypertension is called **hypertensive retinopathy.** The vessels of the retina and choroid layer suffer injury (arteriolosclerosis) because of the constant high blood pressure. These changes can easily be seen by viewing the fundus of the retina with an ophthalmoscope. In fact, ophthalmoscopic examination is an important part of assessing the status of a patient with hypertension, since this is a visual representation of what is happening to other vessels in the body. The retinopathy, which is sclerosis, caused by hypertension can be visibly graded as mild, moderate, or severe. The arterioles become very thin, hardened, and narrowed. Neurons of the retina suffer hypoxia and ischemic damage. Whitish areas of ischemia have been described as cotton wool patches. Tiny areas of dilation or microaneurysms and dot-like hemorrhages are seen. Various types of exudates may be present. Figure 18–13 compares a normal retina to a diseased retina in hypertension. Untreated severe cases of hypertensive retinopathy cause edema of the optic disc, where the nerve exits. This can cause irreparable damage to the retina and blindness. Circulatory disorders of the eye are generally related to _____(1). The most common of the systemic disorders, _____(2) and _____(3), both _____(4) blood vessels. Vascular disease of the retina caused by hypertension is called _____(5). The underlying pathology of these vessels is _____(6). The changes that can be seen include _____(7) and _____(8) of the arterioles, ischemic areas called _____(9), tiny dilations or _____(10), and pinpoint _____(11). Blindness can result in untreated cases where _____(12) of the optic disc has developed.

1. systemic vascular disease
2. hypertension
3. diabetes
4. injure
5. hypertensive retinopathy
6. sclerosis or arteriolosclerosis
7. thinning
8. narrowing
9. cotton wool patches
10. microaneurysms
11. hemorrhages
12. edema

18–60

A leading cause of blindness in this country is diabetes mellitus. This is because of microangiopathy, or disease of tiny vessels, of the retina called **diabetic retinopathy.** (Diabetes also causes cataracts, as discussed in Frame 18–63). The results of diabetic retinopathy are similar to hypertensive retinopathy. The capillaries and arterioles of the choroid and retina undergo changes which include narrowing of their lumens, or the formation of microaneursyms as some areas dilate. Permeability of these vessels is increased, so edema and tiny

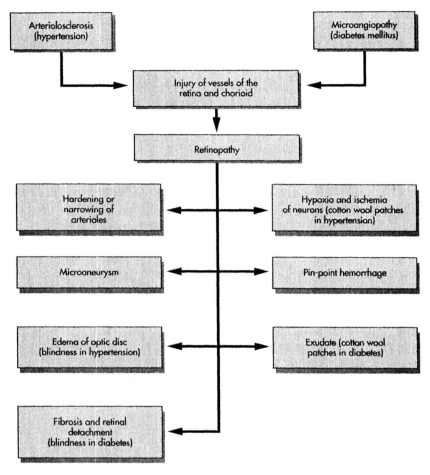

Figure 18–12. Circulatory disorder retinopathy.

1. microangiopathy
2. diabetic retinopathy
3. hypertensive retinopathy
4. significant ischemia
5. fibrosis
6. detachment

local hemorrhages are features of this disorder. Spots of serous exudate are described as cotton wool patches in this disorder also. Blindness results if significant ischemia leads to fibrosis and retinal detachment. Another cause of retinal detachment is the growth or proliferation of new abnormal vessels in the area in response to ischemia. This represents an attempt to reperfuse the area. The disease of vessels in diabetes is called _____(1). When this affects the retina, it is called _____(2). The physical changes in the vessels are very like what is seen in _____(3). Blindness may be caused by _____(4), _____(5), and retinal _____(6).

▶ GLAUCOMA AND CATARACT

18-61

There exists a normal pressure within the eyes known as **intraocular pressure.** In **glaucoma,** that pressure is higher than normal. The increased pressure damages structures within the eye, particularly the neurons of the retina and the optic nerve. The cells undergo atrophy and therefore vision is impaired. If the high pressure remains, the eye can become so damaged that blindness results. Therefore, it is important to diagnose and treat glaucoma as early as possible. The normal intraocular pressure is achieved through the rate of formation and drainage of fluid in the eye. The fluid, or aqueous humor, is secreted by the ciliary body and it drains into venules found at the margins of the iris. This area of drainage is referred to as

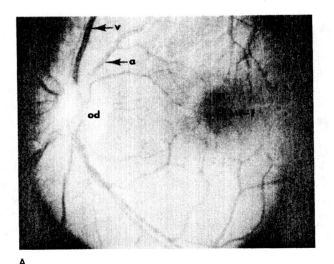

A

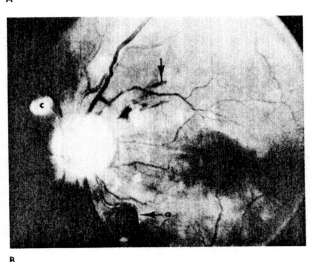

B

Figure 18–13. A. Normal retina showing the optic disk (od), artery, (a), and vein (v). **B.** Retinopathy caused by hypertensive arteriolosclerosis. Note the narrowed tortuous artery (a), spots of hemorrhage *(arrows)*, and cotton wool patches of ischemia (c). *(From Kent and Hart,* Introduction to Human Disease, *3rd ed., Appleton & Lange.)*

the angle. The angle is where the iris meets the corneal–scleral junction. In glaucoma, there is an interruption in drainage of the aqueous humor while normal formation continues. The fluid increases inside the globe, raising the pressure. Pressure within the eye is easily measured with a device called a tonometer, which is placed on the front of the eye. Glaucoma represents a state of _____(1) intraocular _____(2). It develops if there is interference in _____(3) of aqueous humor from the eye. The area of drainage is called the _____(4). Glaucoma injures the intraocular structures, especially the _____(5) and _____(6). Untreated cases may result in _____(7) because of the continued high pressure.

1. increased
2. pressure
3. drainage
4. angle
5. retina
6. optic nerve
7. blindness

18–62

Secondary glaucoma is the result of a primary eye disease such as inflammatory conditions with exudate and adhesions, luxation of the lens so that it falls into the angle, hemorrhage, or a tumor. These physical obstructions block fluid drainage. Primary glaucoma, or that which occurs in the absence of another disorder, is more common than secondary. Primary glaucoma is idiopathic. The two types of primary glaucoma are **open-angle** and **closed-angle.** Open-angle glaucoma is more common than closed-angle. In the open-angle form, there is no physical obstruction of the drainage area that can be identified. The pressure slowly builds over

1. Primary
2. open-angle
3. closed-angle
4. Open-angle
5. obstruction
6. iris
7. obstruction
8. blindness

time in both eyes, although one is usually worse than the other. Atrophy and pressure necrosis of neurons causes blindness in untreated cases. In closed-angle glaucoma, there is a physical obstruction that can be seen. This may be an abnormality in the movement of the iris during contraction, so that its folds cover the drainage angle. Or it may be due to the presence of adhesions. Closed-angle glaucoma is generally characterized by painful intermittent attacks of increased pressure and loss of vision. Glaucoma is treated with drugs that either reduce pressure or decrease formation of aqueous humor. Untreated cases are slowly progressive with loss of peripheral vision preceding blindness. _____(1) glaucoma is more common than secondary glaucoma. There are two forms of primary glaucoma, _____(2) and _____(3). _____(4) is more common than closed-angle. There is no _____(5) that can be found in the open-angle form. In closed-angle, abnormal folding of the _____(6) causes a physical _____(7). Untreated glaucoma causes _____(8).

18-63

1. cataract
2. light
3. retina
4. age-related
5. elderly

The lens of a normal eye is clear to allow refraction and passage of light rays through it and to the retina. A **cataract** is the clouding of the lens so that it becomes opaque and light cannot pass through. Cataracts are the most common reason for pathologically decreased vision in this country. Primary cataracts are an age-related degeneration that affects the elderly. Primary cataracts of old age are called senile cataracts. Senile cataracts are the most common type, as compared to secondary cataracts, and they represent a wearing out of the lens. Secondary cataracts are clouding caused by inflammation, trauma, and metabolic disease such as uncontrolled diabetes mellitus. In diabetes, there is altered carbohydrate metabolism and transport of nutrients. Normally, glucose enters the lens and is reduced to the alcohol sorbitol. Sorbitol is a highly osmotic substance. As sorbitol diffuses out of the lens, water diffuses in. In diabetes, sorbitol production is increased and water entry increases. The fibers of the swollen lens are destroyed over time and the lens becomes opaque. The development of primary or secondary cataracts is slow and causes blurred vision. Complete loss of vision is possible if the lens becomes densely opaque. This is shown in Figure 18–14. Early cataracts can be detected during an ophthalmic exam, while late or mature cataracts can easily be seen grossly. The treatment of cataracts is surgical removal of the lens and replacement with a prosthetic lens, followed by the need for glasses or contact lenses. A cloudy, or opaque, lens is called a _____(1). Cataracts interfere with vision because _____(2) cannot pass through and reach the _____(3). Primary cataracts are a (an) _____(4) degeneration that affect the _____(5), and so they are also called

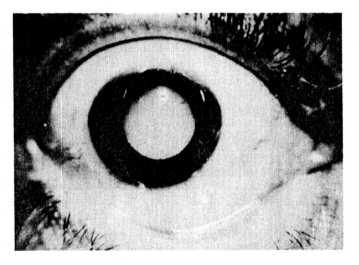

Figure 18–14. A densely opaque, mature senile cataract obstructing vision. *(From Chandrasoma and Taylor, Concise Pathology, 2nd ed., Appleton & Lange.)*

_____(6). Uncontrolled diabetes mellitus can cause _____(7) cataracts because of abnormal _____(8) metabolism.

▶ DISTURBANCES IN VISION

An inability to see well is not a true pathological condition but is a defect in some structures of the globe or the globe itself. Rather than a disease, these conditions are less than optimal function of the eyes and therefore vision is impaired. The medical term for nearsightedness is **myopia.** This means the individual cannot see distant objects very well, or only sees well when close to the object. The reason for this is that light passing through the cornea and lens is refracted or bent abnormally so that it converges, or comes together, just in front of the retina instead of on it. Myopia is caused by an abnormal curvature of the cornea and lens, or by a globe that is elongated (too long) from anterior to posterior. In other words, the shape of these structures is less than optimal. The etiology of myopia is unknown but it tends to be familial. Farsightedness is medically termed **hyperopia.** The individual sees close objects poorly and distant objects more clearly. This is again due to abnormal light refraction, but the light rays converge behind the retina instead of in front of it. Abnormal shape of the cornea, lens, or globe is responsible, as it is in myopia. In hyperopia, the globe is shorter than normal. Myopia and hyperopia are compared to the normal eye in Figure 18–15. While myopia presents in childhood, more cases of hyperopia are seen in older adults as the eye structures lose elasticity. Changes in the lens to adjust its focusing ability is called accommodation. Accommodation relies on elasticity. Accommodation decreases with age, so light convergence on the retina moves accordingly. Both myopia and hyperopia can be corrected with glasses or contact lenses. Myopia is commonly called _____(1), and it means that individuals can see well only when an object is _____(2). Hyperopia is known as _____(3), and it means that individuals can see well only when an object is _____(4). In myopia, the light converges in _____(5) of the retina, and in hyperopia, it converges _____(6) the retina. In nearsightedness, the globe may be _____(7) than normal, while in farsightedness it is _____(8) than normal.

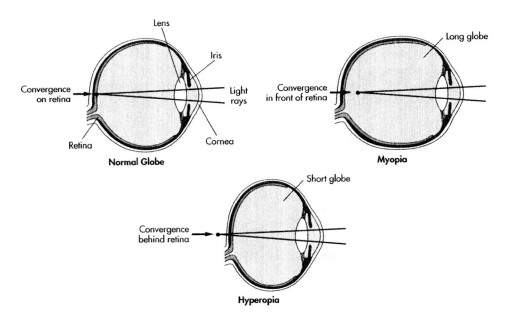

Figure 18–15. Globe shape in myopia and hyperopia.

18-65

1. presbyopia
2. lens
3. elasticity
4. focusing
5. astigmatism

Presbyopia is a decrease in visual ability because of decreased elasticity of the lens in the elderly. It is also caused by impaired accommodation by the lens. As in hyperopia, with presbyopia, light rays converge or meet posterior to the retina. However, hyperopia is caused by a short globe, while presbyopia is a degenerative lens change. Presbyopia results in the need for reading glasses or bifocals and is extremely prevalent in those over 60. **Astigmatism** is another condition resulting from abnormal shape of the cornea, or from irregularities of its surface, or of the lens surface. Vision is poor because of uneven focusing of light. The uneven surfaces cause uneven focusing. This is also corrected with glasses specifically for astigmatism. Impaired vision associated with advanced age is called _____(1). It represents a degeneration of the _____(2), particularly the loss of _____(3). Surface irregularities of the cornea or lens cause uneven _____(4) of light in the condition _____(5).

▶ NEOPLASIA

18-66

1. retinoblastoma
2. retinal neurons, or retinoblasts
3. retina
4. pupil
5. vision
6. death

Tumors of the globe, or intraocular tumors, are rare. About 90 percent are either retinoblastoma or melanoma. **Retinoblastoma** is a primary malignant tumor that occurs in babies and children. It arises from fetal retinal neurons, or retinoblasts. These are the precursor cells of the ganglial cells. A small percentage of cases are hereditary. This mass inside the eye grows and fills the entire globe and may extend to the optic nerve. Some cases (about 30 percent) are bilateral, with tumors inside both eyes. The tumor can be seen through the pupil and causes the pupil to appear white. Vision is lost as the tumor grows. Untreated cases are generally fatal, but treatment (enucleation, or removal of the eye and radiation) produces about a 90 percent survival rate. Long-term survivors are at risk for development of other malignancies, especially osteosarcoma. A malignant eye tumor of children is the _____(1). It originates from fetal _____(2), and so this is a tumor of the _____(3). The growth of the tumor inside the eye makes the _____(4) look white. The presence of the tumor interferes with _____(5). Untreated cases usually end in _____(6).

18-67

1. malignant
2. adults
3. pigmented
4. choroid

The **melanoma** is a primary malignant intraocular tumor that is seen in adults. It arises from pigmented cells of the iris, ciliary body, or choroid. Most melanomas originate from the choroid layer. This tumor is dark, not white, but also grows to fill the inside of the eye. The prognosis depends on which part of the uveal tract gave rise to the tumor. Melanomas of the iris grow slowly and are more easily removed. Melanomas of the choroid require removal of the eye, or enucleation. The 15-year survival rate for this tumor is about 50 percent. Melanoma is a primary _____(1) eye tumor found in _____(2). Its origin is the _____(3) cells of the uveal tract, with most arising from the _____(4).

VI. REVIEW QUESTIONS

1. b–inflammation of the conjunctiva caused by either infection or allergy

1. Conjunctivitis is:
   a. inflammation of the cornea caused by infection only
   b. inflammation of the conjunctiva caused by either infection or allergy
   c. inflammation of the cornea caused by either infection or allergy
   d. inflammation of the conjunctiva caused by infection only

2. Bacterial conjunctivitis may be secondary to (choose all that are correct):
   a. allergic conjunctivitis
   b. keratitis
   c. hyperemia
   d. viral conjunctivitis
   e. trachoma

3. Keratitis most commonly produces:
   a. ulcers of the cornea
   b. pus in the conjunctiva
   c. a hordeolum
   d. severe scarring of the cornea

4. Blindness because of postretinal hematoma and subsequent detachment may be associated with:
   a. severe chemical burns of the cornea
   b. blunt trauma of the eyes
   c. lens luxation
   d. corneal ulcer erosion and penetration

5. The *general* cause of retinopathy due to circulatory disorders is:
   a. ischemia of retinal neurons
   b. edema of the optic nerve
   c. high blood pressure
   d. diabetes
   e. injury of vessels of the eye

6. The underlying pathology in hypertensive retinopathy is:
   a. hypoxia of retinal neurons
   b. arteriolosclerosis of the choroid and retina
   c. microaneurysms
   d. tiny hemorrhages

7. Blindness in untreated cases of hypertensive retinopathy are the result of:
   a. cotton wool patches
   b. hypertension-induced sclerosis
   c. edema of the optic disc
   d. the presence of exudate

8. The underlying pathology in diabetic retinopathy is:
   a. retinal microangiopathy
   b. cataracts
   c. retinal edema
   d. ischemia and fibrosis

9. Blindness in severe cases of diabetic retinopathy is the result of:
   a. severe cataract formation
   b. abnormal carbohydrate metabolism and excess sorbitol formation
   c. microaneurysms and hemorrhage
   d. retinal detachment

10. Glaucoma is _____ and results from _____:
    a. clouding of the lens; excessive aqueous humor formation
    b. decreased intraocular pressure; insufficient aqueous humor formation
    c. increased intraocular pressure; insufficient aqueous humor drainage
    d. clouding of the lens; insufficient aqueous humor drainage

2. a–allergic conjunctivitis; d–viral conjunctivitis

3. a–ulcers of the cornea

4. b–blunt trauma of the eyes

5. e–injury of vessels of the eye

6. b–arteriolosclerosis of the choroid and retina

7. c–edema of the optic disc

8. a–retinal microangiopathy

9. d–retinal detachment

10. c–increased intraocular pressure; insufficient aqueous humor drainage

11. c–increased pressure causing atrophy and pressure
necrosis of retinal neurons

12. b–open-angle glaucoma

13. a–opacification of the lens

14. d–Secondary cataracts in
diabetes are due to excess
deposits of glucose in the
lens.

15. 1. c–astigmatism
2. a–presbyopia
3. b–myopia
4. d–hyperopia

16. False

11. The underlying pathology in glaucoma is:
    a. increased pressure causing arteriolosclerosis of retinal vessels
    b. decreased pressure causing insufficient perfusion and ischemia
    c. increased pressure causing atrophy and pressure necrosis of retinal neurons
    d. clouding of the lens causing lack of light upon the retina and atrophy of neurons

12. Obstruction of drainage of aqueous humor is NOT evident in:
    a. closed-angle glaucoma
    b. open-angle glaucoma
    c. secondary glaucoma
    d. primary glaucoma

13. The underlying pathology in cataracts is:
    a. opacification of the lens
    b. degeneration of the lens
    c. abnormal carbohydrate metabolism in the lens
    d. loss of elasticity of the lens

14. Which of the following statements about cataracts is INCORRECT?
    a. Senile cataracts are primary cataracts of the elderly.
    b. Cataracts prevent refraction and passage of light.
    c. Primary cataracts are an age-related degeneration.
    d. Secondary cataracts in diabetes are due to excess deposits of glucose in the lens.

15. Please match the medical terms that describe visual disturbances in the left column with their meaning in the right column:
    a. presbyopia   1. _____ surface irregularities of the cornea or lens causes uneven focusing
    b. myopia   2. _____ age-related loss of elasticity of the lens
    c. astigmatism 3. _____ light convergence in front of the retina due to a long globe
    d. hyperopia   4. _____ light convergence behind the retina due to a short globe

16. True or false: Retinoblastoma is a primary intraocular malignancy of children. It arises from the pigmented cells of the uveal tract. Melanoma is a primary intraocular malignancy of adults, and it arises from retinal precursor cells. _____

SECTION ▶ VII. DISEASES OF THE EAR

▶ DISEASES OF THE MIDDLE EAR

18-68

Trauma of the middle ear can occur, and its most significant form is puncture of the tympanic membrane, or eardrum. This may be caused by the insertion of a sharp object or an explosion. A small hole generally heals spontaneously. Larger defects leave the middle ear susceptible to infection. Infection of the middle ear is called **otitis media.** Acute otitis media can be caused by bacteria that gain entry into the middle ear. Acute otitis media is seen with some frequency in children, especially as it occurs in conjunction with an upper respiratory infection such as pharyngitis. Viruses or bacteria can enter the middle ear through the eustachian tube, which connects the middle ear with the throat. The pocket of infection behind the eardrum causes it to become inflamed and bulge outward. This is easily recognized during an otoscopic examination. If untreated, the pressure of the exudate may rupture the eardrum, allowing pus to ooze from the ear canal. Other complications of acute otitis media are the development of chronic otitis media, spread of infection to other structures such as the mastoid bone (mastoiditis), and deeper spread of infection into the inner ear (otitis interna) or brain (meningitis or abscess). Acute otitis media presents as severe ear pain and sensitivity. Antibiotics are effective in bacterial infection. If a significant amount of pus is present, it may be drained with a needle inserted through the tympanic membrane (tympanocentesis) or through a small surgical incision (myringotomy). Otitis media is _____(1) of the middle ear. The population that this occurs most frequently in is _____(2). Acute otitis media may accompany a (an) _____(3) infection. Pathogens entering from the throat do so through the _____(4). A red and swollen eardrum, as seen during an examination, is the result of _____(5) behind it. The pressure may cause _____(6) of the eardrum, and this is seen as _____(7) escaping from the ear. Chronic otitis media, mastoiditis, otitis interna, meningitis, or brain abscess are possible _____(8) of acute otitis media.

1. infection
2. children
3. upper respiratory
4. eustachian tube
5. pus or exudate
6. rupture
7. pus
8. complications

.... 18-69 ......

Chronic otitis media can develop after several bouts of acute infection. Purulent drainage from the ear is a feature, as well as constant pain. The tympanic membrane is ruptured or, in some cases, destroyed altogether. Loss of hearing is another feature of chronic otitis media. Diligent treatment is necessary to eliminate the infection. Chronic infection can lead to the development of a cyst in the middle ear called a **cholesteatoma,** which must be surgically removed. The cyst is primarily composed of keratinized epithelial tissue.

.... 18-70 ......

Otosclerosis is increased density of the auditory bones of the middle ear, and it most affects the stapes. The sclerosis develops as a result of deposits of new bone on existing bone. The cause is unknown but there is a genetic component. The movements of the auditory bones, which are so vital to sound wave conduction, is impaired. After a while the tiny bones become fixated, or cannot move. Both ears are affected, although one is often more severely affected. Otosclerosis is the most common cause of conductive hearing loss in middle-aged adults. The sclerotic stapes must be surgically replaced by a prosthesis. Thickening of the auditory bones is the underlying pathology in the condition _____(1). Deposits of _____(2) produce sclerosis. The significance is in the interference in _____(3) of the auditory bones. Movement is necessary to conduct _____(4). Otosclerosis is a common cause of conductive _____(5).

1. otosclerosis
2. new bone
3. movement
4. sound waves
5. hearing loss

▶ DISEASE OF THE INNER EAR

.... 18-71 ......

The most significant primary disease of the inner ear is **Ménière's disease.** This is a disorder of the cochlea, and so it disrupts equilibrium, or one's sense of balance. The cause of Ménière's disease is idiopathic, but it is considered to be of a degenerative nature. The fluid inside the cochlea (the endolymph) undergoes an increase in pressure, and this vestibular apparatus dilates. This produces the clinical presentation of attacks of **vertigo** (dizziness caused by an illusion of movement), **tinnitus** (ringing in the ears), and loss of hearing for certain sound frequencies. Treatment, which is effective, is to decrease endolymphatic pressure with diuretic medications and a low-salt diet. Ménière's disease affects the vestibular structure known as the _____(1), and it causes a disruption of _____(2) so that a normal sense of _____(3) is impaired. The underlying pathology is an increase in the _____(4) of the _____(5) inside the cochlea. Dizziness, or _____(6), and ringing in the ears, or _____(7), are signs of Ménière's disease.

1. cochlea
2. equilibrium
3. balance
4. pressure
5. fluid or endolymph
6. vertigo
7. tinnitus

VII. REVIEW QUESTIONS

1. b—exudate behind the
   eardrum, associated with
   acute otitis media

2. d—the eustachian tube

3. c—increased density of the
   auditory bones because of
   bone deposition, leading to
   loss of movement and
   impaired sound wave conduction

4. b—It affects function of the
   cochlea, which is equilibrium.

1. A red and bulging tympanic membrane, as seen during otoscopic examination, most likely indicates:
   a. exudate behind the eardrum, associated with chronic otitis media
   b. exudate behind the eardrum, associated with acute otitis media
   c. spread of infection during mastoiditis
   d. migration of bacteria through the eustachian tube

2. The literal connection between upper respiratory infection and acute otitis media is:
   a. the pharynx
   b. the nasal passages
   c. the frontal sinuses
   d. the eustachian tube
   e. the inner ear

3. Otosclerosis is:
   a. decreased density of the auditory bones because of bone loss, leading to an inability to conduct sound waves
   b. hardening of the inner ear after chronic otitis interna
   c. increased density of the auditory bones because of bone deposition, leading to loss of movement and impaired sound wave conduction
   d. a complication of chronic otitis media

4. Which of the following statements about Ménière's disease is correct?
   a. It is a secondary complication of chronic middle ear disease.
   b. It affects function of the cochlea, which is equilibrium.
   c. Endolymphatic pressure within the cochlea is decreased.
   d. It is a genetic, untreatable cause of vertigo.

CHAPTER SUMMARY ▶

▶ SECTION II

Developmental defects occur in the forming embryo or fetus, and may be due to malformation of the brain or spinal cord, biochemical errors, or defective genes or chromosomes. Examples of developmental defects are *anencephaly* (the infant is born with most or all of the forebrain missing) and *congenital hydrocephalus* (excess cerebrospinal fluid in the brain due to stenosis of the ducts that drain the fluid from the ventricles of the brain). *Cerebral palsy* is a disorder of the CNS caused by destruction or injury of brain tissue. The condition is most often due to lack of oxygen to the brain, either during pregnancy or after birth. Infection (e.g., meningitis) can also cause cerebral palsy. Retardation, paresis (weakness), and ataxia (incoordination) can be signs of cerebral palsy.

A condition that gets progressively worse over time is called a *degenerative disease*. *Multiple sclerosis* (MS) is a degenerative demyelinating disease in which sclerosed plaques are found in the brain and spinal cord. MS is often classified as an autoimmune disease, although viral infection is also suspected as the cause. *Parkinson's disease* is a degeneration of the basal ganglia in the midbrain, considered to be due to the lack of dopamine production. The cause of Parkinson's disease is idiopathic, with possible hereditary factors. The three main features of Parkinson's are tremors, muscle rigidity, and bradykinesia (slow movement). *Huntington's disease* (Huntington's chorea) is inherited in an autosomal dominant manner. The pathology of Huntington's involves atrophy of parts of the cerebral cortex, causing rapid, jerky, involuntary movement; personality changes; and memory loss. *Amyotrophic lateral sclerosis* (ALS, Lou Gehrig's disease) is characterized by a progressive wasting of muscles, extreme weakness, and eventual death. The condition, the cause of which is unknown, seems to be due to loss of motor neurons in the spinal cord. *Alzheimer's disease* is an age-related degeneration leading to a loss of mental capabilities. Atrophy of parts of the cerebrum and loss of neurons are the only certain pathological findings to date. Features of Alzheimer's disease are loss of short-term memory, personality change, and failure to recognize surroundings or familiar people.

▶ SECTION III

Infectious inflammation of the meninges (the membranous covering of the CNS) is *meningitis*. In *acute bacterial meningitis,* pyogenic bacteria produce a purulent exudate that fills the subarachnoid space. Specific viruses (e.g., influenza, mumps) can also cause acute meningitis. The disease can be fatal if not diagnosed and treated promptly. *Chronic meningitis,* often seen in cases of neurosyphilis, can lead to fibrosis in the meninges, leading to brain ischemia, motor weakness (paresis), and mental disturbances. Chronic meningitis can also be due to tuberculosis or fungal infection. *Encephalitis* is characterized by a widespread infectious inflammation of the brain, most commonly by a virus. In children, the condition can be secondary to chickenpox, measles, and mumps. Common infectious agents which can cause encephalitis include *Toxoplasma gondii,* certain fungi, and herpes simplex type I. The disease can be transmitted by mosquitoes.

▶ SECTION IV

Diseases of the blood vessels supplying the brain are called *cerebrovascular disease* (CVD), and lead to the condition called a *cerebrovascular accident* (CVA) or, commonly, a *stroke*. A stroke results from an acute neurologic deficit due to vascular occlusion (obstruction by thrombi or emboli) or bleeding (due to rupture of an artery). Atherosclerosis of the arteries of the brain is a common cause of CVD. Two forms of the condition are generally seen, *diffuse ischemia of the brain* (due to decreased blood supply to specific areas of the brain) and *cerebral infarct* (due to a sudden and complete obstruction of a major cerebral artery). Depending on which arteries of the brain are infarcted, the affected individual may suffer hemiparesis, hemiplegia, or aphagia. An *intracerebral hemorrhage,* most commonly associated with hypertension, occurs when a vessel in the brain bursts, leading to infarction of the specific area of the brain perfused by the ruptured vessel. Other situations include *intracranial hemorrhage* (bleeding within the skull), *epidural hematoma* (bleeding between the skull and the dura mater), *subdural hematoma* (bleeding between the arachnoid layer of the meninges and the dura mater), and *subarachnoid hemorrhage* (bleeding under the arachnoid layer).

Trauma of the brain is also a major cause of disability and death. A *concussion,* the mildest form of brain trauma, results in no structural injury or physical lesion of the brain. Recovery is complete. A *contusion* is a bruise of the brain created during an impact or blunt trauma. Small vessels rupture, causing edema and increased pressure in the brain. *Epidural* and *subdural hematomas* occur when the trauma ruptures larger vessels. *Penetrating injury of the brain,* most commonly due to gunshots, can lead to infection in survivors because of the open wound.

▶ SECTION V

Even though it is rare, *cancers of the CNS* are significant because the death rate is very high. Secondary tumors, having metastasized from breast, lung, or melignant melanoma, occur as frequently as primary tumors. Removal of CNS tumors is generally difficult. A *glioma* is a malignant tumor that arises from the glial cells of the brain. *Astrocytoma* and *glioblastoma multiforme* are the two forms of astrocytoma, the most common form of glioma. A *meningioma* is a benign tumor that arises from the dura mater and is generally noninfiltrative and slow-growing. A *neuroma* is a benign tumor of the nerve cells and may be a *schwannoma* (arising from the schwann cells) or a *neurofibroma* (arising from the neurofibroblasts). The rare malignant form of a neurofibroma is a neurofibrosarcoma.

A *convulsion* is an involuntary contraction of skeletal muscles and is often the result of excitation of neurons which innervate those muscles. Causes of a convulsion include chemical imbalance, drugs, uremia, and infection of the brain. A *seizure,* seen in the disorder *epilepsy,* is due to disturbances in electrical activity in the brain. Epilepsy may manifest as petit mal (mild seizure with brief loss of consciousness) or grand mal (dramatic involuntary movements, loss of consciousness, and collapse). An aura may precede the seizure. Generalized failure of brain function is a *coma,* in which a vegetative state (i.e., only involuntary functions are maintained by the brain stem) occurs. Many conditions can lead to a coma.

► SECTION VI

Conjunctivitis ("pinkeye") is infection or allergic inflammation of the pink tissue surrounding the anterior external surface of the eye. The condition may be primary in nature or secondary to upper respiratory infection. A *hordeolum* ("stye") is an infected gland of the eyelid. *Photophobia,* or intolerance to light, may accompany conjunctivitis. *Keratitis* is infection of the cornea which manifests as painful ulcers, tearing, and photophobia. Herpesvirus infection is the most common cause of keratitis. Inflammation of the eyes can be caused by physical injury (which may be superficial, blunt, or penetrating) or chemical irritation.

Hypertension and diabetes can affect the blood vessels of the eyes. Hypertension leads to *hypertensive retinopathy,* a condition in which the vessels of the retina and choroid layer become atherosclerotic. *Diabetes mellitus* produces *diabetic retinopathy,* disease of the tiny vessels (microangiopathy) of the eyes. Diabetes is a leading cause of blindness.

In the disease *glaucoma,* the pressure within the eyes (intraocular pressure) is higher than normal, a situation that damages structures within the eye. Secondary glaucoma is the result of a primary eye disease, and primary glaucoma is idiopathic. Open-angle and closed-angle are the two types of primary glaucoma. A *cataract* is the clouding of the lens of the eye so that it becomes opaque. Cataracts may be primary or secondary in nature and are the most common reason for decreased visual acuity.

Myopia ("nearsightedness") is the condition in which the individual cannot see distant objects well. *Hyperopia* ("farsightedness") is the condition in which the individual sees close objects poorly and distant objects clearly. Both conditions are due to abnormal refraction as light passes through the cornea or lens; light is focused in front of (myopia) or behind (hyperopia) the retina. Abnormal shape of the cornea, lens, or globe is responsible for these conditions. *Presbyopia* is a decrease in visual acuity with age. The condition is due to decreased elasticity of the lens, or by impaired accommodation of the lens. *Astigmatism* results from an abnormally or irregularly shaped cornea. Vision is poor because of the uneven focusing of light on the retina.

Retinoblastoma is a primary malignant tumor of the eye that occurs in babies and children. The neoplasia arises from fetal retinal neurons, or retinoblasts, and is generally fatal if untreated. *Melanoma* is a primary malignant intraocular tumor of adults. It arises from pigmented cells of the iris, ciliary body, or choroid.

► SECTION VII

Infection of the middle ear is called *otitis media.* The condition may be caused by bacteria, and it may be seen in conjunction with an upper respiratory infection. Left untreated, the infection can spread into the inner ear or the brain. A *cholesteatoma* is a cyst in the middle ear that develops as a result of chronic otitis media. *Otosclerosis* is increased density of the auditory bones of the middle ear, most often of the stapes. The condition, the cause of which is unknown, develops as a result of deposits of new bone on existing bone. Otosclerosis is the most common cause of conductive hearing loss in middle-aged adults. *Ménière's disease* is a disorder of the cochlea. In this condition, an individual's sense of balance is disrupted. The cause of Ménière's disease is idiopathic, but it is considered to be degenerative in nature. *Vertigo* (dizziness) and *tinnitis* (ringing in the ears) are common symptoms of the disease.

CHAPTER 19

The Skin

▶ OBJECTIVES

SECTION II

Define all highlighted terms.

Characterize the common types of skin lesions, and give an example of each type.

Outline the types of bacterial, viral, fungal, and parasitic skin infections. Describe the specific causative agent, alternate terms, and signs and symptoms for each disease.

Describe the types, causes, and signs and symptoms of the disease dermatitis.

Characterize the causes and signs and symptoms of psoriasis and urticaria.

SECTION III

Define all highlighted terms.

Describe the epithelial neoplasias, seborrheic keratosis, basal cell carcinoma, and squamous cell carcinoma. Outline the causes and signs and symptoms of each.

Describe the pigmented hyperplasias, nevus, dysplastic nevus, malignant melanoma, and superficial spreading melanoma. Outline the causes and signs and symptoms of each.

Identify the terms of the A-B-C-D diagnostic protocol as pertains to nevus observation.

Describe the causes and signs and symptoms of Kaposi's sarcoma.

SECTION IV

Define all highlighted terms.

Describe the difference between sunburn and suntan. Characterize the mechanism of sun-induced damage.

Describe the differences of first-, second-, and third-degree burns.

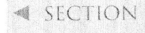

I. ANATOMY AND PHYSIOLOGY IN REVIEW ◀ SECTION 19-1

The skin that covers the human body is considered an organ. It is made up of three layers, which is shown in Figure 19–1. The outermost layer is the **epidermis.** The epidermis is made up of several layers of individual stratified squamous epithelial cells. The innermost cells comprise the **basal layer,** from which new epithelial cells are generated. Covering the outside of the epidermis is **keratin.** This is a coating produced by anuclear keratinized epithelial cells that "seals" and protects the epidermis. The process of keratinization by the epithelial cells represents an extremely important protective mechanism, which greatly contributes to the function of this organ. The proteins that make up keratin are very resistant to injury. The palms of the hands and the soles of the feet have the thickest keratin.

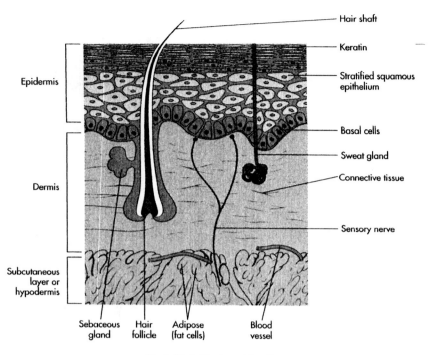

Epidermis

Dermis

Subcutaneous layer or hypodermis

Hair shaft

Keratin

Stratified squamous epithelium

Basal cells

Sweat gland

Connective tissue

Sensory nerve

Sebaceous gland

Hair follicle

Adipose (fat cells)

Blood vessel

Figure 19–1. Structure of the skin.

In the basal layer of the epidermis are **melanocytes,** which are cells that manufacture the skin pigment **melanin.** Melanin is a brown pigment that helps block penetration of the skin layers by sunlight. When the skin is exposed to sunlight, specifically to ultraviolet light, packets of melanin are transferred from the melanocytes through the epidermis and up to the keratin. This causes the characteristic browning effect or tanning in response to the sun. The presence of melanin is like drawing a shade on a window to prevent light from entering. Since outer epithelial cells and keratin are constantly shed and replaced by new cells, the new, unpigmented cells cause a tan to fade.

Underneath the epidermis is the **dermis.** It is in this layer that the accessory structures of the skin are found. These are the hair follicles, the sebaceous (oil) glands, and the sweat glands. Sweat glands occur individually, and sebaceous glands are attached to hair follicles. The sweat glands are important in the homeostatic mechanism of thermoregulation (see Chap. 3), since they aid in heat loss through evaporation and cool the skin. The dermis is composed of fibrous connective tissue and elastic fibers. It also contains blood vessels (also vital in thermoregulation) and the sensory nerves. The innermost layer of the skin is the **subcutaneous layer,** or **hypodermis.** The hypodermis is made of connective tissue and many adipocytes, or fat cells.

The primary function of the skin is **protection.** The skin was listed in Chapter 4 as one of the first lines of defense against microorganisms by acting as a mechanical barrier against entry. For optimal protection against infection, skin must be intact (no open wounds or lacerations) and it must be dry. Chronically moist skin is more prone to penetration by bacteria. It physically protects underlying tissue from the constant environmental abrasion that occurs normally. The skin is able to absorb this insult because of its constant regeneration. The skin also prevents loss of tissue fluid through evaporation. Victims of widespread, severe burns, who have lost a large surface area of skin, must be administered fluids intravenously to prevent dehydration and shock.

19-5

Control of body temperature (thermoregulation) is greatly assisted by the blood vessels and sweat glands, and somewhat less so by the arrector pili muscles that produce "goosebumps." As you learned in Chapter 3, blood vessels dilate to lose heat and constrict to retain heat. The sweat glands aid in heat loss through evaporation and cooling. The fat of the hypodermis provides insulation to help maintain the core body temperature. It also provides a cushion that aids in the mechanical protective function of the skin. A final function of the skin is serving as a sensory organ. The nerves of the dermis convey the sensory messages of touch, cold, heat, pressure, and pain.

II. INFECTIOUS AND INFLAMMATORY DISORDERS ◄ SECTION

► COMMON SKIN LESIONS

19-6

There are several different types of skin injury that will produce the same kind of lesion, such as a blister. That is because the skin is limited in the number of ways it can respond to injury. This can make diagnosis of skin diseases challenging since several diseases are similar in appearance. To help with diagnosis, lesions of the skin have been assigned terminology for identification. The following are the most common types of skin lesions:

1. **Macule.** A flat lesion less than 2 centimeters (cm) in diameter. A macule is pigmented, usually red or brown in color. An example is a freckle.
2. **Patch.** The same appearance as a macule (flat and pigmented) but larger than 2 cm. An example is a measles rash.
3. **Papule.** A lesion raised above the surface of the skin (a small bump or lump) that is less than 1 cm in diameter. A papule is a solid elevation and does not contain any fluid. An example is eczema.
4. **Nodule.** The same kind of a lesion as a papule (raised and solid), but a larger lump at 1 to 5 cm. An example is a mole.
5. **Vesicle.** A raised, bubble-like lesion less than 1 cm in diameter but containing serous or tissue fluid. A common description for a vesicle is a tiny blister. An example is herpesvirus eruptions.

19-7

6. **Bulla.** A large vesicle greater than 1 cm. The common description is a large blister. An example is a burn.
7. **Pustule.** A raised lesion of no specific size, also containing fluid, but the fluid is pus or purulent exudate. Examples are impetigo, acne, or an abscess.
8. **Ulcer.** A depressed lesion (falling below the skin surface) that is a crater-like erosion. An example is syphilitic chancre.
9. **Crust.** Hardened or dried tissue fluid or blood covering a skin defect. An example is a ruptured vesicle.
10. **Scales.** Excess keratin that is flaking or lifting off in small sheets. An example is seborrhea.
11. **Excoriation.** Tiny lacerations of the skin caused by scratching. Several skin diseases are **pruritic,** or itchy, and excoriation is often produced by the patient trying to relieve the itch. An example is contact dermatitis.

Several of the common skin lesions are illustrated in Figure 19–2.

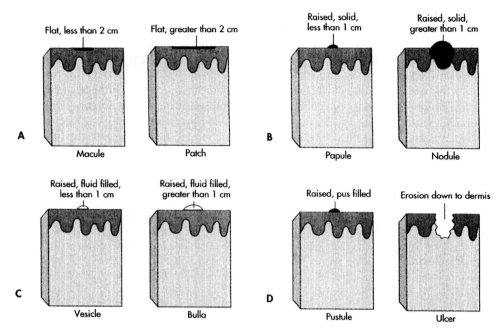

Flat, less than 2 cm

Flat, greater than 2 cm

Raised, solid, less than 1 cm

Raised, solid, greater than 1 cm

A   Macule   Patch   B   Papule   Nodule

Raised, fluid filled, less than 1 cm

Raised, fluid filled, greater than 1 cm

Raised, pus filled

Erosion down to dermis

C   Vesicle   Bulla   D   Pustule   Ulcer

Figure 19–2. Common skin lesions.

1. flat
2. pigmented
3. patch
4. patch
5. papule
6. larger
7. fluid
8. blisters
9. vesicle
10. bulla
11. pus
12. pustule
13. ulcer
14. dried fluid or blood
15. scales
16. lacerations
17. scratching

A macule is a _____(1) lesion that is _____(2). A _____(3) is like a macule except larger. Therefore a red flat area of 3 cm would be called a _____(4). A tiny solid bump (measuring 0.5 cm) is a _____(5). A nodule is a _____(6) solid bump. Both vesicles and bullae are raised lesions that contain _____(7). They are commonly called _____(8). The smaller one is a _____(9) and the larger is a _____(10). Purulent exudate, or _____(11), is found in a raised lesion called a _____(12). A scooped-out erosion is described as a (an) _____(13). A crust is _____(14) that lies over a primary lesion. Heavily flaking keratin is described as _____(15). Excoriations are small _____(16) in the skin caused by _____(17).

▶ BACTERIAL INFECTIONS

A common pathogen that causes bacterial infection of the skin is *Staphylococcus aureus.* Beta-hemolytic streptococcus is also a causative agent of infection. Primary infection affects otherwise normal skin. Infection caused by pyogenic, or pus-producing, organisms, such as *S. aureus,* is called **pyoderma.** Most primary infections are pyodermas, with the appearance of pus. **Acne vulgaris** is a well-known plague among young people, particularly adolescents. Acne is inflamed pustules caused by bacterial infection and is commonly called pimples. The most common location for acne is the face and, less commonly, the chest and back. The excessive secretion of lipid or sebum from sebaceous glands predisposes to acne. At puberty, hormonal changes stimulate the development and activity of these glands. The ducts and associated hair follicles often become plugged with a combination of sebum, keratin, and dirt. These are called blackheads. When pyogenic bacteria that are often present on the skin are trapped and grow in the plugged ducts, an infected pustule results. Occasionally, acne may persist through adulthood and be associated with hormonal changes of the menstrual cycle or aggravated by stress. Chronic severe bouts of acne can cause pitting and scarring. Most cases are self-limiting and can be managed with careful attention to cleanliness of the skin. Severe cases should be treated with antibiotics, which also prevent secondary infection. Pyogenic bacteria causes skin infection that is described as _____(1). A defining feature of pyoderma is the presence of _____(2). A primary pyoderma among young people is _____(3). The skin lesion of acne is inflamed _____(4). Acne develops when secretions from _____(5) mix with other material and _____(6) the ducts of the glands. Trapped _____(7) lead to infection.

1. pyoderma
2. pus
3. acne vulgaris
4. pustules
5. sebaceous glands
6. block
7. bacteria

19–10

Impetigo is a skin infection often seen in children. It is caused by group A streptococcus or *S. aureus*. The face is the most common initial site of impetigo. This disease is characterized by inflamed pustules that rupture and ooze, then crust over. Impetigo is pruritic, which means _____(1), and scratching of the area contaminates the hands, so the infection may spread to other sites on the body (**autoinoculation**). Impetigo is contagious and can be a problem in group situations with children, but it is easily treated with antibiotics. Impetigo is a skin infection most commonly located on the _____(2) of _____(3). The lesions are _____(4) that break open and then develop a _____(5). Autoinoculation may occur, which is the spread of the infection when the _____(6) become contaminated, because the lesions are itchy. Impetigo is _____(7) from one child to another.

1. itchy
2. face
3. children
4. pustules
5. crust
6. hands
7. contagious

19–11

Folliculitis is infection of hair follicles generally caused by *S. aureus*. Purulent exudate is present at the top of the follicle near the surface of the skin and surrounds the hair shaft. If the infection spreads to the tissue around the follicle, a boil develops, which is medically termed a **furuncle**. If the infection spreads farther, so that more tissue and several hair follicles are involved, this much larger boil is called a **carbuncle.** One population in which carbuncles are not uncommon is diabetics. This is because of their general predisposition to infection. The spread of folliculitis is shown in Figure 19–3. The various manifestations of folliculitis may be referred to as a skin abscess, with smaller abscesses called furuncles or boils. Antibiotic treatment is necessary for the advanced stages of folliculitis. Folliculitis is infection that involves the _____(1) and is often caused by _____(2). A boil, which is medically termed a _____(3), develops if the infection _____(4) to surrounding _____(5). Advancement of this infection to involve more tissue and several follicles produces a _____(6).

1. hair follicles
2. *S. aureus*
3. furuncle
4. spreads
5. tissue
6. carbuncle

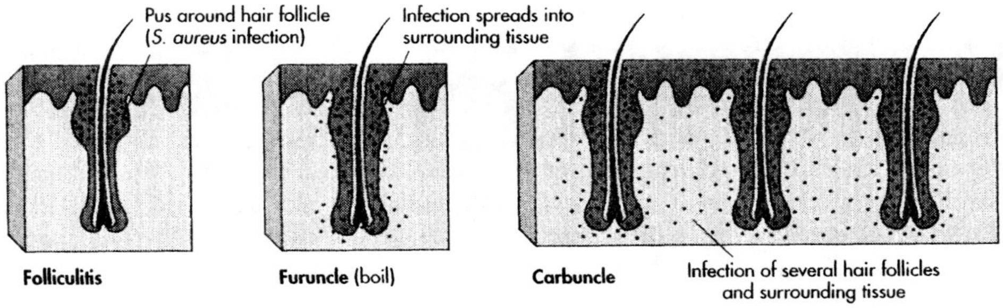

Pus around hair follicle (*S. aureus* infection)
Infection spreads into surrounding tissue

Folliculitis   **Furuncle (boil)**   **Carbuncle**
Infection of several hair follicles and surrounding tissue

Figure 19–3. The spread of folliculitis.

Secondary bacterial infection of the skin is generally a complication of a wound or a primary skin disease. Any area of skin that has already been compromised will experience delayed healing if it becomes infected. Chronic skin diseases such as eczema are often complicated by secondary bacterial infection. The treatment for chronic skin disease usually includes antibiotics for this reason.

▶ VIRAL INFECTIONS

1. maculopapular rash
2. measles
3. vesicles
4. crusted
5. chickenpox
6. herpesvirus

Several viral infections of the skin are caused by the pathogens that were presented in Chapter 5. You should review the characteristics of those infections as necessary. Some childhood viral infections cause acute eruptions of the skin. Measles produce a combination of macules and papules. The appearance is called a **maculopapular rash,** or **exanthem.** Chickenpox causes vesicles that rupture and turn to pruritic crusts. The herpes simplex virus also causes vesicular eruption and crusting, commonly called fever blisters or cold sores. The presence of both red flat lesions and tiny bumps is called a _____(1) rash. This is seen in the childhood disease _____(2). Raised lesions containing tissue fluid, called _____(3), which break open and become _____(4) over, are seen in both _____(5) and _____(6) infection.

1. wart
2. human papillomavirus
3. plantar warts
4. condyloma acuminata
5. venereal
6. contagious
7. squamous papilloma

A wart, medically termed *Verruca vulgaris,* is a chronic viral skin infection caused by the human papillomavirus, or HPV. The virus causes the keratinocytes (keratinized epithelial cells) to proliferate. This forms a raised, benign neoplasm that is called a **squamous papilloma.** Since they are contagious, scratching can spread them to other sites of the body through autoinoculation. Therefore, the presence of multiple warts are not uncommon. The hands and the lower arms are the most common location for verruca vulgaris. **Plantar warts** occur on the soles of the feet. They grow inward instead of in a raised fashion, making them painful and difficult to remove. *Condyloma acuminata* are genital warts appearing in the anogenital area. Some cases can become quite severe. Genital warts are contagious and so are considered a venereal disease. The appearance of verruca vulgaris would commonly be described as a _____(1). The causative agent is the _____(2). Warts on the feet are called _____(3), while those in the genital region are called _____(4). Genital warts are classified as a _____(5) disease because they are _____(6). The raised lesion of a wart is a benign growth referred to as a (an) _____(7).

▶ FUNGAL INFECTIONS

Fungal pathogens that colonize and infect the body surface are called **dermatophytes.** A fungal skin infection is called a **dermatophytosis.** Both pathogenic and nonpathogenic fungi are ubiquitous, that is, present everywhere, so fungal infections are common. While bacterial infection is associated with inflammation, some cases of fungal infection are not inflammatory because of the type of tissue that is colonized. These tissues are the nails, hair, and outer keratin layer of the skin.

The most common type of dermatophytosis is a group of infections collectively called **ringworm.** It is caused by several pathogens of the *Tinea* species, each with its own site predilection. *Tinea pedis* is the agent of athlete's foot. It lives and is spread in the humid environment of areas like locker rooms, where it easily contaminates bare feet. The infection starts in between the toes and can spread from there. Fungal infection of the nails is caused by *Tinea unguium.* Deep, untreated nail infections can cause destruction of the nail. "Jock itch" is a fungal infection of the groin caused by *Tinea cruris.* The familiar ringworm of children that

affects the head and causes hair loss is produced by *Tinea capitis.* Children are also susceptible to the animal tinea that causes ringworm in pets. Ringworm is quite contagious. Moist
areas of the body, or moist skin folds, are most susceptible. Areas that do become inflamed
present as a typical red, ring-shaped lesion that is often itchy and scaly. A dermatophyte is a
_____(1) that infects the skin surfaces. The general term for a fungal skin infec-
tion is _____(2). Ringworm is the most _____(3) kind of dermatophytosis, and it is caused by the _____(4) species of fungus. Ringworm
_____(5) is / is not (choose one) contagious.

1. fungal pathogen
2. dermatophytosis
3. common
4. tinea
5. is

▶ PARASITIC INFESTATION

19–17

Infestation of body surfaces by various types of lice is called **pediculosis.** Lice are classified
as insects, and since they parasitize the surface, not colonize, they *infest* instead of *infect.*
The three recognized types of lice in humans are those that affect the head, the groin, and
the body. Head lice most commonly occur in group situations, such as among schoolchild-
ren. The spread may be direct from child to child, or be through shared items such as combs
or hats. The predominant sign of infestation is pruritus, as lice penetrate the scalp and draw
blood. The tiny white eggs of the lice that are laid on hair shafts are called **nits.** Pubic lice
infest pubic hair, and the general means of spread is sexual contact. Body lice are also contagious and may be found in unsanitary conditions. Of the three, only body lice are associated with the transmission of other pathogens. Epidemics of typhus have historically been a
significant cause of death in those situations in which body lice were present. Lice that parasitize body surfaces produce a condition called _____(1). The manner in
which insects live on the body is called a (an) _____(2) rather than an infection. The three types of human lice infest the _____(3), _____(4),
and the _____(5). A characteristic feature of pediculosis is significant itching,
or _____(6). Body lice can be responsible for spreading other
_____(7) that can cause significant disease.

1. pediculosis
2. infestation
3. head
4. groin
5. body
6. pruritus
7. pathogens

19–18

A different type of insect, a mite, causes the skin disease **scabies.** Scabies is very contagious
and highly pruritic, so it has been commonly named "the itch." Like pediculosis, scabies is
associated with crowded conditions or poor hygiene. Areas of the body with skinfolds are
the most severely infested. Female mites burrow under the skin and lay eggs. The presence
of these intruders causes a hypersensitivity reaction that is responsible for the itch. Secondary bacterial infection is common because of the scratching. Vesicles and pustules may
then develop. Infestation of the skin with _____(1) causes the disease
_____(2). _____(3) is a prominent feature, earning it the nick-
name _____(4). The itching is a _____(5) reaction to the presence of the mites under the _____(6).

1. mites
2. scabies
3. Pruritus
4. "the itch"
5. hypersensitivity
6. skin

▶ DERMATITIS

19–19

Dermatitis literally means inflammation of the skin. Many of the conditions we have already
discussed cause inflammation, but the term dermatitis is used to indicate inflammation caused
specifically by immune-mediated activities. [You have learned that inflammation caused by
infection with pyogenic bacteria is called _____(1).] The word dermatitis is used
to describe several different causes of inflammation. These causes include *contact* (chemical
irritation), *atopic* (allergic), *seborrheic* (scaling and greasy), *light-induced* (UV exposure),
drug-induced (drug reaction), and *exfoliative* (epidermal sloughing). The word **eczema** is
sometimes used in place of dermatitis, particularly in contact dermatitis. Dermatitis may be
acute and, in addition to redness, produce oozing blisters and crusts. Chronic cases cause
thickening of the skin. Pruritus frequently accompanies dermatitis, and continued scratching

1. pyoderma

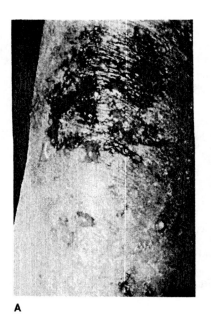
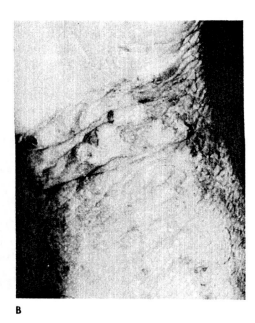

A   B

Figure 19–4. A. Acute dermatitis. **B.** Chronic dermatitis. *(From Kent and Hart,* Introduction to Human Disease, *3rd ed., Appleton & Lange.)*

2. Dermatitis
3. immune
4. eczema
5. thickened
6. itching

19–20

1. allergic
2. hypersensitivity
3. site
4. allergen
5. plants
6. leaves

contributes to thickening of the skin. The appearances of acute and chronic dermatitis are shown in Figure 19–4. _____(2) means inflammation of the skin, but it is used to describe conditions that result because of activity of the _____(3) system. Another term for dermatitis is _____(4). In chronic cases, the skin becomes _____(5) because of prolonged scratching due to _____(6).

Contact dermatitis is an itchy, allergic eczema that develops as a delayed hypersensitivity reaction to certain chemicals that act as allergens. Examples of these allergens include the metal of costume jewelry, cosmetics, dye in clothes, soaps, perfumes, and plants. Contact dermatitis is a localized reaction, causing eruption only at the site of contact. The inflammation is low-grade and becomes chronic with continued exposure. Severe cases present with vesicles or bullae which ooze fluid and crust over. Examples of plants that cause allergic contact dermatitis are poison ivy, poison oak, and poison sumac. Plant resin or oils from the leaves cause inflammation, vesicles, and pruritus at the site of contact. This generally develops within 24 hours after contact with the plant. Oozing from blisters and scratching can transfer the allergens to other parts of the body. Contact dermatitis is a (an) _____(1) type of eczema that has its basis in a delayed _____(2) reaction. Contact dermatitis occurs only at the _____(3) of contact with the offending _____(4). Several kinds of _____(5) cause allergic contact dermatitis because of the resin on their _____(6).

19–21

1. Atopic
2. allergic
3. hypersensitivity or allergic
4. contact
5. genetic

Atopic dermatitis is an allergy that occurs in combination with other hypersensitivity reactions. It may begin in childhood and continue through the adult years. Individuals afflicted with atopic dermatitis usually have other types of allergic reactions such as allergic rhinitis (hayfever), urticaria (hives), or asthma. Atopic dermatitis is believed to be part of a genetic predisposition to some allergens. (This differs from contact dermatitis in which there is no genetic allergy and it may affect anyone.) The pruritus in atopic dermatitis can be quite severe. Children frequently develop vesicles, while adults suffer dry, extremely thick patches of skin. _____(1) dermatitis is a (an) _____(2) reaction that is seen in individuals with other kinds of _____(3) reactions. In contrast to _____(4) dermatitis, which can affect anyone, atopic dermatitis most likely has a _____(5) predisposition.

Seborrheic dermatitis occurs when there is an excess in production of keratin, which leads to sloughing of that layer. This produces scaly lesions. The lesions are also greasy because there is excess secretion of sebum. The locations of seborrheic dermatitis are concentrated around areas with numerous sebaceous glands, such as the face, scalp, axillae, and genital regions. Seborrheic dermatitis of the scalp is commonly called dandruff. This common type of dermatitis often begins in childhood and continues through adulthood. The cause is unknown. The scales that are seen in seborrheic dermatitis are because of _____(1) of the _____(2) layer, which is produced in excess. The lesions are also oily because of excess _____(3) secretion from the _____(4) glands. _____(5) is the common word that describes seborrheic dermatitis of the scalp.

1. sloughing
2. keratin
3. sebum
4. sebaceous
5. Dandruff

▶ OTHER INFLAMMATORY DISORDERS

Psoriasis is a chronic inflammatory skin disease characterized by raised, thickened patches of red scaly lesions. The edges of the patches are sharply defined and the lesions are covered by silvery scales. Figure 19–5 shows the typical presentation of psoriasis. This condition is usually not pruritic. Psoriasis is a proliferation of the epidermis and its severity varies. It is believed to have a hereditary component, but no cause has been identified. Psoriasis has episodes of exacerbation (worsening), followed by remission, or improvement. Factors that trigger the outbreaks include infection or other injury of the skin, and emotional stress. Raised, _____(1) patches of skin, with silver _____(2) overlying the lesions, are characteristic of the skin disease _____(3). _____(4) is generally not a feature. The thickening is caused by _____(5) of the epithelium. The course of psoriasis is periods of _____(6) and then _____(7).

1. thickened
2. scales
3. psoriasis
4. Pruritus
5. proliferation
6. exacerbation
7. remission

Urticaria is the medical term for hives. A hive consists of a raised, edematous area called a **wheal** that is outlined by inflammation, or a red **flare**. The flare is due to vascular congestion that surrounds the edema. Hives, which can be very itchy, occur most commonly as an allergic reaction to an allergen in food or as a drug reaction. The wheal and flare of urticaria is caused by the release of histamine from mast cells in the skin. Hives can last up to 48 hours and then usually fade. Stress worsens the attacks. A hive is medically termed

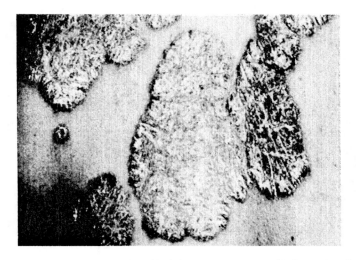

Figure 19–5. Psoriasis. Note the well-defined borders of the lesions, which are covered with silvery scales. *(From Kent and Hart, Introduction to Human Disease, 3rd ed., Appleton & Lange.)*

_____(1). This is a (an) _____(2) reaction to an allergen that may be in _____(3) or some drugs. The appearance of a hive is that of a raised area of edema, called a _____(4), which is surrounded by _____(5) congestion. The surrounding red area is called a _____(6). A hive is produced when mast cells release _____(7) in the skin.

II. REVIEW QUESTIONS

1. Please match the skin lesions in the left column with their correct description in the right column:

    a. pustule
    b. scale
    c. patch
    d. bulla
    e. papule
    f. vesicle
    g. ulcer
    h. nodule
    i. excoriation

    1. _____ raised, solid bump less than 1 cm
    2. _____ raised lesion containing purulent exudate
    3. _____ tiny blister
    4. _____ small lacerations caused by scratching
    5. _____ erosion or crater
    6. _____ flaking keratin
    7. _____ flat, pigmented lesion greater than 2 cm
    8. _____ raised, solid lump greater than 1 cm
    9. _____ large blister

2. Bacterial infection of the skin is called:
    a. impetigo
    b. dermatitis
    c. pyoderma
    d. folliculitis
    e. carbuncle

3. A contagious bacterial skin infection commonly seen in children is:
    a. acne vulgaris
    b. impetigo
    c. verruca vulgaris
    d. exanthem

4. Spread of impetigo from one body site to another is *prompted by:*
    a. excoriation
    b. autoinoculation
    c. oozing pustules
    d. pruritus

5. A carbuncle is:
    a. folliculitis that has spread to involve several hair follicles
    b. a small boil
    c. infection of hair follicles by *S. aureus*
    d. the stage of folliculitis before the development of a furuncle

6. In viral infection that causes eruptions of the skin, measles causes a._____ and chickenpox causes b._____ and c._____

    cold sores   bullae   ulcers
    a maculopapular rash   fever blisters   crusting
    scaling   vesicles

(margin answers)
1. urticaria
2. allergic
3. food
4. wheal
5. vascular
6. flare
7. histamine

1. 1. e–papule
   2. a–pustule
   3. f–vesicle
   4. i–excoriation
   5. g–ulcer
   6. b–scale
   7. c–patch
   8. h–nodule
   9. d–bulla
2. c–pyoderma
3. b–impetigo
4. d–pruritus
5. a–folliculitis that has spread to involve several hair follicles
6. a–a maculopapular rash; b–vesicles; c–crusting

7. A squamous papilloma is:
   a. a benign proliferation of the dermis
   b. a benign proliferation of keratinocytes
   c. a malignant proliferation of the epidermis
   d. a benign neoplasia that is commonly called verruca vulgaris

8. Which of the following is considered a venereal disease because of its sexual transmission?
   a. verruca vulgaris
   b. plantar warts
   c. condyloma acuminata
   d. squamous papilloma

9. Skin infection by a fungal pathogen is called:
   a. pediculosis
   b. a dermatophyte
   c. ringworm
   d. tinea
   e. dermatophytosis

10. The most common dermatophytosis is:
    a. scabies
    b. ringworm
    c. athlete's foot
    d. tinea

11. The type of pediculosis that is associated with the transmission of other pathogens is

    _____.

12. Extreme pruritus is seen with:
    a. scabies
    b. ringworm
    c. pediculosis
    d. dermatophytosis

13. The use of the term "dermatitis" is commonly restricted to skin inflammation caused by:
    a. bacterial infection
    b. excoriations
    c. immune-mediated reactions
    d. parasitic infestations
    e. pruritus

14. A *common* word that can be used to describe the cause of dermatitis is:
    a. itching
    b. infection
    c. hypersensitivity
    d. allergy
    e. hives

15. Dermatitis is also called:
    a. eczema
    b. exanthem
    c. psoriasis
    d. urticaria

7. b–a benign proliferation of keratinocytes
8. c–condyloma acuminata
9. e–dermatophytoses
10. b–ringworm
11. body lice
12. a–scabies
13. c–immune-mediated reactions
14. d–allergy
15. a–eczema

16. For these descriptions of the types of dermatitis, please select the INCORRECT statements:
   a. Poison ivy is an example of contact dermatitis.
   b. Seborrheic dermatitis is an allergic reaction to sebum.
   c. Contact dermatitis affects only the site of contact with an allergen.
   d. Atopic dermatitis is skin allergy in an individual with other kinds of allergies.
   e. Seborrheic dermatitis is associated with scaling.
   f. Genetic predisposition to allergy is associated with the development of atopic dermatitis.

17. Which of the following skin inflammations is *not* pruritic?
   a. hives
   b. contact dermatitis
   c. psoriasis
   d. ringworm
   e. scabies

18. Stress can cause worsening of:
   a. atopic dermatitis
   b. psoriasis
   c. seborrheic dermatitis
   d. dandruff

19. Release of histamine in the skin in response to a food allergen can cause:
   a. hives
   b. urticaria
   c. a wheal and flare
   d. none of the above
   e. all of the above

SECTION ▶ III. NEOPLASIA AND HYPERPLASTIC LESIONS

▶ NEOPLASIA OF THE EPITHELIUM

Skin cancer is the most common neoplasia that occurs in humans. Exposure to ultraviolet radiation or sunlight is thought to be the single most important factor in its etiology. Therefore, it is not surprising that most cases appear on the hands or face of the elderly as a result of years of exposure. The structures of the skin that give rise to neoplasia of the epithelium are the epidermis, sebaceous glands, sweat glands, and hair follicles. Tumors of the accessory structures are much less common than those of the epidermis and will not be discussed. Cancer of the epidermis should be suspected in cases where certain types of lesions are present. One common feature among these lesions is that of a persistent ulcer, with added features such as induration (hardening) around the edges, bleeding, and blurred margins. Some neoplastic lesions present as plaques or nodules. The most common form of neoplasia is _____(1). Its development is strongly linked to exposure to _____(2), which is _____(3). Sites on the body that most commonly give rise to skin cancer are the _____(4) and _____(5). Specific features of certain types of skin _____(6) should alert suspicions of neoplasia.

Seborrheic keratosis is a benign proliferation of the epidermis, specifically of the basal cells. This growth is wart-like in appearance. It is the most common benign epithelial neoplasia. It is a pigmented growth that is usually brown and may be suspected to be malignant melanoma. However, it is not precancerous. Seborrheic keratosis (or senile wart as it is sometimes called) is friable, or breaks up easily. It is very loosely attached to the skin, making its removal easy. This is unlike malignant melanoma. The most common benign proliferation of the epidermis is _____(1). It may be confused with melanoma because it is _____(2). It is fragile, or _____(3), and _____(4) attached and so scrapes off easily. This feature clinically differentiates it from _____(5).

1. seborrheic keratosis
2. pigmented
3. friable
4. loosely
5. malignant melanoma

The most common malignant neoplasia of the epidermis, comprising about 75 percent of cases, is **basal cell carcinoma.** Even though it is histologically classified as a malignancy, the malignancy is very low grade. This means that it does not generally behave in a manner associated with cancer. It rarely metastasizes or causes death. The etiology of basal cell carcinoma is most likely ultraviolet radiation exposure, since most lesions are found on areas exposed to sunlight. The face is a common site of basal cell carcinoma. These tumors present as a nodule that tends to bleed easily because of the number of capillaries contained in them. The tumor is somewhat invasive locally, but grows very slowly. Basal cell carcinoma may also appear in other forms, such as a plaque instead of a nodule. A basal cell carcinoma of the face is shown in Figure 19–6. The prognosis for basal cell carcinoma is excellent with removal of the growth. Basal cell carcinoma is the most _____(1) of the _____(2) neoplasias of the epidermis. The behavior of the malignancy is characterized as _____(3) grade. Therefore, _____(4) and _____(5) due to this cancer are rare. It will invade locally but it _____(6) slowly, so the prognosis is very good upon its removal.

1. common
2. malignant
3. low
4. metastasis
5. death
6. grows

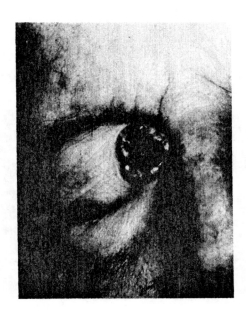

Figure 19–6. Ulcerated form of basal cell carcinoma on the eyelid. *(From Chandrasoma and Taylor,* Concise Pathology, *2nd ed., Appleton & Lange.)*

Squamous cell carcinoma is also a malignant neoplasia of the epidermis. However, it is a higher-grade malignancy than basal cell carcinoma, and local invasion can be aggressive. Its cause is also heavily associated with exposure to sunlight. Squamous cell carcinoma of the lower lip, as discussed in Chapter 12, can also be related to tobacco use. The appearance of squamous cell carcinoma is that of a plaque, an ulcer, or a nodule that bleeds. The growth of squamous cell carcinoma is faster than that of basal cell carcinoma. A large, ulcerated squamous cell carcinoma on the hand is shown in Figure 19–7. Before squamous cell carcinoma reaches a malignant state, a precancerous lesion may be present. This early change is called **actinic keratosis.** It can represent the preinvasive stage, before malignancy reaches into the tissue beneath it. Not all cases of actinic keratosis progress to squamous cell carcinoma, but about half do. In actinic keratosis, there is atypical epidermal proliferation and thickening of the keratin layer. This thickening is called **hyperkeratosis.** If there are additional dysplastic changes of the epidermal cells, and early invasion, this marks the beginning of squamous cell carcinoma. The primary lesion of squamous cell carcinoma is a slowly enlarging nodule that can ulcerate. However, some lesions of squamous cell carcinoma are often indistinct. Any suspicious area of the skin should be biopsied. The percentage of cases that metastasize to lymph nodes seems to be linked to preexisting lesions of the skin. More cases of squamous cell carcinoma metastasize to lymph nodes when the cancer develops in an area injured by chronic infections or ulcers. Squamous cell carcinoma that does not metastasize is still significant because of deep erosion and penetration of underlying tissue. This can lead to infection and, less commonly, bleeding.

1. Squamous cell carcinoma
2. basal cell carcinoma
3. invasion
4. faster
5. atypical
6. keratin
7. hyperkeratosis
8. actinic keratosis
9. lymph nodes
10. injured
11. erosion
12. infection

_____(1) is a more malignant neoplasia of the epidermis than _____(2). Local _____(3) by squamous cell carcinoma can be significant. It also grows _____(4) than basal cell carcinoma. Sometimes there is a lesion of the skin at the site where squamous cell carcinoma later develops. This lesion is _____(5) proliferation of the epidermis along with thickening of the _____(6) layer, which is called _____(7). This early lesion is called _____(8). Metastasis of squamous cell carcinoma to the _____(9) occurs more often if the cancer develops in an area that is already _____(10). In cases that do not metastasize, deep _____(11) can lead to _____(12) or hemorrhage.

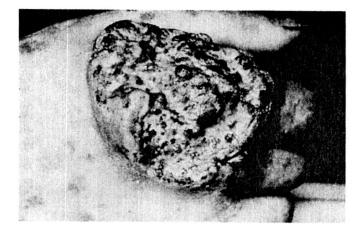

Figure 19–7. Large, ulcerated squamous cell carcinoma on the hand. *(From Kent and Hart,* Introduction to Human Disease, *3rd ed., Appleton & Lange.)*

▶ PIGMENTED HYPERPLASIA AND NEOPLASIA

19–30

A **nevus** is commonly known as a mole. This is a concentrated area of melanocytes, or a benign proliferation of these cells, which causes the lesion to be dark brown. Nevi present at birth [which would be called _____(1)] are birthmarks. Nevi may also develop during puberty or adulthood and be acquired. Nevi are relatively small and have well-defined margins, in contrast to pigmented malignancies. A nevus itself is considered innocuous (harmless). One type of nevus is not so harmless. This is the **dysplastic nevus** that undergoes changes that are likely to be precancerous. The cancer that a dysplastic nevus precedes is malignant melanoma. The tendency of a nevus to become dysplastic and progress to malignancy is believed to be a genetic predisposition, since they are frequently found in families in which other types of cancer occur. About half of all dysplastic nevi turn cancerous. A mole is medically termed a _____(2). It represents a _____(3) proliferation of _____(4). The margins of an ordinary nevus are sharply _____(5), unlike a malignancy. One type of mole that causes some concern is a _____(6), which may become _____(7). This cancer is called _____(8).

1. congenital
2. nevus
3. benign
4. melanocytes
5. defined
6. dysplastic nevus
7. cancerous
8. malignant melanoma

19–31

Malignant melanoma is the most significant skin cancer in terms of mortality among the types of skin cancer. Metastasis to organs does occur, causing death in about 20 percent of the cases. Therefore, its early diagnosis and treatment is imperative. Fortunately, it is the least common type of skin cancer. As the name implies, malignant melanoma arises from melanocytes, or melanin-producing cells. Melanoma may occur on its own or develop from pre-existing dysplastic nevi. The changes in a mole which should be carefully watched for include any Asymmetry of the lesion (uneven surfaces), irregular Borders (blurred margins with the spread of pigment outside the margins), variation in Color within one lesion (pale areas mixed with black, brown, or red), and a larger Diameter than normal for a mole (greater than 6 mm). All of these changes form the "A-B-C-D of diagnosis" in monitoring for melanoma. Other significant changes in a mole are ulceration or bleeding. Malignant melanoma is the skin cancer of greatest concern because of the number of _____(1) it may cause. This is because of _____(2) to internal _____(3). It is fortunate that it is the _____(4) common of the skin cancers. Melanoma may arise from existing _____(5). Changes that might indicate malignant proliferation include:

1. _____(6), which is uneven surfaces.
2. Blurred margins, with leakage of _____(7) beyond the irregular _____(8).
3. Various _____(9) within the lesion.
4. Larger than normal _____(10).
5. The presence of _____(11) or _____(12).

1. deaths
2. metastasis
3. organs
4. least
5. dysplastic nevi
6. Asymmetry
7. pigment
8. borders
9. colors
10. size or diameter
11. ulceration
12. bleeding

19–32

The incidence of melanoma correlates with the amount of exposure to the sun. Lighter-skinned populations are more susceptible because they have less protective pigment. Also, genetic predisposition is a factor because many cases run in families. There are several forms of malignant melanoma. The most common form (**superficial spreading melanoma**) grows aggressively in the epidermis for quite a while and then invades the underlying dermis. Figure 19–8A shows a malignant melanoma lesion on the surface of the skin. Figure 19–8B is a cross-section of skin that shows deep invasion. Metastasis to lymph nodes and to many organs, including the liver and brain, eventually occurs in all untreated forms of this cancer. The prognosis for malignant melanoma depends on the stage in which it is detected. All suspicious areas should be biopsied as soon as possible. Localized melanomas are excised. Metastasis must be treated with radiation and chemotherapy. The 5-year survival rate is approximately 60 percent. The most common of the types of malignant melanoma is _____(1). Invasion of the

1. superficial spreading melanoma
2. dermis

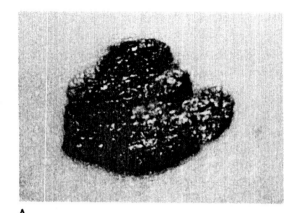

A

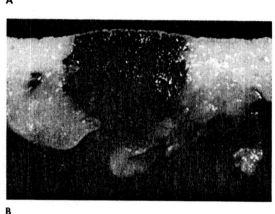

B

Figure 19–8. A. Surface appearance of superficial spreading melanoma. **B.** Cross-section of malignant melanoma showing deep dermal invasion. (**A** from Kent and Hart, Introduction to Human Disease, 3rd ed., Appleton & Lange. **B** from Chandrasoma and Taylor, Concise Pathology, 2nd ed., Appleton & Lange.)

3. growth
4. metastasize
5. liver
6. brain

_____(2) occurs after aggressive _____(3) in the epidermis. All untreated forms of melanoma will _____(4) to organs, including the _____(5) and _____(6).

▶ NEOPLASIA OF THE DERMIS AND CONNECTIVE TISSUE

19–33

1. vessels
2. connective tissue

Kaposi's sarcoma used to be a rare malignancy with low-grade malignant tendencies. However, the incidence of this tumor has risen proportionately with the number of AIDS cases. It is the most common malignancy among AIDS patients. In the early years of AIDS presentation, Kaposi's sarcoma was the unusual cancer that was prevalent in these patients and so helped to lead to the investigation of this disease. Its occurrence in AIDS patients is not well understood, but appears to be related to severe immunosuppression, which allows neoplastic proliferation to develop in response to a virus. Kaposi's sarcoma is neoplasia of the blood vessels and their surrounding connective tissue cells in the dermis. It is a malignant transformation of the vessel-forming cells. The proliferation presents as multiple nodules, which are red with a tendency to bleed, because of the friable abnormal vessels. The usual low-grade malignancy of Kaposi's sarcoma in the general population does not hold true in AIDS patients. In these cases, the malignancy metastasizes widely and causes death. The multiple nature of the primary tumors and the accompanying metastasis cannot be treated with any success. Kaposi's sarcoma is malignant transformation of the cells that form the blood _____(1) and of the _____(2) cells surrounding the vessels in the dermis. In the general population, its occurrence is _____(3) and the malignancy _____(4) grade. However, it is the most _____(5) cancer seen in _____(6) patients. In these cases, the malignancy is _____(7) grade, and widespread _____(8) causes death.

III. REVIEW QUESTIONS

1. It is believed that the single most important causative factor in the development of skin cancer is:
   a. exposure to ultraviolet radiation
   b. genetic predisposition
   c. chronic skin injury
   d. presence or absence of skin pigment

2. The most common benign skin neoplasia is:
   a. basal cell carcinoma
   b. actinic keratosis
   c. seborrheic keratosis
   d. squamous cell carcinoma

3. The most common malignant skin neoplasia is:
   a. dysplastic nevi
   b. basal cell carcinoma
   c. squamous cell carcinoma
   d. malignant melanoma

4. The least common malignant skin neoplasia is:
   a. squamous cell carcinoma
   b. basal cell carcinoma
   c. actinic keratosis
   d. malignant melanoma
   e. dysplastic nevi

5. A brown, wart-like growth that scrapes easily off the skin is most likely:
   a. malignant melanoma
   b. a dysplastic nevus
   c. seborrheic keratosis
   d. basal cell carcinoma

6. The lowest-grade malignancy is seen in:
   a. basal cell carcinoma
   b. actinic keratosis
   c. squamous cell carcinoma
   d. malignant melanoma

7. Aggressive local invasion, with potential metastasis to lymph nodes, is a feature of:
   a. actinic keratosis
   b. squamous cell carcinoma
   c. basal cell carcinoma
   d. seborrheic keratosis

8. Actinic keratosis is:
   a. a likely precursor to malignant melanoma
   b. usually seen in later stages of basal cell carcinoma
   c. also known as hyperkeratosis
   d. epidermal proliferation and keratin thickening that may precede squamous cell carcinoma

9. Squamous cell carcinoma seems more likely to metastasize to lymph nodes if:
   a. deep erosion has led to infection
   b. the cancer develops in a pre-existing skin lesion
   c. actinic keratosis is seen in the later stages
   d. the cancer develops from a dysplastic nevus

10. Death from skin cancer is most likely associated with:
    a. basal cell carcinoma
    b. squamous cell carcinoma
    c. malignant melanoma
    d. actinic keratosis

11. Surveillance for malignant melanoma involves watching for:
    a. specific changes in a mole
    b. the appearance of congenital nevi
    c. the formation and enlargement of a nodule
    d. the formation and erosion of an ulcer

12. Kaposi's sarcoma is:
    a. a common cancer of high malignancy that involves vessels of the dermis
    b. a rare cancer of high malignancy that involves vessels of the dermis
    c. a common cancer of low malignancy in the general population
    d. a common cancer of high malignancy in AIDS patients

SECTION ▶ IV. TRAUMATIC INJURY

▶ ULTRAVIOLET RADIATION INJURY

19–34

Exposure to sunlight causes damage to skin through natural ultraviolet radiation. The two major forms of sun-induced injury are faster aging of the skin and carcinogenesis. With chronic exposure to sunlight, especially with deliberate widespread exposure during sunbathing, several changes occur in the skin. These include areas of hyperpigmentation, atrophy, or thinning, of the epidermis, and degeneration of the connective tissue in the dermis. The atrophy and degeneration lead to loss of the supple elasticity of the skin and wrinkles. The skin is also more brittle, more susceptible to mechanical injury, and slower to heal.

19–35

Sunburn represents first- or second-degree burn injury (see Frame 19–37). It is caused by acute excessive exposure in a short period of time, especially in a light-skinned individual. The redness of the skin is called hyperemia, a term that should be familiar to you. Blisters and peeling of the outer skin layer are common. A **suntan** is acquired with chronic gradual exposure where there is enough time for transfer of melanin from melanocytes to the outer keratinocytes. A suntan is lost when this outer layer is shed. While a suntan does not cause the immediate damage of a sunburn, it still produces accelerated aging over time. The skin is damaged by sunlight because of exposure to natural _____(1). This radiation causes accelerated _____(2) of the skin and _____(3). The effects of chronic sun exposure include hyperpigmentation, _____(4) of the epidermis, and _____(5) of the dermal connective tissue. The skin experiences loss of elasticity and the development of _____(6). During the tanning process, _____(7) is transferred from the melanocytes to the _____(8) of the outer layer. During acute exposure to the sun, when there is lack of protective pigment, a _____(9) may result.

1. ultraviolet radiation
2. aging
3. carcinogenesis
4. atrophy
5. degeneration
6. wrinkles
7. melanin
8. keratinocytes
9. sunburn

19-36

We have already discussed the carcinogenic link between sunlight and skin cancer. The ultraviolet radiation in sunlight penetrates cells of the skin and presumably damages the DNA of cell nuclei. Sunlight can act as both an initiator and a promoter of neoplastic changes, as reproducing cells with damaged DNA undergo the atypical transformations discussed in Chapter 6. The areas of the body at greatest risk for carcinogenesis of the skin are those most exposed (the face, hands, and arms). Those who work outside in their occupations, and light-skinned individuals, are at greater risk than their indoor or darker-skinned counterparts. The most probable underlying pathogenesis in the development of skin cancer is damage of _____(1) in the cell _____(2). When cells with damaged DNA reproduce, they may experience abnormal _____(3) that can lead to neoplasia. As an agent of neoplasia, sunlight can play the role of both _____(4) and _____(5).

1. DNA
2. nucleus
3. transformation
4. initiator
5. promoter

▶ BURN INJURY

19-37

The skin can be injured by burns in a variety of manners, which include sun exposure, flames, hot objects, and hot air. The amount of damage depends on the temperature, the duration of exposure, the mechanism of the burn, and the site of the burn. The significance of a burn, in terms of effect on the body and any complications, depends on how deep the injury is and how much of the body surface is affected. The severity of a burn is graded in terms of "degrees" that correlate to the depth of the burn. The three categories of burn injury are illustrated in Figure 19–9. The least severe type is the **first-degree** burn, where only the epidermis is involved. Only redness and swelling accompany this injury, which heals on its own, without complications. A sunburn is an example of a first-degree burn. **Second-degree** burns cause blistering of the epidermis but don't affect the dermis or the accessory structures

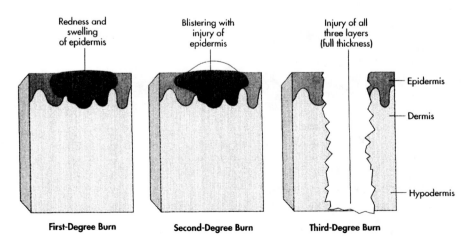

Figure 19–9. Degrees of burn injury.

of the skin (glands and hair follicles). Healing without complications or scarring is generally the rule after the blisters open and the injured areas peel. The clinical importance of a burn injury depends on how _____(1) the injury goes in the layers of the skin and how much body _____(2) has been injured. The depth of a burn injury is clinically measured in terms of _____(3). A _____(4) burn is the least severe. Only the _____(5) is damaged, and the primary manifestations are _____(6) and _____(7). In a second-degree burn, _____(8) of the epidermis occurs, but the damage is still confined to the _____(9) layer of the skin.

A **third-degree** burn is also called a **full-thickness** burn, which is very descriptive of the depth of the injury. There is considerable tissue necrosis of the epidermis, dermis, and subcutaneous tissue. The soft tissue beneath the subcutaneous layer may be severely damaged also, depending on the depth of the burn. Smaller areas of third-degree burns heal slowly and scarring results. Generalized third-degree burns, such as might be incurred in a fire, are most significant in terms of mortality. Death may occur as a result of loss of function of the skin. In this manner, widespread full-thickness burns can be considered a cause of organ failure. Death can result from extreme fluid loss from the soft tissue (causing dehydration and hypovolemic shock) and from generalized infection. The prognosis for survival of generalized third-degree burns depends directly on the amount of surface area that has been destroyed. Third-degree burns involving greater than 9 percent of the surface area must have specialized treatment in an intensive care burn unit. In survivors, extensive scarring can cause crippling. You have learned that excess contracture of scar tissue, which leads to deformity or loss of function, is called _____(1). A descriptive phrase for a third-degree burn is a _____(2) burn. The layers of the skin that are damaged are the _____(3), _____(4), and the _____(5) tissue. The type of burn most associated with death is a _____(6), or widespread, full-thickness burn. Dehydration and hypovolemia can occur due to extreme loss of _____(7) from the denuded areas. Entry of pathogens leads to _____(8) of the areas. These complications represent loss of _____(9) of the skin. Chances of survival depend directly on the amount of _____(10) that is damaged.

IV. REVIEW QUESTIONS

1. Two types of injury caused to the skin by ultraviolet radiation are a. _____ and b. _____.

2. Wrinkling of the skin associated with sunlight is due to (choose all that apply):
   a. hyperkeratosis
   b. degeneration of the dermal connective tissue
   c. hyperpigmentation
   d. atrophy of the epidermis

3. The link between sunlight and skin cancer is likely due to:
   a. blistering and peeling of the outer layer of skin
   b. the production of melanin in response to the sun
   c. damage of nuclear DNA
   d. lack of skin pigment

4. The least severe form of a burn is:
   a. first degree
   b. second degree
   c. third degree

5. The most severe form of a burn is:
   a. first degree
   b. second degree
   c. third degree

6. Death is most likely to occur in a case of:
   a. widespread second-degree burns
   b. localized third-degree burns
   c. widespread first-degree burns
   d. widespread full-thickness burns

7. Three significant complications of generalized third-degree burns are (choose three):
   a. infection
   b. hemorrhage
   c. fluid loss
   d. hyperemia
   e. blistering
   f. cicatrization
   g. sloughing of keratinocytes

5. c–third degree

6. d–widespread full-thickness burns

7. a–infection; c–fluid loss; f–cicatrization

▶ SECTION II

◀ CHAPTER SUMMARY

Because the skin is limited in the ways it can respond to injury, several different types of skin injuries will produce the same type of lesion. Examples of such lesions are *macules, nodules, bullae, ulcers,* and *excoriation.* Infection of the skin by pyogenic bacteria (e.g., *Staphylococcus aureus*) causes *pyoderma. Acne vulgaris* is the condition, often seen in adolescents, of inflamed pustules ("pimples") caused by bacterial infection. *Impetigo,* a contagious bacterial infection primarily of children, is characterized by inflamed pustules that rupture and ooze, then crust over. Infection may spread to other areas of the body by scratching (autoinoculation). *Folliculitis* is bacterial infection of hair follicles, which may spread to tissue around the follicle, producing a *furuncle* ("boil"). Further spread of the infection leads to the development of a *carbuncle,* a condition often seen in diabetics.

Specific viruses can infect the skin. The measles virus produces macules and papules (*maculopapular rash*). Chickenpox and the herpes simplex viruses produce vesicles that rupture and turn to pruritic crusts. *Verruca vulgaris* ("wart") is a chronic skin infection caused by the papillomavirus, which leads to the formation of the benign neoplasm *squamous papilloma. Plantar warts* occur on the soles of the feet, and *Condyloma acuminata* occur in the anogenital area. *Dermatophytes* are fungal pathogens that infect the skin, causing the condition *dermatophytosis.* The most common types of *dermatophytoses* are caused by fungi of the species *Tinea,* and include *T. pedis* ("athlete's foot"), *T. unguium* (fungal nail infection), *T. cruris* ("jock itch"), and *T. capitis* (infection in the hair). *Pediculosis* is infestation of body surfaces, specifically the head and the groin, by lice. Lice infestation is transmitted by direct contact and, as such, is generally associated with crowded conditions. *Scabies,* a contagious and highly pruritic disease, is caused by the female mite depositing eggs under the skin. Scratching may result in secondary bacterial infection, producing vesicles and pustules.

Dermatitis (inflammation of the skin), or eczema, is the result of an immune-mediated reaction. The condition may be acute (with redness and oozing blisters) or chronic (which causes skin thickening). Several types of dermatitis exist: contact, atopic, seborrheic, light-induced, drug-induced, and exfoliative. Each type has its own specific causes and characteristic signs and symptoms. *Psoriasis* is a chronic inflammatory skin disease. The condition is characterized by raised, thickened patches of red scaly lesions. *Urticaria* ("hives") is the presence of a wheal (a raised, edematous area) encircled by a flare (an area of inflammation). The condition, which is caused by the release of histamine from mast cells in the skin, occurs most often as a response to an allergen in food or a drug.

▶ SECTION III

Skin cancer is the most common neoplasm of humans. Most cases appear on the hands and face. Ultraviolet radiation, or sunlight, is thought to be the most important factor in its development. The epidermis, sebaceous glands, sweat glands, and hair follicles most often are the structures from which the neoplasia arises. A persistent ulcer is the common feature among the lesions. *Seborrheic keratosis* ("senile wart") is a benign, non-precancerous proliferation of the basal cells of the epidermis. *Basal cell carcinoma* is the most common malignant neoplasia of the epidermis. The neoplasia, which is likely caused by ultraviolet radiation, rarely metastasizes or causes death. The tumor presents as a nodule that bleeds easily and grows slowly. *Squamous cell carcinoma,* also a malignant neoplasia of the epidermis, is of a higher grade than basal cell carcinoma. This form of neoplasia presents as a plaque, ulcer, or nodule that bleeds. *Actinic keratosis* is a term applied to a squamous cell carcinoma that has not yet reached a malignant state.

A *nevus* ("mole"; plural, nevi) is a concentrated area of melanocytes. A nevus present at birth is called a "birthmark." Nevi are generally innocuous, an exception being the dysplastic nevus, which often precedes *malignant melanoma,* a form of cancer that arises from melanocytes and may metastasize to organs. In monitoring for malignant melanoma, nevi are observed using the A-B-C-D diagnosis protocol, Asymmetry of the lesion, irregular Borders, variation in Color, increase in Diameter. Exposure to the sun is a factor in the incidence of melanoma. Genetic predisposition may also be a factor. *Superficial spreading melanoma* is the most common form of malignant melanoma. *Kaposi's sarcoma* is the most common malignancy among AIDS patients. Its occurrence likely is related to the severe immunosuppression characteristic of these patients. The condition involves neoplasia of the blood vessels and their surrounding connective tissue.

▶ SECTION IV

Exposure to sunlight causes skin damage through ultraviolet radiation. Whereas a *suntan* is acquired with chronic gradual exposure to the sun, a *sunburn* is caused by acute excessive exposure in a short period of time. Blisters and peeling of skin commonly occur in cases of sunburn. Sunlight may act as both an initiator and a promoter of neoplasia, presumably by ultraviolet radiation-induced damage to the DNA in the skin cells. Burns of the skin can occur in a number of ways, and the degree of damage depends on the temperature, duration of exposure, mechanism of the burn, and site of the burn. *Burn severity* is graded in terms of "degrees": *first degree* (only the epidermis is involved), *second degree* (blistering of the epidermis but no dermal or accessory gland involvement), and *third degree* (epidermal necrosis, subcutaneal damage, slow healing, scarring). Third-degree burns are obviously the most serious, and death from hypovolemic shock or generalized infection may occur. The prognosis for survival of third-degree burns depends on the amount of surface area that has been destroyed.

Index

PID. *See* Pelvic inflammatory disease
(PID)
"Piles," 492
Piloerection, 56
"Pink eye," 693–94, 706
"Pink puffer," 414
Pinworm disease, 203
Pitting edema, 76
Pituitary gland, anatomy and
physiology, 600–601
Pituitary gland disorders
adenomas, 605
atrophy, 606
dwarfism, 607
hyperpituitarism, 605–6
hypopituitarism, 606–7
insufficiency, 606
PKD (polycystic kidney disease),
535–36, 558
PKU (phenylketonuria), 244, 273, 275t
Placenta, 563
tumors during pregnancy, 579–80
Plague, 175
Plantar warts, 712, 727
Plaque
atherosclerosis, 347, 370–71
dental, 450, 451
-plasia, 214
Plasma
cells, 46, 115
defined, 24, 304
multiple myeloma, 323–24
Plasmin, 308
Plasmodium, 200–201
Platelet, plugs, 307
Platelets
defined, 37, 306–7
disorders, 326–27
Pleura, 400
Pleural cavity, 400, 423
air in, 435–36
fluids in, 435, 436–37
Pleural diseases, 435–37
effusion, 376, 423–24, 436, 437,
443
secondary neoplasia, 437
Pleural membrane, 435
Pleuritis (pleurisy), 404, 436
Pleurocentesis, 436
Pluripotent stem cells, 304
PMS (premenstrual syndrome),
576–77, 597
Pneumococcus, 163, 404
Pneumoconioses, 425–26, 442
Pneumocystis, 136
Pneumocystis carinii, 202, 405
Pneumocystosis, 202
Pneumocytes
type I, 399
type II, 399

Pneumonia, 402–27, 408t, 440
interstitial, 405, 441
Legionnaire's disease, 404–5,
440–41
lobar, 402, 404, 440
Mycoplasma, 177
nosocomial, 403
primary atypical, 405
primary fungal, 407, 441
viral, 405–6
Pneumonic plague, 175
Pneumonitis, 402
hypersensitivity, 416–17
Pneumothorax, 413, 423, 436, 443
Poisoning
food, 467
uremic, 532, 535, 552–53
"Poker back," 653, 664
Poliomyelitis, 192, 680
Polyarteritis nodosa, 352
Polycystic kidney disease (PKD),
535–36, 558
Polycystic ovary syndrome, 573–74,
597
Polycythemia, 324, 355
primary, 324
secondary, 324
Polycythemia vera, 324
Polydipsia, 76, 106, 283
diabetes mellitus and, 282
Polygenic (multigene) disorders,
247–49, 266
Polymorphonuclear cells, 16, 28
Polymyositis, 658–59, 665
immune, 659
Polypeptides, 240
Polyphagia, 283
Polyps, colon, 484
Polyuria, 73, 79, 283, 535
diabetes insipidus and, 245
diabetes mellitus and, 276, 282
Portal, 502
Portal hypertension, 502–4, 508f
esophageal varices and, 457
Portal system, 446
Portal-systemic anastomoses, 502
Portal-systemic shunting, 503, 528, 529
Portal vein, 499
Positive feedback mechanisms, 600
Post-, 504
Posterior pituitary, 600, 601
Post-hepatic (obstructive) jaundice,
505–6
Postprandial hyperglycemia, 277
Postrenal failure, 534
Poststreptococcal glomerulonephritis,
163, 538
Potassium, 62
hyperkalemia and, 87–88
hypokalemia and, 85

Potential diabetes, 277
Pott's disease, 643
PPD (purified protein derivative) test,
174
Pre-, 504
Precipitation, antigen, 119
Prediabetes, 277
Predisposing factors, 1
Preeclampsia, 579
Pregnancy, 563
Pregnancy disorders, 577–80
ectopic, 168, 567, 577
"pregnancy-induced hypertension,"
578
toxemia, 578–79
tumors, 579–80
Pre-hepatic (hemolytic) jaundice,
504–5
Premature birth, newborn respiratory
distress syndrome, 438–39
Premenstrual syndrome (PMS),
576–77, 597
Prepuce, 564
Prerenal failure, 534
Presbyopia, 700, 706
Pressure, malignant neoplasia and, 229
Pressure gradients, 399
Pressure necrosis, 172
malignant neoplasia and, 229, 237
Primary dysfunction, 4
Primary filtrate, 533
Primary (first) response, 113–14, 115
Primary intention (primary union), 39
Productive cough, 402
Progesterone, 562, 563, 570
Prognosis, 5
Progression, in carcinogenesis, 223
Prokaryotic cells, 161
Prolactin, 600
Prolactinoma, 605, 628
Promoters, viruses as, 221
Promotion, in carcinogenesis, 223
Prostaglandin, 565
fever and, 67
Prostate, 565
Prostate cancer, 589–91, 598
frequency of, 234
Prostate disease, 587–91, 598
Prostate-specific antigen (PSA), 591
Prostatic acid phosphatase (PAP), 591
Prostatic hyperplasia, benign, 588–89
Prostatitis, 587–88
Prostration, influenza virus and, 406
Protein denaturation, defined, 13
Protein-losing enteropathy, 78
Protein metabolism, liver and, 498
Proteins
function, 271
as pH regulators, 66
Proteinuria, 535, 537